D1454904

Dear Doctor:

Boehringer Ingelheim Pharmaceuticals, Inc. is pleased to present you with the 30th Edition of the *Washington Manual of Medical Therapeutics*. We believe that this Manual will be a useful addition to your medical library.

Representative
Boehringer Ingelheim Pharmaceuticals, Inc.

Boehringer Ingelheim Pharmaceuticals, Inc. assumes no responsibility for the content and judgments contained herein.

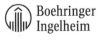 Boehringer
Ingelheim

The Washington Manual of Medical Therapeutics

30th Edition

Department of Medicine
Washington University
School of Medicine
St. Louis, Missouri

Shubhada N. Ahya, M.D.
Kellie Flood, M.D.
Subramanian Paranjothi, M.D.
Editors

Robyn A. Schaiff, Pharm.D.
Associate Editor for
Pharmacotherapeutics

LIPPINCOTT WILLIAMS & WILKINS
A **Wolters Kluwer** Company
Philadelphia • Baltimore • New York • London
Buenos Aires • Hong Kong • Sydney • Tokyo

Acquisitions Editor: Richard Winters
Developmental Editor: Delois Patterson
Production Editor: Alyson Langlois, Silverchair Science + Communications
Manufacturing Manager: Colin Warnock
Cover Designer: Patricia Gast
Compositor: Silverchair Science + Communications
Printer: RR Donnelly, Crawfordsville

Printed in the USA

ISBN 0-7817-2359-0

Care has been taken to confirm the accuracy of the information presented and to describe generally accepted practices. However, the authors, editors, and publisher are not responsible for errors or omissions or for any consequences from application of the information in this book and make no warranty, expressed or implied, with respect to the currency, completeness, or accuracy of the contents of the publication. Application of this information in a particular situation remains the professional responsibility of the practitioner.

The authors, editors, and publisher have exerted every effort to ensure that drug selection and dosage set forth in this text are in accordance with current recommendations and practice at the time of publication. However, in view of ongoing research, changes in government regulations, and the constant flow of information relating to drug therapy and drug reactions, the reader is urged to check the package insert for each drug for any change in indications and dosage and for added warnings and precautions. This is particularly important when the recommended agent is a new or infrequently employed drug.

Some drugs and medical devices presented in this publication have Food and Drug Administration (FDA) clearance for limited use in restricted research settings. It is the responsibility of health care providers to ascertain the FDA status of each drug or device planned for use in their clinical practice.

10 9 8 7 6 5 4 3 2 1

To Daniel Goodenberger, M.D., an unparalleled clinician and teacher, whose commitment and devotion to the education of medical students and house staff serve as an inspiration for all physicians and medical educators

Contents

Preface

This edition celebrates the 30th edition of *The Washington Manual of Medical Therapeutics*. *The Washington Manual*, as it is affectionately known, will have a sister manual, *The Washington Manual of Ambulatory Therapeutics*, available in the fall of 2001. The introduction of the new outpatient manual with this edition, unlike previous editions, has allowed the 30th edition to have an updated, inpatient focus with special attention to disorders seen primarily in the hospital setting. This has resulted in the incorporation of the content from the previous edition's Mineral and Metabolic Bone Diseases and Lipid Disorders chapters into the newly modified Endocrine Diseases, Fluid and Electrolyte Management, and Ischemic Heart Disease chapters. All of the chapters have been extensively revised to ensure that they are consistent with current medical practice.

We are proud to include a new chapter, Transplant Medicine. With this addition, The Immunocompromised Host, a chapter from the 29th edition, has been changed to HIV Infection and AIDS. Non-HIV immunocompromised states are now addressed in the Medical Management of Malignant Disease and Transplant Medicine chapters.

However, in keeping with the tradition of *The Washington Manual of Medical Therapeutics* since its inception in 1943 by the Department of Medicine at Washington University in St. Louis, the purpose of the 30th edition remains to clearly and concisely present a rational therapeutic approach to medical problems encountered by practitioners, house officers, and students of internal medicine.

Although there may be several effective therapies for any disease process, the therapeutic approach presented here reflects the current practices of physicians at the Washington University School of Medicine. *The Washington Manual of Medical Therapeutics* again has been written primarily by subspecialty fellows and junior faculty—physicians who can recall what is practical in the middle of the night—as well as senior faculty.

We are grateful for the assistance of the pharmacy staff at Barnes-Jewish Hospital, especially that of Robyn A. Schaiff, who has served as the Associate Editor for Pharmacotherapeutics since the 29th edition and whose expertise has been invaluable in previous editions. The editorial assistance provided by Katie Sharp and the editorial staff of Lippincott Williams & Wilkins has been greatly appreciated. We would like to thank Alison Whelan, an editor of the 27th edition of the manual, for her guidance and support.

We have had the pleasure of serving as chief residents for the Karl-Flance, Kipnis-Daughaday, and Wood-Moore firms of the Department of Medicine at Washington University, under the guidance of our firm chiefs William Clutter, Gerald Medoff, and Daniel Goodenberger, as well as Kenneth Polonsky, Chairman of Medicine.

We would especially like to thank our parents and families—Narendra, Geeta, and Vivek; Joe and Penny; and Namita, Jothi, and Bala—for their support.

S.N.A.
K.F.
S.P.

The Washington Manual of Medical Therapeutics

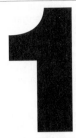

Patient Care in Internal Medicine

Yoon Kang and
Alison J. Whelan

General Care of the Hospitalized Patient

Although a general approach to common problems can be outlined, **therapy must be individualized.** All diagnostic and therapeutic procedures should be explained carefully to the patient, including the potential risks, benefits, and alternatives. This explanation minimizes anxiety and gives the patient and the physician the appropriate expectations.

I. **Hospital orders**
   A. **Admission orders** should be written promptly after evaluation of a patient. Each set of orders should bear the **date and time** of writing and the legible signature of the physician. All orders should be clear, concise, organized, and legible.
   B. To ensure that no important therapeutic measures are overlooked, the **content and organization** of admission orders should follow the following routine (e.g., the mnemonic ADC VAAN DISML).
      1. **A**dmitting diagnosis, location, and physician responsible for the patient
      2. **D**iagnoses pertinent to nursing care
      3. **C**ondition of the patient
      4. **V**ital signs: type (temperature, heart rate, respiratory rate, and BP), frequency, and parameters for notification of the physician (e.g., systolic BP <90) specified
      5. **A**ctivity limitations
      6. **A**llergies, sensitivities, and previous drug reactions
      7. **N**ursing instructions (e.g., Foley catheter to gravity drainage, wound care, daily weights)
      8. **D**iet
      9. **I**ntravenous fluids, including composition and rate
      10. **S**edatives, analgesics, and other per-request medications
      11. **M**edications, including dose, frequency, and route of administration
      12. **L**aboratory tests and radiographic studies
   C. **Orders should be re-evaluated frequently** and altered as patient status dictates. **In changing an order,** the old order must be specifically canceled before a new one is written.
   D. **DVT prophylaxis** with heparin SC or sequential stockings should be considered for all hospitalized patients.
   E. **Orders for medications to be taken prn** require careful consideration to avoid adverse drug interactions. The minimum dosing interval should be specified (e.g., q4h).
   F. **Fall precautions** should be written for patients who have a history of falls or are at high risk of a fall (i.e., those with dementia, syncope, orthostatic hypotension). **Seizure precautions** should be considered for patients with a history of seizures or those at risk of seizing. Precautions include **padded bed rails** and an **oral airway and tongue blade at the bedside. Restraining**

orders are written for patients who are at risk of injuring themselves or interfering with their treatment due to **disruptive or dangerous behaviors.** Restraining orders must be **reviewed every 24 hours.**

G. **Discharge planning** begins at the time of admission. An assessment of the patient's **social situation** and potential **discharge needs** such as home oxygen should be made. **Early coordination** with nursing, social work, and case coordinators/managers is needed to facilitate efficient discharge.

II. Drug therapy

A. **Adverse drug reactions** occur frequently, and the rate increases in proportion to the number of drugs taken. Adverse reactions may be allergic, idiosyncratic, or dose-related magnification of known effects. Following the principles below may decrease the incidence of adverse drug reactions.

1. **Record a careful history** of previous drug reactions, the drug involved, and adverse reaction clearly on the chart.
2. **Use as few drugs** as possible.
3. **Consider drug interactions.** A new medication should be added only after careful consideration of the patient's current medical regimen. See Appendix C for a list of commonly used medications and their interactions.
4. **Consider the metabolism,** route of excretion, and major adverse effects associated with each drug used. Individualize dosages according to the patient's age, weight, and kidney and liver function.
5. **Report unusual drug reactions** to the U.S. Food and Drug Administration. The MEDWATCH program provides an easy method for voluntary reporting of adverse drug reactions.

B. **Prescriptions** should include the name of the patient, date, name of the drug, dosage, route of administration, amount dispensed, dosage schedule instructions, and signature of the physician. The number of refills should be limited, especially for patients who appear to be self-injurious. **For narcotics,** write out all numbers in parentheses [e.g., dispense 30 (thirty), refills 2 (two)].

Acute Inpatient Care

New or recurrent symptoms that require evaluation and management frequently develop in hospitalized patients. Evaluation should generally include a directed history, including a complete description of the symptom (i.e., palliating and precipitating factors, quality of the symptom, associated symptoms, and the course of the symptom, including acuity of onset, severity, duration, and previous episodes); physical examination; review of the medical problem list; review of medications with attention to recent medication discontinuation, addition, or dosage adjustment; and consideration of recent procedures. Further evaluation should be directed by initial evaluation, the acuity and severity of the complaint, and the diagnostic possibilities. An approach to selected common complaints is presented in this section.

I. **Chest pain** is a common complaint in the hospitalized patient, and the severity of chest discomfort and the gravity of its cause are not necessarily correlated. Chest pain should be evaluated to **distinguish potentially life-threatening conditions,** such as myocardial infarction, aortic dissection, and pulmonary embolus, from less serious causes. **Initial history** should be taken in the context of the patient's other medical conditions, particularly previous cardiac or vascular history, cardiac risk factors, and factors that would predispose to a pulmonary embolus. Ideally, the **physical examination** is conducted during an episode of pain and includes vital signs with bilateral BPs, a careful cardiopulmonary and abdominal examination, and inspection and palpation of the chest for possible trauma, herpes zoster rash, and for reproducibility of the pain. **Assessment of oxygenation status, chest radiography, and ECG** are appropriate in most patients. **Management of chest pain** is guided by the diagnostic possibilities. If **cardiac ischemia** is a concern, initial therapy should include supplemental oxygen, chewed aspirin, and sublingual administration of nitroglycerin, 0.4 mg, or morphine sulfate (MSO_4), 1–2 mg IV, or both. Treatment of ischemic heart disease is discussed in Chap. 5. A combination of **Maalox and diphenhydramine** (30 ml of each in a 1:1 mix) can also be administered if the chest pain may be caused by a GI source. Costochondritis typically responds to **nonsteroidal anti-inflammatory drug (NSAID) therapy.**

II. **Dyspnea** is most often caused by a cardiopulmonary abnormality such as congestive heart failure, cardiac ischemia, bronchospasm, pulmonary embolus, and/or infection and must be promptly and carefully evaluated. Initial evaluation should include a review of the **medical history** for underlying pulmonary or cardiovascular disease, a directed history, and **a detailed cardiopulmonary examination including vital signs** with comparison of current findings to those documented earlier. Assessment of the patient's oxygenation status is useful in most patients. Other diagnostic and therapeutic measures should be directed by the findings in the initial evaluation and the severity of the suspected diagnoses.

III. **Fever** accompanies many illnesses and is a valuable **marker of disease activity.** It can cause increased tissue catabolism, increased oxygen consumption, dehydration, exacerbation of heart failure, delirium, and convulsions. Therefore, the **cause of fever should be ascertained as quickly as possible.** Infection is a primary concern; drug reaction, malignancy, vasculitis, and tissue infarction are other possibilities but are diagnoses of exclusion.

A. **Evaluation.** The differential diagnosis for fever is very broad, and the pace and complexity of the workup depend on the **diagnostic considerations** taken in the context of the **clinical stability and immune status of the host.**

1. **History** should include chronology of the symptoms, associated symptoms, medications, potential exposures, and a complete social and travel history. **Physical examination** should include **oral or rectal temperature** monitoring from a consistent site. In the hospitalized patient, special attention should be paid to any rash, new murmur, abnormal fluid accumulation, intravascular lines, and indwelling devices such as gastric tubes or Foley catheters. In the **neutropenic patient,** the skin, oral cavity, and perineal area should be examined carefully for **breaches of mucosal integrity.**

2. Diagnostic evaluation generally includes **chest radiography, CBC with differential, serum chemistries with liver function tests, urinalysis, and blood and urine cultures.** Cultures of abnormal fluid collections, sputum, cerebrospinal fluid, and stool should be sent if clinically indicated.

B. **Treatment of fever** is indicated to prevent harmful sequelae and for patient discomfort. **Heat stroke** and **malignant hyperthermia** are medical emergencies that require prompt recognition and treatment (see Chap. 26).

1. **Antipyretic drugs** can be given regularly until the underlying disease process has been controlled. Aspirin and acetaminophen are the drugs of choice [325–650 mg PO or per rectum (PR) q4h]. Aspirin should be avoided in adolescents with possible viral infections because this combination has been associated with Reye's syndrome.

2. **Hypothermic (cooling) blankets** may be effective but require careful monitoring of rectal temperatures. Often, they produce excessive shivering and patient discomfort. The blanket should be discontinued when a patient's temperature falls below 39°C.

3. **Empiric antibiotics** should be considered in **hemodynamically unstable** patients in whom infection is a primary concern and in **neutropenic and asplenic** patients (see Chap. 21).

IV. **Mental status changes** have a broad differential diagnosis that includes neurologic (e.g., stroke, delirium), metabolic (e.g., hypoxemia, hypoglycemia), toxic (e.g., drug effects, alcohol withdrawal), and other etiologies. Infection (e.g., urinary tract infections, pneumonia, etc.) is a common cause of mental status changes in the elderly and patients with underlying neurologic disease and must be considered. **Medical history** should particularly focus on medications, underlying dementia or neurologic disorder, and history of alcohol use. Directed history should be obtained from the patient, but family and nursing personnel may provide useful additional details. **Physical examination** should generally include vital signs, a search for sites of infection, and cardiopulmonary and detailed neurologic examinations including mental status evaluation. **Blood glucose and arterial oxygen saturation** determinations are reasonable in most patients. Serum electrolytes, creatinine, CBC, urinalysis, and chest radiograph may also be useful. Further evaluation such as CT scan of the head and lumbar puncture should be directed by the initial findings and diagnostic possibilities. Management of specific disorders is discussed in Chap. 25.

  V. **Nausea/vomiting, diarrhea, and constipation** are discussed in Chap. 17.

  VI. **Rash** may develop as a recurrence of a chronic skin condition, manifestation of a systemic illness, or a contact dermatitis or drug reaction. Stevens-Johnson drug reactions are discussed in Chap. 11 (see Dermatologic Therapy).

  VII. **Acute hypertensive episodes** in the hospital are most often caused by inadequately treated essential hypertension. Evaluation and treatment decisions should consider baseline BP, presence of symptoms (e.g., chest pain or shortness of breath), and current and baseline antihypertensive medications. Hypertension associated with **withdrawal syndromes** (e.g., alcohol, cocaine, etc.) and **rebound hypertension** associated with sudden withdrawal of antihypertensive medications (i.e., clonidine, β-adrenergic antagonists) should be considered. These entities should be treated as discussed in Chap. 4. **Volume expansion** and **inadequate pain control** may exacerbate hypertension and should be appropriately recognized and treated.

  VIII. **Pain** is subjective, and therapy must be individualized. Such objective measurements as tachycardia are not reliable. A placebo response does not distinguish organic from psychogenic pain. **Acute pain** usually requires only temporary therapy. For **chronic pain,** nonnarcotic preparations should be used when possible. Anticonvulsants and antidepressants are more useful than narcotics for **neuropathic pain.** Occasionally, pain is refractory to conventional therapy, and nonpharmacologic modalities such as nerve blocks, sympathectomy, and relaxation therapy may be appropriate.

    A. Acetaminophen has antipyretic and analgesic actions but does not have anti-inflammatory or antiplatelet properties.

      1. Preparations and dosage. Acetaminophen, 325–1000 mg q4–6h (maximum dose, 4 g/day), is available in tablet, caplet, liquid, and rectal suppository form. It should be avoided or used with caution at low doses in patients with liver disease.

      2. Adverse effects. The principal advantage of acetaminophen is its lack of gastric toxicity. Hepatic toxicity may be serious, however, and acute overdose with 10–15 g can cause fatal hepatic necrosis (see Chap. 26).

    B. Aspirin has analgesic, antipyretic, and anti-inflammatory effects.

      1. Preparations and dosages. Aspirin is given in a dosage of 325–1000 mg PO q4h prn (maximum dose, 3g/day) for relief of pain. Rectal suppositories (300–600 mg q3–4h) may be irritating to the mucosa and have variable absorption. Enteric-coated tablets and nonacetylated salicylates may cause less injury to the gastric mucosa than do buffered or plain aspirin. The nonacetylated salicylates also lack antiplatelet effects.

      2. Adverse effects. Dose-related side effects include tinnitus, dizziness, and hearing loss. **Dyspepsia and GI bleeding** can develop and may be severe. **Hypersensitivity reactions,** including bronchospasm, laryngeal edema, and urticaria, are uncommon, but patients with asthma and nasal polyps are more susceptible. Patients with allergic or bronchospastic reactions to aspirin should not be given NSAIDs. **Chronic excessive use** can result in interstitial nephritis and papillary necrosis. Aspirin should be used with caution in patients with hepatic or renal disease.

      3. Antiplatelet effects. These effects may last for up to 1 week after a single dose. Aspirin should be avoided in patients with known bleeding disorders, in those who are receiving anticoagulant therapy, and during pregnancy. Discontinuation of aspirin before elective surgery should be considered.

C. NSAIDs have analgesic, antipyretic, and anti-inflammatory properties mediated by inhibition of cyclooxygenase. All NSAIDs have **similar efficacy and toxicities,** with a side effect profile similar to that of the salicylates. **NSAIDs should be used with caution in patients with impaired renal or hepatic function** (see Chap. 24). **Ketorolac tromethamine** is an analgesic that can be given IM or IV and is often used postoperatively; however, parenteral therapy should not exceed 5 days. Nephrotoxicity is more pronounced with IM than with PO administration.

D. Cyclooxygenase-2 (cox-2) inhibitors act primarily on cox-2, which is the inducible form of cyclooxygenase and an important mediator of pain and inflammation. Cox-2 inhibitors have **no significant effects on platelet aggregation or on the gastric mucosa.** The agents that are currently available include **celecoxib and rofecoxib. Meloxicam** is also available but is less selective for cox-2. Cox-2 inhibitors should not be used in patients who have allergic or bronchospastic reactions to aspirin or other NSAIDs, and **celecoxib is contraindicated in patients with allergic-type reactions to sulfonamides.**

E. Opioid analgesics are pharmacologically similar to opium or morphine and are the drugs of choice when analgesia without antipyretic action is desired. Table 1-1 lists equianalgesic dosages.

    1. Preparations and dosages

        a. Constant pain requires continuous (around-the-clock) analgesia with supplementary (prn) doses for breakthrough pain. Each patient should be maintained at the lowest dosage that provides adequate analgesia. If frequent prn doses are required, the maintenance dose should be increased, or the dosing interval should be decreased.

        b. If adequate analgesia cannot be achieved at the maximum recommended dose of one narcotic or if the side effects are intolerable, the patient should be changed to another preparation beginning at one-half the equianalgesic dose.

        c. Oral medications should be used when possible. Parenteral or transdermal administration is useful in the setting of dysphagia, emesis, or decreased GI absorption. The lowest starting dose should be given, with a gradual increase in the amount of drug given until adequate analgesia is obtained.

        d. Continuous IV administration provides steady blood levels and allows rapid dose adjustment. Agents with short half-lives, such as morphine, should be used. **Patient-controlled analgesia** often is

Table 1-1. Equianalgesic doses of opioid analgesics

Drug	Onset (mins)	Duration (hrs)	IM (mg)	PO (mg)
Fentanyl	7–8	1–2	0.1	NA
Levorphanol	30–90	6–8	2	4
Hydromorphone	15–30	4–5	1.5–2.0	7.5
Methadone	30–60	6–8	10	20
Morphine	15–30	4–6	10	60*
Oxycodone	15–30	4–6	15	30
Meperidine	10–45	2–4	75	300
Codeine	15–30	4–6	120	200

NA = not applicable.
Note: Equivalences are based on single-dose studies.
*An IM:oral ratio of 1:2–3 is used for repetitive dosing.

used to control pain in a postoperative or terminally ill patient. Patient-controlled analgesia often enhances pain relief, decreases anxiety, and decreases the total dose requirement.

2. **Selected drugs**

   a. Immediate (MSIR) and sustained-release (MS Contin) **morphine sulfate** preparations (MSIR, 5–30 mg PO q2–8h; MS Contin, 15–120 mg PO q12h; or a rectal suppository) can be used. Elixir may be useful in patients with dysphagia. Larger doses of morphine may be necessary to control pain as tolerance develops.

   b. **Hydromorphone** [2–4 mg PO q4–6h; 1–2 mg IM, IV, or SC q4–6h] is a potent morphine derivative. It can be given IV with caution. It is also available as a 3-mg rectal suppository.

   c. **Meperidine** (50–150 mg PO, SC, or IM q2–3h) causes less biliary spasm, urinary retention, and constipation than morphine but results in more respiratory depression and is a **myocardial depressant. It is contraindicated in patients who are taking monoamine oxidase inhibitors (MAOIs) and in patients with renal failure** (accumulation of active metabolites causes CNS excitement and seizures). Repetitive dosing is more likely to cause seizures; therefore, chronic administration is not recommended. Coadministration of **hydroxyzine** (25–100 mg IM q4–6h) may decrease nausea and potentiate the analgesic effect of meperidine.

   d. **Methadone** is very effective when administered orally and suppresses the symptoms of withdrawal from other opioids due to its extended half-life. Despite its long elimination half-life, its analgesic duration of action is much shorter.

   e. **Oxycodone and propoxyphene** usually are prescribed orally in combination with aspirin or acetaminophen. Available tablets include oxycodone with acetaminophen (5 mg/325 mg PO q6h), oxycodone with aspirin (4.5 mg/325 mg PO q6h), and propoxyphene with acetaminophen (50 mg/325 mg or 100 mg/650 mg q6h).

   f. **Codeine** can also be given in combination with aspirin or acetaminophen. It is an effective cough suppressant at a dosage of 10–15 mg PO q4–6h.

   g. **Fentanyl** is available in a **transdermal patch** with sustained release over 72 hours. Initial onset of action is delayed. A high incidence of respiratory depression occurs with fentanyl.

   h. **Mixed agonist-antagonist agents** (butorphanol, nalbuphine, oxymorphone, pentazocine) offer few advantages and produce more adverse effects than do the other agents.

3. **Precautions. Opioids are contraindicated in acute disease states** in which the pattern and degree of pain are important diagnostic signs (e.g., head injuries, abdominal pain). They may also increase intracranial pressure. **Opioids should be used with caution** in patients with hypothyroidism, Addison's disease, hypopituitarism, anemia, respiratory disease (e.g., chronic obstructive pulmonary disease, asthma, kyphoscoliosis, severe obesity), severe malnutrition, debilitation, or chronic cor pulmonale. The **dosage should be adjusted** for patients with impaired hepatic function. Drugs that potentiate the adverse effects of opioids include phenothiazines, antidepressants, benzodiazepines, and alcohol. **Tolerance** develops with chronic use and coincides with the development of physical dependence. **Physical dependence** is characterized by a withdrawal syndrome (anxiety, irritability, diaphoresis, tachycardia, GI distress, and temperature instability) when the drug is stopped abruptly. It may occur after only 2 weeks of therapy. Administration of an opioid antagonist (e.g., naloxone) may precipitate withdrawal after only 3 days of therapy. Withdrawal can be minimized by tapering the medication slowly over several days.

4. **Adverse and toxic effects.** Although individuals may tolerate some preparations better than others, at equianalgesic doses few differences are seen.
   a. **CNS effects** include sedation, euphoria, and pupillary constriction.
   b. **Respiratory depression** is dose related and is especially pronounced after IV administration.
   c. **Cardiovascular effects** include peripheral vasodilatation and hypotension, especially after IV administration.
   d. **GI effects** include constipation, nausea, and vomiting. Patients who are receiving opioid medications should be provided with stool softeners and laxatives. Nausea and vomiting can be limited by keeping the patient in a recumbent position. Benzodiazepines, dopamine antagonists (i.e., prochlorperazine, metoclopramide, etc.), and ondansetron can be used as antiemetics. Opioids may precipitate toxic megacolon in patients with inflammatory bowel disease.
   e. **Urinary retention** may be caused by increased bladder, ureter, and urethral sphincter tone.
   f. **Pruritus** occurs most commonly with spinal administration.
F. **Tramadol** is similar to opioids but has less potential for addiction and abuse.
   1. **Preparations and dosages.** Between 50 and 100 mg PO q4–6h can be used. For elderly patients and those with renal or liver dysfunction, dosage reduction is recommended.
   2. **Adverse effects.** CNS effects include sedation, and concomitant use of alcohol, sedatives, or narcotics should be avoided. Nausea, dizziness, constipation, and headache also may occur. Respiratory depression has not been described at prescribed dosages but may occur with overdose. **Tramadol should not be used in patients who are taking an MAOI.**
G. **Anticonvulsants [gabapentin (Neurontin), valproate], amitriptyline, and mexiletine** are PO agents used for neuropathic pain. Mexiletine should be avoided in the elderly.

Sedative and Psychoactive Drug Therapy

I. **Anxiety/insomnia**
A. **Principles of management. Sedative-hypnotic and anxiolytic drugs** are among the medications most widely prescribed in the United States, owing primarily to the popularity of benzodiazepines in the treatment of insomnia and anxiety.
   1. **Insomnia** may be attributed to a variety of underlying medical or psychiatric disorders. Possible causes of insomnia to consider include mood and anxiety disorders, substance abuse disorders, common medications (i.e., beta-blockers, steroids, bronchodilators, etc.), sleep apnea, hyperthyroidism, and nocturnal myoclonus. **Behavioral and relaxation techniques** should be attempted before drug therapy for insomnia is initiated.
   2. **Anxiety** may be seen in anxiety disorder, depression, substance abuse disorders, hyperthyroidism, and complex partial seizures. Accurate determination of the underlying cause of anxiety is essential for effective treatment. The use of antianxiety medications for transient anxiety-provoking situations should be **short term.**
   3. **Physical dependence** develops with regular use of benzodiazepines, and efforts should be made to limit duration of use to 4 weeks for insomnia; certain primary anxiety disorders may warrant longer-term use. Abrupt termination of prolonged treatment at usual therapeutic doses can result in a withdrawal syndrome consisting of agitation, irri-

tability, insomnia, tremor, palpitations, headache, GI distress, and perceptual disturbance. **Seizures and delirium** may also occur with sudden discontinuation of benzodiazepines.

   4. **Sedative-hypnotic** medications potentiate the effects of other CNS depressants such as alcohol and opiates.

B. **Benzodiazepines** are effective as anxiolytics, hypnotics, anticonvulsants, and muscle relaxants. Use should be short term, as they produce tolerance and dependence. The potential for abuse is considerable. Table 1-2 provides a list of selected benzodiazepines and their dosages.

   1. **Pharmacology.** Most benzodiazepines undergo oxidation to active metabolites in the liver. The metabolites of **lorazepam, oxazepam,** and **temazepam** are inactive; therefore, these agents may be useful in the elderly and those with liver disease. Although the metabolite of **triazolam** is also inactive, this drug can produce significant rebound insomnia and has a greater likelihood of seizures with withdrawal; triazolam should be used with extreme caution in the elderly. **Benzodiazepine toxicity** is increased by malnutrition, advanced age, hepatic disease, and concomitant use of alcohol, other CNS depressants, isoniazid, and cimetidine. **Benzodiazepines with long half-lives** may accumulate substantially, even with single daily dosing. This effect is a particular concern in the elderly, in whom the half-life may be increased twofold to fourfold.

   2. **Indications and dosage**

      a. **Relief of anxiety and insomnia** is achieved at the doses outlined in Table 1-2. Therapy should be started at the lowest recommended dosage with intermittent dosing schedules. **Temazepam** should be taken 1–2 hours before bedtime.

      b. **The acute treatment of status epilepticus** includes parenteral diazepam or lorazepam (see Chap. 25).

      c. **Skeletal muscle spasm** is relieved by benzodiazepines. Diazepam, 2–10 mg PO tid–qid, can be used for brief periods in the treatment of sciatica, temporomandibular joint pain, and other disorders with associated muscle spasm.

Table 1-2. Selected benzodiazepines

Drug	Route	Dosage	Half-life (hrs)
Alprazolam	PO	0.75–4.0 mg/24 hr (in 3 doses)	11–15
Chlordiazepoxide	PO	15–100 mg/24 hr (in divided doses)	6–30
Clorazepate	PO	7.5–60 mg/24 hr (in 1–4 doses)	30–100
Diazepam	PO	6–40 mg/24 hr (in 1–4 doses)	20–50
	IV	2.5–20 mg (slowly)	20–50
Flurazepam	PO	15–30 mg qhs	50–100
Lorazepam*	PO	1–10 mg/24 hr (in 2–3 doses)	10–20
	IV or IM	0.05 mg/kg (4 mg max)	10–20
Midazolam	IV	0.035–0.100 mg/kg	1–12
	IM	0.08 mg/kg	1–12
Prazepam	PO	20–60 mg/24 hr (in 3–4 divided doses)	36–70
Oxazepam*	PO	30–120 mg/24 hr (in 3–4 doses)	5–10
Temazepam*	PO	15–30 mg qhs	9–12
Triazolam*	PO	0.125–0.250 mg qhs	2–3

*Metabolites are inactive.

    d. Before procedures such as cardioversion, diazepam, 2–5 mg IV, or midazolam, 1–3 mg IV, over 2–5 minutes, relieves anxiety and reduces the patient's memory of the procedure.

    e. Delirium tremens and early signs of alcohol withdrawal may require high doses of benzodiazepines. Chlordiazepoxide or lorazepam is frequently used (see Chap. 25).

  3. Toxicity

    a. Side effects include drowsiness, dizziness, fatigue, and incoordination. Patients must be warned about psychomotor impairment and the hazard of driving after even a single dose of these agents. They should also be alerted to the possibility of developing anterograde amnesia.

    b. The elderly are more sensitive to these agents and may experience falls, paradoxical agitation, and delirium.

    c. IV administration of diazepam and midazolam can be associated with hypotension and respiratory or cardiac arrest in individuals without underlying disease. **Respiratory depression** can occur even with oral doses in **patients with respiratory compromise.**

    d. Tolerance to the benzodiazepines can develop. **Dependence** may develop after only 2–4 weeks of therapy. The **withdrawal syndrome** begins 1–10 days after a rapid decrease in dosage or abrupt cessation of therapy and may last for several weeks. Although the severity and incidence of withdrawal symptoms appear to be related to dose and duration of treatment, withdrawal symptoms have been reported after brief therapy at doses in the recommended range. Symptoms may range from mild dysphoria and insomnia to abdominal and muscular cramps, vomiting, diaphoresis, tremors, and seizures. Short-acting and intermediate-acting drugs should be decreased by 10–20% every 5 days, with a slower taper in the final few weeks; long-acting preparations can be tapered more quickly.

C. Buspirone is an anxiolytic with few side effects and lacks abuse and dependence potential. It has no sedative or hypnotic effect and does not interact with ethanol. Neither tolerance nor withdrawal occurs. Side effects include nausea, headache, and insomnia. The usual starting dosage is 5 mg PO tid, titrating to 10 mg tid as needed. Initial response is seen in 2 weeks, with optimal benefit in 4–6 weeks.

D. Zolpidem is an imidazopyridine hypnotic agent that is useful for the treatment of insomnia. It has no withdrawal syndrome, rebound insomnia, or tolerance and because of its rapid onset is useful for initiating and maintaining sleep. Side effects include headache, daytime somnolence, and GI upset. Zolpidem should be **avoided in patients with obstructive sleep apnea.** The starting dose is 5 mg for the elderly and 10 mg for other patients, titrating to 20 mg as needed. Doses should be reduced in cirrhosis.

E. Zaleplon is another nonbenzodiazepine hypnotic that is useful for insomnia. This agent has a half-life of approximately 1 hour and has no active metabolites. Side effects include drowsiness, dizziness, and impaired coordination. Zaleplon should be used with caution in those with compromised respiratory function. The starting dose is 5 mg for the elderly or patients with hepatic dysfunction and 10–20 mg for other patients.

F. Tricyclic antidepressants (TCAs) with sedative actions (i.e., doxepin and amitriptyline) are useful in generalized anxiety disorder, and imipramine can be used for panic disorder. An initial **hyperstimulatory reaction** may occur with the use of TCAs in anxiety disorders.

G. Trazodone is an antidepressant that may be useful for the treatment of severe anxiety or insomnia and is generally not used for depression. It is highly sedating, causes postural hypotension, and is associated with ventricular ectopy and priapism. No deaths or cardiovascular complications have been reported in patients who take trazodone alone. A number of potential drug interactions can occur with trazodone (see Appendix C).

H. Melatonin may have some benefit in preventing insomnia associated with jet lag and in one study was found to be superior to placebo in improving sleep efficiency in the elderly.

I. Over-the-counter antihistamines can be used for sedation and anxiety, particularly in patients with a history of drug dependence, but are only minimally effective in inducing sleep. Anticholinergic side effects limit the use of these agents.

II. Depression

A. Principles of management. Patients with a known history of depression or in whom depression is suspected should be evaluated for the presence of **suicidal or homicidal ideations.** Patients with active ideations or a plan of action, or both, should be monitored by a **1:1 sitter.** Psychiatric and medical conditions that may mimic or worsen depression, such as other mood disorders, substance abuse, and hypothyroidism, should be considered. **Psychiatric consultation** should be obtained for patients with psychotic features or suicidal or homicidal ideations and to determine the patient's capacity to make health care decisions.

B. Pharmacotherapy is the most effective and well-studied treatment for moderate to severe depression without psychotic symptoms (Table 1-3). Available antidepressants all have similar overall efficacy. Depressive symptoms can recur. **In elderly patients,** the initial dose is usually one-half the usual starting dose, and response to therapy is often delayed. Antidepressants have the potential to provoke manic episodes in patients with underlying bipolar affective disorder; therefore, patients who present with depression should be screened for a history of manic episodes.

1. TCAs

a. Pharmacologic properties. TCAs block the reuptake of norepinephrine and serotonin. They are potent antihistamines and anticholinergics and should be used with caution or, in selected cases, avoided in patients with glaucoma, cardiovascular disease, or prostatic hypertrophy. These compounds are metabolized by the liver, and their metabolism may differ greatly in individuals. TCAs are used infrequently due to the availability of new antidepressants with safer side effect profiles and should generally be avoided in the elderly.

b. Choice of drug should be individualized on the basis of history of prior treatment response, the side effect profile, and the degree of sedation associated with the drug. Plasma levels of specific tricyclic agents may aid in patient management. **Amitriptyline** is useful for depressed patients who may benefit from sedation. However, this agent should not be used to treat insomnia unless the symptom is a manifestation of depression, and because of its profound **anticholinergic** effects, amitriptyline is generally avoided in the elderly. The usual starting dosage of amitriptyline is 50 mg PO qhs. This dosage can be increased by 25 to 50 mg every 2–3 days as needed to a maximum of 200–300 mg/day in divided doses. Patients usually require 2–4 weeks to achieve a significant clinical response.

c. Drug overdosage from TCAs is a common cause of drug overdose death in the United States. Because these antidepressants are given to patients at high risk of suicide, prescriptions should be limited to a total of 1 g, without refills, in the early stages of therapy and when a patient appears to be suicidal.

d. Side effects and toxicities. (See Chap. 26 for management of overdose.) **Anticholinergic effects** include blurred vision, constipation, dry mouth, tachycardia, and urinary retention. These effects are increased by drugs that impair hepatic metabolism and by other anticholinergic drugs such as antihistamines. **Cardiovascular effects** include postural hypotension and myocardial depression. Arrhythmias, tachycardia, and ECG changes such as prolongation of the QRS or QT intervals and ST-T wave changes may occur. **These drugs should be**

Table 1-3. Selected antidepressant medications

Drug	Usual initial dose (mg)*	Daily dose range (mg)
Tricyclics		
Amitriptyline	50	100–300
Desipramine	50	100–300
Imipramine	50	100–300
Nortriptyline	25	75–150
Tetracyclic		
Maprotiline	75	150–225
Selective serotonin reuptake inhibitors		
Citalopram	20	20–40
Fluoxetine	20	20–80
Paroxetine	20	20–60
Sertraline	50	50–200
Others		
Trazodone	50	150–400
Bupropion	100	450
Mirtazapine	15	15–45
Venlafaxine	75	75–375

*Use one-half the dose in elderly patients.

used with caution or avoided in patients with cardiovascular disease. TCAs have potential **interactions with many drugs** (see Appendix C). **Hypersensitivity reactions** include rashes, leukopenia, and cholestatic jaundice. **Sedation** occurs in varying degrees, depending on the specific preparation. Other **CNS effects** include anxiety, confusion, tremor, and lowering of the seizure threshold. TCAs should only be used in the **first trimester of pregnancy.** Serum levels can be monitored during therapy with nortriptyline and desipramine.

2. **Selective serotonin reuptake inhibitors (SSRIs)** are chemically unrelated to the tri- and tetracyclic antidepressants and are the most widely used antidepressants due to their tolerability and safety (see Table 1-3). These agents act by inhibiting presynaptic uptake of serotonin. They are metabolized by the liver. **SSRIs should never be used in combination with the MAOIs or within 14 days of MAOI use.** Generally, morning dosing is recommended. **Citalopram** is the most selective of the SSRIs for the serotonin reuptake pump. Its elimination half-life of 1.5 days (increased up to 3–4 days in the elderly) allows for once-daily dosing. Randomized double-blind, placebo-controlled trials have shown significant improvement in depressive symptoms as early as 1 week after initiation of therapy, with the most benefit at doses of 20–40 mg/day. In comparator trials, the efficacy of citalopram is at least that of other SSRIs and most TCAs. The most common adverse effects with citalopram include nausea, dry mouth, somnolence or insomnia, and increased sweating. Citalopram has less inhibitory effect on cytochrome P450 enzymes than do other SSRIs. **Fluoxetine** can be used in the treatment of depression and may also be useful in the treatment of obsessive-compulsive disorder. Fluoxetine is available in a **liquid formulation.**

The onset of action occurs 2–4 weeks after initiation of therapy. Fluoxetine has an average half-life of 7 days, making it less appropriate for use in the elderly and requiring discontinuation **5 weeks before the initiation of an MAOI. Manifestations of toxicity** include agitation, seizures, and vomiting. **Paroxetine** can inhibit norepinephrine reuptake and has more anticholinergic activity than do other SSRIs. The usual dose range is 20–60 mg. It can be sedating and has a high potential for drug interactions but may be useful in depressed patients with insomnia. Paroxetine can also increase bleeding times in patients who are taking oral anticoagulants. **Sertraline** can be mildly activating and is best dosed in the morning. The usual dose range is 50–200 mg/day, which should be taken with food. **Fluvoxamine** is an SSRI, chemically unrelated to other SSRIs and clomipramine, and is indicated for the treatment of obsessive-compulsive disorder. Fluvoxamine has a dose range of 100–300 mg/day and has multiple drug interactions. **Common side effects** of SSRIs include anxiety, headache, insomnia, nausea, sexual dysfunction, and weight loss. **Less common but clinically significant side effects** include hyponatremia, hypercholesterolemia, and bruising. Withdrawal syndromes may occur with this class.

3. **Trazodone** is an antidepressant that may be useful for the treatment of severe anxiety or insomnia. It is not typically used for depression due to its side effect profile, which includes sedation, arrhythmias, postural hypotension, and priapism. **Nefazodone** is a trazodone analog with fewer side effects and is useful in suicidal patients. Nefazodone and trazodone carry a **high risk for drug interactions.**

4. **Bupropion** is a phenylethylamine compound that is currently indicated for the treatment of depression and, in its sustained-release form, also as an aid to smoking cessation. It is hepatically metabolized with several active metabolites. Side effects include agitation, restlessness, insomnia, and dose-related risk of seizures; caution should be used in patients with a history of seizure disorder or in those who are withdrawing from anxiolytics or alcohol. When used in combination with dopaminergic agents, bupropion may potentiate the likelihood of hallucinations or delirium. It has fewer anticholinergic effects than the TCAs and does not cause sexual dysfunction. The initial dosage for depression is 100 mg bid and can be increased to 100 mg three times a day in 4–7 days. The dose of the sustained-release preparation that is used in smoking cessation therapy is 150–300 mg/day. **A 2-week washout period is required before the initiation of an MAOI.**

5. **Venlafaxine** blocks serotonin and norepinephrine reuptake. This agent may be more effective than the SSRIs for severely depressed patients. It carries a low risk of drug interactions. Side effects include nausea, anorexia, dizziness, sexual dysfunction, and dose-related increases in diastolic BP. Withdrawal may be seen with abrupt discontinuation. Initial dose is 75 mg with a maximum dose of 225–375 mg/day in divided doses. An extended-release formulation is also available for once-daily dosing. **A 2-week washout period is required when switching to an MAOI.**

6. **Mirtazapine** antagonizes serotonergic receptors as well as central presynaptic α_2-adrenergic receptors. The initial dosage is 15 mg qhs with a maximum dose of 45 mg. Studies have shown that concomitant administration of alcohol and diazepam with mirtazapine may exaggerate the impairment of motor skills seen with alcohol and diazepam alone despite minimal effects on actual plasma levels of mirtazapine. Patients should be advised to avoid benzodiazepines and alcohol while taking mirtazapine. Other side effects of mirtazapine include sedation, appetite stimulation, and elevation in liver function tests. **Neutropenia and agranulocytosis** have also been seen. **A 2-week washout period is required before an MAOI is initiated.**

7. **Psychostimulants** such as methylphenidate and dextroamphetamine may improve mood. They may be useful for short-term management of social withdrawal or psychomotor retardation in the depressed elderly patient.

8. **MAOIs** (phenelzine, tranylcypromine, isocarboxazid) are used to treat depression and anxiety disorders. MAOIs may interact with tyramine-containing foods and other drugs to produce a **hypertensive crisis.** Drugs that precipitate this reaction include sympathomimetic amines (e.g., those in decongestants and anorectal preparations), meperidine, methyldopa, and levodopa. Food interactions include beer, broad beans, canned figs, certain cheeses, chicken liver, chocolate, herring, processed meats, red wine, and yeast. **Treatment** requires immediate administration of an α-adrenergic antagonist such as phentolamine, 5 mg IV given slowly every 4–6 hours, until the BP is stabilized. Norepinephrine should be available in case of an exaggerated hypotensive response. MAOIs **should not be used with CNS depressants or SSRIs.** Seizures, hyperpyrexia, circulatory collapse, and death have been reported after a single dose of **meperidine** in patients receiving MAOIs.

9. **Electroconvulsive therapy** is the most effective treatment of major depression and catatonia and can also be used for mania and acute-onset psychosis. Generally, its use is limited to cases in which pharmacologic therapy has failed or for patients who are severely suicidal. Electroconvulsive therapy is performed under anesthesia and can be administered safely to all age groups and in the presence of most medical illnesses. The **only absolute contraindication is increased intracranial pressure.** Relative contraindications include recent myocardial infarction, severe pulmonary disease, severe congestive heart failure, severe hypertension, and venous thrombosis; the risks must be weighed against those of suicide, starvation, and immobility. **Adverse effects** include headaches, confusion, memory loss, myalgias, and minor arrhythmias. Death occurs in approximately 1 in 10,000 patients and is generally associated with cardiac disease, advanced age, and hypertension.

10. **Mood stabilizers** include lithium and select anticonvulsants. **Lithium** is used to treat bipolar affective disorder. Because lithium has a narrow therapeutic index, cautious monitoring of serum levels during therapy is necessary. Renal function must be monitored, and the dose must be reduced in patients with impaired renal function. The therapeutic range is 0.6–1.2 mEq/L. **Common side effects** include tremor, polydipsia, polyuria, weight gain, GI discomfort, and benign reversible T-wave depression on ECG. **Adverse reactions** include goiter, nephrogenic diabetes insipidus, leukocytosis, hypercalcemia, and multiple drug interactions (see Appendix C). Serum levels above 1.5 mEq/L are accompanied by ataxia, CNS depression, seizures, GI disturbance, arrhythmias, and hypotension. Treatment of toxicity is supportive. If renal function is adequate, excretion can be accelerated with osmotic diuresis and sodium bicarbonate infusion. Hemodialysis effectively removes lithium and is indicated for severe toxicity. **Divalproex sodium** is also indicated for the treatment of bipolar affective disorder. Side effects include sedation, nausea, weight gain, increased liver enzymes, pancreatitis, and thrombocytopenia. Multiple drug interactions can occur, particularly with other anticonvulsants and anxiolytics. Blood levels can be monitored, and the generally accepted therapeutic level is 50–150 mg/ml. Although other anticonvulsants, including carbamazepine, lamotrigine, gabapentin, and topiramate, can be used for bipolar affective disorder, their efficacy is still under investigation.

III. **Neuroleptics or antipsychotic drugs** are used in the treatment of psychotic symptoms and to control nausea, vomiting, and intractable hiccups. These agents vary widely in their potency and side effects. Addiction does not occur, and overdosage rarely results in death.

A. Newer-generation neuroleptics have fewer side effects, are better tolerated, and are more efficacious than older-generation agents. Although these newer agents can cause extrapyramidal symptoms, tardive dyskinesia, and parkinsonism, the incidence of these effects is reduced compared to older-generation agents (see sec. **III.B**). These newer agents may be useful in the management of psychosis complicating dementia (see sec. **III.B.2.e**). **Risperidone** is a benzisoxazole derivative with serotonin and dopamine antagonism. Side effects include sedation, hypotension, amenorrhea secondary to hyperprolactinemia, and weight gain. Prolongation of the QT interval is also possible. **Olanzapine** is a thienobenzodiazepine that acts on dopamine, serotonin, histamine, α_1-adrenergic, and muscarinic receptors. Side effects include sedation and weight gain. The usual dose range is 5–20 mg. **Quetiapine** is a debenzothiazepine derivative that acts on dopamine, serotonin, and α_1- and α_2-receptors. Side effects include sedation and hypotension. The usual dose range is 150–750 mg/day in divided doses. **Yearly eye examinations** are recommended in patients taking quetiapine due to an increased incidence of cataracts. **Clozapine** is a dibenzodiazepine derivative that acts on multiple receptors. Side effects include sedation, hypotension, tachycardia, weight gain, sialorrhea, dose-dependent seizures, and, rarely, agranulocytosis. **A WBC count must be obtained every 1–2 weeks to monitor for leukopenia.** The dose is titrated slowly to a target of 300–450 mg/day in divided doses.

B. Older-generation neuroleptics

    1. Pharmacologic properties. These drugs have anticholinergic and anti–α-adrenergic effects. The plasma half-life is 10–20 hours for most drugs in this class, although clinical duration of action may be shorter. These agents should be used cautiously in patients with impaired hepatic function. The absorption of oral preparations is hindered by use of antacids.

    2. Indications and dosages

        a. Acute psychotic symptoms. The usual drug of choice is **haloperidol**, 1–5 mg (reduced in the elderly) PO, IM, or IV. This dose can be repeated hourly until the desired effect is achieved. Prolongation of the QT interval has been reported with the use of haloperidol. The risk is increased in the setting of electrolyte abnormalities, and efforts should be made to maintain electrolytes (primarily potassium and magnesium) within the normal range.

        b. Chronic antipsychotic therapy. These medications can be used in the treatment of schizophrenia, schizoaffective disorder, psychotic depression, mania, and dementias (with the exception of Lewy body dementia) with psychotic manifestations. These drugs can also be used in depression and anxiety disorders. Maintenance doses for selected antipsychotics include chlorpromazine, 50–400 mg/day; prochlorperazine, 20–60 mg/day; fluphenazine, 1–15 mg/day; and haloperidol, 1–15 mg/day. Long-acting injectable preparations are available for fluphenazine and haloperidol.

        c. Nausea and vomiting. Prochlorperazine is usually given in a dosage of 5–10 mg PO, IM, or IV qid or as a rectal suppository, 25 mg bid. Dystonic reactions may occur, especially in young patients.

        d. Intractable hiccups can be controlled with **chlorpromazine** in the lowest effective dose (i.e., 10–25 mg PO q4–6h; 25–50 mg IM q3–4h; 25–100 mg PR q6–8h). Pathologic processes associated with intractable hiccups such as pulmonary diseases and subdiaphragmatic abscesses should be considered.

        e. In the management of agitation and psychosis in patients with delirium or dementia, behavioral interventions (i.e., repeated reorientation, bright light during the day, avoiding restraints, providing the patients with their glasses and/or hearing aids), with or without concomitant use of high-potency antipsychotic agents, are essential. Low-dose **haloperidol** is the drug of choice in acute delirium in elderly patients who display behavior that is self-endangering or hinders medical care. Initial doses start at 0.25 mg PO or IM and can be titrated up as needed to the lowest effective dose. Haloperidol rarely causes hypotension, cardiovascular compromise, or excessive sedation in low dosages. Gradual withdrawal of the medication should be attempted once the target symptoms respond and the patient's condition is stable. In patients with chronic agitation or psychosis associated with dementia, the newer-generation neuroleptics are preferred (see sec. **III.A**). **Sundown syndrome** refers to the appearance of worsening confusion in the evening and is associated with dementia, delirium, and unfamiliar environments. If behavioral interventions, such as increased lighting and attention and maintenance of a familiar environment, are ineffective, short-term antipsychotic therapy may be beneficial.

C. Adverse reactions. In general, lower-potency drugs such as chlorpromazine are more sedating and produce more anticholinergic side effects; high-potency agents, such as haloperidol, produce less sedation and fewer anticholinergic effects but cause more extrapyramidal reactions.

  1. **Postural hypotension** occasionally may be acute and severe after IM administration. If significant hypotension occurs, administering IV fluids and placing the patient in the Trendelenburg position are usually sufficient. If **vasopressors** are required, norepinephrine or phenylephrine should be used. Dopamine may exacerbate the psychotic state.

  2. **Anticholinergic effects** include dry mouth, blurred vision, urinary retention, constipation, and tachycardia.

  3. **Extrapyramidal reactions** include **acute dystonic reactions** that are characterized by torticollis, opisthotonus, tics, grimacing, dysarthria, or oculogyric crisis occurring soon after therapy is initiated. Effective treatment is **diphenhydramine**, 25–50 mg, or **benztropine**, 1 mg PO, IM, or IV. Repeat doses may be required. **Parkinsonian reactions** occur early in therapy and may require treatment with antiparkinsonian drugs, such as benztropine (1–2 mg PO or IM). **Akathisia** is a sense of motor restlessness in which the patient feels a constant need to move about. It occurs early in therapy and can be managed with dose reduction or substitution of a less potent agent. β-Adrenergic antagonists, benzodiazepines, and anticholinergics have also been used in combination with the antipsychotic agent. **Tardive dyskinesia** is a late adverse effect characterized by involuntary movement of the lips, tongue, jaw, and extremities. The condition may be reversible with discontinuation of the antipsychotic agent.

  4. **Neuroleptic malignant syndrome** is an infrequent, potentially lethal complication of antipsychotic drug therapy. Clinical manifestations include rigidity, akinesia, altered sensorium, fever, tachycardia, and alteration in BP. Severe muscle rigidity can cause rhabdomyolysis and acute renal failure. Laboratory abnormalities include elevations in creatine kinase, liver function tests, and WBC count (see Chap. 25).

  5. **Less common adverse reactions** of antipsychotic drugs include **photosensitivity, urticaria, and maculopapular rashes** that usually resolve after the offending agent is discontinued. **Cholestatic jaundice** occurs rarely, most often during the first month of therapy, and generally subsides after withdrawal of the drug. **Transient leukopenia** may develop; agranulocytosis is rare during the first 3 months of therapy. Leukocyte counts should be obtained when infections develop in patients who are taking these medications.

  6. **Clozapine toxicity** includes tachycardia, hypotension, and seizures. Clozapine may also cause severe agranulocytosis; patients who take clozapine must be enrolled in the clozapine program, which includes weekly monitoring of the WBC count.

Therapy of Surgical Patients

Medical care of the surgical patient includes appropriate management of underlying illnesses and assistance in avoiding perioperative medical complications. Elective surgery carries less risk of postoperative complications than does emergency surgery, because the patient's general medical condition can be improved by treating malnutrition, metabolic and electrolyte abnormalities, hypoxemia, and anemia. However, in emergency situations, excessive delay of surgery to stabilize the patient may not be beneficial.

I. **Cardiovascular considerations**

A. **Preoperative assessment of risk** is performed to minimize perioperative cardiac complications in patients undergoing noncardiac surgery. An appropriate assessment allows a rational evaluation of risks and benefits in elective surgery (*J Am Coll Cardiol* 27:910, 1996; *Ann Intern Med* 127:309, 1997).

   1. **Clinical risk assessment.** History, physical examination, and ECG assessment are important components of preoperative risk evaluation. Clinical markers that predict perioperative risk of cardiac events can be grouped into major, intermediate, and minor predictors (Table 1-4). The presence of **major predictors** mandates intensive management that may delay or cancel elective surgery; **intermediate predictors** identify patients who have increased risk for cardiac events and may require further testing; **minor predictors** alone are not associated with increased perioperative risk (*J Am Coll Cardiol* 27:910, 1996). Preoperative risk is influenced also by functional capacity as measured by metabolic equivalents (METs), presence of comorbid illnesses, advanced age, and risk associated with type of surgery. High surgical risk procedures include prolonged or emergency operations and vulvular or vasculary surgery, whereas intermediate surgical risk procedures include head and neck surgery, carotid endarterectomy, intraperitoneal and intrathoracic surgery. Endoscopic and dermatologic procedures, breast surgery, and cataract removal are all considered low risk. The algorithm in Fig. 1-1 summarizes recommendations for preoperative management based on clinical risk group. Groups with high and low clinical risk highly predict severity of coronary stenosis (*Circulation* 94:1563, 1996). Intermediate-risk groups have uncertain severity of coronary disease; this group may benefit most from further noninvasive testing. Preoperative evaluation and intraoperative management should be aimed at eliminating these factors and reducing the risk of a cardiac event (myocardial infarction, unstable angina, congestive heart failure, arrhythmia, and death). Moderate or excellent functional capacity (>4 METs) includes the ability to run a short distance, climb a flight of stairs, or walk up a hill. Inability to perform at this level of activity indicates poor functional capacity (<4 METs).

   2. **Noninvasive tests of cardiac function. In the preoperative evaluation,** such noninvasive tests are most useful when the presence, type, or severity of coronary artery disease is unknown. Patients with intermediate clinical risk should undergo noninvasive testing if they have poor functional capacity or are undergoing major surgery. Exercise stress testing is most useful in evaluating patients with new, unexplained chest pain and those with uncertain or poorly characterized coronary disease (*N Engl J Med* 333:1752, 1996). Dobutamine stress echocardiography and dipyridamole thallium also can be used to evaluate patients at intermediate clinical risk (*Ann Intern Med* 124:770, 1996). Preoperative cardiac catheterization should be performed in patients with markedly positive stress tests and patients with high clinical risk who would be considered for revascularization independent of the scheduled noncardiac surgery.

Table 1-4. Clinical predictors of increased perioperative cardiovascular risk

Major predictors

Unstable coronary syndromes

Recent myocardial infarction (>1 wk, <1 mo) with evidence of important ischemic risk by clinical symptoms or noninvasive study

Unstable or severe angina (Canadian class III or IV)

Decompensated congestive heart failure

Significant arrhythmias

High-grade atrioventricular block

Symptomatic ventricular arrhythmias in the presence of underlying cardiac disease

Supraventricular arrhythmias with uncontrolled ventricular rate

Severe valvular disease

Intermediate predictors

Mild angina pectoris (Canadian class I or II)

Previous myocardial infarction by history or pathologic Q waves

Compensated or previous congestive heart failure

Diabetes mellitus

Minor predictors

Advanced age (>70 yrs)

Abnormal ECG (LVH, LBBB, ST-T segment abnormalities)

Rhythm other than sinus

Low functional capacity (e.g., unable to climb 1 flight of stairs with groceries)

History of stroke

Uncontrolled systemic hypertension

LBBB = left bundle branch block; LVH = left ventricular hypertrophy.
Source: Modified from LA Fleisher, KA Eagle. Screening for cardiac disease in patients having noncardiac surgery. *Ann Intern Med* 124:769, 1996.

B. Hemodynamic monitoring. Such monitoring with pulmonary artery or intra-arterial catheters aids in the management of high-risk patients with a history or presence of congestive heart failure (including S3 gallop or jugular venous distenstion), aortic stenosis, recent angina, or myocardial infarction. Prudence mandates invasive monitoring of most elderly patients and those at risk for development of intraoperative hypotension (i.e., those having vascular procedures). Monitoring should be continued for 48 hours postoperatively until fluids have been mobilized into the vascular space.

C. Medical therapies

 1. **Angiotensin-converting enzyme inhibitors and digoxin** should be considered in the preoperative treatment of patients with signs and symptoms of systolic heart failure. A preoperative echocardiogram may be useful in patients with congestive heart failure.

 2. **Antianginal drugs** should be continued in the perioperative period. If oral medications cannot be taken, alternate routes of administration should be used (e.g., topical nitrates or IV administration of nitrates or β-adrenergic antagonists). Intraoperative nitroglycerin is indicated in high-risk patients who are receiving an oral nitrate and have active signs of ischemia without hypotension. In patients with substantial risk of cardiac disease, preoperative therapy with β-adrenergic antagonists

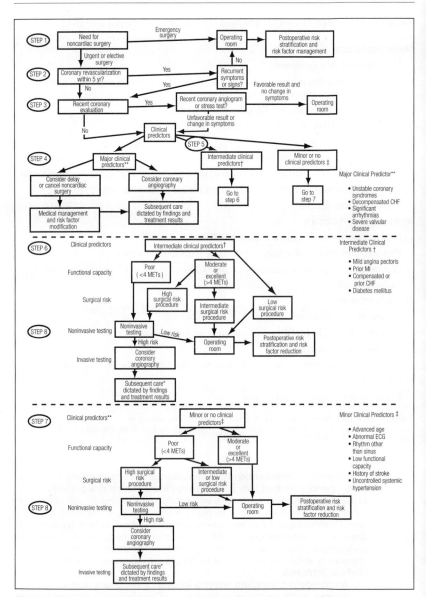

Fig. 1-1. Stepwise approach to preoperative cardiac assessment. *Subsequent care may include cancellation or delay in surgery, coronary revascularization followed by noncardiac surgery, or intensified care. (CHF, congestive heart failure; METs, metabolic equivalents; MI, myocardial infarction.) (From KA Eagle, BH Brundage, BR Chaitman, et al. Guidelines for perioperative cardiovascular evaluation for noncardiac surgery. Report of the American College of Cardiology/American Heart Association Task Force on Practice Guidelines. Committee on Perioperative Cardiovascular Evaluation for Noncardiac Surgery. *Circulation* 83:1278–1317, 1996, with permission.)

should be considered to decrease cardiac effects of perioperative stress (*Ann Intern Med* 124:768, 1996) and decrease subsequent mortality (*N Engl J Med* 335:1713, 1996).

   3. **Antiarrhythmic drugs** in usual doses should be given on the morning of surgery to patients with a history of arrhythmias. Lidocaine may be useful in patients with a family history of sudden death or symptomatic ventricular arrhythmias. **The half-life of lidocaine is prolonged by most general anesthetics,** and toxicity may occur. Serum levels of lidocaine should be monitored in most cases.

D. Specific conditions

   1. **Aortic stenosis,** if suspected, necessitates that patients have preoperative echocardiographic evaluation. In cases of symptomatic stenosis, aortic valve replacement or percutaneous balloon valvuloplasty should precede elective surgery. Similarly, patients with severe **mitral stenosis** may benefit from valve replacement or valvuloplasty before surgery.

   2. **Aortic and mitral regurgitation** should be identified because these patients benefit from afterload reduction and **antibiotic prophylaxis.**

   3. **Permanent transvenous pacemakers** should be placed when indicated, before elective surgery (see Chap. 7). **Temporary transvenous pacemakers** or transthoracic pacing units should be used preoperatively in patients who have indications for a permanent pacemaker and in whom this cannot be done safely before surgery.

   4. **Stable hypertension** with diastolic BPs of less than 110 mm Hg does not increase the risk of cardiovascular complications (*Med Clin North Am* 77:352, 1993). Antihypertensive medication should be continued through the morning of surgery. Particular care should be taken to avoid withdrawal of beta-blockers and clonidine. If oral medications cannot be taken for a prolonged period, IV or transdermal alternatives can be substituted (see Chap. 4).

   5. **Patients with prosthetic valves** are at risk for complications from chronic anticoagulation (see Chap. 19) and bacterial endocarditis (see Chap. 14).

E. Common postoperative complications

   1. **Hypertension. Sedation, analgesia, and oxygen** are most effective for the treatment of hypertension in the immediate postoperative period. Marked hypertension should be controlled with IV nitroprusside or nitroglycerin (see Chap. 4). Enalapril, 0.625–1.25 mg IV; labetalol, 20–40 mg IV; nicardipine, 5 mg IV; or hydralazine, 5–10 mg IV or IM, also may be effective. Diuretics can be used with caution 24–48 hours postoperatively after mobilization of fluid into the vascular space has occurred or with evidence of volume overload compromising oxygenation.

   2. **Ventricular premature contractions** are best treated by correcting fluid and electrolyte abnormalities. Specific antiarrhythmic therapy is reserved for patients with hemodynamic compromise or life-threatening arrhythmias (see Chap. 7).

   3. **Supraventricular tachycardias** are best treated by correcting the precipitating causes, such as medications, fever, hypoxemia, and electrolyte abnormalities, hypokalemia and hypomagnesemia in particular. Acute management may require the use of medications (e.g., adenosine) or direct current cardioversion (see Chap. 7). Rate control should be established with oral or IV **digoxin, beta-blockers, or calcium channel blockers.** Class Ia and III antiarrhythmics should be reserved for refractory and poorly tolerated rhythms. Rate-controlling agents used perioperatively in patients without underlying heart disease can usually be discontinued before hospital discharge.

   4. **Heart failure** usually is caused by exogenous fluid administration. Diuretics are the treatment of choice. The possibility of postoperative myocardial ischemia or infarction should be considered.

5. **Myocardial infarction** tends to occur within 6 days of a procedure. Painless infarction is common. In patients without evidence of coronary artery disease, surveillance ECGs are generally restricted to those in whom symptoms or signs develop perioperatively that are suggestive of myocardial ischemia. In patients with known or suspected coronary artery disease who are undergoing procedures with a high incidence of cardiovascular morbidity, a baseline ECG should be obtained preoperatively, with subsequent ECGs immediately after surgery and on the first 2 postoperative days. Troponin levels may also be useful in patients with clinical evidence of myocardial ischemia.

II. **Pulmonary considerations.** The risk of pulmonary complications is greatest in the setting of acute or chronic lung disease, cigarette smoking, obesity, abdominal or thoracic surgery, advanced age, and anesthesia time longer than 3 hours. Patients should be advised to stop smoking 3–4 weeks before an elective procedure.

A. **Preoperative evaluation** of patients with known pulmonary disease or symptoms suggestive of pulmonary disease should include spirometry, arterial blood gas analysis, and (occasionally) radioisotope determination of regional lung function. Spirometry is useful for diagnosing the presence and severity of underlying lung disease, but correlations between specific pulmonary function test results and risk for postoperative pulmonary complications are poor. For patients with **asthma exacerbations,** elective surgery should be postponed until the acute episode is treated. General anesthesia can induce bronchospasm; therefore, patients with reactive airway disease should be treated preoperatively with aggressive bronchodilator therapy to maximize lung function. **Preoperative antibiotics** should be reserved for patients with evidence of infected sputum.

B. **Postoperative management** should include frequent monitoring of oxygen saturation, arterial blood gases as needed, and bedside spirometry monitoring in patients with asthma and chronic obstructive pulmonary disease. **Sedative and narcotic medications should be used cautiously** to minimize respiratory depression, but adequate pain relief must be attained. Deep breathing exercises (e.g., incentive spirometry) and encouragement of coughing are useful in the prevention and management of atelectasis. Incentive spirometry is most effective if patients are instructed in appropriate technique preoperatively. Postural drainage and chest physical therapy may also be useful. Antibiotics and bronchodilators may be required to treat infection and bronchospasm.

III. **Anticoagulation** for the prevention of deep venous thrombosis is discussed in Chap. 19.

IV. **Chronic glucocorticoid therapy.** Patients who are receiving such therapy may require stress doses of hydrocortisone perioperatively (see Chap. 23).

General Eye Care

I. **The complete physical examination** should include assessment of the external eye and eyelid; pupillary size, shape, and reactivity; extraocular muscle function; and visual fields and acuity. A direct funduscopic examination should also be performed.

II. **Ocular symptoms. Changes in vision** should be evaluated by an ophthalmologist. Sudden loss of vision requires evaluation by an ophthalmologist in the first few hours. **Burning and itching** usually are caused by relatively minor eye disorders. **A foreign body sensation** should be evaluated first by eversion of the upper eyelid and examination of the lids, sclera, and conjunctiva for a foreign body, which can be removed carefully with a cotton swab dipped in saline. If no foreign body is seen, the eye should be irrigated with normal saline. If the sensation persists, the patient should be referred to an ophthalmologist.

III. Ocular trauma requires urgent ophthalmologic evaluation.

IV. Red eye is a common problem that may be caused by conjunctivitis, corneal injury or ulceration, foreign body, acute glaucoma, endophthalmitis (intraocular infections), iritis, scleritis, and episcleritis. If alterations in visual acuity are present, the patient should be referred to an ophthalmologist. Patients with corneal injury or ulceration, acute glaucoma, endophthalmitis, iritis, or scleritis also require referral.

  A. Conjunctivitis refers to inflammation with or without infection of the ocular mucosa and is manifested by itching, burning, and discharge without decreased vision. Prolonged or severe cases or patients with any decrease in vision should be referred to an ophthalmologist. Contact lenses should not be worn until symptoms have resolved and the lenses have been replaced or washed thoroughly and sterilized.

   1. Viral conjunctivitis is characterized by watery discharge and preauricular adenopathy with an associated upper respiratory infection and often is bilateral. Symptoms usually resolve in 7–10 days but may last up to 3 weeks. Individuals should be cautioned to avoid contact with other people (e.g., shaking hands, sharing towels or pillows). Warm compresses provide symptomatic relief of any mattering or crusting, especially in the early morning hours. Ocular decongestants such as naphazoline or tetrahydrozoline generally are not recommended, owing to side effects such as rebound hyperemia and hypersensitivity.

   2. Bacterial conjunctivitis presents with purulent discharge and usually is unilateral. Broad-spectrum antibiotic preparations, such as trimethoprim sulfate and polymyxin B sulfate (Polytrim) gtt qid or bacitracin zinc and polymyxin B sulfate ophthalmic ointment (Polysporin) qid, usually are effective. Sulfacetamide, 10% ophthalmic drops qid (e.g., Sulamyd), also can be used but is associated with a much higher incidence of allergic reaction. Tobramycin or gentamicin eyedrops should be reserved for more serious infections. **Gonococcal and chlamydial conjunctivitis** require antibiotics (PO or IM) sufficient to treat systemic disease (see Chap. 14). Appropriate cultures should be obtained if gonococcal or chlamydial infection is suspected.

   3. Allergic conjunctivitis presents with itching, whitish mucous discharge, and boggy conjunctival edema. Allergic upper respiratory symptoms also may be present. Cold compresses provide symptomatic relief. Naphazoline combined with an antihistamine (e.g., pheniramine) may relieve the itching. Olopatadine, 1 gtt bid, is a combination antihistamine and decongestant. Cromolyn sodium eyedrops may also be effective. **Ophthalmic glucocorticoid drops or systemic glucocorticoids should not be used.** Systemic antihistamines may decrease pruritus.

   4. Toxic or hypersensitive conjunctivitis mimics viral and allergic inflammations. Antibiotics, ocular decongestants, contact lens solutions, and eye makeup are common causes. Treatment involves discontinuation of the offending agent.

  B. Corneal injury may be caused by trauma or infection.

   1. Corneal and conjunctival abrasions should be assessed with fluorescein staining. A sterile fluorescein strip is placed under the lower eyelid. The fluorescein will spread across the eye in the tears. After a second, the strip is removed, and the eye is rinsed with sterile saline or eyewash. Defects in the conjunctiva or corneal layer stain bright yellow-green when examined with a Wood's lamp. **Minor defects** should be irrigated and treated with ophthalmic antibiotic ointment. If a patch is worn, it should be removed after no more than a few hours to allow for reassessment. **Referral to an ophthalmologist should take place within 24 hours.** Analgesics may be required. **Extensive abrasions** require urgent evaluation. **Abrasions from vegetable matter or contaminated material** must be evaluated daily by an ophthalmologist for signs of infection until healing occurs. **Contact lens wearers** should have abrasions evaluated by an ophthalmologist. **Topical glucocorticoids or anesthetic drops should never be used for treatment of abrasions.**

2. **Corneal ulcerations should be referred to an ophthalmologist immediately.** Antibiotics should be withheld until the ophthalmologic evaluation occurs, **and under no circumstance should steroid drops be prescribed.**

V. **Glaucoma** is characterized by progressive visual field loss caused by nerve damage from increased intraocular pressure.

   A. **Open-angle glaucoma** is the most common form of glaucoma and is caused by a malfunction of the trabecular meshwork despite normal angle structures by gonioscopic examination. It is asymptomatic, and the etiology is multifactorial. Risk factors associated with an increased tendency toward the development of open-angle glaucoma include a family history of the disease, age, black race, diabetes, hypertension, and myopia. Treatment includes topical cholinergic or adrenergic agonists, β-adrenergic antagonists, topical carbonic anhydrase inhibitors (brinzolamide, dorzolamide), and topical prostaglandin inhibitors (latanoprost). Systemic carbonic anhydrase inhibitors can be added if topical agents do not reduce intraocular pressure adequately (see sec. **VII**).

   B. **Angle-closure glaucoma** results from obstruction of the outflow of aqueous humor through the trabecular meshwork. Common signs include conjunctival hyperemia, corneal edema, and a fixed middilated pupil. An acute rise in pressure may result in pupil dilatation; eye or face pain, or both; nausea; vomiting; loss of visual acuity; and/or seeing colored halos around lights. **An acute angle-closure attack should be treated promptly in coordination with an ophthalmologist.** Therapeutic agents include acetazolamide, 250 mg PO or IV; 0.05% timolol, 1 gtt bid; and 0.5% apraclonidine, 1 gtt bid, in addition to other topicals. **Ophthalmologic referral** for mild cases is necessary within 12 hours.

VI. **Ophthalmic medications**

   A. **Ophthalmic antibiotics** are available as drops or ointments. Topical ophthalmic Polytrim or 10% Sulamyd, 1 gtt qid or ointment qid, usually is sufficient. Polysporin is a good alternative. Tobramycin and gentamicin drops should be reserved for specific indications. Neosporin ointment causes ocular hypersensitivity and should be avoided.

   B. **Ophthalmic steroids should be prescribed only by an ophthalmologist.** These steroids can cause cataracts, glaucoma, ocular perforation, and exacerbation of infections.

   C. **Dilating drops** include a single drop of 0.5% tropicamide, which usually is adequate for direct bedside ophthalmoscopy. **Acute angle-closure attacks** can be induced (rarely) by pupillary dilation, and usually occur several hours after instillation of the mydriatic drops (see sec. **V.B**). This problem can be avoided by using weak agents, such as 1 gtt of 2.5% phenylephrine (Neo-Synephrine) or 0.5% tropicamide. **Artificial tear substitutes** provide symptomatic relief for dry eyes.

   D. **Ocular decongestants,** such as tetrahydrozoline and naphazoline, are mild adrenergic agents that are available in combination with an ocular antihistamine (pheniramine) or with phenylephrine. They relieve minor irritation and vasoconstrict surface blood vessels. Overuse may result in hypersensitivity reactions or rebound hyperemia. Pupillary dilation may precipitate an acute angle-closure glaucoma attack.

VII. **Systemic side effects from ocular medication.** Ophthalmic medications often are an unsuspected cause of patient complaints.

   A. **Cholinergic agonists** for glaucoma (pilocarpine, carbachol) often cause a dull aching in the brow. Cholinergic toxicity can cause rhinorrhea, salivation, diaphoresis, cramping and other GI complaints, and CNS effects.

   B. **Anticholinesterases** for glaucoma and strabismus (echothiophate, isoflurophate, demecarium) can cause side effects that are similar to those of the cholinergics. Many patients experience mild side effects, especially paresthesias. **Echothiophate inhibits serum pseudocholinesterase; therefore, it must be discontinued several weeks before surgery to avoid possible succinylcholine toxicity.** Red blood cell pseudocholinesterase levels can be measured if necessary.

C. **Adrenergic agonists** for glaucoma (epinephrine, dipivefrin) can cause adrenergic activation with cardiovascular side effects, especially arrhythmias. Dipivefrin is a prodrug that is activated mostly in the eye and, therefore, produces fewer of these complications.

D. β-**Adrenergic antagonists** for glaucoma (timolol, levobunolol, betaxolol, metipranolol) are absorbed through the mucosa, and many patients achieve significant plasma levels after a topical dose. Typical side effects include bronchospasm, bradycardia, congestive heart failure, mood alterations, and neurologic findings. Betaxolol and metipranolol are cardioselective and have fewer systemic side effects.

E. **Carbonic anhydrase inhibitors** for glaucoma (acetazolamide, methazolamide) almost always cause a metabolic acidosis and paresthesias. Mood disturbances, fatigue, anorexia, GI upset, and diarrhea are common. Occasionally, renal calculi can occur, and these agents should not be used in patients with a history of nephrolithiasis. Hypokalemia may occur, particularly if these agents are used concomitantly with thiazide diuretics. Rarely, idiosyncratic aplastic anemia has been reported. Methazolamide causes less of a metabolic acidosis than does acetazolamide.

F. **Cycloplegics** for uveitis (atropine, scopolamine, cyclopentolate) are parasympathetic antagonists that can produce systemic toxicity. Facial flushing, disorientation, GI upset, and tachycardia are encountered rarely. Small children are more likely to absorb a toxic dose of atropine when it is used for cycloplegia of the lens and ciliary body before refraction.

G. **Adrenergics** used for dilating the pupil (phenylephrine) can have a high level of systemic absorption. Hypertension following dilation of the pupil occurs in a small percentage of patients who receive the 10% solution. Rarely, hemorrhagic complications secondary to a hypertensive crisis have been associated with phenylephrine.

VIII. **Presurgical evaluation of eye patients.** Eye surgery can be performed using local retrobulbar anesthesia, general anesthesia, topical anesthesia, or subtenon's anesthesia. As retinal procedures and orbital operations can require 2–6 hours and often are done under general anesthesia, cardiac risk assessment is important (see Fig. 1-1 and Table 1-4). **Complications of the local anesthetic agent** include seizures, hypotension, bradycardia, cardiovascular collapse, and respiratory depression or arrest. Coagulopathies can result in retrobulbar hemorrhage, a potentially disastrous complication. However, with the varied anesthesia options, it may be possible to continue anticoagulation in patients in whom it is medically necessary. Coordination with the operating ophthalmologist is advised.

Dermatologic Therapy

I. **Principles of management.** The initial approach to any dermatologic lesion includes a careful history and physical examination. Questions to be considered when taking the **history** include onset of the lesion(s), time course and manner of progression, symptoms associated with the lesion such as pruritus or photosensitivity, systemic symptoms (i.e., fever, malaise, arthralgias), new detergents, lotions, soaps, and current or recently added medications. Features of the lesion(s) that should be determined based on **physical examination** include size, shape, and distribution (i.e., generalized vs. focal distribution, with or without mucosal involvement), type of primary lesion, and presence of secondary lesions.

A. **Primary lesions** arise from previously normal skin. **Macules** are flat, nonpalpable colored lesions that are less than 2 cm in diameter; a **patch** is a macule that is 2 cm or more. **Papules** are raised, palpable solid lesions that are up to 1 cm in diameter. **Nodules** are papules that are 1–5 cm in diameter, and **tumors** are nodules that are greater than 5 cm in diameter. **Plaques** are raised lesions with a flat top that are greater than 1 cm in diameter. A **wheal** is a raised, erythematous area of localized skin edema that may be a papule or plaque. A **vesicle** is a raised, serous fluid-filled lesion that is less than 1 cm in diameter, whereas a **bulla** is a vesicle that is more than 1 cm in diameter and a **pustule** is a vesicle filled with leukocytes. A **cyst** is an encapsulated lesion filled with liquid or semisolid contents. **Telangiectasia** are dilated small blood vessels with a red or bluish hue.

1. **Herpes simplex infection** typically causes groups of vesicles around the mouth or genitalia and can be verified by Tzanck smear or culture.

2. **Pemphigus vulgaris** causes flaccid bullae and erosions on the skin and in the mouth. **Bullous pemphigoid** manifests as tense bullae on red skin and usually does not affect the mouth. Both are primary skin disorders and can be diagnosed by biopsy.

B. **Secondary lesions** result from alterations in primary lesions. **Erosions** are a loss of epidermis that result in a superficial disruption of skin integrity, whereas **ulcers** are epithelial loss causing deeper surface disruption. **Excoriations** are linear erosions caused by scratching. **Fissures** are linear cracks in the skin. **Crust** is dried exudate that consists of serum, pus, or blood. **Scale** refers to the flaky appearance of skin caused by an overabundance of stratum corneum. Examples of scaling disorders are eczema, psoriasis, and superficial fungal infections. These skin disorders may be accompanied by pruritus, inflammation, alterations in hydration, and susceptibility to irritation. Identification and treatment of specific underlying conditions should always be attempted.

C. **Other common dermatologic terms. Lichenification** is thickening and roughening of skin characterized by increased skin fold markings. **Atrophy** is skin loss and may appear as an area of thin, shiny skin with loss of normal skin fold markings (epidermal atrophy) or may be a depression in the skin (loss of dermal or subcutaneous tissue with intact epidermis). **Scar** is a change in skin caused by trauma or inflammation that may be erythematous, hypopigmented, or hypertrophic.

D. **Restoration of proper hydration**

1. **Dry skin** is a common problem in older patients and in many patients with dermatoses. **Bathing** should be followed by application of a moisturizer immediately after blotting dry with a towel. Extrafatted soaps, such as Basis, should be used. Soap should be used only on the face, axillae, crural areas, feet, and obviously dirty areas. **Lubricating emollients** should be applied frequently and should be rubbed thoroughly into the skin. Available products include Aquaphor, Eucerin, lanolin, Nivea, white petrolatum, and urea-containing products.

2. **Excessive moisture** in intertriginous areas requires careful drying followed by application of a powder (not cornstarch) or dry dressing of absorptive material. In severe cases with maceration, exudation, and erosion, a dressing with or without hydrocortisone cream or an empiric, topical antiyeast agent, or both, should be applied (see sec. **II.D**). The skin surfaces should be kept separated with absorptive materials.

E. **Pruritus and burning** can lead to uncontrolled scratching and can perpetuate an underlying condition. Pruritus typically accompanies eczema. Patients with pruritus should also be inspected for infestations such as scabies. **Pruritus without dermatitis** warrants further investigation because it is often a symptom that accompanies kidney or liver disease and is occasionally associated with malignancy.

1. **Topical** steroids may improve pruritus (Table 1-5).

2. **Systemic antihistamines** (H_1-receptor antagonists) such as diphenhydramine or hydroxyzine, 25–50 mg q6h, often provide added relief for

Table 1-5. Commonly used topical glucocorticoids

Ointments and creams	Lotions and solutions
Low strength	
Hydrocortisone 1%	Hydrocortisone lotion 1%
Desonide 0.05%	
Medium strength	
Triamcinolone acetonide 0.1%	Triamcinolone acetonide lotion 0.1%
Flurandrenolide 0.05%	Fluocinolone acetonide solution 0.01%
Fluocinolone acetonide 0.025%	Betamethasone valerate lotion 0.1%
Betamethasone valerate 0.1%	
Betamethasone dipropionate 0.05%	
High strength	
Halcinonide 0.1%	Fluocinonide solution 0.05%
Fluocinonide 0.01% and 0.025%	
Desoximetasone 0.25%	
Highest strength*	
Clobetasol propionate 0.05%	
Betamethasone dipropionate 0.05% in optimized vehicle (e.g., Diprolene)	

*May produce adrenal suppression.

patients with pruritus. These agents are also useful in the treatment of urticaria (see Chap. 11).

F. Control of inflammation. Inflammation is manifested by erythema, scale, edema, and/or vesicles. Table 1-5 categorizes commonly used **topical steroid preparations** according to type of base and strength of preparation.

  1. Base. Ointments and creams are more lubricating than are gels, lotions, and solutions. Ointments are more occlusive and, therefore, more potent. Ointment bases are best for dry scaling disorders, whereas a cream would be more appropriate for a weeping eczematous dermatitis. Lotions, gels, and solutions are easy to use in hairy areas, including the scalp.

  2. Strength. The choice of topical steroid depends on the severity of the inflammation, the site to be treated, and the expected duration of treatment. Fluorinated steroids are significantly more potent than hydrocortisone or nonfluorinated preparations and should not be used on the face. A 1% hydrocortisone preparation is appropriate for the groin, face, and intertriginous areas and can be used safely for extended periods. Triamcinolone 0.1% is more potent than hydrocortisone and is typically used for the treatment of chronic dermatitis on the torso and extremities of adults. High-potency steroids such as betamethasone dipropionate or clobetasol are effective in treating severely inflamed skin but have the potential to cause atrophy. High-potency topical steroids can also cause suppression of the pituitary-adrenal axis.

  3. Dosage. Dosage of topical steroids depends on the clinical situation. Application should be performed bid–qid. When cream or ointment is used, roughly 25–40 g is needed to cover the entire body of an adult.

  4. Occlusion. Occlusion with plastic wrap increases the potency of the products but should be reserved for severe resistant lesions. Occlusion can cause sweat retention, atrophy, maceration, folliculitis, and suppression of the pituitary-adrenal axis if extensive areas of skin are involved.

G. Skin protection

1. **Cotton and rubber gloves** can be used to avoid excessive contact with water or chemical irritants. Cotton absorbs palmar sweat and should be cleaned or changed frequently.

2. **Barrier creams and ointments** that contain silicone may prevent contact of irritating chemicals with sensitive skin but are not substitutes for mechanical barriers.

II. Treatment of specific conditions

A. Eczema is a term that refers to inflamed skin. **Contact dermatitis** is a form of eczema caused by external allergens or irritants. Specific causes include nickel in jewelry, adhesives in bandages or monitoring devices, chemicals in laundry detergents or soaps, topical ointments, and other skin irritants. Contact dermatitis is manifested by erythema, scale, and/or edematous papules and plaques. Vesicles and bullae may also form. Identification of the causative agent and discontinuation of skin contact are important for treatment. Mild dermatitis responds to high-potency topical glucocorticoids. More extensive cases and those that involve the face should be treated with prednisone, 0.5–1.0 mg/kg/day for the first 3 days and tapered over 10 days. Severe cases (i.e., extensive poison ivy) may require up to 3 weeks of prednisone. Pruritus may be severe (see sec. **I.E**).

B. Chronic dermatitis (e.g., atopic or stasis dermatitis, dyshidrotic eczema) is seen in the setting of venous insufficiency, in atopic patients, and in the elderly, whose skin is prone to becoming dry in the winter. It is characterized by lichenification, scaling, intense pruritus, and hyperpigmentation. Chronic dermatitis is often worsened by scratching. Effective therapy includes hydration, reduction of pruritus, and control of inflammation. The frequent use of emollients, systemic antihistamines, and topical steroid ointments is beneficial. Successful treatment of stasis dermatitis requires reduction of lower extremity edema. Stasis ulcers may form at a site of trauma in the area of the dermatitis. The utility of topical and systemic antibiotics is controversial.

C. Urticaria and angioedema. See Chap. 11 for a discussion of these skin disorders.

D. Intertrigo. In intertriginous areas where the skin is occluded and moist, maceration may be seen instead of scale. This form of dermatitis is termed *intertrigo* and develops in the body folds (most frequently under the breasts and abdominal pannus) from skin rubbing against skin. The area may be colonized by yeast or bacteria. Treatment consists of a low-potency topical steroid to reduce inflammation and symptoms in combination with nystatin, ketoconazole, or econazole cream if **fungal skin infection** is suspected. The skin surfaces must be kept clean, separated, cool, and dry.

E. Toxic epidermal necrolysis (TEN) is a drug reaction manifested by blistering and erosion of greater than 30% of the body surface area and is one of the few true dermatologic emergencies. Affected areas of skin often resemble second-degree burns. TEN typically affects the oral and ocular mucosa and may be fatal. The most common offending drugs include the sulfa antibiotics, penicillin, carbamazepine, barbiturates, phenytoin, lamotrigine, and allopurinol. Treatment includes immediate discontinuation of the suspected offending drug, isolation to minimize exogenous infections, and replacement of fluid and electrolyte losses. At early stages, systemic corticosteroid use may also be considered, although their use is controversial.

F. Stevens-Johnson syndrome. See Chap. 11.

2

Nutritional Therapy

Samuel Klein

An understanding of the fundamental aspects of clinical nutrition is important for the management of many hospitalized patients. Illness and injury can alter nutritional requirements and the ability to ingest, absorb, and process nutrients. The disruption in nutrient equilibrium can affect intermediary metabolism, organ function, body composition, and ultimately clinical outcome.

I. Basic principles

A. Energy stores.
Triglycerides present in adipose tissue are the body's major fuel reserve. During starvation, adipose tissue triglyceride becomes the major source of energy, and breakdown of body protein is decreased to conserve vital enzymatic, mechanical, and structural functions. The duration of survival during starvation depends largely on the amount of available body fat and lean tissue mass. Death from starvation is associated with body weight loss (loss of >35% of body weight), protein depletion (loss of >30% of body protein), fat depletion (loss of >70% of body fat stores), and body size [body mass index (BMI) of 13 kg/m² for men and 11 kg/m² for women] (see sec. **II.B.2**).

B. Nutrient requirements

1. **Energy.** Total daily energy expenditure (TEE) can be divided into resting energy expenditure (normally ≈ 70% of TEE), thermic effect of food (normally ≈ 10% of TEE), and energy expenditure of physical activity (normally ≈ 20% of TEE). Malnutrition and hypocaloric feeding decrease resting energy expenditure to values 15–20% below those expected for actual body size, whereas metabolic stress, such as inflammatory diseases or trauma, often increase energy requirements. However, it is rare for illnesses or injury to increase resting energy expenditure by more than 50% of preillness values. It is impossible to determine daily energy requirements precisely in hospitalized patients by using predictive equations because of the complexity of factors that affect metabolic rate. However, judicious use of predictive equations provides a reasonable estimate for most patients, although the calculated energy requirements should be modified as needed based on the patient's clinical course.

   a. **BMI approach.** A simple method for estimating total daily energy requirements in hospitalized patients based on BMI is shown in Table 2-1. In general, energy given per kilogram of body weight is inversely related to BMI. The lower range within each category should be considered in insulin-resistant, critically ill patients, unless they are depleted in body fat, to decrease the risk of hyperglycemia and infection associated with overfeeding (see sec. **II.B.2**).

   b. The **Harris-Benedict equation** provides a reasonable estimate of resting energy expenditure (in kcal/day) in healthy adults:

   $$\text{Men} = 66 + (13.7 \times \text{W}) + (5 \times \text{H}) - (6.8 \times \text{A})$$

   $$\text{Women} = 665 + (9.6 \times \text{W}) + (1.8 \times \text{H}) - (4.7 \times \text{A})$$

   where W = weight in kilograms, H = height in centimeters, and A = age in years. This equation takes into account the effect of body size

Table 2-1. Estimated energy requirements for hospitalized patients based on body mass index (BMI)

BMI (kg/m^2)	Energy requirements (kcal/kg/day)
<15	35–40
15–19	30–35
20–29	20–25
≥30	15–20[a]

Note: These values are recommended for critically ill patients and all obese patients; add 20% of total calories in estimating energy requirements in non–critically ill patients.
[a]Do not exceed 2000 kcal/day for critically ill patients.

and lean tissue mass (which is influenced by gender and age) on energy requirements and can be used to estimate total daily energy needs in hospitalized patients. An **adjusted body weight** rather than actual body weight should be used in obese patients (BMI ≥30 kg/m^2) to avoid overfeeding. Adjusted body weight = ideal body weight + [(actual body weight − ideal body weight) × (0.25)]. **Ideal body weight** can be estimated based on height. For men, 106 lb is allotted for the first 5 ft, then 6 lb is added for each inch above 5 ft; for women, 100 lb is given for the first 5 ft, with 5 lb added for each additional inch. Providing total daily energy equal to the Harris-Benedict calculation plus an additional 20% is a reasonable goal for nonobese, non–critically ill patients who have increased metabolic demands. Providing total daily energy equal to the Harris-Benedict calculation should be considered in obese and critically ill patients. An additional 300–500 kcal should be added to Harris-Benedict estimates in patients who are underweight (BMI <18.5 kg/m^2).

c. **The Fick equation** can be used to calculate energy expenditure in patients who have a pulmonary artery catheter in place:

Resting energy expenditure (kcal/day) =
$$(SaO_2 - SvO_2) \times CO \times Hb \times 95.18$$

where SaO_2 and SvO_2 are the percent oxygen saturation in arterial and venous blood (in fractions), respectively; CO is cardiac output (in L/minute); and Hb is hemoglobin (in g/dl).

2. **Protein.** Protein intake of 0.8 g/kg/day meets the requirements of 97% of the adult population. Individual protein requirements are affected by several factors, such as the amount of nonprotein calories provided, overall energy requirements, protein quality, and the patient's nutritional status. Inadequate amounts of any of the essential amino acids result in inefficient utilization. Table 2-2 lists approximate protein requirements during different clinical conditions.

3. **Essential fatty acids.** Most fatty acids can be synthesized by the liver, but humans lack the desaturase enzyme needed to produce the n-3 and n-6 fatty acid series. Linoleic acid should constitute at least 2% and linolenic acid at least 0.5% of the daily caloric intake to prevent the occurrence of essential fatty acid deficiency. The plasma pattern of increased triene:tetraene ratio (>0.4) can be used to detect essential fatty acid deficiency before the presence of clinical manifestations (i.e., dermatitis).

4. **Carbohydrate.** Certain tissues, such as bone marrow, erythrocytes, leukocytes, renal medulla, eye tissues, and peripheral nerves, cannot metabolize fatty acids and require glucose (≈ 40 g/day) as a fuel, whereas other tissues, such as the brain, prefer glucose (≈ 120 g/day) as a fuel.

Table 2-2. Recommended daily protein intake

Clinical condition	Protein requirements (g/kg IBW/day)[a]
Normal	0.8
Metabolic "stress" (illness/injury)	1.0–1.5
Acute renal failure (undialyzed)	0.8–1.0
Hemodialysis	1.2–1.4
Peritoneal dialysis	1.3–1.5

IBW = ideal body weight.
[a]Additional protein intake may be needed to compensate for excess protein loss in specific patient populations, such as those with burn injury, open wounds, and protein-losing enteropathy or nephropathy. Lower protein intake may be necessary in patients with chronic renal insufficiency not treated by dialysis and certain patients with liver disease and hepatic encephalopathy.

5. **Major minerals.** Major minerals are important for ionic equilibrium, water balance, and normal cell function. The following are the daily recommended intakes (enteral and parenteral values, respectively) for sodium (0.5–5.0 g and 60–150 mEq), potassium (2–5 g and 60–100 mEq), magnesium (300–400 mg and 8–24 mEq), calcium (800–1200 mg and 5–15 mEq), and phosphorus (800–1200 mg and 12–24 mEq).
6. **Micronutrients (trace elements and vitamins).** Trace elements and vitamins are essential constituents of enzyme complexes. The recommended dietary intake for trace elements, fat-soluble vitamins, and water-soluble vitamins (Table 2-3) is set at two standard deviations above the estimated mean so that it will cover the needs of 97% of the healthy population. Therefore, the recommended dietary intake exceeds the micronutrient requirements of most persons.
7. **Special considerations**
   a. **Mineral and vitamin supplementation in patients with severe malabsorption.** Patients who have an inadequate length of functional small bowel because of intestinal resection or intestinal disease require additional vitamins and minerals if they are not receiving home parenteral nutrition. Table 2-4 provides guidelines for supplementation in these patients.
   b. **Patients with excessive GI tract losses** require additional fluids and electrolytes. An assessment of fluid losses through diarrhea, ostomy output, and fistula volume should be made to help determine fluid requirements. Knowledge of fluid losses is also useful in calculating intestinal mineral losses by multiplying fluid loss by an estimate of intestinal fluid electrolyte concentration (Table 2-5).

II. **Assessment of nutritional status.** The assessment of nutritional status can be divided into techniques that identify specific nutrient deficiencies and those used to assess protein-energy malnutrition. At present there is no "gold standard" for evaluating the nutritional status of hospitalized patients. The best overall approach involves a careful clinical evaluation, which includes a nutritional history and physical examination in conjunction with appropriate laboratory studies to evaluate further the abnormal findings obtained during clinical examination.
   A. **Specific nutrient deficiencies.** A careful history and physical examination, routine blood tests, and selected laboratory tests can be used to diagnose specific macronutrient, major mineral, vitamin, and trace mineral deficiencies (see Table 2-3).
   B. **Protein-energy malnutrition.** Commonly used indicators of protein-energy malnutrition correlate with clinical outcome. However, all these indicators are influenced by illness or injury, and therefore it is often difficult to separate the contribution of malnutrition from the severity of illness itself on

Table 2-3. Trace mineral, fat-soluble vitamin, and water-soluble vitamin requirements and assessment of deficiency

Nutrient	Recommended daily enteral intake in normal adults	Recommended daily parenteral intake in normal adults	Symptoms or signs of deficiency	Laboratory evaluation
Chromium	30–200 µg	10–20 µg	Glucose intolerance, peripheral neuropathy, encephalopathy	Serum chromium
Copper	2 mg	0.3 mg	Anemia, neutropenia, osteoporosis, diarrhea	Serum copper; plasma ceruloplasmin
Iodine	150 µg	70–140 µg	Hypothyroidism, goiter	Urine iodine, thyroid-stimulating hormone
Iron	10–15 mg	1.0–1.5 mg	Microcytic hypochromic anemia	Serum iron and total iron-binding capacity, serum ferritin
Manganese	1.5 mg	0.2–0.8 mg	Hypercholesterolemia, dementia, dermatitis	Serum manganese
Selenium	500–200 µg	20–40 µg	Cardiomyopathy, muscle weakness	Serum selenium, blood glutathione peroxidase activity
Zinc	15 mg	2.5–4.0 mg	Growth retardation, delayed sexual maturation, hypogonadism, alopecia, acro-orificial skin lesion, diarrhea, mental status changes	Plasma zinc
K (phylloquinone)	50–100 µg	100 µg	Easy bruising/bleeding	Prothrombin time
A (retinol)	5000 IU	3300 IU	Night blindness, Bitot's spots, keratomalacia, follicular hyperkeratosis, xerosis	Serum retinol
D (ergocalciferol)	400 IU	200 IU	Rickets, osteomalacia, osteoporosis, bone pain, muscle weakness, tetany	Serum 25-hydroxyvitamin D

E (alpha tocopherol)	10–15 IU	10 IU	Hemolysis, retinopathy, neuropathy, abnormal clotting	Serum tocopherol: total lipid (triglyceride and cholesterol) ratio
B_1 (thiamine)	1.0–1.5 mg	3 mg	Beriberi, cardiac failure, Wernicke's encephalopathy, peripheral neuropathy, fatigue, ophthalmoplegia	RBC transketolase activity
B_2 (riboflavin)	1.1–1.8 mg	3.6 mg	Cheilosis, sore tongue and mouth, eye irritation, seborrheic dermatitis	RBC glutathione reductase activity
B_5 (pantothenic acid)	5–10 mg	10 mg	Fatigue, weakness, paresthesias, tenderness of heels and feet	Urinary pantothenic acid
B_3 (niacin)	12–20 mg	40 mg	Pellagra (dermatitis, diarrhea, dementia), sore mouth and tongue	Urinary N-methyl-nicotinamide
B_6 (pyridoxine)	1–2 mg	4 mg	Seborrheic dermatitis, cheilosis, glossitis, peripheral neuritis, convulsions, hypochromic anemia	Plasma pyridoxal phosphate
B_7 (biotin)	100–200 μg	60 μg	Seborrheic dermatitis, alopecia, mental status change, seizures, myalgia, hyperesthesia	Plasma biotin
B_9 (folic acid)	400 μg	400 μg	Megaloblastic anemia, glossitis, diarrhea	Serum folic acid, RBC folic acid
B_{12} (cobalamin)	3 μg	5 μg	Megaloblastic anemia, paresthesias, decreased vibratory or position sense, ataxia, mental status changes, diarrhea	Serum cobalamin, serum methyl-malonic acid
C (ascorbic acid)	60 mg	100 mg	Scurvy, petechia, purpura, gingival inflammation, acid and bleeding, weakness, depression	Plasma ascorbic acid, leukocyte ascorbic acid

RBC = red blood cell.

Table 2-4. Guidelines for vitamin and mineral supplementation in patients with severe malabsorption

Supplement	Dose	Route
Prenatal multivitamin with minerals[a]	1 tablet qd	PO
Vitamin D[a]	50,000 U 2–3 times/wk	PO
Calcium[a]	500 mg elemental calcium tid–qid	PO
Vitamin B_{12}[b]	1 mg qd	PO
	100–500 μg q1–2mo	SC
Vitamin A[b]	10,000–50,000 U qd	PO
Vitamin K[b]	5 mg/day	PO
	5–10 mg/wk	SC
Vitamin E[b]	30 U/day	PO
Magnesium gluconate[b]	108–169 mg elemental magnesium qid	PO
Magnesium sulfate[b]	290 mg elemental magnesium 1–3 times/wk	IM/IV
Zinc gluconate or zinc sulfate[b]	25 mg elemental zinc qd plus 100 mg elemental zinc/L intestinal output	PO
Ferrous sulfate[b]	60 mg elemental iron tid	PO
Iron dextran[b]	Daily dose based on formula or table	IV

[a]Recommended routinely for all patients.
[b]Recommended for patients with documented nutrient deficiency or malabsorption.

outcome. The assessment techniques listed below can be used to determine subjectively whether patients are well nourished, moderately malnourished, or severely malnourished (see sec. **IV.A**).

  1. **History.** The patient or appropriate family members, or both, should be interviewed to provide insight into the patient's current nutritional state and future ability to consume an adequate amount of nutrients. The nutritional history should evaluate the following.
    a. **Body weight.** The presence of mild (<5%), moderate (5–10%), or severe (>10%) unintentional body weight loss in the last 6 months should be established. In general, a 10% or greater unintentional loss in body weight in the last 6 months is associated with a poor clinical outcome (*Am J Med* 69:491, 1980).

Table 2-5. Electrolyte concentrations in gastrointestinal fluids

Location	Na (mEq/L)	K (mEq/L)	Cl (mEq/L)	HCO_3 (mEq/L)
Stomach	65	10	100	—
Bile	150	4	100	35
Pancreas	150	7	80	75
Duodenum	90	15	90	15
Mid–small bowel	140	6	100	20
Terminal ileum	40	8	60	70
Rectum	40	90	15	30

b. **Food intake.** A change in habitual diet pattern (number, size, and contents of meals) should be determined. If present, the reason for altered food intake (e.g., change in appetite, mental status or mood, ability to prepare meals, ability to chew or swallow, GI symptoms) should be investigated.

c. **Evidence of malabsorption**

d. **Specific nutrient deficiencies**

e. **Level of metabolic stress**

f. **Functional status.** Any change in function should be determined (bedridden, suboptimally active).

2. **Physical examination.** The physical examination corroborates and adds to the findings obtained by history and should include an assessment of the following.

a. **BMI,** which is defined as weight (in kg) divided by [height (m)]^2 or weight (in lb) $\times$ 704 divided by [height (in.)]^2. Patients can be classified by BMI as underweight (<18.5 kg/m^2), normal weight (18.5–24.9 kg/m^2), overweight (25.0–29.9 kg/m^2), class I obesity (30.0–34.9 kg/m^2), class II obesity (35.0–39.9 kg/m^2), or class III obesity ($\geq$40.0 kg/m^2) [*Obes Res* 6(Suppl 2):S53, 1998]. Patients who are extremely underweight (BMI <14 kg/m^2) are at high risk of death and should be considered for admission to the hospital for nutritional support.

b. **Tissue depletion** can be assessed by the loss of body fat and skeletal muscle wasting.

c. **Muscle function** should be assessed by strength testing of individual muscle groups.

d. **Fluid status** can be assessed by signs and symptoms of either dehydration (hypotension, tachycardia, postural changes, mucosal xerosis, decreased axillary sweat, or dry skin) or excess body fluid (i.e., edema or ascites).

3. **Laboratory studies** should be performed to determine specific nutrient deficiencies when clinically indicated (see Table 2-3). The concentration of several plasma proteins (e.g., albumin, prealbumin, retinol-binding protein, and transferrin) has been shown to correlate with clinical outcome. For example, a low serum albumin concentration is associated with an increased incidence of medical complications and death (*Crit Care Med* 10:305, 1982). However, illness or injury, not malnutrition, is responsible for hypoalbuminemia in sick patients (*Gastroenterology* 99:1845, 1990). Inflammation and injury decrease albumin synthesis, increase albumin degradation, and increase albumin transcapillary losses from the plasma compartment. In addition, certain GI, renal, and cardiac diseases can increase albumin losses through the GI tract and kidney, and albumin can be lost through surface tissues that have been damaged by wounds, burns, and peritonitis.

III. **Enteral nutrition**

A. **General principles.** Whenever possible, oral/enteral rather than parenteral feeding should be used in patients who need nutritional support. Oral/enteral nutrition helps maintain the structural and functional integrity of the GI tract by preventing atrophy of the intestinal mucosa and pancreas, preserving mucosal digestive and pancreatic secretory enzyme activity, maintaining GI immunoglobulin A secretion, and preventing cholelithiasis. In addition, oral/enteral nutrition is usually less expensive than parenteral nutrition. However, the intestinal tract cannot be used effectively in patients who have persistent nausea or vomiting, intolerable postprandial abdominal pain or diarrhea, mechanical obstruction, severe hypomotility, severe malabsorption, or high-output fistulas that do not permit feedings proximal or distal to the fistula.

B. **Feeding regimens**

1. **Hospital diets** include a regular diet and diets modified in either nutrient content (amount of fiber, fat, protein, or sodium) or consistency (liquid, pureed, soft). Food intake can often be increased by encouraging

patients to eat, providing assistance at mealtime, avoiding unpalatable diets, allowing some food to be supplied by relatives and friends, and limiting missed meals for medical tests and procedures.

2. **Defined liquid formulas** include feeding modules, monomeric formulas, oligomeric formulas, and polymeric formulas. **Feeding modules** (e.g., Polycose, ProMod, Microlipid) consist of single nutrients, such as protein (intact protein, hydrolyzed protein, or crystalline amino acids), carbohydrate (glucose polymers), or fat (long-chain or medium-chain triglyceride), which can be used to supplement a specific diet or be part of a modular enteral system composed of several nutrient modules. **Elemental (monomeric) formulas** (e.g., Vivonex) contain nitrogen in the form of free amino acids and small amounts of fat (<5% of total calories) and are hyperosmolar (550–650 mOsm/kg). These formulas are not palatable and require either tube feeding or mixing with other foods or flavorings for oral ingestion. Absorption of monomeric formulas is not clinically superior to that of oligomeric or polymeric formulas in patients with adequate pancreatic digestive function. **Semielemental (oligomeric) formulas** (e.g., Vital, Propeptide, Peptamen) contain hydrolyzed protein in the form of small peptides and sometimes free amino acids. **Polymeric formulas** contain nitrogen in the form of whole proteins and include blenderized food, milk-based, and lactose-free formulas. Milk-based formulas (e.g., Carnation Instant Breakfast, Meritine) contain milk as a source of protein and fat and tend to be more palatable than other defined formula diets. Milk-based formulas can be problematic for some lactose-intolerant patients but are often tolerated when infused continuously because this approach decreases the rate of lactose delivered to the intestine. Lactose-free formulas are the most commonly used polymeric formulas in hospitalized patients. These formulas are available as standard iso-osmolar solutions, containing approximately 1 kcal/ml, 16% calories as protein, 55% calories as carbohydrate, and 30% calories as fat (e.g., Osmolite, Ensure, Isocal). Most patients can be fed with standard iso-osmolar lactose-free formulas. Predigested (elemental and semielemental) formulas are more expensive than standard formulas and do not usually provide additional clinical benefits, even in patients with limited digestive and absorptive function, such as those with pancreatic insufficiency treated with enzyme replacement and those with short-bowel syndrome. Other formulas are also available that have modified nutrient content, such as high-nitrogen (e.g., Promote) or high-calorie (e.g., Two Cal HN) formulas for patients who require fluid restriction and fiber-enriched formulas (e.g., Jevity) for patients with constipation or loose stools or those receiving long-term enteral tube feeding.

3. **Oral rehydration solutions.** Oral rehydration solutions stimulate sodium and water absorption by taking advantage of the sodium-glucose cotransporter present in the brush border of intestinal epithelium. Oral rehydration therapy can be useful in patients with severe GI fluid and mineral losses, such as those with short-bowel syndrome [*Clin Ther* 12(Suppl A):129, 1990] and HIV infection (*Nutrition* 5:390, 1989). In patients with short-bowel syndrome, it is particularly important that the sodium concentration of the solution is between 90 and 120 mEq/L to avoid intestinal sodium secretion and negative sodium and water balance. The characteristics of several oral rehydration solutions are listed in Table 2-6.

C. **Enteral tube feeding.** Enteral tube feeding is useful in patients who have a functional GI tract but who cannot or will not ingest adequate nutrients. The type of tube feeding approach selected (nasogastric, nasoduodenal, nasojejunal, gastrostomy, jejunostomy, pharyngostomy, and esophagostomy tubes) depends on physician experience, clinical prognosis, gut patency and motility, risk of aspirating gastric contents, patient preference, and anticipated duration of feeding.

Table 2-6. Characteristics of selected oral rehydration solutions

Product	Na (mEq/L)	K (mEq/L)	Cl (mEq/L)	Citrate (mEq/L)	kcal/L	CHO (g/L)	mOsm
Equalyte	78	22	68	30	100	25	305
CeraLyte 70	70	20	98	30	165	40	235
CeraLyte 90	90	20	98	30	165	40	260
Pedialyte	45	20	35	30	100	20	300
Rehydralyte	74	19	64	30	100	25	305
Gatorade	20	3	NA	NA	210	45	330
WHO[a]	90	20	80	30	80	20	200
Washington University[b]	105	0	100	10	85	20	250

NA = not applicable.
Note: Mix formulas with sugar-free flavorings as needed for palatability.
[a]WHO (World Health Organization) formula: mix 3/4 tsp sodium chloride, 1/2 tsp sodium citrate, 1/4 tsp potassium chloride, and 4 tsp glucose (dextrose) in 1 L (4 1/4 cups) of distilled water.
[b]Washington University formula: mix 3/4 tsp sodium chloride, 1/2 tsp sodium citrate, and 3 tbsp + 1 tsp Polycose powder in 1 L (4 1/4 cups) of distilled water.

1. **Short-term (<6 weeks) tube feeding** can be achieved by placement of a soft, small-bore nasogastric or nasoenteric feeding tube. These tubes are made of silicone or polyurethane and do not cause the tissue irritation and necrosis associated with larger polyvinyl chloride tubes. Because many patients are able to eat with the tube in place, tube feeding can be used to supplement oral intake. Although nasogastric feeding is usually the most appropriate route, orogastric feeding in patients with nasal injury or gross nasal deformity and nasoduodenal or nasojejunal feeding in patients with gastroparesis can also be used.

2. **Long-term (>6 weeks) tube feeding** usually requires a gastrostomy or jejunostomy tube that can be placed endoscopically, radiologically, or surgically, depending on the clinical situation and local expertise. **Percutaneous endoscopic gastrostomy** can be performed within 30 minutes and is successfully completed in over 90% of attempts (*Am J Surg* 149:102, 1985). Gastrostomy tubes can be placed percutaneously without endoscopy by inserting the catheter directly into the stomach via a peel-away sheath introduced over a previously placed J wire guide (*Am J Surg* 184:132, 1984). This approach permits tube placement in patients with an obstructing lesion of the esophagus or hypopharynx that prevents passage of an endoscope or gastrostomy tube. Jejunal tube placement can be achieved by threading a tube through an existing gastrostomy or by direct percutaneous endoscopic jejunostomy in patients with previous partial or total gastrectomy (*Gastrointest Endosc* 33:372, 1987). **Surgical gastrostomy and jejunostomy** can be performed by open and laparoscopic techniques and are particularly useful when endoscopic and radiologic approaches are technically impossible or cannot be performed safely because of overlying bowel.

3. **Feeding schedules.** Patients who have feeding tubes in the stomach can often tolerate **intermittent bolus or gravity feedings,** in which the total amount of daily formula is divided into four to six equal portions. Bolus feedings are given by syringe as rapidly as tolerated, and gravity feedings are infused over 30–60 minutes. The patient's upper body should be elevated by 30–45 degrees during and for at least 2 hours after feeding. Tubes should be flushed with water after each feeding.

Intermittent feedings are useful for patients who cannot be positioned with continuous head-of-the-bed elevation or who require greater freedom from feeding. However, patients who experience nausea and early satiety with bolus gravity feedings may require continuous infusion at a slower rate. **Continuous feeding** can often be started at 40–50 ml/hour and advanced by 10 ml/hour every 6 hours until the feeding goal (see sec. **I.B**) is reached. Patients who have gastroparesis often tolerate gastric tube feedings when they are started at a slow rate (e.g., 10 ml/hour) and advanced by small increments (e.g., 10 ml/hour q8–12h). However, patients with severe gastroparesis require passage of the feeding tube tip past the ligament of Treitz. Continuous feeding should always be used when feeding directly into the duodenum or jejunum to avoid distention, abdominal pain, and dumping syndrome.

4. **Complications**
   a. **Mechanical complications. Nasogastric feeding tube misplacement** occurs more commonly in unconscious than in conscious patients. Intubation of the tracheobronchial tree has been reported in up to 15% of patients; intracranial placement can occur in patients with skull fractures. **Erosive tissue damage** can lead to nasopharyngeal erosions, pharyngitis, sinusitis, otitis media, pneumothorax, and GI tract perforation. **Tube occlusion** is often caused by inspissated feedings or pulverized medications given through small-diameter (<10 French) tubes. Frequent flushing of the tube with 30–60 ml water and avoiding administration of pill fragments or "thick" medications help prevent occlusion. Techniques used to unclog tubes include the use of a small-volume syringe (10 ml) to flush warm water or pancreatic enzymes (Viokase dissolved in water) through the tube. Commercially made products can be obtained that either dissolve or mechanically remove the obstruction.
   b. **Hyperglycemia.** Management of blood glucose in tube-fed patients with diabetes can be challenging. Subcutaneously administered insulin can usually maintain good control. Intermediate-duration insulin can often be used safely once tube feedings reach 1000 kcal/day. Providing intermediate-duration insulin every 12 hours is appropriate for patients given continuous (24 hour/day) feeding. A sliding scale algorithm for regular insulin supplementation may be necessary to cover glucose excursions and should be designed to meet each patient's specific needs based on type of diabetes, tube feeding regimen, and concurrent medical therapies that may affect blood glucose concentration.
   c. **Pulmonary aspiration.** The etiology of pulmonary aspiration can be difficult to determine in tube-fed patients because aspiration can occur from refluxed tube feedings or oropharyngeal secretions that are unrelated to feedings. Assessing the color of respiratory secretions after adding several drops of blue food coloring to the feeding formula has been used to aid in determining whether tube feedings are contributing to recovered secretions. **However, recent case reports suggest that food coloring can be absorbed by the GI tract in critically ill patients, which can lead to serious complications (i.e., refractory hypotension, metabolic acidosis) and death.** (*N Engl J Med* 343:1047, 2000) Prevention of reflux by decreasing gastric acid secretion, keeping the head of the bed elevated during feedings, and avoiding gastric feeding in high-risk patients (e.g., those with gastroparesis, gastric outlet obstruction, or frequent vomiting; dysphagia is not a contraindication for gastric tube feeding) is the best management approach.
   d. **GI complications** include nausea, vomiting, abdominal pain, diarrhea, and intestinal ischemia/necrosis. Diarrhea is common in patients who receive tube feeding and occurs in up to 50% of critically ill patients.

Diarrhea is often associated with antibiotic therapy (*JPEN J Parenter Enteral Nutr* 15:277, 1991) and the use of liquid medications that contain nonabsorbable carbohydrates, such as sorbitol (*Am J Med* 88:91, 1990). If diarrhea from tube feeding persists after proper evaluation of possible causes, a trial of antidiarrheal agents or fiber is justified.

IV. Parenteral nutrition

A. General principles. Patients who are unable to consume "adequate" nutrients for a "prolonged" period of time by oral or enteral routes require parenteral nutritional therapy to prevent the adverse effects of malnutrition. However, the decision to use parenteral nutrition can be difficult because the precise definition of "adequate" and "prolonged" is not clear and depends on the patient's amount of body fat and lean tissue mass, the presence of pre-existing medical illnesses, and the level of metabolic stress. In general, parenteral nutrition should be considered if energy intake has been, or is anticipated to be, inadequate (<50% of daily requirements) for more than 7 days. However, the efficacy of this approach has not been tested in clinical trials.

B. Central parenteral nutrition (CPN)

1. Catheters. The infusion of hyperosmolar (usually >1500 mOsm/L) nutrient solutions requires a large-bore, high-flow vessel to minimize vessel irritation and damage. Percutaneous subclavian vein catheterization with advancement of the catheter tip to the junction of the superior vena cava and right atrium is the most commonly used technique for CPN access. The internal jugular, saphenous, and femoral veins are also used. Although these sites either decrease or eliminate the risk of pneumothorax, they are less desirable because of decreased patient comfort and difficulty in maintaining sterility. **Peripherally inserted central venous catheters (PICC),** which also eliminate the risk of pneumothorax, can be used to provide CPN in patients with adequate antecubital vein access.

2. Macronutrient solutions

a. Crystalline amino acid solutions, containing 40–50% essential and 50–60% nonessential amino acids, usually with little or no glutamine, glutamate, aspartate, asparagine, tyrosine, and cysteine, are used to provide protein needs (see Table 2-2). Infused amino acids are oxidized and should be included in the estimate of energy provided as part of the parenteral formulation. Some amino acid solutions have been modified for specific disease states, such as those enriched in branched-chain amino acids, advocated for use in patients who have hepatic encephalopathy, or those that contain mostly essential amino acids, advocated for patients with renal insufficiency.

b. Glucose (dextrose) in IV solutions is hydrated; each gram of dextrose monohydrate provides 3.4 kcal. At least 150 g glucose per day is needed to maximize protein balance by providing energy to tissues that require and prefer glucose as a fuel.

c. Lipid emulsions are available as a 10% (1.1 kcal/ml) or 20% (2.0 kcal/ml) solution and provide energy and a source of essential fatty acids. Emulsion particles are similar in size and structure to chylomicrons and are metabolized like nascent chylomicrons after acquiring apoproteins from contact with circulating endogenous high-density lipoprotein particles. Lipid emulsions are as effective as glucose in conserving body nitrogen economy once absolute tissue requirements for glucose are met. The optimal percentage of calories that should be infused as fat is not known, but 20–30% of total calories is reasonable for most patients. The rate of infusion should not exceed 1.0 kcal/kg/hour (0.11 g/kg/hour) because most complications associated with lipid infusions have been reported when providing more than this amount (*Curr Opin Gastroenterol* 7:306, 1991). A rate of 0.03–0.05 g/kg/minute is adequate for most patients who are receiving continuous CPN. Lipid emulsions should not be given to patients who have triglyceride concentrations of

>400 mg/dl. Moreover, patients at risk for hypertriglyceridemia should have serum triglyceride concentrations checked at least once during lipid emulsion infusion to ensure adequate clearance. Lipids may not be necessary in obese patients; underfeeding obese patients by the amount of lipid calories that would normally be given (e.g., 20–30% of calories) facilitates mobilization of endogenous fat stores for fuel and may improve insulin sensitivity and glucose control.

3. **Complications.** The incidence of most complications associated with the use of CPN is reduced with careful management and supervision, preferably by an experienced nutrition support team if available (*JAMA* 243:1906, 1980).

   a. **Mechanical complications** such as pneumothorax, brachial plexus injury, subclavian and carotid artery puncture, hemothorax, thoracic duct injury, and chylothorax occur during central line insertion. Even when the subclavian vein is cannulated successfully, other mechanical complications can still occur. The catheter may be advanced upward into the internal jugular vein, or the tip can be sheared off completely if it is withdrawn back through an introducing needle. Air embolism can occur during insertion or whenever the connection between the catheter and IV tubing is disrupted.

   b. **Metabolic complications,** such as fluid overload, hypertriglyceridemia, hypercalcemia, hypoglycemia, hyperglycemia, and specific nutrient deficiencies, are usually caused by overzealous or inadequate nutrient administration. Blood glucose above 200 mg/dl should be avoided because it is associated with leukocyte and complement dysfunction and increases the risk of infection. Blood glucose goals for most patients are 100–200 mg/dl initially and 100–150 mg/dl when stable. Blood glucose should be kept below 120 mg/dl in pregnant patients to avoid complications of gestational diabetes and large-for-gestational-age births. Management principles for patients with hyperglycemia or diabetes are outlined in Table 2-7.

   c. **Thrombosis and pulmonary embolus.** Radiologically evident subclavian vein thrombosis occurs commonly ($\approx$ 25–50%), but clinically significant manifestations, such as upper extremity edema, superior vena cava syndrome, or pulmonary embolism, are rare. Fatal microvascular pulmonary emboli caused by nonvisible precipitate, containing calcium and phosphorus, in total nutrient admixtures underscore the importance of maintaining strict pharmacy standards regarding physical-chemical compatibility. Moreover, inline filters should be used with all parenteral nutrient solutions. The smallest pulmonary capillaries are 5 μm in diameter, and the size limit for visual detection of microprecipitates is 50–100 μm (*Clin Nutr* 10:114, 1995).

   d. **Infectious complications.** Catheter-related sepsis is the most common life-threatening complication in patients who receive CPN and is most commonly caused by *Staphylococcus epidermidis* and *Staphylococcus aureus*. In immunocompromised patients (e.g., with AIDS, immunosuppressive therapy, chemotherapy, absolute neutrophil count <200) and those with long-term (>2 weeks) CPN, *Enterococcus*, *Candida* species, *Escherichia coli*, *Pseudomonas*, *Klebsiella*, *Enterobacter*, *Acinetobacter*, *Proteus*, and *Xanthomona* should be considered. The principles of evaluation and management of suspected catheter-related infection in patients receiving CPN are outlined in Table 2-8.

   e. **Hepatobiliary complications.** Hepatic abnormalities associated with CPN include biochemical (elevated serum aminotransferase and alkaline phosphatase) and histologic (steatosis, steatohepatitis, lipidosis and phospholipidosis, cholestasis, fibrosis, and cirrhosis) alterations [L Schiff, ER Schiff (eds), *Disease of the Liver* (7th ed). Philadelphia: JB Lippincott, 1993:1505–1516]. Although these abnormalities are

Table 2-7. Management of hyperglycemia in patients receiving parenteral nutrition

If blood glucose is >200 mg/dl or patient has diabetes:

Consider obtaining better control of blood glucose before starting central parenteral nutrition (CPN).

If CPN is started: (1) Limit dextrose to <200 g/day, (2) add 0.1 units of regular insulin for each gram of dextrose in CPN solution (e.g., 15 units for 150 g), (3) discontinue other sources of IV dextrose, and (4) order SC sliding-scale regular insulin with blood glucose monitoring by fingerstick every 4–6 hrs or sliding-scale IV regular insulin infusion with blood glucose monitoring by fingerstick every 1–2 hrs as follows:

Blood glucose (mg/dl)	SC regular insulin (units) or	IV regular insulin (units/hr)
150–199	2.0	—
200–249	2–3	2.5
250–300	4–6	3.0
301–350	6–8	4.0
351–400	8–12	6.0
>400	—	8.0

If blood glucose remains >200 mg/dl and patient has been receiving:

SC insulin: add 50% of sliding-scale regular insulin given in last 24 hrs to next day's CPN solution; double amount of SC insulin sliding-scale dose for blood glucose values >200 mg/dl.

IV insulin: add 50% of IV insulin given in last 24 hrs to next day's CPN solution; increase sliding-scale IV insulin infusion rate by 50% for blood glucose values >200 mg/dl.

If patient's blood glucose remains >200 mg/dl, consider (1) discontinuing CPN until better glucose control can be established, (2) decreasing dextrose content in CPN, or (3) initiating insulin drip if not already started.

Dextrose in CPN can be increased when blood glucose control (100–150 mg/dl) is achieved. Insulin:dextrose ratio in CPN formulation should be maintained while CPN dextrose content is changed.

Source: Adapted from MM McMahon, RA Rizza. Nutrition support in hospitalized patients with diabetes mellitus. *Mayo Clin Proc* 71:587–594, 1996.

usually benign and transient, more serious and progressive disease may develop in a small subset of patients, usually after 16 weeks of CPN therapy. The biliary complications associated with the use of CPN include acalculous cholecystitis, gallbladder sludge, and cholelithiasis and usually occur in patients receiving CPN for more than 3 weeks. Efforts to prevent hepatobiliary complications by providing a portion (20–40%) of calories as fat, cycling CPN so that the glucose infusion is stopped for at least 8–10 hours/day, encouraging enteral intake to stimulate gallbladder contraction and maintain mucosal integrity, and avoiding excessive calories should be routine in all patients who are receiving long-term CPN. If abnormal liver biochemistries or other evidence of liver damage occur, an evaluation for other possible causes of liver disease should be performed. Parenteral nutrition does not need to be discontinued, but the same principles used in preventing hepatic complications can be applied therapeutically. When cholestasis is present, copper and manganese should be deleted from the CPN formula to prevent accumulation in the liver and basal ganglia. A 4-week trial of metronidazole or ursodeoxycholic acid has been reported to be helpful in some patients.

Table 2-8. Management of suspected catheter-related infection

1. Initial evaluation
   a. Evaluate catheter insertion site and culture any drainage
   b. Obtain blood cultures from peripheral vein and central vein catheter
   c. Consider culture of hub, skin, infusate
   d. Culture catheter tip, if removed
   e. CBC and differential
   f. Look for other causes of infection (e.g., urinalysis, chest radiography, sputum, wounds)
   g. Evaluate if catheter can be replaced or if it is "irreplaceable" because of limited access
2. Stop total parenteral nutrition for 48–72 hrs
3. Indications for central venous catheter removal
   a. Immediate removal
      (1) Purulent discharge or abscess at insertion site
      (2) Septic shock without another etiology for the source of infection
   b. Removal of "replaceable" catheters after culture results are obtained
      (1) Persistent or recurrent catheter-related bacteremia
      (2) *Candida* species or *Pseudomonas* infection
      (3) Polymicrobial infection
      (4) *Staphylococcus aureus* infection
4. Antibiotic therapy
   a. Empiric antibiotic therapy administered through central venous catheter until culture results are back
      (1) Vancomycin, 1 g q12h (adjust dose for creatinine/glomerular filtration rate)
      (2) Cefepime, 1 g q12h (if gram-negative infection suspected)
   b. Specific antibiotic therapy administered through central venous catheter once culture results are available
   c. If a catheter is "irreplaceable," consider trial of antibiotic therapy with line in place
   d. Duration of antibiotic therapy usually ranges from 2–6 wks depending on patient, organism, and whether central line has been left in place
5. Repeat blood cultures in 48 and 72–96 hrs to ensure clearance of bacteremia
6. Fever should resolve within 72–96 hrs if appropriate antibiotics are given; remove catheter if fever persists

---

     f. Metabolic bone disease has been observed in patients receiving long-term (>3 months) CPN. The clinical manifestations of bone disease are seen in asymptomatic patients who have radiologic evidence of demineralization, those who have bone pain, and those who experience bone fracture (*Annu Rev Nutr* 11:93, 1991). Histologic examination has found osteomalacia or osteopenia, or both. The cause or causes of metabolic bone disease are not known, but several mechanisms have been proposed, including aluminum toxicity, vitamin D toxicity, and negative calcium balance.
  C. Peripheral parenteral nutrition (PPN) is often considered to have limited usefulness because of the high risk of thrombophlebitis. However, appropriate

adjustments in the management of peripheral parenteral nutrition can increase the life of a single infusion site to more than 10 days. The following guidelines are recommended: (1) Provide at least 50% of total energy as a lipid emulsion piggy-backed with the dextrose–amino acid solution, (2) add 500–1000 units heparin and 5 mg hydrocortisone (to decrease phlebitis) per L, (3) place a fine-bore 22- or 23-gauge polyvinyl pyrrolidone–coated polyurethane catheter in as large a vein as possible in the proximal forearm using sterile technique, (4) place a 5-mg glycerol trinitrate ointment patch (or $1/4$ in. of 2% nitroglycerin ointment) over the infusion site, (5) infuse the solution with a volumetric pump, (6) keep the total infused volume below 3500 ml/day, and (7) filter the solution with an inline 1.2-μm filter (*Nutrition* 10:49, 1994).

D. Long-term home parenteral nutrition (HPN) is usually given through a tunneled catheter or an implantable subcutaneous port that is inserted in the subclavian vein and exits on the anterior chest. Nutrient formulations can be infused overnight to permit daytime activities. IV lipids may not be necessary in patients who are able to ingest and absorb adequate amounts of fat.

V. Monitoring nutrition support in the hospital is needed to ensure that nutritional therapy is safe and adequate. When nutrition support is initiated, other sources of glucose (e.g., peripheral IV dextrose infusions) should be stopped and the volume of other IV fluids adjusted to account for CPN. Vital signs should be checked every 8 hours. In certain patients, body weight, fluid intake, and fluid output should be followed daily. Serum electrolytes (including phosphorus) should be measured every 1 or 2 days after CPN is started until values are stable and then rechecked weekly. Serum glucose should be checked up to every 4–6 hours by fingerstick until blood glucose concentrations are stable and then rechecked weekly. If lipid emulsions are being given, serum triglycerides should be measured during lipid infusion in patients at risk for hypertriglyceridemia to demonstrate adequate clearance (triglyceride concentrations <400 mg/dl). Careful attention to the catheter and catheter site can help prevent catheter-related infections. Gauze dressings should be changed every 48–72 hours or when contaminated or wet, but transparent dressings can be changed weekly. Tubing that connects the parenteral solutions with the catheter should be changed every 24 hours. A 0.22-μm filter should be inserted between the IV tubing and the catheter when lipid-free CPN is infused and should be changed with the tubing. A 1.2-μm filter should be used when a total nutrient admixture containing a lipid emulsion is infused. When a single-lumen catheter is used to deliver CPN, the catheter should not be used to infuse other solutions or medications, with the exception of compatible antibiotics, and it should not be used to monitor central venous pressure. Adjustment of the nutrient formulation is often needed as medical therapy or clinical status changes.

VI. Refeeding the severely malnourished patient

    A. Complications. Initiating nutritional therapy in patients who are severely malnourished and have had minimal nutrient intake can have adverse clinical consequences known as the **"refeeding syndrome,"** which includes the following features.

        1. Hypophosphatemia, hypokalemia, and hypomagnesemia. Rapid and marked decreases in these electrolytes occur during initial refeeding because of insulin-stimulated increases in cellular mineral uptake from extracellular fluid. For example, plasma phosphorus concentration can fall below 1 mg/dl and cause death within hours of initiating nutritional therapy if adequate phosphate is not given (*Am J Clin Nutr* 34:393, 1981).

        2. Fluid overload and congestive heart failure are associated with decreased cardiac function and insulin-induced increased sodium and water reabsorption in conjunction with nutritional therapy containing water, glucose, and sodium.

        3. Cardiac arrhythmias. Patients who are severely malnourished often have bradycardia. Sudden death from ventricular tachyarrhythmias can occur during the first week of refeeding in severely malnourished patients and may be associated with a prolonged QT interval (*Ann Intern Med* 102:49, 1985) or plasma electrolyte abnormalities.

   4. **Glucose intolerance.** Starvation causes insulin resistance, so that refeeding with high-carbohydrate meals or large amounts of parenteral glucose can cause marked elevations in blood glucose concentration, glucosuria, dehydration, and hyperosmolar coma. In addition, carbohydrate refeeding in patients who are depleted in thiamine can precipitate Wernicke's encephalopathy.

B. Clinical recommendations. Careful evaluation of cardiovascular function and plasma electrolytes (history, physical examination, ECG, and blood tests) and correction of abnormal plasma electrolytes are important before initiation of feeding. Refeeding by the oral or enteral route involves the frequent or continuous administration of small amounts of food or an isotonic liquid formula. Parenteral supplementation or complete parenteral nutrition may be necessary if the intestine cannot tolerate feeding. During initial refeeding, fluid intake should be limited to approximately 800 ml/day plus insensible losses. However, adjustments in fluid and sodium intake are needed in patients who have evidence of fluid overload or dehydration. Changes in body weight provide a useful guide for evaluating the efficacy of fluid administration. Weight gain greater than 0.25 kg/day, or 1.5 kg/week, probably represents fluid accumulation in excess of tissue repletion. Initially, approximately 15 kcal/kg, containing approximately 100 g carbohydrate and 1.5 g protein/kg actual body weight, should be given daily. The rate at which the caloric intake can be increased depends on the severity of the malnutrition and the tolerance to feeding; however, in general, increases of 2–4 kcal/kg q24–48h are appropriate. Sodium should be restricted to approximately 60 mEq or 1.5 g/day, but liberal amounts of phosphorus, potassium, and magnesium should be given to patients who have normal renal function. All other nutrients should be given in amounts needed to meet the recommended dietary intake (see Table 2-3). Body weight, fluid intake, urine output, and plasma glucose and electrolyte values should be monitored daily during early refeeding (first 3–7 days) so that nutritional therapy can be appropriately modified when necessary.

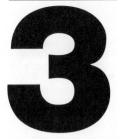

Fluid and Electrolyte Management

Gary G. Singer

General Management of Fluids

I. **Maintenance therapy** can be provided enterally or intravenously for patients who are unable to take food or liquid by mouth. This section assumes normal renal function and the absence of electrolyte or acid-base disturbances.

  A. **Minimum water requirements** for daily fluid balance can be approximated from the sum of the urine output necessary to excrete the daily solute load (500 ml/day) plus the insensible water losses from the skin and respiratory tract (500 ml/day), minus the amount of water produced from endogenous metabolism (250–350 ml/day). It is not uncommon to administer 2–3 L water/day to produce a urine volume of greater than 1000–1500 ml/day, because there is no advantage to minimizing urine output. **Weighing the patient daily** is the best means of assessing net gain or loss of total body fluid, since GI, renal, and insensible fluid losses of patients are unpredictable. Table 3-1 lists commonly used IV fluid preparations.

  B. **The electrolytes** that are usually administered during maintenance fluid therapy are Na^+ and K^+ salts. Requirements depend on minimum obligatory and ongoing losses. The kidneys are normally capable of compensating for wide fluctuations in dietary Na^+ intake—renal Na^+ excretion can fall to less than 5 mmol/day in the absence of Na^+ intake. It is customary to provide 50–150 mmol Na^+ daily (as NaCl). Generally, K^+ supplementation (20–60 mmol/day) is included if renal function is adequate. Carbohydrate in the form of dextrose (100–150 g/day) is given to minimize protein catabolism and prevent ketoacidosis.

  C. **A maintenance IV fluid regimen** can be provided by the administration of 2–3 L (90–125 ml/hour) 0.45% NaCl with 5% dextrose and 20 mmol/L KCl. Calcium, magnesium, phosphorus, vitamins, and protein replacement are necessary after 1 week of parenteral therapy (see Chap. 2). However, in very ill patients, this hypotonic solution can lead to severe hyponatremia (see Salt and Water, sec. **IV.A**).

II. **Replacement of abnormal water and electrolyte losses**

  A. **Insensible water losses** from the skin and respiration depend on respiratory rate, ambient temperature, humidity, and body temperature. Water losses increase by 100–150 ml/day for each degree of body temperature over 37°C. Fluid losses from sweating can vary enormously (100–2000 ml/hour) and depend on physical activity as well as body and ambient temperatures. Mechanical ventilation with humidified gases minimizes losses from the respiratory tract. Replacement of insensible water losses should be with 5% dextrose or hypotonic saline.

  B. **Gastrointestinal losses** vary in composition and volume depending on their source. Laboratory measurement of fluid composition can be performed to increase the accuracy of electrolyte replacement.

Table 3-1. Commonly used parenteral solutions

IV solution	Osmolality (mOsm/kg)	[Glucose] (g/L)	[Na$^+$] (mmol/L)	[Cl$^-$] (mmol/L)
5% D/W	278	50	0	0
10% D/W	556	100	0	0
50% D/W	2778	500	0	0
0.45% NaCl[a]	154	—[b]	77	77
0.9% NaCl[a]	308	—[b]	154	154
3% NaCl	1026	—	513	513
Lactated Ringer's[c]	274	—[b]	130	109

D/W = dextrose in water.
Note: One 50-ml ampule of 7.5% NaHCO$_3$ contains 44.6 mmol each of Na$^+$ and HCO$_3^-$. One 50-ml ampule of 8.4% NaHCO$_3$ contains 50 mmol each of Na$^+$ and HCO$_3^-$.
[a]NaCl 0.45% and 0.9% are half-normal and normal saline, respectively.
[b]Also available with 5% dextrose.
[c]Also contains 4 mmol/L K$^+$, 1.5 mmol/L Ca^{2+}, and 28 mmol/L lactate.

   C. Renal losses of Na$^+$ may be significant, particularly in the setting of diuretic use, the recovery phase of acute tubular necrosis (ATN), postobstructive diuresis, interstitial renal disease, or mineralocorticoid deficiency. Kaliuresis may occur with the recovery phase of ATN, renal tubular acidosis (RTA), diuretic use, hyperaldosteronism, and catabolic states. If prolonged losses occur, measurement of the urine sodium and potassium may help guide replacement.
   D. Rapid internal fluid shifts can occur with peritonitis, pancreatitis, portal vein thrombosis, extensive burns, severe nephrotic syndrome, ileus or intestinal obstruction, bacterial enteritis, crush injuries, and rhabdomyolysis, as well as during the postoperative period. Replacement of sequestered fluid with isotonic saline may be necessary in these situations.

Salt and Water

 I. Total body water and Na$^+$. Water comprises approximately 60% of body weight in men and 50% in women. Total body water is distributed in two major compartments: two-thirds intracellular fluid (ICF) and one-third extracellular fluid (ECF). The latter is further subdivided into intravascular and interstitial spaces in a ratio of 1:4. **Osmolality** is the solute or particle concentration of a fluid. Solutes that are restricted to the ECF (Na$^+$ and accompanying anions) or the ICF (K$^+$ salts and organic phosphate esters) determine the **effective osmolality or tonicity** of that compartment. Osmotic equilibrium occurs because water diffuses rapidly across cell membranes; this prevents differences in tonicity (ICF vs. ECF). The majority (85–90%) of total body Na$^+$ is extracellular. Water and Na$^+$ balance are regulated independently. Changes in [Na$^+$] generally reflect disturbed water homeostasis and ICF volume, whereas alterations in Na$^+$ content are manifest as ECF volume contraction or expansion and imply abnormal Na$^+$ balance.
 II. ECF volume depletion
   A. Manifestations. Symptoms are usually nonspecific and secondary to electrolyte imbalances and tissue hypoperfusion. These include thirst, fatigue, weakness, muscle cramps, and postural dizziness. More severe degrees of volume contraction can lead to syncope and coma. Diminished skin turgor and dry mucous membranes are poor markers of decreased interstitial fluid.

Signs of intravascular volume contraction include decreased jugular venous pressure, postural hypotension, and postural tachycardia. Mild degrees of volume depletion are often not clinically detectable. Weight loss can help estimate the magnitude of the volume deficit. Larger fluid losses often present as hypovolemic shock, manifest as hypotension, tachycardia, peripheral vasoconstriction, and hypoperfusion—cyanosis, cold and clammy extremities, oliguria, and altered mental status. A thorough history and physical examination are generally sufficient to determine the presence and cause of ECF volume contraction. Laboratory data confirm and support the clinical diagnosis. Measurement of the fractional excretion of Na^+ and BUN/creatinine ratio may provide additional diagnostic information (see Chap. 12). ECF volume contraction often leads to a relative elevation in hematocrit (hemoconcentration) and plasma albumin concentration.

- **B. Etiology.** ECF volume depletion reflects a deficit in total body Na^+ content as a result of renal or extrarenal losses that exceed Na^+ intake. Renal losses may be secondary to diuretics (pharmacologic or osmotic), interstitial renal disease (Na^+ wasting), or mineralocorticoid deficiency. Excessive renal losses of Na^+ and water may also occur during the diuretic phase of ATN and after the relief of bilateral urinary tract obstruction. Nonrenal causes of hypovolemia include fluid loss from the GI tract (vomiting, nasogastric suction, fistula drainage, diarrhea), skin and respiratory losses, third-space accumulations (burns, pancreatitis, peritonitis), and hemorrhage.
- **C. Treatment.** The therapeutic goal is to restore normovolemia with fluid similar in composition to that which was lost, as well as to replace ongoing losses. Mild volume contraction can usually be corrected via the oral route. More severe cases of hypovolemia require IV therapy. Patients with significant hemorrhage, anemia, or IV volume depletion may require blood transfusion or colloid-containing solutions (albumin, dextran). Isotonic or normal saline (0.9% NaCl or 154 mmol/L Na^+) is the solution of choice in normonatremic and mildly hyponatremic individuals and should also be used initially in patients with hypotension or shock. Severe hyponatremia may require hypertonic saline (3.0% NaCl or 513 mmol/L Na^+). Hypokalemia may be present initially or may ensue as a result of increased urinary K^+ excretion and should be corrected by adding appropriate amounts of KCl to replacement solutions. Finally, the appropriate management of hypovolemia must include correction of the underlying cause.

III. ECF volume excess
- **A. Manifestations.** Because 75–80% of the ECF is extravascular, ECF volume excess results in expansion of the interstitial compartment, that is, **edema.** Incipient edema may only be detected by the presence of weight gain. Overt edema is apparent only after 3–4 L of fluid have accumulated. Clinical findings include dyspnea, tachypnea, tachycardia, pulmonary rales, elevated jugular venous pressure, hepatojugular reflux, presence of an S3 gallop, and peripheral or presacral edema.
- **B. Etiology.** ECF volume expansion is caused by salt intake in the presence of renal Na^+ retention. The latter may be caused by a primary renal disorder such as renal failure or the nephrotic syndrome. Alternatively, enhanced Na^+ reabsorption may be secondary to decreased effective circulating or arterial volume that results from heart failure or hypoalbuminemia (e.g., hepatic cirrhosis).
- **C. Treatment** must address not only the ECF volume excess but also the underlying pathologic process. Treatment of the nephrotic syndrome and the cardiovascular volume overload associated with renal failure are discussed in Chap. 12. Treatment of heart failure and cirrhosis are discussed in Chaps. 6 and 17, respectively.

IV. Hyponatremia is defined as a plasma $[Na^+]$ of less than 135 mmol/L. In the absence of hyperglycemia, this usually reflects a hypo-osmolar state and an increased ICF volume. To maintain homeostasis and a normal plasma $[Na^+]$, the ingestion of solute-free water must eventually lead to the loss of the same volume of electrolyte-free water. Three steps are required for the kidney to excrete a water load: (1) glomerular filtration and delivery of water (and electrolytes) to the diluting sites of the nephron, (2) active reabsorption of Na^+ and Cl^- without water in the thick ascending limb of the loop of Henle, and (3) maintenance of a dilute urine due to impermeability of the collecting duct to water in the absence of vasopressin (antidiuretic hormone). Abnormalities of any of these steps can result in impaired free water excretion and eventual hyponatremia.

A. Hyponatremia with a low plasma osmolality. Most causes of hyponatremia are associated with a low plasma osmolality (high ICF volume). In general, hypotonic hyponatremia is caused either by a primary water gain or Na^+ loss. The ECF volume, reflecting total body Na^+ content, may be decreased, normal, or increased in hyponatremia.

   1. Hyponatremia associated with ECF volume depletion may result from renal or nonrenal causes of net Na^+ loss (see sec. II.B). A decreased effective arterial volume stimulates thirst. It also stimulates vasopressin release from the posterior pituitary gland, which impairs the capacity to excrete a dilute urine. Hyponatremia develops as a consequence of electrolyte-free water retention. Furthermore, certain causes of hypovolemic hyponatremia (e.g., diuretics or vomiting) may be associated with a large K^+ deficit, resulting in transcellular ion exchange (K^+ exits and Na^+ enters cells), which contributes to hyponatremia.

   2. Hyponatremia associated with ECF volume excess is usually a consequence of edematous states, such as CHF, hepatic cirrhosis, and the nephrotic syndrome. These disorders all have in common a decreased effective circulating arterial volume, leading to increased thirst and vasopressin levels. The increase in total body Na^+ is exceeded by the rise in total body water. The degree of hyponatremia often correlates with the severity of the underlying condition and is therefore an important prognostic factor. Oliguric acute and chronic renal failure may be associated with hyponatremia if water intake exceeds the kidney's limited ability to excrete equivalent volumes.

   3. Hyponatremia associated with a normal ECF volume

   a. The syndrome of inappropriate antidiuretic hormone secretion (SIADH) is the commonest cause of normovolemic hyponatremia. This disorder is caused by the nonphysiologic release of vasopressin from the posterior pituitary or an ectopic source, resulting in impaired renal free water excretion. Common causes of SIADH include neuropsychiatric disorders, pulmonary diseases, and malignant tumors. SIADH is characterized by (1) hypo-osmotic hyponatremia, (2) an inappropriately concentrated urine (urine osmolality >100 mOsm/kg), (3) euvolemia, and (4) normal renal, adrenal, and thyroid function.

   b. Glucocorticoid deficiency and hypothyroidism may present with hyponatremia and should not be confused with SIADH. Although decreased mineralocorticoids may contribute to the hyponatremia of Addison's disease, it is the cortisol deficiency that leads to hypersecretion of vasopressin directly (cosecreted with corticotropin-releasing factor) and indirectly (secondary to volume depletion). The mechanisms by which hypothyroidism leads to hyponatremia include decreased cardiac output and glomerular filtration rate (GFR) and increased vasopressin secretion in response to hemodynamic stimuli.

   c. Pharmacologic agents may cause hyponatremia by one of at least three mechanisms: (1) stimulation of vasopressin release (e.g., nicotine, carbamazepine, tricyclic antidepressants, antipsychotic agents, antineoplastic drugs, narcotics), (2) potentiation of antidiuretic action of vasopressin [e.g., chlorpropamide, methylxanthines, nonsteroidal anti-inflammatory drugs (NSAIDs)], or (3) vasopressin analogs [e.g., oxytocin, desmopressin acetate (DDAVP)].

   d. **Physical and emotional stress** are often associated with vaso-
      pressin release, possibly secondary to nausea or hypotension, or
      both, associated with stress-induced vasovagal reactions.
   e. **Acute hypoxia or hypercapnia** also stimulates vasopressin secretion.
   f. **Primary polydipsia** refers to a condition of compulsive water con-
      sumption that may overwhelm the normally large renal excretory
      capacity of 12 L/day. These patients often have psychiatric illnesses
      and may be taking medications, such as phenothiazines, that
      enhance the sensation of thirst by causing a dry mouth.
B. **Hyponatremia with a normal or high plasma osmolality**
   1. **Pseudohyponatremia** is hyponatremia associated with a normal
      plasma osmolality. It occurs as a result of a decrease in the aqueous
      phase of plasma. Plasma is 93% water, with the remaining 7% consist-
      ing of plasma proteins and lipids. Because Na^+ ions are dissolved in
      plasma water, increasing the nonaqueous phase will artificially lower
      the $[Na^+]$ measured per L of plasma (except when Na^+-sensitive glass
      electrodes are used). The plasma osmolality and the $[Na^+]$ measured
      per L of plasma water remain normal. Therefore, this type of
      hyponatremia has no clinical significance, except to ascertain the cause
      of the hyperproteinemia or hyperlipidemia.
   2. **Hyponatremia associated with a hyperosmolar state** is usually caused
      by an increase in the concentration of a solute that is largely restricted
      to the ECF compartment. The resulting osmotic gradient causes water
      to shift from the ICF to the ECF, and hyponatremia ensues. Hypertonic
      hyponatremia is usually caused by hyperglycemia or, occasionally, IV
      administration of mannitol. Quantitatively, the plasma $[Na^+]$ falls by
      1.4 mmol/L for every 100 mg/dl rise in the plasma glucose concentra-
      tion. Isotonic or slightly hypotonic hyponatremia may complicate trans-
      urethral resection of the prostate or bladder (*Br J Urol* 66:71, 1990).
C. **Manifestations.** The clinical features of **acute** hyponatremia are related to
   osmotic water shift leading to increased ICF volume, specifically brain cell
   swelling. Therefore, the symptoms are primarily neurologic, and their
   severity is dependent on the rapidity of onset and absolute decrease in
   plasma $[Na^+]$. Patients may be asymptomatic or may complain of nausea
   and malaise. As the plasma $[Na^+]$ falls, the symptoms progress to include
   headache, lethargy, confusion, and obtundation. Stupor, seizures, and
   coma do not usually occur unless the plasma $[Na^+]$ falls acutely below 120
   mmol/L. In **chronic** hyponatremia, adaptive mechanisms designed to
   defend cell volume occur and tend to minimize the increase in ICF volume
   and its symptoms.
D. **Diagnosis** (Fig. 3-1). The underlying cause of hyponatremia can often be
   ascertained from an accurate history and physical examination, including
   an assessment of ECF volume status and effective circulating arterial volume. Three laboratory findings often provide useful information and can
   narrow the differential diagnosis of hyponatremia: (1) the plasma osmolality, (2) the urine osmolality, and (3) the urine $[Na^+] + [Cl^-]$.
   1. **Plasma osmolality.** Because ECF tonicity is determined primarily by
      the $[Na^+]$, most patients with hyponatremia have a decreased plasma
      osmolality. If the plasma osmolality is not low, pseudohyponatremia and
      hypertonic hyponatremia must be ruled out.
   2. **Urine osmolality and volume.** The appropriate renal response to hypo-
      osmolality is to excrete the maximum volume of dilute urine, that is,
      urine osmolality and specific gravity of less than 100 mOsm/kg and
      1.003, respectively. This occurs in patients with primary polydipsia. If
      this is not present, it suggests impaired free water excretion due to the
      action of vasopressin on the kidney. The secretion of vasopressin may
      be a physiologic response to hemodynamic stimuli, or it may be inap-
      propriate in the presence of hyponatremia and euvolemia. The maximal

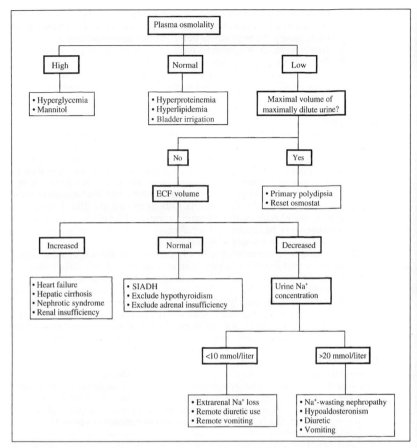

Fig. 3-1. Algorithm depicting clinical approach to hyponatremia. (ECF = extracellular fluid; SIADH = syndrome of inappropriate antidiuretic hormone.) [From GG Singer, BM Brenner. Fluid and Electrolyte Disturbances. In AS Fauci, et al. (eds). *Harrison's Principles of Internal Medicine* (15th ed). New York: McGraw-Hill, 2001, with permission.]

urine output is a function of the minimum urine osmolality achievable and the mandatory solute excretion. Metabolism of a normal diet generates 600–900 mOsm/day, and the minimum urine osmolality in humans is not more than 50 mOsm/kg. Therefore, the maximum daily urine output will be 12 L or more (600 ÷ 50 = 12). A solute excretion rate of greater than 900 mOsm/day is, by definition, an **osmotic diuresis.** A low-protein, low-salt diet may yield as few as 100 mOsm/day, which translates into a maximal urine output of 2 L/day at a minimum urine tonicity of 50 mOsm/kg. Moreover, net Na^+ loss and ECF volume contraction lead to vasopressin release, further impairing free water excretion.

3. **Urine Na^+ + Cl^- concentrations.** Because Na^+ is the major ECF cation and is largely restricted to this compartment, ECF volume contraction represents a deficit in total body Na^+ content. Therefore, volume depletion in patients with normal underlying renal function results in

enhanced tubule Na^+ reabsorption and a urine $[Na^+] + [Cl^-]$ of less than 20 mmol/L. The finding of a urine $[Na^+] + [Cl^-]$ of greater than 20 mmol/L in hypovolemic hyponatremia implies diuretic therapy, hypoaldosteronism, or occasionally vomiting.

E. Treatment. The goals of therapy are threefold: (1) raise the plasma $[Na^+]$ (lowering the ICF volume) by restricting water intake and promoting water loss, (2) replace the Na^+ and K^+ deficit(s), and (3) correct the underlying disorder. Mild asymptomatic hyponatremia is generally of little clinical significance and requires no treatment.

   1. ECF volume contraction. Management of asymptomatic hyponatremia should include Na^+ repletion, generally in the form of saline that is isotonic to the patient, to avoid rapid changes in ICF volume.

   2. Edematous states. Hyponatremia tends to reflect the severity of the underlying disease and is usually asymptomatic. Treatment should include restriction of Na^+ and water intake, correction of hypokalemia, and promotion of water loss in excess of Na^+. The latter may require the use of loop diuretics with replacement of a proportion of the urinary Na^+ loss to ensure net free water excretion. Dietary water restriction should be less than the urine output. Correction of the K^+ deficit may raise the plasma $[Na^+]$. Water restriction is also a component of the therapeutic approach to hyponatremia associated with primary polydipsia, renal failure, and SIADH.

   3. The rate of correction of hyponatremia depends on the absence or presence of neurologic dysfunction (*Lancet* 352:220, 1998). This, in turn, is related to the rapidity of onset and magnitude of the fall in plasma $[Na^+]$. The risks of correcting hyponatremia too rapidly are ECF volume excess and the development of osmotic demyelination or **central pontine myelinolysis.** This disorder, in its most overt form, is characterized by flaccid paralysis, dysarthria, and dysphagia. The diagnosis is occasionally suspected clinically and can be confirmed by appropriate neuroimaging studies (CT scan or MRI). In addition to rapid or overcorrection of hyponatremia, risk factors for osmotic demyelination include hypokalemia and malnutrition, especially secondary to alcoholism.

   4. Acute hyponatremia tends to present with altered mental status or seizures, or both, and requires more rapid correction. Severe **symptomatic** hyponatremia should be treated with hypertonic saline, and the plasma $[Na^+]$ should be raised by 1–2 mmol/L/hour with an absolute limit of 5 mmol/L. Once again, the plasma $[Na^+]$ should be raised by no more than 8 mmol/L during the first 24 hours. The quantity of Na^+ that is required to increase the plasma Na^+ concentration by a given amount can be estimated by multiplying the desired change in plasma $[Na^+]$ by the total body water (e.g., 5 mmol/L $\times$ 30 L = 150 mmol = 300 ml 3% NaCl). In **asymptomatic** patients, the plasma $[Na^+]$ should be raised by no more than 0.3 mmol/L/hour and equal to or less than 8 mmol/L over the first 24 hours.

   5. Water restriction in primary polydipsia and IV saline therapy in ECF volume–contracted patients may also lead to overly rapid correction of hyponatremia as a result of vasopressin suppression and a brisk water diuresis. This can be prevented by administration of water or use of a vasopressin analog to slow down the rate of free water excretion.

   6. The hyponatremia of SIADH can be treated by limiting the intake of water or promoting its excretion, or both. The standard first-line therapy is water restriction. If this fails or if the patient is symptomatic, agents that enhance water excretion can be tried. Loop diuretics impair the ability to excrete concentrated urine and, when combined with Na^+ replacement in the form of salt tablets, can enhance free water excretion. In SIADH, the urine osmolality is relatively fixed. Therefore, the maximum urine output is a direct function of the solute excretion rate, which can be increased by dietary modification (high salt, high protein) or by administering urea, leading to increased urine output and water excretion. Drugs that interfere with the collecting tubule's ability to respond to vasopressin include lithium and demeclocycline. These agents are rarely used and should only be considered in severe hyponatremia that is unresponsive to more conservative measures.

V. **Hypernatremia** is defined as a plasma [Na$^+$] of greater than 145 mmol/L and represents a state of hyperosmolality. Maintenance of osmotic equilibrium in hypernatremia results in ICF volume contraction. Hypernatremia may be caused by a primary Na$^+$ gain or water deficit. The two components of an appropriate response to hypernatremia are increased water intake stimulated by thirst and the excretion of the minimum volume of maximally concentrated urine, reflecting vasopressin secretion in response to an osmotic stimulus.

  A. **Impaired thirst.** The degree of hyperosmolality is typically mild unless the thirst mechanism is abnormal or access to water is limited. The latter occurs in infants, the physically handicapped, patients with impaired mental status, in the postoperative state, and in intubated patients in the ICU. Rarely, impaired thirst may be caused by **primary hypodipsia**, as a result of damage to the hypothalamic osmoreceptors that control thirst. Primary hypodipsia may be caused by a variety of pathologic changes, including granulomatous disease, vascular occlusion, and tumors.

  B. **Hypernatremia due to water loss** accounts for the majority of cases of hypernatremia. Because water is distributed between the ICF and the ECF in a 2:1 ratio, a given amount of solute-free water loss results in the same percentage change but, quantitatively, a twofold greater absolute reduction in the ICF compartment than the ECF compartment.

    1. **Nonrenal water loss** may be due to evaporation from the skin and respiratory tract (insensible losses) or loss from the GI tract. Insensible losses are increased with fever, exercise, heat exposure, and severe burns, and in mechanically ventilated patients. Diarrhea is the commonest GI cause of hypernatremia. Specifically, osmotic diarrheas (induced by lactulose, sorbitol, or malabsorption of carbohydrate) and viral gastroenteritides result in water loss exceeding that of Na$^+$ and K$^+$.

    2. **Renal water loss** is the most common cause of hypernatremia and is caused by either osmotic diuresis or diabetes insipidus. The most frequent cause of an osmotic diuresis is hyperglycemia and glucosuria in poorly controlled diabetes mellitus. IV administration of mannitol and increased production of urea (high-protein diet) can also result in an osmotic diuresis. Hypernatremia secondary to nonosmotic urinary water loss is usually caused by (1) central or neurogenic diabetes insipidus characterized by impaired vasopressin secretion or (2) **nephrogenic diabetes insipidus (NDI)** that results from resistance to the actions of vasopressin. The commonest cause of **central diabetes insipidus** (CDI) is destruction of the neurohypophysis as a result of trauma, neurosurgery, granulomatous disease, neoplasms, vascular accidents, or infection. In many cases, CDI is idiopathic and may occasionally be hereditary. **NDI** may be either inherited or acquired. The latter can be further subdivided into disorders associated with renal medullary disease or with impaired vasopressin action. The causes of sporadic NDI are numerous and include drugs (especially lithium), hypercalcemia, hypokalemia, and conditions that impair medullary hypertonicity (e.g., papillary necrosis or osmotic diuresis).

  C. **Hypernatremia due to Na$^+$ gain** occurs infrequently. This is most commonly seen in patients with diabetic ketoacidosis (DKA) and an osmotic diuresis (urine [Na$^+$] ≈ 50 mmol/L) treated with isotonic saline. Inadvertent administration of hypertonic NaCl or NaHCO$_3$ or replacing sugar with salt in infant formula can lead to hypernatremia.

D. Transcellular water shift from ECF to ICF occurs in rare circumstances (e.g., secondary to seizures or rhabdomyolysis). Hypernatremia is accompanied by ECF volume contraction with no change in body weight.

E. Manifestations. The major symptoms of hypernatremia are neurologic and include altered mental status, weakness, neuromuscular irritability, focal neurologic deficits, and occasionally coma or seizures. Patients may also complain of polyuria or thirst. For unknown reasons, patients with polydipsia from CDI tend to prefer ice-cold water. The signs and symptoms of volume depletion are often present in patients with a history of excessive sweating, diarrhea, or an osmotic diuresis. As with hyponatremia, the severity of the clinical manifestations is related to the acuity and magnitude of the rise in plasma [Na^+]. Chronic hypernatremia is generally less symptomatic as a result of adaptive mechanisms designed to defend cell volume.

F. Diagnosis (Fig. 3-2). A complete history and physical examination often provide clues as to the underlying cause of hypernatremia. The history should include a list of current and recent medications, and the physical examination is incomplete without a thorough mental status and neurologic assessment.

    1. Assessment of urine volume and osmolality is essential in the evaluation of hyperosmolality. The appropriate renal response to hypernatremia is the excretion of the minimum volume (500 ml/day) of maximally concentrated urine (urine osmolality >800 mOsm/kg). These findings suggest extrarenal or remote renal water loss or administration of hypertonic Na^+ salt solutions. A primary Na^+ excess can be confirmed by the presence of ECF volume expansion and natriuresis (urine [Na^+] usually >100 mmol/L). Many causes of hypernatremia are associated with polyuria and a submaximal urine osmolality. The solute excretion rate (urine volume × urine osmolality) is helpful in determining the basis of the polyuria. To maintain a steady state, total solute excretion must equal solute production. As mentioned previously, a daily solute excretion in excess of 900 mOsm defines an osmotic diuresis (see sec. IV.D.2). This can be confirmed by measuring the urine glucose and urea.

    2. CDI and NDI generally present with polyuria and hypotonic urine (urine osmolality <250 mOsm/kg). The degree of hypernatremia is usually mild unless the patient has an associated thirst abnormality. The clinical history, physical examination, and pertinent laboratory data can often rule out causes of acquired NDI. CDI and NDI can be distinguished by administering the vasopressin analog DDAVP (10 μg intranasally) after careful water restriction. The urine osmolality should increase by at least 50% in CDI and will not change in NDI. Unfortunately, the diagnosis is sometimes difficult due to partial defects in vasopressin secretion and action.

G. Treatment. The therapeutic goals are (1) to stop ongoing water loss and (2) to correct the water deficit. The ECF volume should be restored in hypovolemic patients. The quantity of water required to correct the deficit can be calculated from the following equation:

$$\text{Water deficit} = \left(\frac{\text{plasma}[Na^+] - 140}{140} \right) \times \text{total body water (L)}$$

    1. The rate of correction. As in hyponatremia, rapid correction of hypernatremia is potentially dangerous due to a rapid shift of water into brain cells, increasing the risk of seizures or permanent neurologic damage. Therefore, the water deficit should be corrected slowly over at least 48–72 hours. When calculating the rate of water replacement, ongoing losses should be taken into account, and the plasma [Na^+] should be lowered by 0.5 mmol/L/hour and by no more than 12 mmol/L over the first 24 hours. The safest route of administration of water is by

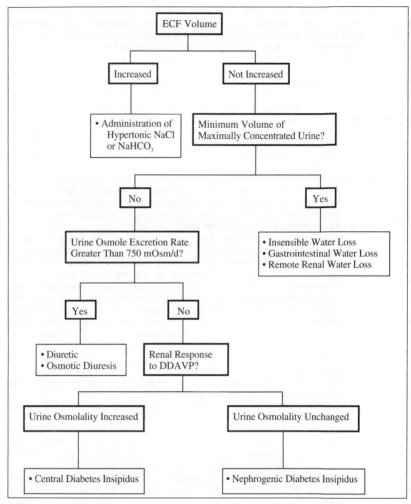

Fig. 3-2. Algorithm depicting clinical approach to hypernatremia. (DDAVP = desmopressin acetate; ECF = extracellular fluid.) [From GG Singer, BM Brenner. Fluid and Electrolyte Disturbances. In AS Fauci, et al. (eds). *Harrison's Principles of Internal Medicine* (15th ed). New York: McGraw-Hill, 2001, with permission.]

mouth or via a nasogastric tube. Alternatively, half-isotonic or quarter-isotonic saline can be given IV.

2. **CDI.** The appropriate treatment of CDI consists of administering DDAVP intranasally.

3. **NDI.** The concentrating defect in NDI may be reversible by treating the underlying disorder or eliminating the offending drug. Symptomatic polyuria caused by NDI can be treated with a low-Na$^+$ diet and thiazide diuretics. This results in mild volume depletion, enhanced proximal reabsorption of salt and water, and decreased delivery to the site of action of vasopressin, the collecting duct. NSAIDs potentiate vasopressin action and thereby increase urine osmolality and decrease urine volume.

Potassium

Potassium is the major intracellular cation. The normal plasma [K$^+$] is 3.5–5.0 mmol/L, whereas that inside cells is approximately 150 mmol/L. Therefore, the amount of K$^+$ in the ECF constitutes less than 2% of the total body K$^+$ content. The Na$^+$–K$^+$–ATPase pump actively transports Na$^+$ out and K$^+$ in the cell in a 3:2 ratio, and the passive outward diffusion of K$^+$ is quantitatively the most important factor that generates the resting membrane potential. The K$^+$ intake of individuals on an average Western diet is approximately 1 mmol/kg/day, 90% of which is absorbed by the GI tract. Maintenance of the steady state necessitates matching K$^+$ ingestion with excretion.

Renal excretion is the major route of elimination of excess K$^+$. Ninety percent of filtered K$^+$ is reabsorbed by the proximal convoluted tubule and loop of Henle. Net distal K$^+$ secretion or reabsorption occurs in the setting of K$^+$ excess or depletion, respectively. The cell responsible for K$^+$ secretion in the distal convoluted tubule and cortical collecting duct (CCD) is the principal cell. Virtually all regulation of renal K$^+$ excretion and total body K$^+$ balance occurs in the distal nephron. The driving force for K$^+$ secretion is a favorable electrochemical gradient across the luminal membrane of the principal cell. The generation of a lumen-negative transepithelial potential difference favors K$^+$ secretion and depends on the relative rates of reabsorption of Na$^+$ and its accompanying anion (primarily Cl$^-$). Equimolar reabsorption of Na$^+$ and Cl$^-$ at equivalent rates is electroneutral, whereas reabsorption of Na$^+$ in excess of Cl$^-$ is electrogenic.

Potassium secretion is regulated by two physiologic stimuli, aldosterone and hyperkalemia. Aldosterone is secreted in response to high renin and angiotensin II or hyperkalemia. The plasma [K$^+$], independent of aldosterone, can directly affect K$^+$ secretion. In addition to the [K$^+$] in the lumen of the CCD, renal K$^+$ loss depends on the urine flow rate, a function of daily solute excretion. Because excretion is equal to the product of concentration and volume, increased distal flow rate can significantly enhance urinary K$^+$ output.

I. Hypokalemia

A. Manifestations. The clinical features of K$^+$ depletion vary greatly, and their severity depends in part on the degree of hypokalemia. Symptoms seldom occur unless the plasma [K$^+$] is less than 3.0 mmol/L. Fatigue, myalgia, and muscular weakness of the lower extremities are common complaints. More severe hypokalemia may lead to progressive weakness, hypoventilation, and eventually complete paralysis. Profound K$^+$ depletion is associated with an increased risk of arrhythmias and also rhabdomyolysis. Smooth-muscle function may also be affected and manifest as paralytic ileus. The ECG changes of hypokalemia do not correlate well with the plasma [K$^+$]. Early changes include flattening or inversion of the T wave, a prominent U wave, ST segment depression, and a prolonged QU interval. Severe K$^+$ depletion may result in a prolonged PR interval, decreased voltage and widening of the QRS complex, and an increased risk of ventricular arrhythmias. Hypokalemia may also predispose to digitalis toxicity.

Hypokalemia is often associated with acid-base disturbances related to the underlying disorder. In addition, K$^+$ depletion results in enhanced proximal HCO$_3^-$ reabsorption, increased renal ammoniagenesis, and increased distal H$^+$ secretion. This contributes to the generation of metabolic alkalosis that is frequently present in hypokalemic patients. NDI can occur with K$^+$ depletion and is manifest as polydipsia and polyuria.

B. Etiology. Hypokalemia, defined as a plasma [K$^+$] of less than 3.5 mmol/L, may result from one or more of the following: decreased net intake, shift into cells, or increased net loss.

    1. Diminished intake is seldom the sole cause of K$^+$ depletion because urinary excretion can be effectively decreased to less than 15 mmol/day.

However, dietary K^+ restriction may exacerbate the hypokalemia secondary to increased GI or renal loss.

2. Transcellular shift. Movement of K^+ into cells may transiently decrease the plasma $[K^+]$ without altering total body K^+ content. The magnitude of the change is relatively small, often less than 1 mmol/L, but may amplify the hypokalemia due to K^+ wasting. Metabolic alkalosis is always associated with hypokalemia as a result of K^+ redistribution as well as excessive renal K^+ loss. Insulin therapy for DKA may lead to hypokalemia. Furthermore, uncontrolled hyperglycemia often leads to K^+ depletion from an osmotic diuresis. Stress-induced catecholamine release and administration of β_2-adrenergic agonists directly induce cellular uptake of K^+, as well as promote insulin secretion by the pancreas. Anabolic states can potentially result in hypokalemia caused by a K^+ shift into cells. This may occur after rapid cell growth, seen in patients with pernicious anemia or neutropenia treated with vitamin B_{12} or granulocyte-macrophage colony-stimulating factor, respectively. It can also be seen in patients on total parenteral nutrition and after treatment for DKA.

3. Nonrenal K^+ loss. Moderate to severe K^+ depletion is often associated with vomiting or nasogastric suction and is primarily due to increased renal K^+ excretion. Loss of gastric contents results in volume depletion and metabolic alkalosis, both of which promote kaliuresis. Hypovolemia stimulates aldosterone release, which augments K^+ secretion by the principal cells. In addition, bicarbonaturia enhances the electrochemical gradient favoring K^+ loss in the urine. Hypokalemia subsequent to increased GI loss can occur in patients with profuse diarrhea, villous adenomas, vasoactive intestinal polypeptide (VIP)omas, or laxative abuse. Excessive sweating that leads to hypovolemia may result in K^+ depletion from increased integumentary and renal K^+ losses (secondary to ECF volume contraction).

4. Renal K^+ loss accounts for most cases of chronic hypokalemia. This may be caused by factors that increase the K^+ concentration in the lumen of the CCD or augment distal flow rate. Diuretic use and abuse are common causes of K^+ depletion (*Kidney Int* 28:988, 1985). As described previously, distal nephron K^+ secretion is driven by a lumen-negative transepithelial potential difference, affected by aldosterone and the relative rates of reabsorption of Na^+ and its accompanying anion(s). Mineralocorticoid excess commonly results in hypokalemia. **Primary hyperaldosteronism** is caused by dysregulated aldosterone secretion by an adrenal adenoma, carcinoma, or adrenocortical hyperplasia. **Hyperreninemia** (and secondary hyperaldosteronism) is commonly seen in renovascular and malignant hypertension. Renin-secreting tumors are a rare cause of hypokalemia. Hyperreninemia also occurs secondary to decreased effective circulating arterial volume. Enhanced distal nephron secretion of K^+ may result from increased production of nonaldosterone mineralocorticoids in congenital adrenal hyperplasia. The syndrome of apparent mineralocorticoid excess, due to 11β-hydroxysteroid dehydrogenase deficiency or suppression, is associated with the ingestion of licorice and the use of chewing tobacco and carbenoxolone. The presentation of Cushing's syndrome may include hypokalemia. Increased distal delivery of Na^+ with a nonreabsorbable anion (without Cl^-) enhances the electrochemical force that drives K^+ secretion. Typically, this is seen with vomiting, DKA, toluene abuse, and high doses of penicillin derivatives. Classic distal (type 1) RTA is associated with hypokalemia due to increased renal K^+ loss, and amphotericin B causes hypokalemia due to increased distal nephron permeability to Na^+ and K^+, and renal K^+ wasting.

C. Diagnosis (Fig. 3-3). In most cases, the etiology of K^+ depletion can be determined by a careful history. Diuretic and laxative abuse as well as surreptitious vomiting may be difficult to identify but should be excluded. After

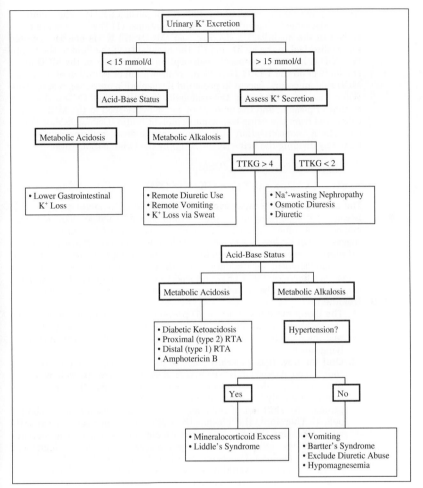

Fig. 3-3. Algorithm depicting clinical approach to hypokalemia. (RTA = renal tubular acidosis; TTKG = transtubular K^+ concentration gradient.) [From GG Singer, BM Brenner. Fluid and Electrolyte Disturbances. In AS Fauci, et al. (eds). *Harrison's Principles of Internal Medicine* (15th ed). New York: McGraw-Hill, 2001, with permission.]

eliminating decreased intake and intracellular shift as potential causes of hypokalemia, examination of the renal response can help to clarify the source of K^+ loss. The appropriate response to K^+ depletion is to excrete less than 15 mmol/day K^+ in the urine. Hypokalemia with minimal renal K^+ excretion suggests that K^+ was lost via the skin or GI tract, or a remote history of vomiting or diuretic use. Renal K^+ wasting may be caused by factors that either increase the $[K^+]$ in the CCD or increase the distal flow rate. The ECF volume status, BP, and associated acid-base disorder may help to differentiate the causes of excessive renal K^+ loss.

The transtubular K^+ concentration gradient (TTKG) is a rapid and simple test designed to evaluate the driving force for net K^+ secretion (*Lancet* 352:135, 1998). The TTKG is the ratio of the $[K^+]$ in the lumen of the CCD

$([K^+]_{CCD})$ to that in peritubular capillaries or plasma $([K^+]_p)$. The validity of this measurement depends on three assumptions: (1) Few solutes are reabsorbed in the medullary collecting duct (MCD), (2) K^+ is neither secreted nor reabsorbed in the MCD, and (3) the osmolality of the fluid in the terminal CCD is known. In general, reabsorption of Na^+ salts in the MCD has a small effect on the TTKG. Significant reabsorption or secretion of K^+ in the MCD seldom occurs, except in profound K^+ depletion or excess, respectively. When vasopressin is acting, the osmolality in the terminal CCD is the same as that of plasma, and the amount of water reabsorbed in the MCD can be calculated from the urine-to-plasma osmolality ratio (OSM_U/OSM_P). Therefore, the K^+ concentration in the lumen of the distal nephron can be estimated by dividing the urine $[K^+]$ $([K^+]_U)$ by the OSM_U/OSM_P ratio:

$$[K^+]_{CCD} = [K^+]_U \div OSM_U / OSM_P$$

$$TTKG = [K^+]_{CCD} \div [K^+]_P = ([K^+]_U \div OSM_U / OSM_P) \div [K^+]_P$$

The urine osmolality must exceed that of plasma to calculate the TTKG. Because it is dependent on the state of total body K^+ balance, there is no normal range of values for the TTKG. Hypokalemia with a TTKG greater than 4 suggests renal K^+ loss due to increased distal K^+ secretion. Plasma renin and aldosterone levels are often helpful in differentiating the various causes of hyperaldosteronism. Bicarbonaturia and the presence of other nonreabsorbed anions also increase the TTKG and lead to renal K^+ wasting. Finally, hypomagnesemia should be looked for as a cause of refractory hypokalemia.

D. Treatment
   1. **The therapeutic goals** are to (1) prevent life-threatening complications (arrhythmias, respiratory failure, and hepatic encephalopathy), (2) correct the K^+ deficit, (3) minimize ongoing losses, and (4) treat the underlying cause.
   2. **Oral therapy.** It is generally safer to correct hypokalemia via the oral route. The degree of K^+ depletion does not correlate well with the plasma $[K^+]$. A decrement of 1 mmol/L in the plasma $[K^+]$ may represent a total body K^+ deficit of 200–400 mmol. Furthermore, factors that promote K^+ shift out of cells may result in underestimation of the K^+ deficit. Therefore, the plasma $[K^+]$ should be monitored frequently when assessing the response to treatment. KCl is usually the preparation of choice and promotes more rapid correction of hypokalemia and metabolic alkalosis. Potassium bicarbonate and citrate tend to alkalinize the patient and would be more appropriate for hypokalemia associated with chronic diarrhea or RTA.
   3. **IV therapy.** Patients with severe hypokalemia or those who are unable to take anything by mouth require IV replacement therapy with KCl. The maximum concentration of administered K^+ should be no more than 40 mmol/L via a peripheral vein or 60 mmol/L via a central vein. The rate of infusion should not exceed 20 mmol/hour unless paralysis or malignant ventricular arrhythmias are present. Ideally, KCl should be mixed in normal saline because dextrose solutions may initially exacerbate hypokalemia because of insulin-mediated movement of K^+ into cells. Rapid IV administration of K^+ should be used judiciously and requires close observation of the clinical manifestations of hypokalemia (ECG and neuromuscular examination).

II. Hyperkalemia
   A. Manifestations. The most serious effect of hyperkalemia is cardiac toxicity, which does not correlate well with the plasma $[K^+]$. The earliest ECG changes include increased T-wave amplitude, or peaked T waves. More severe degrees of hyperkalemia result in a prolonged PR interval and QRS duration, atrioventricular conduction delay, and loss of P waves. Progressive widening of the QRS complex and merging with the T wave produce a sine-

wave pattern. The terminal event is usually ventricular fibrillation or asystole. Hyperkalemia partially depolarizes the cell membrane, which impairs membrane excitability and is manifest as weakness that may progress to flaccid paralysis and hypoventilation if the respiratory muscles are involved. Hyperkalemia also inhibits renal ammoniagenesis and reabsorption of NH_4^+ in the loop of Henle. Thus, net acid excretion is impaired and results in metabolic acidosis, which may further exacerbate the hyperkalemia because of K^+ movement out of cells.

B. Etiology. Hyperkalemia, defined as a plasma $[K^+]$ of greater than 5.0 mmol/L, occurs primarily as a result of decreased renal loss, especially if chronic.

1. **Increased K^+ intake** is rarely the sole cause of hyperkalemia. Iatrogenic hyperkalemia may result from overzealous parenteral K^+ replacement or in patients with renal insufficiency.

2. **Pseudohyperkalemia** represents an artificially elevated plasma $[K^+]$ due to K^+ movement out of cells immediately before or following venipuncture. Contributing factors include repeated fist clenching, hemolysis, and marked leukocytosis or megakaryocytosis. Pseudohyperkalemia should be suspected in an otherwise asymptomatic patient with no obvious underlying cause. The plasma (not serum) $[K^+]$ is normal.

3. **Transcellular shift.** Tumor lysis syndrome and rhabdomyolysis lead to K^+ release from cells. Metabolic acidoses, with the exception of those due to the accumulation of organic anions, can be associated with mild hyperkalemia resulting from intracellular buffering of H^+. Insulin deficiency and hypertonicity (e.g., hyperglycemia) promote K^+ shift from the ICF to the ECF. Exercise-induced hyperkalemia is due to release of K^+ from muscles and is usually rapidly reversible, often associated with rebound hypokalemia. Treatment with beta-blockers may contribute to the elevation in plasma $[K^+]$ seen with other conditions. Hyperkalemic periodic paralysis is a rare cause of hyperkalemia. Depolarizing muscle relaxants such as succinylcholine can increase the plasma $[K^+]$, especially in patients with massive trauma, burns, or neuromuscular disease.

4. **Decreased renal K^+ excretion** is virtually always associated with chronic hyperkalemia and is due to either impaired secretion or diminished distal solute delivery. Decreased K^+ secretion results from either impaired Na^+ reabsorption or increased Cl^- reabsorption.

   a. **Impaired Na^+ reabsorption.** Decreased aldosterone synthesis may be due to primary adrenal insufficiency (Addison's disease) or congenital adrenal enzyme deficiency. Heparin inhibits production of aldosterone and can lead to severe hyperkalemia in a subset of patients with underlying renal disease or diabetes mellitus or those who are receiving K^+-sparing diuretics, angiotensin-converting enzyme (ACE) inhibitors, or NSAIDs. Pseudohypoaldosteronism is a rare disorder characterized by hyperkalemia, high renin and aldosterone levels, and end-organ resistance to aldosterone. The kaliuretic response to aldosterone is impaired by K^+-sparing diuretics. Spironolactone is a competitive mineralocorticoid antagonist, whereas amiloride and triamterene block the apical Na^+ channel of the principal cell. Two other drugs that impair K^+ secretion by blocking distal nephron Na^+ reabsorption are trimethoprim and pentamidine. NSAIDs inhibit renin secretion and the synthesis of vasodilatory renal prostaglandins. The resultant decrease in GFR and K^+ secretion is often manifest as hyperkalemia. ACE inhibitors block the conversion of angiotensin I to angiotensin II, resulting in impaired aldosterone release. Patients at increased risk of ACE inhibitor–induced hyperkalemia include those with diabetes mellitus, renal insufficiency, decreased effective circulating arterial volume, bilateral renal artery stenosis, or concurrent use of K^+-sparing diuretics or NSAIDs. A similar effect may be seen with the use of angiotensin II receptor antagonists. Hyperkalemia frequently complicates acute oliguric renal failure due to increased K^+ release from cells and decreased excretion. In chronic renal insufficiency, adaptive mechanisms eventually fail to maintain K^+ balance when the GFR falls below 10–15 ml/minute or oliguria ensues.

b. **Increased Cl^- reabsorption (Cl^- shunt).** Hyperkalemia is commonly seen in mild renal insufficiency, diabetic nephropathy, or chronic tubulointerstitial disease. Patients frequently have an impaired kaliuretic response to exogenous mineralocorticoid administration, suggesting that enhanced distal Cl^- reabsorption may account for many of the findings of hyporeninemic hypoaldosteronism. A similar mechanism may be partially responsible for the hyperkalemia associated with cyclosporine nephrotoxicity (*J Am Soc Nephrol* 2:1279, 1992). Hyperkalemic distal (type 4) RTA may be caused by either hypoaldosteronism or a Cl^- shunt.

c. **Decreased distal flow rate** is seldom the only cause of impaired K^+ excretion but may significantly contribute to hyperkalemia in protein-malnourished (low urea excretion) and ECF volume–contracted (decreased distal NaCl delivery) patients. A classic example is the cachectic patient with AIDS who has an opportunistic infection.

C. **Diagnosis** (Fig. 3-4). With rare exceptions, chronic hyperkalemia is always caused by impaired K^+ excretion. If the etiology is not readily apparent and the patient is asymptomatic, pseudohyperkalemia should be excluded by drawing blood without fist clenching. Oliguric acute renal failure and severe chronic renal insufficiency should also be ruled out. The history should focus on medications that impair K^+ handling and potential sources of K^+ intake. Evaluation of the ECF compartment, effective circulating volume, and urine output are essential components of the physical examination. The appropriate renal response to hyperkalemia is to excrete at least 200 mmol K^+ per day. In most cases, diminished renal K^+ loss is caused by impaired K^+ secretion, which can be revealed by finding a low TTKG (see sec. **I.C**). A TTKG of less than 7 implies a decreased driving force for K^+ secretion caused by either hypoaldosteronism or resistance to the renal effects of mineralocorticoid. This can be determined by evaluating the kaliuretic response to administration of mineralocorticoid [e.g., fludrocortisone (Florinef), 50–200 µg PO]. Primary adrenal insufficiency can be differentiated from hyporeninemic hypoaldosteronism by examining the renin-aldosterone axis. Renin and aldosterone levels should be measured in the supine and upright positions, after days of Na^+ restriction (Na^+ intake <10 mmol/day) in combination with a loop diuretic to induce mild volume contraction. Aldosterone-resistant hyperkalemia can result from the various causes of impaired distal Na^+ reabsorption or, alternatively, from a Cl^- shunt. The former leads to salt wasting, ECF volume contraction, and high renin and aldosterone levels. In contrast, enhanced distal Cl^- reabsorption is associated with volume expansion and suppressed renin and aldosterone secretion.

D. **Treatment.** The approach to therapy depends on changes on the ECG and the degree of hyperkalemia.

1. **Acute therapy.** Severe hyperkalemia is a medical emergency and requires treatment directed at minimizing membrane depolarization over a few minutes, shifting K^+ into cells over the next 30–90 minutes, and longer-term objectives that promote K^+ loss. Exogenous K^+ intake and antikaliuretic drugs should be discontinued.

a. **Administration of calcium gluconate** decreases membrane excitability. The usual dose is 10 ml of a 10% solution infused over 2–3 minutes. The effect begins within minutes but is short lived (30–60 minutes), and the dose can be repeated if no change in the ECG is seen after 5–10 minutes.

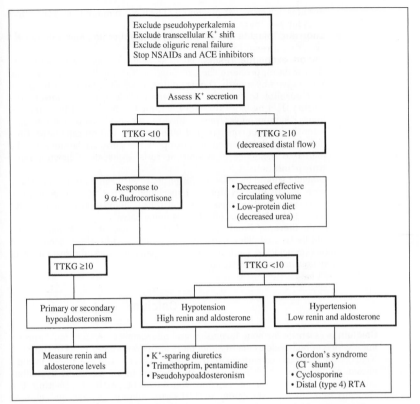

Fig. 3-4. Algorithm depicting clinical approach to hyperkalemia. (ACE = angiotensin-converting enzyme; NSAIDs = nonsteroidal anti-inflammatory drugs; RTA = renal tubular acidosis; TTKG = transtubular K^+ concentration gradient.) [From GG Singer, BM Brenner. Fluid and Electrolyte Disturbances. In AS Fauci, et al. (eds). *Harrison's Principles of Internal Medicine* (15th ed). New York: McGraw-Hill, 2001, with permission.]

b. Insulin causes K^+ to shift into cells and temporarily lowers the plasma $[K^+]$. Although **glucose** alone stimulates insulin release, a more rapid response generally occurs when exogenous insulin is administered (with glucose to prevent hypoglycemia). A commonly recommended combination is 10–20 units of regular insulin and 25–50 g glucose. Hyperglycemic patients should not be given glucose. If effective, the plasma $[K^+]$ will fall by 0.5–1.5 mmol/L in 15–30 minutes, and the effect will last for several hours.

c. Alkali therapy with IV NaHCO$_3$ can also shift K^+ into cells. This is safest when administered as an isotonic solution of 3 ampules/L 5% dextrose (134 mmol/L NaHCO$_3$) and ideally should be reserved for severe hyperkalemia associated with metabolic acidosis. Patients with end-stage renal disease seldom respond to this intervention and may not tolerate the Na^+ load and resultant volume expansion.

d. β_2-adrenergic agonists, when administered parenterally or in nebulized form, promote cellular uptake of K^+. The onset of action is 30 minutes, lowering the plasma [K$^+$] by 0.5–1.5 mmol/L, and the effect lasts for 2–4 hours.

e. Loop and thiazide diuretics, often in combination, may enhance K$^+$ excretion if renal function is adequate.

f. Cation exchange resins, such as sodium polystyrene sulfonate (Kayexalate), promote the exchange of Na$^+$ for K$^+$ in the GI tract. When given by mouth, the usual dose is 25–50 g mixed with 100 ml 20% sorbitol to prevent constipation. This generally lowers the plasma [K$^+$] by 0.5–1.0 mmol/L within 1–2 hours and lasts for 4–6 hours. Sodium polystyrene sulfonate can also be administered as a retention enema consisting of 50 g resin in 150 ml tap water. Enemas should be avoided in postoperative patients because of the increased incidence of colonic necrosis, especially following renal transplantation.

g. Dialysis should be reserved for patients with renal failure and those with severe life-threatening hyperkalemia that is unresponsive to more conservative measures. Peritoneal dialysis also removes K$^+$ but is only 15–20% as effective as hemodialysis.

2. Chronic therapy. Finally, the underlying cause of the hyperkalemia should be treated. This may involve dietary modification, correction of metabolic acidosis, cautious volume expansion, and administration of exogenous mineralocorticoid.

Calcium

Calcium is essential for bone formation and neuromuscular function. Approximately 99% of body calcium is in bone; most of the remaining 1% is in the ECF. Nearly 50% of serum calcium is ionized (free), whereas the remainder is complexed, primarily to albumin. Changes in serum albumin, especially hypoalbuminemia, alter total serum calcium concentration without affecting the clinically relevant ionized calcium level. If serum albumin is abnormal, clinical decisions should be based on ionized calcium levels, which must lie within a narrow range (4.6–5.1 mg/dl) for normal neuromuscular function. Calcium metabolism is regulated by parathyroid hormone (PTH) and metabolites of vitamin D. PTH increases serum calcium by stimulating bone resorption, increasing renal calcium reabsorption, and promoting renal conversion of vitamin D to its active metabolite, calcitriol (1,25-dihydroxycholecalciferol; 1,25-dihydroxyvitamin D$_3$ [1,25(OH)$_2$D$_3$]). PTH also increases renal phosphate excretion. Serum calcium regulates PTH secretion by a negative feedback mechanism; hypocalcemia stimulates and hypercalcemia suppresses PTH release. Vitamin D is absorbed from food and synthesized in skin that is exposed to sunlight. The liver converts it to 25-hydroxyvitamin D$_3$ [25(OH)D$_3$], which in turn is converted by the kidney to 1,25(OH)$_2$D$_3$. The latter metabolite increases serum calcium by promoting intestinal calcium absorption, and it plays a role in bone formation and resorption. It also enhances phosphate absorption by the intestine. Synthesis of 1,25(OH)$_2$D$_3$ is stimulated by PTH and hypophosphatemia and is inhibited by increased serum phosphorus.

I. Hypercalcemia almost always is caused by increased entry of calcium into the ECF (from bone resorption or intestinal absorption) and decreased renal calcium clearance. More than 90% of cases are due to primary hyperparathyroidism or malignancy.

A. Primary hyperparathyroidism causes most cases of hypercalcemia in ambulatory patients. It is a common disorder, especially in elderly women, in whom the annual incidence is approximately 2 in 1000. Nearly 85% of cases are due to an adenoma of a single gland, 15% to hyperplasia of all four glands, and 1% to parathyroid carcinoma. Most patients have asymptomatic hypercalcemia that is found incidentally. Patients may have symptoms of hypercalcemia (see sec. **D**), nephrolithiasis, osteopenia that primarily affects cortical bone, or, rarely, a specific bone disorder, osteitis fibrosa.

B. Malignancy is responsible for most cases of hypercalcemia among hospitalized patients, acting via two major mechanisms. In local osteolytic hypercalcemia, tumor cell products, such as cytokines, act locally to stimulate osteoclastic bone resorption. This form of malignant hypercalcemia occurs only with extensive bone involvement by tumor, most often due to breast carcinoma, myeloma, and lymphoma. In humoral hypercalcemia of malignancy, tumor products act systemically to stimulate bone resorption and, in many cases, to decrease calcium excretion. PTH-related peptide, which acts via PTH receptors but is not detected by PTH immunoassays, is an important mediator of this syndrome; tumor-derived growth factors may also play a role. Humoral hypercalcemia of malignancy is caused most often by squamous carcinoma of the lung, head and neck, or esophagus, or by renal, bladder, or ovarian carcinoma. Patients with malignant hypercalcemia almost always have advanced, clinically obvious disease.

C. Other causes of hypercalcemia are uncommon (sarcoidosis, vitamin D toxicity, hyperthyroidism, lithium use, milk-alkali syndrome, and immobilization) and are usually clinically evident. Thiazide diuretics cause persistent hypercalcemia in patients with increased bone turnover (e.g., mild primary hyperparathyroidism). **Familial hypocalciuric hypercalcemia** is a rare, autosomal dominant disorder characterized by asymptomatic hypercalcemia from childhood and a family history of hypercalcemia.

D. Clinical manifestations generally are present only if serum calcium exceeds 12 mg/dl and tend to be more severe if hypercalcemia develops rapidly. Renal manifestations include polyuria and nephrolithiasis. GI symptoms include anorexia, nausea, vomiting, and constipation. Neurologic findings include weakness, fatigue, confusion, stupor, and coma. ECG manifestations include a shortened QT interval. Polyuria, nausea, and vomiting cause marked dehydration, resulting in impaired calcium excretion and rapidly worsening hypercalcemia. If serum calcium rises above 13 mg/dl, renal failure and ectopic soft-tissue calcification may develop.

E. Diagnosis of hypercalcemia requires distinction of primary hyperparathyroidism from malignancy. Increases in serum albumin can raise the total calcium level slightly, without affecting the clinically relevant ionized calcium concentration. Therefore, the serum ionized calcium should be measured to determine whether hypercalcemia actually is present.

   1. The history and physical examination should focus on (1) the duration of hypercalcemia, (2) a history of renal stones, (3) clinical evidence of any of the unusual causes of hypercalcemia, and (4) symptoms and signs of malignancy (which almost always precede malignant hypercalcemia). If hypercalcemia has been present for more than 6 months without obvious cause, primary hyperparathyroidism is almost certain.

   2. The serum PTH level should be measured. Assays measuring intact PTH should be used, as these are independent of renal function. Serum PTH levels are elevated in more than 90% of patients with primary hyperparathyroidism and invariably are suppressed in patients with hypercalcemia due to malignancy or other causes, except familial hypocalciuric hypercalcemia.

   3. Hypercalcemia due to malignancy or uncommon causes is almost always evident from the history, physical examination, and routine laboratory tests; serum intact PTH levels are not elevated in these disorders. In a patient with chronic asymptomatic hypercalcemia, an elevated serum PTH, and no clinical evidence of malignancy, the diagnosis of primary hyperparathyroidism is secure. Some patients with the rare familial hypocalciuric hypercalcemia could present in this manner and can be distinguished by documenting low urinary calcium clearance. Malignancy or other causes should be sought if hypercalcemia is severe or develops rapidly and the serum PTH is not elevated.

F. **Acute management of hypercalcemia** includes measures that increase calcium excretion and decrease resorption of calcium from bone. The following regimen is warranted if severe symptoms are present or serum calcium is greater than 12 mg/dl. The goal is alleviation of symptoms rather than brisk normalization of serum calcium. The first step is replacement of ECF volume (see sec. **I.F.1**), followed by saline diuresis. An inhibitor of bone resorption should be given early; pamidronate is the drug of choice. If pamidronate is not effective, plicamycin can be used, but the latter is more toxic and should be given only to those with malignant hypercalcemia. Calcitonin can be used in patients with renal failure or can be added to a bisphosphonate to achieve rapid control of severe hypercalcemia. In oliguric renal failure that cannot be treated with IV saline, hemodialysis with a calcium-free dialysate lowers serum calcium temporarily.

1. **ECF volume restoration** with 0.9% saline constitutes initial therapy in severely hypercalcemic patients, who usually are dehydrated. The goal of this therapy is restoration of the normal GFR. The initial infusion rate should be 300–500 ml/hour and should be reduced after the ECF volume deficit has been partially corrected. At least 3–4 L should be given in the first 24 hours, and a positive fluid balance of at least 2 L should be achieved.

2. **Saline diuresis** with 0.9% saline infusion (100–200 ml/hour) promotes calcium excretion after ECF volume is restored. Therapy should be monitored carefully, with frequent evaluation for evidence of heart failure. Serum electrolytes, calcium, and magnesium should be measured q6–12h. Adequate replacement of potassium and magnesium is essential (see Potassium and Magnesium). Furosemide, 20–40 mg IV bid–qid, adds little to the effect of saline diuresis and may prevent adequate restoration of ECF volume. It should not be given unless clinical evidence of heart failure develops. Thiazide diuretics must be avoided, as they impair calcium excretion.

3. **Pamidronate** is a bisphosphonate that inhibits bone resorption. A single dose of 60 mg in 500 ml 0.9% saline or 5% dextrose in water (D5W) is infused over 4 hours; for severe hypercalcemia (>13.5 mg/dl), 90 mg in a liter should be infused over 24 hours. Hypocalcemic response is seen within 2 days and peaks in nearly 7 days, and it may persist for 2 weeks or longer. Treatment can be repeated if hypercalcemia recurs. Side effects include hypomagnesemia, hypophosphatemia, and transient low-grade fever.

4. **Calcitonin** inhibits bone resorption and increases renal calcium excretion. Salmon calcitonin, 4–8 IU/kg IM or SC q6–12h, lowers serum calcium 1–2 mg/dl within several hours in 60–70% of patients. The hypocalcemic effect wanes after several days due to tachyphylaxis. Calcitonin is less potent than are other inhibitors of bone resorption but has no serious toxicity, is safe in renal failure, and may have an analgesic effect in patients with skeletal metastases. It can be used early in the treatment of severe hypercalcemia to achieve a rapid response; concomitant use of a bisphosphonate ensures a prolonged effect. Side effects include flushing, nausea, and, rarely, allergic reactions.

5. **Plicamycin (mithramycin),** an inhibitor of bone resorption, is used as a second-line agent in malignant hypercalcemia. It is less effective and less well tolerated than is pamidronate. A dose of 25 g/kg in 500 ml D5W, infused over 4–6 hours, gradually reduces serum calcium over 2–4 days; its effect lasts for 5–15 days. Side effects include thrombocytopenia, coagulation factor deficiency, renal failure, and hepatic dysfunction. Frequent monitoring for toxicities is mandatory during plicamycin therapy, and the drug is **contraindicated** in patients with a bleeding diathesis,

renal failure, or hepatic dysfunction, or during myelotoxic chemotherapy. As a result, plicamycin is rarely used to treat hypercalcemia.

6. **Glucocorticoids** lower serum calcium by inhibiting cytokine release, by direct cytolytic effects on some tumor cells, by inhibiting intestinal calcium absorption, and by increasing urinary calcium excretion. They are effective in hypercalcemia due to myeloma, other hematologic malignancies, sarcoidosis, and vitamin D intoxication. Other tumors rarely respond. The initial dose is prednisone, 20–50 mg PO bid, or its equivalent. Serum calcium may take 5–10 days to fall. After serum calcium stabilizes, the dose should be gradually reduced to the minimum needed to control symptoms of hypercalcemia. Toxicity (see Chap. 24) limits the usefulness of glucocorticoids for long-term therapy.

7. **Oral phosphate** inhibits calcium absorption and promotes calcium deposition in bone and soft tissue. It should be used only if the serum phosphorus level is lower than 3 mg/dl and renal function is normal, to minimize the risk of soft-tissue calcification. Doses of 0.5–1.0 g elemental phosphorus PO tid (see Phosphorus) modestly lower serum calcium in some patients. Serum calcium, phosphorus, and creatinine should be monitored frequently, and the dose should be reduced if serum phosphorus exceeds 4.5 mg/dl or if the product of serum calcium and phosphorus (measured in mg/dl) exceeds 60. Side effects include diarrhea, nausea, and soft-tissue calcification. IV phosphate should never be used to treat hypercalcemia.

8. **Dialysis.** Hemodialysis using dialysate with little or no calcium and peritoneal dialysis are very effective means of treating hypercalcemia, particularly in patients with CHF or renal insufficiency.

G. **Chronic management of hypercalcemia**

1. **Parathyroidectomy** for primary hyperparathyroidism is the only effective therapy. The natural history of asymptomatic hyperparathyroidism is not fully known, but in many patients the disorder has a benign course, with little change in clinical findings or serum calcium concentration for years. The possibility of progressive loss of bone mass and increased risk of fracture are the main concerns, but the likelihood of these outcomes appears to be low. Deterioration of renal function is possible but unlikely in the absence of nephrolithiasis. Currently, it is impossible to predict which patients will develop complications.

   a. **Indications for surgery include** (1) symptoms caused by hypercalcemia, (2) nephrolithiasis, (3) reduced bone mass (more than 2 standard deviations below the mean for age), (4) serum calcium in excess of 12 mg/dl, (5) age younger than 50 years, and (6) infeasibility of long-term follow-up. Surgery is a reasonable choice in healthy patients even if they do not meet these criteria, because it has a high success rate, with low morbidity and mortality. However, asymptomatic patients can be followed by assessing clinical status and serum calcium and creatinine levels at 6- to 12-month intervals. Bone mass at the hip should be assessed annually, using dual-energy radiography. Surgery should be recommended if any of the aforementioned criteria develop or if progressive decline in bone mass or renal function occurs.

   b. **Parathyroidectomy** performed by a surgeon experienced in the procedure has a success rate of 90–95%. Often a brief (1- to 2-day) period of mild, asymptomatic hypocalcemia ensues. In rare patients with overt bone disease, hypocalcemia may be severe and prolonged (the so-called hungry bone syndrome), requiring therapy. Other complications include permanent hypoparathyroidism and injury to the recurrent laryngeal nerve. Re-exploration is associated with a lower success rate and a greater risk of complications and should be performed at a referral center. Parathyroid localization procedures are not indicated before initial neck exploration but may be helpful before re-exploration.

   c. **Medical therapy** has not been shown to affect the clinical outcome of primary hyperparathyroidism. However, in postmenopausal women with primary hyperparathyroidism, estrogen replacement therapy preserves bone mass with minimal effects on serum ionized calcium or PTH levels. In patients with symptomatic hypercalcemia who refuse or cannot tolerate surgery, physical activity should be encouraged, along with a diet that contains at least 2–3 L of fluid and 8–10 g salt per day. Dietary calcium need not be restricted, and thiazide diuretics must not be used. Oral phosphate therapy may lower serum calcium but also raises serum PTH levels; its benefits do not clearly outweigh risks, and it should be used only if symptomatic hypercalcemia cannot be corrected surgically.

2. **Treatment of malignant hypercalcemia** may control symptoms while antineoplastic therapy takes effect but rarely succeeds for a long period unless the cancer responds to treatment. Because patients usually have extensive, unresectable disease, with a median survival of less than 3 months, the initial decision should be whether therapy is warranted. Treatment of hypercalcemia may palliate symptoms such as anorexia, nausea, and malaise. After acute management of hypercalcemia, physical activity and adequate fluid intake (at least 2–3 L/day) should be encouraged. Nausea should be treated, and a salt intake of 8–10 g/day is advisable; dietary calcium restriction is not beneficial. Repeated doses of IV pamidronate (see sec. **I.F.3**) can be given when hypercalcemia recurs. Plicamycin can be used if pamidronate is ineffective. Prednisone, 20–50 mg PO bid, usually controls hypercalcemia in multiple myeloma and other hematologic malignancies (see sec. **I.F.6**). Oral phosphate can be tried if the serum phosphorus level is low and renal function is normal.

3. **Hypercalcemia due to other disorders** should be treated with prednisone and a low-calcium diet (<400 mg/day). The effects of vitamin D itself may take up to 2 months to abate, but the toxicity of its metabolites is more short lived. Hypercalcemia due to sarcoidosis often responds to prednisone, and a dose of 10–20 mg/day may be sufficient for long-term control.

II. **Hypocalcemia** (low total serum calcium) most commonly is caused by hypoalbuminemia. If serum free (ionized) calcium is normal, no disorder of calcium metabolism is present. If ionized calcium cannot be measured, the total serum calcium can be corrected by adding 0.8 mg/dl for every 1 g/dl decrease of serum albumin below 4 g/dl, to determine whether true hypocalcemia is present. **Causes of low serum free calcium levels** include renal failure, hypoparathyroidism (either idiopathic or postsurgical), severe hypomagnesemia, hypermagnesemia, acute pancreatitis, rhabdomyolysis, tumor lysis syndrome, vitamin D deficiency, pseudohypoparathyroidism (PTH resistance), and, rarely, multiple citrated blood transfusions. A low serum free calcium level is common in critically ill patients, sometimes without evident cause. Drugs may cause hypocalcemia, including antineoplastic agents (cisplatin, cytosine arabinoside), antimicrobials (pentamidine, ketoconazole, foscarnet), and agents used to treat hypercalcemia (see sec. **I.F**).

   A. **Clinical manifestations** vary with the degree and rate of onset. Chronic hypocalcemia may be asymptomatic. Alkalosis augments calcium binding to albumin and increases the severity of symptoms. Increased excitability of nerves and muscles causes paresthesias and tetany, including carpopedal spasms. **Trousseau's sign** is development of carpal spasm when a BP cuff is inflated above systolic pressure for 3 minutes. **Chvostek's sign** is twitching of facial muscles when the facial nerve is tapped anterior to the ear. The presence of these signs is known as **latent tetany.** Severe hypocalcemia may cause lethargy or confusion or, rarely, laryngospasm, seizures, or heart failure. The ECG may show a prolonged QT interval. Chronic hypocalcemia may cause cataracts and calcification of the basal ganglia.

B. In the **diagnosis,** the **history and physical examination** should focus on (1) previous neck surgery (as hypoparathyroidism may develop immediately or gradually over years), (2) disorders associated with idiopathic hypoparathyroidism (e.g., hypothyroidism, adrenal failure, candidiasis, vitiligo), (3) family history of hypocalcemia (which may be present in cases of familial hypocalcemia, hypoparathyroidism, or pseudohypoparathyroidism), (4) drugs that cause hypocalcemia or hypomagnesemia, (5) conditions that cause vitamin D deficiency, and (6) findings of pseudohypoparathyroidism (short stature, short metacarpals). **Laboratory studies** should include measurement of serum free calcium, phosphorus, magnesium, creatinine, and PTH. The serum phosphorus level is elevated in hypocalcemia resulting from most causes, although in hypocalcemia from vitamin D deficiency, it usually is low. Serum PTH is elevated in disorders other than hypoparathyroidism and magnesium deficiency.

C. **Acute management** for symptomatic hypocalcemia should be on an emergency basis with 2 g **calcium gluconate** (180 mg elemental calcium or 20 ml 10% calcium gluconate) IV over 10 minutes, followed by infusion of 6 g calcium gluconate in 500 ml D5W over 4–6 hours (10 ml 10% calcium gluconate = 1 g). Serum calcium should be measured q4–6h. The infusion rate should be adjusted to avoid recurrent symptomatic hypocalcemia and to maintain the serum calcium level at between 8 and 9 mg/dl. The underlying cause should be treated or long-term therapy started, and the IV infusion then should be gradually tapered. **Hypomagnesemia,** if present, must be treated to correct hypocalcemia (see sec. **III.C**). In patients who take digoxin, the ECG should be monitored, as hypocalcemia potentiates digitalis toxicity. **Calcium and bicarbonate are not compatible IV admixtures.**

D. **Long-term management** of hypoparathyroidism and pseudohypoparathyroidism requires calcium supplements and vitamin D or its active metabolite to increase intestinal calcium absorption. Because PTH cannot limit urinary calcium excretion in these diseases, hypercalciuria and nephrolithiasis are potential side effects. **The objective is to maintain serum calcium levels at slightly below the normal range (8.0–8.5 mg/dl),** which usually prevents manifestations of hypocalcemia and minimizes hypercalciuria. While the dose of vitamin D is being titrated, serum calcium should be measured twice a week. When a maintenance dose is achieved, serum and 24-hour urinary calcium levels should be monitored every 3–6 months, because unexpected fluctuations may occur. If urine calcium exceeds 250 mg/24 hours, the dose of vitamin D should be reduced. If hypercalciuria develops at serum calcium levels of less than 8.5 mg/dl, hydrochlorothiazide (50 mg PO qd) can be used to reduce urinary calcium excretion.

   1. **Oral calcium supplements. Calcium carbonate** (Os-Cal, 250 or 500 mg elemental calcium per tablet; Tums Extra-Strength, 400 mg elemental calcium per 5 ml; or various generic formulations) is the least expensive compound. The initial dosage is 1–2 g elemental calcium PO tid during the transition from IV to oral therapy. For long-term therapy, the typical dosage is 0.5–1.0 g PO tid with meals. Calcium carbonate is well absorbed when taken with food, even in patients with achlorhydria. Side effects include dyspepsia and constipation.

   2. **Vitamin D.** Dietary deficiency can be corrected by 400–1000 IU/day, but treatment of other hypocalcemic disorders requires much larger doses of vitamin D or use of an active metabolite. In patients with severe hyperphosphatemia, serum phosphorus should be lowered to less than 6.5 mg/dl with oral phosphate binders (see Phosphorus) before vitamin D is started. **Calcitriol** (0.25 or 0.5 μg per capsule) has a rapid onset of action. The initial dosage is 0.25 μg PO qd, and most patients are main-

tained on 0.5–2.0 µg PO qd. The dose can be increased at 2- to 4-week intervals. **Vitamin D** (50,000 IU or 1.25 mg per capsule) requires weeks to achieve full effect. The initial dosage is 50,000 IU PO qd, and usual maintenance dosages are 25,000–100,000 IU PO qd. The dose can be increased at 4- to 6-week intervals. Calcitriol is much more expensive than vitamin D, but its lower risk of toxicity makes it the best choice for most patients.

   3. **Development of hypercalcemia.** In the event that hypercalcemia develops, vitamin D and calcium supplements should be stopped until serum calcium falls to a normal concentration; then both should be restarted at lower doses. Hypercalcemia due to calcitriol usually resolves within 1 week, and serum calcium should be monitored q24–48h. Hypercalcemia due to vitamin D may require more than 2 months to resolve. Symptomatic vitamin D–induced hypercalcemia should be treated with prednisone (see sec. **I.F.6**). In mild vitamin D toxicity, serum calcium can be monitored at weekly intervals until the level returns to normal.

Phosphorus

Phosphorus is critical for bone formation and cellular energy metabolism. Approximately 85% of body phosphorus is in bone, and most of the remainder is within cells; only 1% is in the ECF. Thus, serum phosphorus levels may not reflect total body phosphorus stores. Phosphorus exists in the body as phosphate, but serum concentration is expressed as mass of phosphorus (1 mg/dl phosphorus = 0.32 mM phosphate). The normal range is 3.0–4.5 mg/dl, with somewhat higher values in children and postmenopausal women. Serum phosphorus is best measured in the fasting state, because there is diurnal variation, with a morning nadir, and because carbohydrate ingestion and glucose infusion lower serum phosphorus, whereas a high-phosphate meal raises it. Major regulatory factors include **PTH,** which lowers serum phosphorus by increasing renal excretion; **1,25(OH)$_2$D$_3$,** which increases serum phosphorus by enhancing intestinal phosphate absorption; insulin, which lowers serum levels by shifting phosphate into cells; dietary phosphate intake; and renal function.

I. **Hyperphosphatemia** most often is caused by renal failure but also occurs in hypoparathyroidism, pseudohypoparathyroidism, rhabdomyolysis, tumor lysis syndrome, and metabolic and respiratory acidosis, and after excess phosphate administration.

   A. **Clinical manifestations.** Symptoms and signs are those attributable to hypocalcemia (see Calcium, sec. **II.A**) and metastatic calcification of soft tissues, including blood vessels, cornea, skin, kidney, and periarticular tissue. Severe hyperphosphatemia may result in tissue ischemia or calciphylaxis. Chronic hyperphosphatemia contributes to renal osteodystrophy (see Chap. 12).

   B. **Management**
   1. **Dietary phosphate** should be restricted to 600–900 mg/day.
   2. **Oral phosphate binders.** In patients with renal failure (see Chap. 12), **calcium carbonate** is given at an initial dosage of 0.5–1.0 g elemental **calcium PO tid with meals.** The dosage can be increased at intervals of 2–4 weeks to a maximum of 3 g tid. The goal of therapy is to maintain serum phosphorus levels between 4.5 and 6.0 mg/dl. Serum calcium and phosphorus levels should be measured frequently and the dose adjusted to keep the serum calcium level at less than 11 mg/dl and the calcium-phosphorus product at less than 60, to minimize the risk of ectopic calcification. If hyperphosphatemia persists despite doses of calcium that cause hypercalcemia, small doses of aluminum gels can be added, for example, **aluminum hydroxide** (600 mg per tablet or 320 mg/5 ml) or

aluminum carbonate (600 mg per tablet or 400 mg/5 ml), 5–10 ml or one to two tablets PO tid with meals. Side effects of aluminum gels include **nausea and constipation; prolonged use in renal failure may cause aluminum toxicity** (see Chap. 12). **Calcium citrate** should not be used concurrently with aluminum gels because citrate increases aluminum absorption and can precipitate acute aluminum toxicity. **Sevelamer** is a phosphate binder that avoids the complications of hypermagnesemia, hypercalcemia, and aluminum toxicity. It is a nonabsorbable cationic polymer that binds phosphate through ion exchange and also lowers total cholesterol concentrations. Its major side effects are GI.

3. **Saline diuresis.** Acute hyperphosphatemia in patients who do not have renal failure is reduced by saline diuresis.

4. **Dialysis** is not very effective at removing phosphate due to the large intracellular stores. Extended or nocturnal hemodialysis is the only mode of dialysis that has been proven to lower phosphate levels.

II. **Hypophosphatemia** may be caused by impaired intestinal absorption, increased renal excretion, or redistribution of phosphate into cells. **Severe hypophosphatemia** (<1 mg/dl; causes include alcohol abuse and withdrawal, respiratory alkalosis, malabsorption, oral phosphate binders, refeeding after malnutrition, hyperalimentation, severe burns, and DKA therapy) usually indicates total body phosphate depletion. However, during therapy for DKA, hypophosphatemia seldom reflects severe phosphate depletion and very rarely causes clinical manifestations. **Moderate hypophosphatemia** (1.0–2.5 mg/dl) is common in hospitalized patients and may not indicate total body phosphate depletion. In addition, moderate hypophosphatemia may be caused by (1) infusion of glucose, (2) dietary vitamin D deficiency or malabsorption, and (3) increased renal phosphate loss due to hyperparathyroidism, the diuretic phase of ATN, renal transplantation, familial X-linked hypophosphatemia, Fanconi's syndrome, oncogenic osteomalacia, and ECF volume expansion.

A. **Clinical manifestations.** Signs and symptoms typically occur only if total body phosphate depletion is present and the serum phosphorus level is less than 1 mg/dl. Muscular abnormalities include weakness, rhabdomyolysis, impaired diaphragmatic function, respiratory failure, and heart failure. Neurologic abnormalities include paresthesias, dysarthria, confusion, stupor, seizures, and coma. Hemolysis, platelet dysfunction, and metabolic acidosis rarely occur. Chronic hypophosphatemia causes rickets in children and osteomalacia in adults.

B. **Diagnosis.** The cause is usually apparent, but, if not, measurement of urine phosphorus levels helps define the mechanism. Excretion of more than 100 mg/day during hypophosphatemia indicates excessive renal loss. Family history, serum calcium and PTH, and urine amino acids help distinguish among renal causes. Low serum $25(OH)D_3$ suggests dietary vitamin D deficiency or malabsorption.

C. **Management**

1. **Moderate hypophosphatemia** (1.0–2.5 mg/dl) is usually asymptomatic and requires no therapy except correction of the underlying cause. Persistent hypophosphatemia should be treated with oral phosphate supplements, 0.5–1.0 g elemental phosphorus PO bid–tid. Preparations include Neutra-Phos (250 mg elemental phosphorus and 7 mEq each sodium and potassium per capsule) and Neutra-Phos K (250 mg elemental phosphorus and 14 mEq potassium per capsule). The contents of capsules should be dissolved in water. Fleet Phospho-Soda (815 mg phosphorus and 33 mEq sodium/5 ml) is an alternative oral agent. For patients who require long-term therapy, bulk powder is more economical; a 64-g bottle of Neutra-Phos dissolved in 1 gal water provides 250 mg elemental phosphorus/75 ml. Serum phosphorus, calcium, and creatinine should be measured daily as the dose is adjusted. Side effects include diarrhea, which is often dose limiting, and nausea.

Hypocalcemia and ectopic calcification are rare unless hyperphosphatemia occurs.

2. **Severe hypophosphatemia** (<1 mg/dl) may require IV phosphate therapy when associated with serious clinical manifestations. **IV phosphate should not be used in the treatment of DKA,** unless evidence exists of pre-existing phosphate depletion from another cause. IV preparations include potassium phosphate (1.5 mEq potassium per mmol phosphate) and sodium phosphate (1.3 mEq sodium per mmol phosphate). An infusion of phosphate, 0.08–0.16 mmol/kg (elemental phosphorus, 2.5–5.0 mg/kg) in 500 ml 0.45% saline, is given intravenously over 6 hours. If hypotension occurs, the infusion rate should be slowed. Further doses should be based on symptoms and on the serum calcium, phosphorus, and potassium levels, which should be measured q6h. IV infusion should be stopped when the serum phosphorus level is greater than 1.5 mg/dl or when oral therapy is possible. Because of the need to replenish intracellular stores, 24–36 hours of phosphate infusion may be required. Extreme care must be used to avoid hyperphosphatemia, which may cause hypocalcemia, ectopic soft-tissue calcification, renal failure, hypotension, and death. In renal failure, IV phosphate should be given only if absolutely necessary. Hypophosphatemic patients frequently are hypokalemic and hypomagnesemic, and these disorders must be corrected as well. (Conversion equations for phosphate therapy are as follows: 1 mmol phosphate = 31 mg phosphorus; 1 mg phosphorus = 0.032 mmol phosphate.)

Magnesium

Magnesium plays an important role in neuromuscular function. Approximately 60% of body magnesium is in bone, and most of the remainder is within cells. Only 1% is in the ECF, and serum magnesium levels often do not reflect total body magnesium content. Because clinical effects of magnesium disorders are determined primarily by tissue magnesium content, **serum magnesium levels** have limited diagnostic value. Normal serum concentrations are 1.3–2.2 mEq/L.

I. **Hypermagnesemia** occurs in renal failure, usually after therapy with magnesium-containing antacids or laxatives, and during treatment of preeclampsia with IV magnesium.

A. **Clinical manifestations.** Signs and symptoms are seen only if the serum magnesium level is greater than 4 mEq/L. Neuromuscular abnormalities usually include areflexia, lethargy, weakness, paralysis, and respiratory failure. Cardiac findings include hypotension; bradycardia; prolonged PR, QRS, and QT intervals; complete heart block; and asystole. Hypocalcemia may occur.

B. **Therapy.** Hypermagnesemia can be prevented by avoiding the use of magnesium preparations in renal failure. Asymptomatic hypermagnesemia requires only withdrawal of this therapy. Severe symptomatic hypermagnesemia should be treated with 10% calcium gluconate, 10–20 ml IV (1–2 g) over 10 minutes, to antagonize temporarily the effects of magnesium. Prompt supportive therapy is critical, including mechanical ventilation for respiratory failure and a temporary pacemaker for bradyarrhythmias. In severe renal failure, hemodialysis is required for definitive therapy. In the absence of severe renal failure, 0.9% saline with 2 g calcium gluconate/L can be given at 150–200 ml/hour to promote magnesium excretion.

II. **Magnesium deficiency** may be caused by decreased intestinal absorption due to malnutrition, malabsorption, prolonged diarrhea, or nasogastric aspiration, or by increased renal excretion due to hypercalcemia, osmotic diuresis, and several drugs, including loop diuretics, aminoglycosides, amphotericin B, cisplatin, and cyclosporine. It often complicates alcoholism and alcohol withdrawal.

A. Clinical manifestations. Magnesium deficiency often causes hypokalemia and hypocalcemia, which contribute to the clinical picture. Neurologic abnormalities include lethargy, confusion, tremor, fasciculations, ataxia, nystagmus, tetany, and seizures. ECG abnormalities include prolonged PR and QT intervals. Atrial and ventricular arrhythmias may occur, especially in patients treated with digoxin.

B. Diagnosis. Magnesium deficiency should be suspected in the clinical situations described in sec. **II.A** In these settings, hypomagnesemia is sufficient to establish the diagnosis of magnesium deficiency. However, routine measurement of serum magnesium without clinical suspicion of magnesium deficiency has little diagnostic value, and a normal serum level does not exclude total body magnesium deficiency. The etiology of hypomagnesemia usually is evident, but, if it is not, measurement of urine magnesium levels helps define the mechanism. Magnesium excretion of more than 2 mEq/day during hypomagnesemia indicates excessive renal loss.

C. Therapy. In patients with normal renal function, excess magnesium is readily excreted, and there is little risk of causing hypermagnesemia with recommended doses. However, magnesium must be given with extreme care in renal failure because of the risk of hypermagnesemia.

    1. Mild or chronic hypomagnesemia can be treated with 240 mg elemental magnesium PO qd–bid. Magnesium oxide preparations include Mag-Ox 400 (240 mg elemental magnesium per 400-mg tablet) and Uro-Mag (84 mg elemental magnesium per 140-mg tablet). The major side effect is diarrhea.

    2. Severe symptomatic hypomagnesemia can be treated with 1–2 g magnesium sulfate (4 mEq/ml) IV over 15 minutes, followed by an infusion of 6 g magnesium sulfate in 1 L or more IV fluid over 24 hours. Because of the need to replenish intracellular stores, the infusion should be continued for 3–7 days. Serum magnesium should be measured q24h and the infusion rate adjusted to maintain a serum magnesium level of less than 2.5 mEq/L. Tendon reflexes should be tested frequently, as hyporeflexia suggests hypermagnesemia. Reduced doses and more frequent monitoring must be used even in mild renal failure. (The conversion equation for magnesium therapy is as follows: 1 mmol = 2 mEq = 24 mg elemental magnesium.)

Acid-Base Disturbances

The normal ECF $[H^+]$ is 40 nmol/L (pH 7.40) and is maintained within a narrow range. Perturbations in acid-base balance occur as a consequence of the gain or loss of H^+ or HCO_3^-. Individuals who consume a typical Western diet generate approximately 1 mmol/kg H^+ daily as a result of the metabolism of sulfur-containing (cysteine and methionine) and cationic (arginine and lysine) amino acids. To achieve H^+ balance, the dietary acid load must be excreted (and HCO_3^- regenerated). Acid-base homeostasis is essential for normal cellular function and consists of three integral components: (1) Chemical buffering by ECF (HCO_3^-) and ICF (proteins and organic and inorganic phosphates) buffers minimizes changes in H^+ concentration, (2) changes in alveolar ventilation alter carbon dioxide tension (PCO_2), and (3) regulation of renal H^+ excretion controls ECF $[HCO_3^-]$. The latter is accomplished by proximal HCO_3^- reabsorption and the generation of new HCO_3^- as a result of titratable acid ($H_2PO_4^-$) and NH_4^+ excretion. The major adaptive response to an acid load is to stimulate ammoniagenesis and distal H^+ secretion, thereby increasing NH_4^+ excretion.

I. **Arterial blood gases (ABG).** Normal ABG values are pH, 7.40 ± 0.03 ($[H^+]$ 40 ± 3 nmol/L); PCO_2, 40 ± 5 mm Hg; and $[HCO_3^-]$, 24 ± 4 mmol/L. The relationship between these parameters is defined by the Henderson-Hasselbalch equation:

$$pH = 6.10 + \log([HCO_3^-]/0.03 \times PCO_2)$$

or, more simply, by the Henderson equation:

$$[H^+] = 24 \times (PCO_2/[HCO_3^-])$$

For every 0.1 increase/decrease in pH, multiply/divide the $[H^+]$ by 0.8 as follows:

pH	6.80	6.90	7.00	7.10	7.20	7.30	7.40	7.50	7.60	7.70	7.80
$[H^+]$	160	125	100	80	63	50	40	32	26	20	16
					(nmol/L)						

Intermediate values can be estimated by interpolation.

II. **Primary acid-base disturbances.** The Henderson formula predicts that **acidemia** (high $[H^+]$, low pH) can result from either a decreased $[HCO_3^-]$ or an increased PCO_2. Likewise, **alkalemia** (low $[H^+]$, high pH) is the consequence of an increased $[HCO_3^-]$ or a decreased PCO_2. The compensatory responses (Table 3-2) tend to return the plasma $[H^+]$ toward normal. A normal $[H^+]$ implies either a mixed acid-base disorder or no acid-base disturbance.

A. **Metabolic acidosis** results from a primary decrease in plasma $[HCO_3^-]$ due to either HCO_3^- loss or the accumulation of acid. A compensatory fall in PCO_2 occurs as a result of alveolar hyperventilation.

B. **Metabolic alkalosis** is characterized by a primary increase in plasma $[HCO_3^-]$ due to either H^+ loss or HCO_3^- gain. The compensatory change is a rise in PCO_2 caused by decreased alveolar ventilation.

C. **Respiratory acidosis** is defined as a primary increase in PCO_2 (alveolar hypoventilation). The renal compensatory response is enhanced H^+ secretion. This occurs over 3–5 days and results in an increased plasma $[HCO_3^-]$.

D. **Respiratory alkalosis** is manifest as hyperventilation that leads to a primary decrease in PCO_2. Chronically, a small compensatory decrease in renal NH_4^+ excretion occurs, leading to a fall in plasma $[HCO_3^-]$. The plasma pH is usually in the normal range.

Table 3-2. Expected compensatory responses to primary acid-base disorders

Disorder	Primary change	Compensatory response
Metabolic acidosis	$\downarrow[HCO_3^-]$	$\downarrow PCO_2$ by 1.0–1.3 mm Hg for every 1 mmol/L $\downarrow[HCO_3^-]$
		PCO_2 should equal last two digits of pH $\times$ 100
Metabolic alkalosis	$\uparrow[HCO_3^-]$	$\uparrow PCO_2$ 0.6–0.7 mm Hg for every 1 mmol/L $\uparrow[HCO_3^-]$
Respiratory acidosis	$\uparrow PCO_2$	
Acute		$\uparrow[HCO_3^-]$ 1.0 mmol/L for every 10 mm Hg $\uparrow PCO_2$
Chronic		$\uparrow[HCO_3^-]$ 3.0–3.5 mmol/L for every 10 mm Hg $\uparrow PCO_2$
Respiratory alkalosis	$\downarrow PCO_2$	
Acute		$\downarrow[HCO_3^-]$ 2.0 mmol/L for every 10 mm Hg $\downarrow PCO_2$
Chronic		$\downarrow[HCO_3^-]$ 4.0–5.0 mmol/L for every 10 mm Hg $\downarrow PCO_2$ (pH usually in normal range)

III. **Useful diagnostic tests**

A. **The plasma unmeasured anion gap (AG)** is the difference between the measured cations and the measured anions. Because the $[K^+]$ is usually unimportant quantitatively, it is often omitted from the calculation:

$$AG = [NA^+] - ([Cl^-] + [HCO_3^-])$$

The AG is normally 12 ± 2 mmol/L and is helpful in the differential diagnosis of metabolic acidosis. The normal AG is largely accounted for by anionic plasma proteins (i.e., albumin). A high AG generally signifies the overproduction of an organic acid or renal failure (see sec. **IV.B.1**). An increased AG may also be seen in metabolic alkalosis associated with ECF volume contraction. The causes of a low AG include hypoalbuminemia, halide (Br^- or I^-) intoxication, severe hyperlipidemia, and some cases of multiple myeloma (cationic immunoglobulin G paraprotein).

B. **The plasma osmolal gap** is the difference between the measured and the calculated plasma osmolality:

$$\text{Plasma osmolality (calculated)} = 2 \times [NA^+] + [glucose]/18 + BUN/2.8$$
$$\text{(mmol/L)} \qquad \text{(mg/dl)} \qquad \text{(mg/dl)}$$

A high plasma osmolal gap reflects the presence of an unmeasured nonionized compound, usually an alcohol such as methanol, ethanol, isopropanol, or ethylene glycol. This test is useful in distinguishing between the various causes of an increased AG metabolic acidosis (see sec. **IV.B.1**). Administration of IV mannitol or glycine is also detected as a high osmolal gap.

C. **The urine AG (UAG or urine net charge)** is useful when evaluating a normal AG metabolic acidosis (see sec. **IV.B.2**). The UAG is the difference between the major measured anions and cations:

$$UAG = ([NA^+] + [K^+]) - [Cl^-]$$

Because NH_4^+ is the major unmeasured urinary cation, a negative UAG reflects high NH_4^+ excretion. Conversely, a positive UAG signifies either low NH_4^+ excretion or the loss of NH_4^+ with a non-Cl^- anion. If the latter is suspected, the urine osmolal gap (UOG) can help detect the presence of NH_4^+ in the urine.

D. **UOG** is the difference between the measured and the calculated urine osmolality:

$$UOG = \text{urine osmolality} - 2 \times ([NA^+] + [K^+]) - [glucose]/18 - BUN/2.8$$
$$\text{(mmol/L)} \qquad \text{(mg/dl)} \qquad \text{(mg/dl)}$$

The UOG is not affected by unmeasured anions (e.g., hippurate and beta-hydroxybutyrate) and largely reflects the presence of NH_4^+ salts—the urine $[NH_4^+]$ is half the osmolal gap.

IV. **Metabolic acidosis**

A. **Diagnosis.** After a thorough history and physical examination, the presence of metabolic acidosis is confirmed by finding a high $[H^+]$ and a low $[HCO_3^-]$. If the ventilatory compensation is inappropriate, a superimposed respiratory disorder is also present. In the absence of causes for a low AG (see sec. **III.A**), a normal AG metabolic acidosis suggests either loss of HCO_3^- or gain of H^+ without a detectable accompanying plasma anion. The UAG and UOG should be determined to assess NH_4^+ excretion (see secs. **III.C** and **III.D**). Laboratory studies that are helpful in evaluating an increased AG metabolic acidosis include serum ketones (and beta-hydroxybutyrate), lactate, creatinine, and a plasma osmolal gap (see sec. **III.B**). The ratio of the change in AG to the change in $[HCO_3^-]$ (Δ/Δ) is usually approximately 1:1. If the Δ/Δ is less than 1:1, a mixed normal and high AG metabolic acidosis should be suspected. Conversely, a Δ/Δ of greater than 1:1 suggests a concurrent metabolic alkalosis.

B. Etiology and chronic treatment
  1. Increased AG acidosis
    a. Ketoacidosis is due to relative insulin deficiency as a result of insulin-dependent diabetes mellitus, inhibition of insulin release, hypoglycemia, or liver disease. **DKA** is described in Chap. 22. **Alcoholic ketoacidosis** occurs when ethanol consumption is accompanied by impaired insulin release (β-adrenergic) and is usually due to vomiting, malnutrition, and ECF volume depletion. If enough ethanol remains in the blood, an osmolal gap, along with the increase in the AG, will be present. The osmolal gap should be equal to [ethanol] (in mg/dl)/4.6 unless there is an associated ingestion of another toxic alcohol. Because beta-hydroxybutyrate initially predominates in the serum, the nitroprusside ketone reaction (Acetest), which detects acetoacetate and acetone, can underestimate the severity of the acidosis. Lactic acidosis may coexist, but lactate levels usually do not exceed 3 mmol/L. Serum glucose is typically normal or low. Treatment is directed at correction of ECF volume contraction. Thiamine should also be administered. The acidosis, unless severe, usually corrects with these measures. Hypokalemia, hypophosphatemia, and hypomagnesemia may occur, especially after 12–24 hours of therapy.
    b. Lactic acidosis results from overproduction or decreased utilization of lactic acid. The former results from tissue hypoperfusion or impaired oxygenation, for example, cardiopulmonary arrest, shock, pulmonary edema, severe hypoxemia, carbon monoxide poisoning, or vascular insufficiency (mesenteric or limb ischemia). Hyperphosphatemia, hyperuricemia, and moderate hyperkalemia can accompany the acidosis. Conditions that cause a marked increase in the metabolic rate may also cause a lactic acidosis, for example, generalized seizures, anaerobic exercise, severe asthma, and hypothermic shivering. Other conditions associated with lactic acidosis include malignancy, diabetes mellitus, hypoglycemia, D-lactate–producing bacteria in the short-bowel syndrome, and various intoxications. Among the latter are cyanide, ethanol, methanol, and salicylate.
    c. Renal failure results in an AG acidosis when the GFR falls below 20–30 ml/minute (see Chap. 12). The AG is due to retained sulfate, phosphate, and organic anions. The AG does not account for the entire decrease in the serum HCO_3^- because the acidosis is in part secondary to decreased NH_4^+ excretion.
    d. Intoxication with methanol and ethylene glycol causes an increased AG metabolic acidosis along with an osmolal gap. Paraldehyde may cause an increased AG acidosis, but without an osmolal gap. Salicylate intoxication usually results in respiratory alkalosis and metabolic acidosis. The metabolic acidosis may be due to increased lactate and ketoacid levels, as well as, to a minor degree, salicylic acid and its acid intermediates themselves. Diagnosis and treatment are described in Chap. 26.
  2. Normal AG acidosis
    a. Renal HCO_3^- loss or proximal (type 2) RTA is due to impaired proximal tubular HCO_3^- reabsorption and ammoniagenesis. Proximal RTA may be isolated or can occur in association with other transport defects (Fanconi's syndrome) manifest as glycosuria, aminoaciduria, hypouricemia, and hypophosphatemia. Causes include inherited disorders (cystinosis, galactosemia, Wilson's disease), toxins (heavy metals, outdated tetracycline, ifosfamide), multiple myeloma, autoimmune diseases (systemic lupus erythematosus, Sjögren's syndrome, chronic active hepatitis), amyloidosis, and acetazolamide. Bone disease (osteomalacia and osteopenia) is commonly associated with type 2 RTA. However, nephrocalcinosis seldom occurs. The diagnosis is made by administering

NaHCO$_3$ intravenously and documenting bicarbonaturia as the plasma [HCO$_3^-$] approaches normal: a urine pH of greater than 7.0 and a fractional excretion of HCO$_3^-$ greater than 15%. The fractional excretion of HCO$_3^-$ can be calculated using the following formula:

$$\text{Fractional excretion of } [HCO_3^-] = \frac{\text{urine } [HCO_3^-] \times \text{plasma Cr}}{\text{plasma } [HCO_3^-] \times \text{urine Cr}} \times 100$$

Treatment should include attempts to correct the underlying cause. Large amounts of alkali (10–15 mmol/kg/day) are required. Citrate may cause fewer GI side effects than HCO$_3^-$. Administration of potassium salts minimizes the degree of hypokalemia associated with alkali therapy. Thiazide diuretics can be used to promote proximal tubule HCO$_3^-$ reabsorption by inducing mild ECF volume depletion.

b. **Enhanced NH4⁺ excretion** (negative UAG and/or high UOG) indicates an appropriate renal response to metabolic acidosis and suggests two possible etiologies: GI HCO$_3^-$ loss or acid gain. The latter may result from the ingestion of HCl, NH$_4$Cl, lysine, arginine-HCl, or organic anions that are rapidly excreted in the urine (e.g., hippurate produced by patients who abuse toluene). GI loss of HCO$_3^-$ may be due to diarrhea, urinary diversion (ureterosigmoidostomy, long or obstructed ileal conduit), cholestyramine (especially in the presence of renal failure), or ingestion of calcium or magnesium chloride. GI losses may also be due to small bowel, biliary, or pancreatic drainage or fistulas.

c. **Impaired NH4⁺ excretion** or distal RTA (positive UAG and/or UOG <100 mOsm/kg) is associated with a heterogeneous group of disorders and results from either decreased [NH$_3$] in the medullary interstitium (urine pH <5.3) or impaired distal H⁺ secretion (urine pH >5.8). Historically, these conditions have been referred to as type 1 (distal or classic) and type 4 (hyperkalemic) RTA according to the plasma [K⁺]. However, the pathophysiologic classification allows a rational approach to diagnosis and helps identify the possible etiologies. A low [NH$_3$] in the renal medulla may be due to either decreased ammoniagenesis (usually associated with renal failure or hyperkalemia) or impaired medullary function due to various tubulointerstitial diseases (e.g., autoimmune diseases and hypergammaglobulinemia, nephrocalcinosis, analgesic use, chronic infection or obstruction). Low distal H⁺ secretion can result from (1) low H⁺ adenosine triphosphatase pump activity (autoimmune or medullary interstitial diseases), (2) impaired voltage augmentation of H⁺ secretion associated with hypoaldosteronism or mineralocorticoid resistance (see Potassium, sec. **II.B.4**), or (3) back-leak of H⁺ due to increased membrane permeability (e.g., amphotericin B). Treatment of distal RTA should be directed at reversing the underlying disorder(s). Correction of the metabolic acidosis consists of HCO$_3^-$ replacement (usually 1–2 mmol/kg/day) with NaHCO$_3$ or sodium citrate. Hypokalemia should be corrected, and chronic potassium citrate replacement may be necessary for patients with nephrolithiasis or nephrocalcinosis. Treatment of hyperkalemia (see Potassium, sec. **II.D**) consists of dietary K⁺ restriction (40–60 mmol/day) and possibly a loop diuretic. Chronic Kayexalate therapy may also be necessary. Mineralocorticoid administration (fludrocortisone, 100–200 μg PO qd) should be considered in patients with primary adrenal insufficiency.

C. **Treatment with NaHCO$_3$** is appropriate for patients with a normal AG metabolic acidosis. In addition, correcting severe acidemia to a pH of 7.20 decreases the risk of arrhythmias and enhances cardiac contractility. The plasma [HCO$_3^-$] should be raised to approximately 5 mmol/L if the PCO$_2$ is less than 20 mm Hg. Calculation of the HCO$_3^-$ deficit assumes a volume of distribution of 50% of total body weight. The HCO_3^- distribution space increases with the severity of the acidosis and may exceed 100% of total body weight in very severe metabolic acidosis. Rapid infusion of $NaHCO_3$ should only be considered for severe acidemia, and the tonicity of the $NaHCO_3$ administered depends on the patient's tonicity. Parenteral $NaHCO_3$ should always be prescribed with caution because of the potential adverse effects, including pulmonary edema, hypokalemia, and hypocalcemia.

V. Metabolic alkalosis

A. Etiology. A primary increase in the plasma $[HCO_3^-]$ may be due to either HCO_3^- gain (H^+ loss) or ECF volume contraction. To maintain electroneutrality, the addition of HCO_3^- must be accompanied by either Cl^- loss or Na^+ gain. In general, Cl^- depletion results from either vomiting (or nasogastric suction, villous adenoma, Cl^--losing diarrhea) or diuretics (thiazide or loop). This leads to ECF volume contraction, K^+ depletion, ICF acidosis, and increased NH_4^+ excretion (new HCO_3^- generation). Other causes of metabolic alkalosis that are associated with a decreased ECF volume include administration of nonreabsorbable anions (penicillin or carbenicillin), posthypercapnia, Bartter's syndrome, and Mg^{2+} depletion. Exogenous administration of $NaHCO_3$, metabolism of organic anions (e.g., citrate, acetate, lactate, or ketoacid anions), or milk-alkali syndrome can result in metabolic alkalosis. Impaired renal HCO_3^- excretion is required to maintain metabolic alkalosis. This occurs as a result of a decreased GFR and enhanced tubular HCO_3^- reabsorption (due to effective circulating volume depletion, hypokalemia, and hyperaldosteronism). Metabolic alkalosis may also be associated with hypokalemia due to primary mineralocorticoid excess or secondary hyperaldosteronism (renal artery stenosis, malignant hypertension, renin-secreting tumor).

B. Diagnosis begins with a complete history, focusing on eating habits (vomiting) and drug use (diuretics). The physical examination should include an assessment of BP and ECF volume status. The two commonest causes of metabolic alkalosis, vomiting and diuretic use, are associated with ECF volume contraction. In contrast, patients with primary hyperreninemia or primary hyperaldosteronism tend to have a normal or expanded ECF compartment and are often hypertensive. The urine electrolytes are generally useful in identifying the etiology of metabolic alkalosis when the history is unrevealing. A low urine $[Cl^-]$ (<20 mmol/L) and decreased ECF volume suggest vomiting or remote diuretic use. Recent vomiting is associated with an alkaline urine (pH >7.0), a high TTKG (see Potassium, sec. **I.C**), and a urine $[Na^+]$ of greater than 20 mmol/L. The urine $[Na^+]$ and $[Cl^-]$ are both greater than 20 mmol/L after (recent) diuretics. Without ECF volume contraction, the presence of hypertension, urine $[Na^+]$ and $[Cl^-]$ greater than 20 mmol/L, and a high TTKG are indicative of mineralocorticoid excess.

C. Treatment should be aimed at correcting the underlying disorder and replacing the deficits of NaCl and KCl. In the setting of ECF volume depletion, the latter is accomplished by giving isotonic NaCl. KCl should be administered to correct the K^+ deficit and intracellular acidosis. Metabolic alkalosis due to certain causes may be saline resistant, for example, edematous states, renal failure, mineralocorticoid excess, and severe K^+ or Mg^{2+} depletion. These conditions are often associated with a normal or expanded ECF volume, and NaCl administration would be hazardous and ineffective. The K^+ or Mg^{2+} deficits should be repleted, and hyperaldosteronism can be managed with a K^+-sparing diuretic (amiloride or spironolactone). Acetazolamide promotes bicarbonaturia, but renal K^+ loss is enhanced. Metabolic alkalosis associated with renal failure can be corrected with hemodialysis against a bath with a low $[HCO_3^-]$. Finally, severe alkalemia (pH >7.70) with ECF volume excess or renal failure, or both, can be treated with isotonic (150 mmol/L) HCl administered via a central vein (*Surgery* 75:194, 1974).

VI. Respiratory acidosis

  A. Diagnosis is established by the detection of an increased $[H^+]$ and an elevated PCO_2 on ABG. Hypercapnia almost always results from alveolar hypoventilation due to one of the following causes: (1) respiratory center depression (drugs, sleep apnea, obesity, CNS disease), (2) neuromuscular disorders (myasthenia gravis, Guillain-Barré syndrome, hypokalemia, myopathy), (3) upper airway obstruction, (4) pulmonary disease (chronic obstructive pulmonary disease, asthma, pulmonary edema, pneumothorax, pneumonia), or (5) mechanical hypoventilation. It is important to determine whether the change in $[H^+]$ is appropriate for the change in PCO_2 to differentiate acute from chronic respiratory disturbances: For every mm Hg increase in PCO_2 from 40 mm Hg, the $[H^+]$ should increase by 0.8 or 0.3 nmol/L in acute or chronic respiratory acidosis, respectively. The renal response occurs over several days, resulting in increased net acid excretion and an increased plasma $[HCO_3^-]$ (see Table 3-2).

  B. Treatment is directed at correcting the underlying disorder and improving ventilation (see Chap. 9). Administration of $NaHCO_3$ may exacerbate pulmonary edema, enhance hypercapnia, and lead to metabolic alkalosis. However, mechanically ventilated patients with severe status asthmaticus and acidosis (pH <7.15) may benefit from small doses of $NaHCO_3$ (44–88 mmol). Specifically, a higher plasma $[HCO_3^-]$ allows the $[H^+]$ to be controlled at a higher PCO_2 with a lower minute ventilation and peak airway pressures, thereby minimizing barotrauma.

VII. Respiratory alkalosis

  A. Diagnosis. Respiratory alkalosis results from the temporary removal of carbon dioxide exceeding its generation, as a result of increased alveolar ventilation. The diagnosis is confirmed by finding a low $[H^+]$ and a decreased $[HCO_3^-]$ on ABG. Causes of respiratory alkalosis include (1) hypoxemia (pulmonary disease, anemia, heart failure, high altitude), (2) respiratory center stimulation [CNS disorders, liver failure, gram-negative sepsis, drugs (salicylates, progesterone, theophylline, catecholamines), pregnancy, psychogenic], (3) pulmonary disease (pneumonia, edema, emboli, interstitial fibrosis), and (4) mechanical hyperventilation. The compensatory renal response should be assessed (see Table 3-2) and, if inappropriate, a mixed acid-base disturbance suspected.

  B. Treatment. Metabolic alkalosis is a diagnosis of great concern, and therapy should be directed at the underlying disorder.

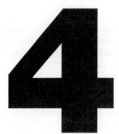

Hypertension

Aubrey R. Morrison

Definitions and Diagnostic Evaluation

Hypertension is defined as the presence of a BP elevation to a level that places patients at increased risk for target organ damage in several vascular beds, including the retina, brain, heart, kidneys, and large conduit arteries (Table 4-1). Hypertension characterized by a BP of greater than 140/90 mm Hg is a common condition that **affects an estimated 50 million Americans.** Of these patients, 90% have essential hypertension; the remainder have secondary hypertension caused by renal parenchymal disease, renovascular disease, pheochromocytoma, Cushing's syndrome, primary hyperaldosteronism, coarctation of the aorta, and uncommon autosomal dominant or recessive diseases of the adrenal-renal axis that result in salt retention. Disease-associated morbidity and mortality, including atherosclerotic cardiovascular disease, stroke, heart failure (HF), and renal insufficiency, increase with higher levels of systolic and diastolic BP. Isolated systolic hypertension of the elderly is also associated with increased cardiovascular and cerebrovascular complications.

I. **Detection and classification.** BP measurements should be performed on multiple occasions under nonstressful circumstances (e.g., rest, sitting, empty bladder, comfortable temperature) to obtain an accurate assessment of BP in a given patient. Hypertension should not be diagnosed on the basis of one measurement alone, unless it is greater than 210/120 mm Hg or accompanied by target organ damage. Three or more abnormal readings should be obtained, preferably over a period of several weeks, before therapy is considered. Care should be used also to exclude pseudohypertension, which usually occurs in elderly individuals with stiff, noncompressible vessels. A palpable artery that persists after cuff inflation (Osler's sign) should alert the physician to this possibility. Home and ambulatory BP monitoring can be used to assess a patient's true average BP, which correlates better with target organ damage. Circumstances in which ambulatory BP monitoring might be of value include (1) suspected "white-coat hypertension" (increases in BP associated with the stress of physician office visits), (2) high normal BP (130–139 mm Hg systolic, 85–89 mm Hg diastolic) with target organ damage, (3) evaluation of possible "drug resistance," and (4) episodic hypertension. Hypertension is present if a patient's average BP is greater than 140 mm Hg systolic or greater than 90 mm Hg diastolic (Table 4-2).

II. **Initial clinical evaluation.** BP elevation usually is discovered in asymptomatic individuals during screening. Optimal detection and evaluation of hypertension require accurate noninvasive BP measurement, which should be obtained in a seated patient with the arm level with the heart. A calibrated, appropriately fitting BP cuff should be used because falsely high readings can be obtained if the cuff is too small. Two readings should be taken, separated by 2 minutes. Systolic BP should be noted with the appearance of Korotkoff sounds (phase I) and diastolic BP with the disappearance of sounds (phase V). In certain

Table 4-1. Manifestations of target organ disease

Organ system	Manifestations
Large vessels	Aneurysmal dilatation
	Accelerated atherosclerosis
	Aortic dissection
Cardiac	
Acute	Pulmonary edema, myocardial infarction
Chronic	Clinical or ECG evidence of CAD; LVH by ECG or echocardiogram
Cerebrovascular	
Acute	Intracerebral bleeding, coma, seizures, mental status changes, TIA, stroke
Chronic	TIA, stroke
Renal	
Acute	Hematuria, azotemia
Chronic	Serum creatinine >1.5 mg/dl, proteinuria >1+ on dipstick
Retinopathy	
Acute	Papilledema, hemorrhages
Chronic	Hemorrhages, exudates, arterial nicking

CAD = coronary artery disease; LVH = left ventricular hypertrophy; TIA = transient ischemic attack.

patients, the Korotkoff sounds do not disappear but are present to 0 mm Hg. In this case, the initial muffling of Korotkoff sounds (phase IV) should be taken as the diastolic BP (*Hypertension* 11:211A, 1988). One should be careful to avoid spuriously low BP readings due to an auscultatory gap, which is caused by the disappearance and reappearance of Korotkoff sounds in hypertensive patients and may account for up to a 25-mm Hg gap between true and measured BP. Hypertension should be confirmed in both arms, and the higher reading should be used. The history should seek to discover secondary causes of hypertension and note the presence of medications that can affect BP (e.g., decongestants, oral contraceptives, appetite suppressants, nonsteroidal anti-inflammatory agents, exogenous thyroid hormone, recent alcohol consumption, and illicit stimulants). A diagnosis of secondary hypertension should be considered in the following situations: (1) age at onset younger than 30 or older than 60 years, (2) hypertension that is difficult to control after therapy has been initiated, (3) stable hypertension that becomes difficult to control, (4) clinical occurrence of a hypertensive crisis (see Therapeutic Considerations, sec. **I.D**), and (5) the presence of signs or symptoms of a secondary cause such as hypokalemia or metabolic alkalosis that is not explained by diuretic therapy. In patients who present with significant hypertension at a young age, a careful family history may give clues to forms of hypertension that follow simple mendelian inheritance. The physical examination should include investigation for target organ damage or a secondary cause of hypertension by noting the presence of carotid bruits, a third or fourth heart sound, cardiac murmurs, neurologic deficits, elevated jugular venous pressure, rales, retinopathy, unequal pulses, enlarged or small kidneys, cushingoid features, and abdominal bruits.

III. Laboratory evaluation. All newly diagnosed hypertensive patients should have a laboratory assessment, which may include a urinalysis, hematocrit, plasma

Table 4-2. Classification of blood pressure for adults age 18 years and older[a]

Category	Systolic pressure (mm Hg)	Diastolic pressure (mm Hg)
Normal[b]	<130	<85
High normal	130–139	85–89
Hypertensive[c]		
Stage 1	140–159	90–99
Stage 2	160–179	100–109
Stage 3	>180	>110

[a]Not taking antihypertensive drugs and not acutely ill. When systolic and diastolic pressures fall into different categories, the higher category should be selected to classify the individual's BP status. Isolated systolic hypertension is defined as a systolic BP of 140 mm Hg or more and a diastolic BP of less than 90 mm Hg and staged appropriately (e.g., 170/85 mm Hg is defined as stage 2 isolated systolic hypertension). In addition to classifying stages of hypertension on the basis of average BP levels, the clinician should specify presence or absence of target organ disease and additional risk factors. This specificity is important for risk classification and management.
[b]Optimal blood pressure with respect to cardiovascular risk is less than 120 mm Hg systolic and less than 80 mm Hg diastolic. However, unusually low readings should be evaluated for clinical significance.
[c]Based on the average of two or more readings taken at each of two or more visits after an initial screening.
Source: Sixth Report of the Joint National Committee on Detection, Evaluation, and Treatment of High Blood Pressure. *Arch Intern Med* 157:2413–2446, 1997.

glucose, serum potassium, serum creatinine, calcium, uric acid, chest radiography, and ECG. Fasting serum cholesterol and triglyceride levels should be obtained to screen for hyperlipidemia. This battery of tests helps to identify patients with possible target organ damage and provides a baseline for assessing adverse effects of therapy. Assessment of cardiac function or left ventricular hypertrophy (LVH) by echocardiography may be of value for certain patients.

Therapeutic Considerations

I. **General considerations and goals.** The goal of treatment for hypertension is to prevent long-term sequelae (i.e., target organ damage). Barring an overt need for immediate pharmacologic therapy, most patients should be given the opportunity to achieve a reduction in BP over an interval of 3–6 months by applying nonpharmacologic modifications. The primary goal is to reduce BP to less than 140/90 mm Hg while concurrently controlling other modifiable cardiovascular risk factors. As isolated systolic hypertension is also associated with increased cerebrovascular and cardiac events, the therapeutic goal in this subset of patients should be to lower BP to less than 140 mm Hg systolic. Treatment should be more aggressive for those patients in whom target organ damage or other cardiovascular risk factors are present. Discretion is warranted in prescribing medication to lower BP that may affect cardiovascular risk adversely in other ways (e.g., glucose control, lipid metabolism, uric acid levels). In the absence of hypertensive crisis (see sec. **I.D**), BP should be reduced gradually to avoid end-organ (e.g., cerebral) ischemia. Patient education is an essential component of the treatment plan and promotes patient compliance. Physicians should emphasize that (1) lifelong treatment usually is required, (2) symptoms are an unreliable gauge of severity of hypertension, and (3) prognosis improves with proper management. Cultural and other individual differences among patients must be considered in planning a therapeutic regimen. Although classification of adult blood pressure is somewhat arbitrary, it may nevertheless be useful in making clinical decisions (see Table 4-2).

A. Normal BP is defined as <130/<85; pharmacologic intervention is not indicated.

B. High-normal BP is defined as BP of 130–139/85–89, whereas **stage 1 hypertension** is BP 140–159/90–99. In these patients with no more than one cardiovascular risk factor excluding diabetes mellitus and no target organ damage, BP can be followed for up to 6 months with nonpharmacologic therapy. If treatment is ineffective or there is evidence of end-organ damage or diabetes, or both, with or without additional risk factors, pharmacologic therapy should be initiated.

C. In stages 2 (160–179/100–109) and 3 (>180/>110) hypertension, pharmacologic therapy should be initiated in addition to lifestyle modification. Patients with BP levels greater than 180/110 mm Hg often require more than one medication and frequent intervals of follow-up before adequate control is achieved. Patients with an average BP of 200/120 or greater require immediate therapy and, if symptomatic end-organ damage is present, require hospitalization.

D. Hypertensive crisis includes hypertensive emergencies and urgencies (see Special Considerations, sec. **III**). It usually develops in patients with a previous history of elevated BP but may arise in patients who were previously normotensive. The severity of a hypertensive crisis correlates not only with the absolute level of BP elevation but also with the rapidity of development, because autoregulatory mechanisms have not had sufficient time to adapt.

   1. Hypertensive urgencies are defined as a substantial increase in BP, usually with a diastolic BP of greater than 120–130 mm Hg, and occur in approximately 1% of hypertensive patients. Hypertensive urgencies (i.e., upper levels of stage 3 hypertension, hypertension with optic disk edema, progressive end-organ complications rather than damage, and severe perioperative hypertension) warrant BP reduction within several hours (*Arch Intern Med* 157:2412, 1997).

   2. Hypertensive emergencies include **accelerated hypertension** defined as a systolic BP typically exceeding 210 and diastolic BP greater than 130 presenting with headaches, blurred vision, or focal neurologic symptoms and **malignant hypertension,** which requires the presence of papilledema. Hypertensive emergencies require immediate BP reduction (not necessarily to normal ranges) to prevent or minimize end-organ damage [i.e., hypertensive encephalopathy, intracranial hemorrhage, unstable angina pectoris, acute myocardial infarction (MI), acute left ventricular failure with pulmonary edema, dissecting aortic aneurysm, progressive renal failure, or eclampsia].

E. Isolated systolic hypertension. Isolated systolic hypertension—defined as a systolic BP greater than 140 mm Hg—occurs frequently in the elderly (beginning after the fifth decade and increasing with age). Nonpharmacologic therapy should be attempted initially. If it fails, medication should be used to lower systolic BP to less than 160 mm Hg if it is initially greater than 180 mm Hg, and to lower the systolic BP by 20 mm Hg in those with a systolic BP of 160–180 mm Hg. Patient tolerance of antihypertensive therapy should be assessed frequently.

II. Nonpharmacologic therapy. Lifestyle modifications should be encouraged in all hypertensive patients regardless of whether they require medication. These changes may have beneficial effects on other cardiovascular risk factors. Some of these lifestyle modifications include cessation of smoking, reduction in body weight if overweight, judicious consumption of alcohol, and adequate nutritional intake of minerals and vitamins.

III. Pharmacologic therapy

A. Diuretics (Table 4-3) are effective agents in the therapy of hypertension, and data have accumulated to demonstrate their safety and benefit in reducing the incidence of stroke and cardiovascular events. Chlorthalidone, a thiazide diuretic, may be more effective than α-adrenergic antagonists (doxazosin) in the treatment of hypertension and may also have less risk of cardiovascular disease and stroke in patients with hypertension and at least one risk factor for coronary heart disease (*JAMA* 283:1967, 2000). However, diuretics have shown a less consistent decrease in ischemic cardiac events at higher doses (e.g., >50 mg hydrochlorothiazide) and may increase ventricular arrhythmias.

1. **The mechanism of action** is to initiate a natriuresis and subsequently to decrease intravascular volume. Diuretics may initially cause an increase in peripheral resistance and a decrease in cardiac output, but, with chronic administration, these parameters return to normal. Diuretics may also produce mild vasodilation by inhibiting sodium entry into vascular smooth-muscle cells. Indapamide in particular has a pronounced vasodilating effect.

2. **Several classes of diuretics** are available, generally categorized by their site of action in the kidney. Thiazide and thiazide-like diuretics (e.g., hydrochlorothiazide, chlorthalidone) block sodium reabsorption predominantly in the distal convoluted tubule by inhibition of the thiazide-sensitive Na/Cl cotransporter. Loop diuretics (e.g., furosemide,

Table 4-3. Commonly used antihypertensive agents by functional class

Drugs by class	Properties	Initial dose	Usual dosage range
β-Adrenergic antagonists			
Atenolol[a,b]	Selective	50 mg PO qd	25–100 mg
Betaxolol	Selective	10 mg PO qd	5–40 mg
Bisoprolol[a]	Selective	5 mg PO qd	2.5–20.0 mg
Metoprolol	Selective	50 mg PO bid	50–450 mg
Metoprolol XL	Selective	50–100 mg PO qd	50–400 mg
Nadolol[a]	Nonselective	40 mg PO qd	20–240 mg
Propranolol[b]	Nonselective	40 mg PO bid	40–240 mg
Propranolol LA	Nonselective	80 mg PO qd	60–240 mg
Timolol[b]	Nonselective	10 mg PO bid	20–40 mg
Carteolol[a]	ISA	2.5 mg PO qd	2.5–10.0 mg
Penbutolol	ISA	20 mg PO qd	20–80 mg
Pindolol	ISA	5 mg PO qd	10–60 mg
Labetalol	α- and β-antagonist properties	100 mg PO bid	200–1200 mg
Carvedilol	α- and β-antagonist properties	6.25 mg PO bid	12.5–50 mg
Acebutolol[a]	ISA, selective	200 mg PO bid, 400 mg PO qd	200–1200 mg

Drugs by class	Properties	Initial dose	Usual dosage range
Calcium channel antagonists			
Amlodipine	DHP	5 mg PO qd	2.5–10.0 mg
Diltiazem	—	30 mg PO qid	90–360 mg
Diltiazem SR	—	60–120 mg PO bid	120–360 mg
Diltiazem CD	—	180 mg PO bid	180–360 mg
Diltiazem XR	—	80 mg qd	180–480 mg
Isradipine	DHP	2.5 mg PO bid	2.5–10.0 mg
Nicardipine[b]	DHP	20 mg PO tid	60–120 mg
Nicardipine SR	DHP	30 mg PO bid	60–120 mg
Nifedipine	DHP	10 mg PO tid	30–120 mg
Nifedipine XL (or LL)	DHP	30 mg PO qd	30–90 mg
Nisoldipine	DHP	20 mg PO qd	20–40 mg
Verapamil[b]	—	80 mg PO tid	80–480 mg
Verapamil COER	—	80 mg PO qd	180–480 mg
Verapamil SR	—	120–140 mg PO qd	120–480 mg
Angiotensin-converting enzyme inhibitors			
Benazepril[a]	—	10 mg PO bid	10–40 mg
Captopril[a]	—	25 mg PO bid–tid	50–450 mg
Enalapril[a]	—	5 mg PO qd	2.5–40.0 mg
Fosinopril	—	10 mg PO qd	10–40 mg
Lisinopril[a]	—	10 mg PO qd	5–40 mg
Moexipril	—	7.5 mg PO qd	7.5–30.0 mg
Quinapril[a]	—	10 mg PO qd	5–80 mg
Ramipril[a]	—	2.5 mg PO qd	1.25–20.0 mg
Trandolapril	—	1–2 mg PO qd	1–4 mg
Angiotensin II receptor blocker			
Candesartan	—	8 mg PO qd	8–32 mg
Irbesartan	—	150 mg PO qd	150–300 mg
Losartan	—	25 mg PO qd	25–100 mg
Telmisartan	—	20 mg PO qd	20–80 mg
Valsartan	—	80 mg PO qd	80–160 mg
Diuretics			
Bendroflumethiazide	Thiazide diuretic	5 mg PO qd	2.5–15.0 mg
Benzthiazide	Thiazide diuretic	25 mg PO bid	50–100 mg
Chlorothiazide	Thiazide diuretic	500 mg PO qd (or IV)	125–1000 mg
Chlorthalidone	Thiazide diuretic	25 mg PO qd	12.5–50.0 mg

Table 4-3. (continued)

Drugs by class	Properties	Initial dose	Usual dosage range
Hydrochlorothiazide	Thiazide diuretic	25 mg PO qd	12.5–50.0 mg
Hydroflumethiazide	Thiazide diuretic	50 mg PO qd	50–100 mg
Indapamide	Thiazide diuretic	1.25 mg PO qd	2.5–5.0 mg
Methyclothiazide	Thiazide diuretic	2.5 mg PO qd	2.5–5.0 mg
Metolazone	Thiazide diuretic	2.5 mg PO qd	1.25–5.00 mg
Polythiazide	Thiazide diuretic	2.0 mg PO qd	1–4 mg
Quinethazone	Thiazide diuretic	50 mg PO qd	25–100 mg
Trichlormethiazide	Thiazide diuretic	2.0 mg PO qd	1–4 mg
Bumetanide	Loop diuretic	0.5 mg PO qd (or IV)	0.5–5.0 mg
Ethacrynic acid	Loop diuretic	50 mg PO qd (or IV)	25–100 mg
Furosemide	Loop diuretic	20 mg PO qd (or IV)	20–320 mg
Torsemide	Loop diuretic	5 mg PO qd (or IV)	5–10 mg
Amiloride	Potassium-sparing diuretic	5 mg PO qd	5–10 mg
Spironolactone	Potassium-sparing diuretic	50 mg PO qd	25–100 mg
Triamterene	Potassium-sparing diuretic	50 mg PO bid	50–200 mg
α-Adrenergic antagonists			
Doxazosin	—	1 mg PO qd	1–16 mg
Prazosin	—	1 mg PO bid–tid	1–20 mg
Terazosin	—	1 mg PO qhs	1–20 mg
Centrally acting adrenergic agents			
Clonidine[b]	—	0.1 mg PO bid	0.1–1.2 mg
Clonidine patch	—	TTS 1/wk (equivalent to 0.1 mg/day release)	0.1–0.3 mg
Guanfacine	—	1 mg PO qd	1–3 mg
Guanabenz	—	4 mg PO bid	4–64 mg
Methyldopa[b]	—	250 mg PO bid–tid	250–2000 mg
Direct-acting vasodilators			
Hydralazine	—	10 mg PO qid	50–300 mg
Minoxidil	—	5 mg PO qd	2.5–100.0 mg
Miscellaneous			
Reserpine[b]	—	0.5 mg PO qd	0.01–0.25 mg

DHP = dihydropyridine; ISA = intrinsic sympathomimetic activity; TTS = transdermal therapeutic system.
[a]Adjusted in renal failure.
[b]Available in generic form.

bumetanide, ethacrynic acid, and torsemide) block sodium reabsorption in the thick ascending loop of Henle through inhibition of the Na/K/2Cl cotransporter and are the most effective agents in patients with renal insufficiency (creatinine >2.5 mg/dl). Spironolactone, a potassium-sparing agent, acts by competitively inhibiting the actions of aldosterone on the kidney. Triamterene and amiloride are potassium-sparing drugs that inhibit the epithelial Na^+ channel in the distal nephron to inhibit reabsorption of Na^+ and secretion of potassium ions. Potassium-sparing diuretics are weak agents when used alone; thus, they are often combined with a thiazide for added effects.

3. **Side effects** of diuretics vary by class. Thiazide diuretics can produce weakness, muscle cramps, and impotence. Metabolic side effects include hypokalemia, hypomagnesemia, hyperlipidemia (with increases in low-density lipoproteins and triglyceride levels), hypercalcemia, hyperglycemia, hyperuricemia, hyponatremia, and, rarely, azotemia. Thiazide-induced pancreatitis also has been reported. Metabolic side effects may be limited when thiazides are used in low doses (e.g., hydrochlorothiazide, 12.5–25.0 mg/day). Loop diuretics can cause electrolyte abnormalities, such as hypomagnesemia, hypocalcemia, and hypokalemia, and also can produce irreversible ototoxicity (usually dose related and more common with parenteral therapy). Spironolactone can produce hyperkalemia; gynecomastia may occur in men, and breast tenderness has been noted in women. Triamterene (usually in combination with hydrochlorothiazide) can cause renal tubular damage and renal calculi. Unlike thiazides, potassium-sparing and loop diuretics do not cause adverse lipid effects.

B. **Sympatholytic agents**
   1. β-**Adrenergic antagonists** (see Table 4-3) are effective antihypertensive agents and are part of medical regimens that have been proven to decrease the incidence of stroke, MI, and HF. These agents may offer advantages in selected populations, including patients with increased adrenergic drive (i.e., those with a wide pulse pressure and tachycardia), LVH, and a previous MI. Low doses of β-adrenergic antagonists can be useful in patients with stable HF; however, because of the potential for clinical deterioration, their use should be limited to closely supervised settings (see Chap. 6, Heart Failure, sec. **II.C.2**).
      a. The **mechanism of action** of β-adrenergic antagonists is competitive inhibition of the effects of catecholamines at β-adrenergic receptors, which decreases heart rate and cardiac output. These agents also decrease plasma renin and cause a resetting of baroreceptors to accept a lower level of BP. β-Adrenergic antagonists cause release of vasodilatory prostaglandins, decrease plasma volume, and also may have a CNS-mediated antihypertensive effect.
      b. **Classes of** β-**adrenergic antagonists** can be subdivided into those that are cardioselective, with primarily β_1-blocking effects, and those that are nonselective, with β_1- and β_2-blocking effects. At low doses, the cardioselective agents can be given with caution to patients with mild chronic obstructive pulmonary disease, diabetes mellitus, or peripheral vascular disease. At higher doses, these agents lose their β_1 selectivity and may cause unwanted effects in these patients. β-Adrenergic antagonists also can be categorized according to the presence or absence of partial agonist or intrinsic sympathomimetic activity (ISA). β-Adrenergic antagonists with ISA cause less bradycardia than do those without it.
      c. **Side effects** include high-degree atrioventricular block, HF, Raynaud's phenomenon, and impotence. Lipophilic β-adrenergic antagonists, such as propranolol, have a higher incidence of CNS side effects, such as insomnia and depression, than do the more hydro-

philic agents. Propranolol also can cause nasal congestion. β-Adrenergic antagonists can cause adverse effects on the lipid profile; increased triglyceride and decreased high-density lipoprotein (HDL) levels occur mainly with nonselective β-adrenergic antagonists but generally do not occur when β-adrenergic antagonists with ISA are used. Pindolol, a selective β-adrenergic antagonist with ISA may actually increase HDL and nominally increase triglycerides. Because beta-receptor density is increased with chronic antagonism, abrupt withdrawal of these agents can precipitate angina pectoris, increases in BP, and other effects attributable to an increase in adrenergic tone (*Br Heart J* 45:637, 1981).

2. **Selective α-adrenergic antagonists,** such as prazosin, terazosin, and doxazosin, have replaced nonselective α-adrenergic antagonists, such as phenoxybenzamine (see Table 4-3), in the treatment of essential hypertension.

   a. The **mechanism of action** of selective α_1-adrenergic antagonists is to block postsynaptic alpha receptors, producing arterial and venous vasodilation.

   b. **Side effects** of these agents include a "first-dose effect," which results from a greater decrease in BP with the first dose than with subsequent doses. Selective α_1-adrenergic antagonists can cause syncope, orthostatic hypotension, dizziness, headache, and drowsiness. In most cases, side effects are self-limited and do not recur with continued therapy. Selective α_1-adrenergic antagonists may improve lipid profiles by decreasing total cholesterol and triglyceride levels and increasing HDL levels. Additionally, these agents can improve the negative effects on lipids induced by thiazide diuretics and β-adrenergic antagonists (*Am Heart J* 121:1307, 1991). However, doxazosin specifically may be less effective in lowering systolic blood pressure than thiazide diuretics and may additionally be associated with a higher risk of cardiovascular disease, particularly HF, and stroke in patients with hypertension and at least one additional risk factor for coronary heart disease (*JAMA* 283:1967, 2000).

3. **Agents with mixed properties** (labetalol, carvedilol) have α- and β-adrenergic antagonist actions (see Table 4-3). In addition, carvedilol may have antioxidant properties. These agents are effective in both white and black hypertensive patients.

   a. The **mechanism of action** of these drugs is to antagonize the effects of catecholamines at β receptors and peripheral α_1 receptors. The effects of labetalol on alpha receptors decrease with chronic administration and are essentially gone within a few months.

   b. **Side effects** of labetalol include hepatocellular damage, postural hypotension, a positive antinuclear antibody test (ANA), a lupus-like syndrome, tremors, and potential hypotension in the setting of halothane anesthesia. Labetalol has negligible effects on lipids. Carvedilol appears to have a similar side effect profile to other β-adrenergic antagonists. Rarely, reflex tachycardia may occur because of the initial vasodilatory effect of labetalol and carvedilol.

4. **Centrally acting adrenergic agents** (see Table 4-3) are potent antihypertensive agents. In addition to its oral dosage forms, clonidine is available as a transdermal patch that is applied weekly.

   a. The **mechanism of action** of centrally acting adrenergic agents is to stimulate the presynaptic α_2-adrenergic receptors in the CNS. This stimulation leads to a decrease in peripheral sympathetic tone, which reduces systemic vascular resistance. Also, it causes a modest decrease in cardiac output and heart rate. Renal blood flow is not compromised by centrally acting adrenergic agents, but fluid retention may occur.

b. **Side effects** may include bradycardia, drowsiness, dry mouth, orthostatic hypotension, galactorrhea, and sexual dysfunction. Transdermal clonidine causes a rash in up to 20% of patients. These agents can precipitate HF in patients with decreased left ventricular function, and abrupt cessation can precipitate an acute withdrawal syndrome (AWS) of elevated BP, tachycardia, and diaphoresis (see Special Considerations, sec. II). Methyldopa produces a positive direct antibody (Coombs') test in up to 25% of patients, but significant hemolytic anemia is much less common. If a hemolytic anemia develops secondary to methyldopa, the drug should be withdrawn. Severe cases of hemolytic anemia may require treatment with glucocorticoids. Methyldopa also causes positive ANA test results in approximately 10% of patients and can cause an inflammatory reaction in the liver that is indistinguishable from viral hepatitis; fatal hepatitis has been reported. Guanabenz and guanfacine decrease total cholesterol levels, and guanfacine also can decrease serum triglyceride levels.

5. **Other sympatholytics** (reserpine, guanethidine, guanadrel). These agents (see Table 4-3) were among the first effective antihypertensive agents available. Currently, these drugs are not regarded as first- or second-line therapy because of their significant side effects.

a. The **mechanism of action** of these agents is to inhibit the release of norepinephrine from peripheral neurons. Reserpine, which is more lipophilic than are other drugs in this class, also affects the CNS. Reserpine depletes biogenic amines from being packaged into storage vesicles within neurons, thereby allowing norepinephrine to be degraded by cytoplasmic monoamine oxidase. Guanethidine and guanadrel directly inhibit the release of norepinephrine from peripheral nerve terminals.

b. **Side effects** of reserpine include severe depression in approximately 2% of patients. Sedation and nasal stuffiness also are potential side effects. Guanethidine can cause severe postural hypotension by effecting a decrease in cardiac output, a decrease in peripheral resistance, and venous pooling in the extremities. Patients who are receiving guanethidine with orthostatic hypotension should be cautioned to arise slowly and to wear support hose. Guanethidine also can cause ejaculatory failure and diarrhea.

C. **Calcium channel antagonists** (see Table 4-3) are effective agents in the treatment of hypertension. Generally, they are effective in both black and white hypertensive patients, have no significant CNS side effects, and can be used to treat diseases, such as angina pectoris, that can coexist with hypertension. Concern has risen that the use of short-acting dihydropyridine calcium channel antagonists may increase the number of ischemic cardiac events (*JAMA* 274:620, 1995); however, long-acting agents are safe in the management of hypertension (*Am J Cardiol* 77:81, 1996).

1. **The mechanism of action** is to cause arteriolar vasodilation by selective blockade of the slow inward calcium channels in vascular smooth-muscle cells. These agents also cause an initial natriuresis, which may dissipate with time.

2. **Classes of calcium channel antagonists** include diphenylalkylamines (e.g., verapamil), benzothiazepines (e.g., diltiazem), and dihydropyridines (e.g., nifedipine). The dihydropyridines include many newer second-generation drugs (e.g., amlodipine, felodipine, isradipine, and nicardipine), which are more vasoselective and have longer plasma half-lives than nifedipine. Verapamil and diltiazem have negative cardiac inotropic and chronotropic effects. Nifedipine also has a negative inotropic effect, but, in clinical use, it is much less pronounced than that of verapamil or diltiazem because of peripheral vasodilatation and reflex tachycardia. Less negative inotropic effects have been observed with the

second-generation dihydropyridines. All calcium channel antagonists
are metabolized in the liver; thus, in patients with cirrhosis, the dosing
interval should be adjusted accordingly. Some of these drugs also inhibit
the metabolism of other hepatically cleared medications (e.g., cyclosporine; see Appendix C). Verapamil and diltiazem should be used with
caution in patients with cardiac conduction abnormalities and can cause
or worsen HF in patients with decreased left ventricular function.

3. **Side effects** of verapamil include constipation, nausea, headache, and
orthostatic hypotension. Diltiazem can cause nausea, headache, and
rash. Dihydropyridines can cause lower-extremity edema, flushing,
headache, and rash. Calcium channel antagonists have no significant
effects on glucose tolerance, electrolytes, or lipid profiles. In general,
calcium channel antagonists should not be initiated in patients immediately following MI because of increased mortality in all but the most
stable patients without evidence of HF (see Chap. 5). Additionally, in
patients with hypertension and non–insulin-dependent diabetes mellitus, dihydropyridines (nisoldipine) may be associated with a higher incidence of fatal and nonfatal MIs (*N Engl J Med* 338:645, 1998).

D. **Inhibitors of the renin-angiotensin system** (see Table 4-3) are effective
antihypertensive agents in a broad array of patients.

1. **Angiotensin-converting enzyme (ACE) inhibitors** may have beneficial
effects in patients with concomitant HF or kidney disease. One study has
also suggested that ACE inhibitors (ramipril) may significantly reduce
the rate of death, MI, and stroke in patients without HF or low ejection
fraction (*N Engl J Med* 342:145, 2000). Additionally, they can reduce
hypokalemia, hypercholesterolemia, hyperglycemia, and hyperuricemia
caused by diuretic therapy and are particularly effective in states of
hypertension associated with a high renin state (e.g., scleroderma renal
crisis) (*Med Clin North Am* 71:979, 1987). Fosinopril is unique in that
50% of the drug is eliminated by the liver under normal conditions, but
this percentage increases in the presence of renal insufficiency.

   a. **Mechanism of action.** ACE inhibitors block the production of angiotensin II, a vasoconstrictor, by inhibiting ACE competitively, thereby
leading to arterial and venous vasodilation and to natriuresis. Furthermore, ACE inhibitors, by inhibiting the formation of angiotensin
II, reduce aldosterone secretion, thus producing a mild natriuresis
and a decrease in K^+ secretion. Additionally, ACE inhibitors increase
levels of vasodilating bradykinins. Some agents (i.e., captopril)
directly stimulate production of renal and endothelial vasodilatory
prostaglandins. Despite these vasodilating effects, ACE inhibitors do
not cause significant reflex tachycardia, perhaps owing to a resetting
of the baroreceptor reflex.

   b. **Side effects** associated with the use of ACE inhibitors are infrequent.
They do not cause levels of lipids, glucose, or uric acid to increase. ACE
inhibitors can cause a dry cough (up to 20% of patients), angioneurotic
edema, and hypotension. ACE inhibitors that contain a sulfhydryl
group (e.g., captopril) may cause taste disturbance, leukopenia, and a
glomerulopathy with proteinuria. Because ACE inhibitors cause preferential vasodilation of the efferent arteriole in the kidney, worsening
of renal function may occur in patients who have decreased renal perfusion or who have pre-existing severe renal insufficiency. ACE inhibitors can cause hyperkalemia and should be used with caution in
patients with a decreased glomerular filtration rate, in those who are
taking potassium supplements, or in those who are receiving potassium-sparing diuretics.

2. **Angiotensin-receptor antagonists (ARBs)** are a class of antihypertensive drugs that are effective in diverse patient populations (*N Engl J
Med* 334:1649, 1996). Several of these agents are now approved for the

management of mild to moderate hypertension (see Table 4-3). Additionally, ARBs (losartan) may be a useful alternative in patients with HF who are unable to tolerate ACE inhibitors (*Lancet* 355:1582, 2000).

   a. **The main mechanisms of action** of these drugs are to antagonize the vasoconstrictor effects on smooth muscle and the secretory effects on the zona glomerulosa of angiotensin II at the angiotensin II type 1 receptor. These actions result in decreased peripheral vascular resistance.

   b. **Side effects** of losartan occur rarely but include angioedema, allergic reaction, and rash. The cough seen with ACE inhibitors occurs much less frequently with losartan. The side effect profile is otherwise similar to that of the ACE inhibitors. Losartan specifically is uricosuric. These agents do not appear to affect lipids.

E. **Direct-acting vasodilators,** potent antihypertensive agents (see Table 4-3), now are reserved for refractory hypertension or specific circumstances, such as the use of hydralazine in pregnancy. Hydralazine in combination with nitrates is useful in treating patients with hypertension and HF (see Chap. 6).

   1. **The mechanism of action** of these agents (e.g., minoxidil and hydralazine) is to produce direct arterial vasodilation. Minoxidil hyperpolarizes and relaxes smooth muscle by stimulating an adenosine triphosphate–dependent K^+ channel. The mechanism of action of hydralazine is unknown. Although these drugs lower BP when used alone, their sustained antihypertensive action is limited because of reflex sodium and fluid retention and sympathetic hyperactivity producing tachycardia. Often, concomitant diuretic or β-adrenergic antagonist use is required to ameliorate these unwanted effects. These agents should be used with caution or avoided in patients with ischemic heart disease because of the reflex sympathetic hyperactivity that they induce.

   2. **Side effects** of hydralazine therapy may include headache, nausea, emesis, tachycardia, and postural hypotension. Asymptomatic patients may have a positive ANA test result, and a hydralazine-induced systemic lupus–like syndrome may develop in approximately 10% of patients. Patients who may be at increased risk for this latter complication include (1) those treated with excessive doses (e.g., >400 mg/day), (2) those with impaired renal or cardiac function, and (3) those with the slow acetylation phenotype. Hydralazine should be discontinued if clinical evidence of a lupus-like syndrome develops and a positive ANA test result is present. The syndrome usually resolves with discontinuation of the drug, leaving no adverse long-term effects. Side effects of minoxidil include weight gain, hypertrichosis, hirsutism, ECG abnormalities, and pericardial effusions.

F. **Parenteral antihypertensive agents** are indicated for the immediate reduction of BP in patients with hypertensive emergencies. Judicious administration of these agents (Table 4-4) may be appropriate also in patients with hypertension complicated by HF or MI. These drugs are indicated also for individuals who have perioperative hypertensive urgency or are in need of emergency surgery. If possible, an accurate baseline BP should be determined before the initiation of therapy. In the setting of hypertensive emergency, the patient should be admitted to an ICU for close monitoring, and an intra-arterial monitor should be used when available. Although parenteral agents are indicated as a first line in hypertensive emergencies, oral agents may also be effective in this group (see sec. **III.G**); the choice of drug and route of administration must be individualized. If parenteral agents are used initially, oral medications should be administered shortly thereafter to facilitate rapid weaning from parenteral therapy.

   1. **Sodium nitroprusside,** a direct-acting arterial and venous vasodilator, is the drug of choice for most hypertensive emergencies (see Table 4-4). It reduces BP rapidly and is easily titratable, and its action is short lived

Table 4-4. Intravenous antihypertensive drug preparations

Drug	Administration	Onset	Duration of action	Dosage	Adverse effects and comments
Sodium nitroprusside	IV infusion	Immediate	2–3 mins	0.5–10.0 µg/kg/min (initial dose, 0.25 µg/kg/min for eclampsia and renal insufficiency)	Hypotension, nausea, vomiting, apprehension. Risk of thiocyanate and cyanide toxicity increased in renal and hepatic insufficiency, respectively; levels should be monitored. Must shield from light.
Diazoxide	IV bolus	1–5 mins	6–12 hrs	50–100 mg q5–10min, up to 600 mg	Hypotension, tachycardia, nausea, vomiting, fluid retention, hyperglycemia. May exacerbate myocardial ischemia, heart failure, or aortic dissection.
	IV infusion			10–30 mg/min	May require concomitant use of a β-adrenergic antagonist.
Labetalol	IV bolus	5–10 mins	3–6 hrs	20–80 mg q5–10min up to 300 mg	Hypotension, heart block, heart failure, bronchospasm, nausea, vomiting, scalp tingling, paradoxic pressor response. May not be effective in patients receiving α- or β-antagonists.
	IV infusion			0.5–2.0 mg/min	
Nitroglycerin	IV infusion	1–2 mins	3–5 mins	5–100 µg/min	Headache, nausea, vomiting; tolerance may develop with prolonged use.
Esmolol	IV bolus	1–5 mins	10 mins	500 µg/kg/min for first 1 min	Hypotension, heart block, heart failure, bronchospasm.
	IV infusion			50–300 µg/kg/min	
Phentolamine	IV bolus	1–2 mins	3–10 mins	5–10 mg q5–15min	Hypotension, tachycardia, headache, angina, paradoxic pressor response.

Trimethaphan	IV infusion	1–5 mins	10 mins	0.5–4.0 mg/min	Hypotension, urinary retention, ileus, respiratory arrest, mydriasis, cycloplegia, dry mouth. More effective if patient's head is elevated.
Hydralazine (for treatment of eclampsia)	IV bolus	10–20 mins	3–6 hrs	10–20 mg q20min (if no effect after 20 mg, try another agent)	Hypotension, fetal distress, tachycardia, headache, nausea, vomiting, local thrombophlebitis, infusion site should be changed after 12 hrs.
Methyldopate (for treatment of eclampsia)	IV bolus	30–60 mins	10–16 hrs	250–500 mg	Hypotension.
Nicardipine	IV infusion	1–5 mins	3–6 hrs	5mg/hr; increased by 1.0–2.5 mg/hr q15min, up to 15 mg/hr	Hypotension, headache, tachycardia, nausea, vomiting.
Enalaprilat	IV bolus	5–15 mins	1–6 hrs	0.625–2.50 mg q6h	Hypotension.

Source: DA Calhoun, S Oparil. Treatment of hypertensive crisis. *N Engl J Med* 323:1177, 1990.

when discontinued. Patients should be monitored very closely to avoid an exaggerated hypotensive response. Therapy for more than 48–72 hours with a high cumulative dose or renal insufficiency may cause accumulation of thiocyanate, a toxic metabolite. Thiocyanate toxicity may cause paresthesias, tinnitus, blurred vision, delirium, or seizures. Serum thiocyanate levels should be kept at less than 10 mg/dl. Patients on high doses (>2–3 mg/kg/minute) or those with renal dysfunction should have serum levels of thiocyanate drawn after 48–72 hours of therapy. In patients with normal renal function or those receiving lower doses, levels can be drawn after 5–7 days. Hepatic dysfunction may result in accumulation of cyanide, which can cause metabolic acidosis, dyspnea, vomiting, dizziness, ataxia, and syncope. Hemodialysis should be considered for thiocyanate poisoning. Nitrites and thiosulfate can be administered intravenously for cyanide poisoning.

2. **Nitroglycerin** given as a continuous IV infusion (see Table 4-4) may be appropriate in situations in which sodium nitroprusside is relatively contraindicated, such as in patients with severe coronary insufficiency or advanced renal or hepatic disease. It is the preferred agent for patients with moderate hypertension in the setting of acute coronary ischemia or after coronary artery bypass surgery because of its more favorable effects on pulmonary gas exchange and collateral coronary blood flow. In patients with severely elevated BP, sodium nitroprusside remains the agent of choice. Nitroglycerin reduces preload more than afterload and should be used with caution or avoided in patients who have inferior MI with right ventricular infarction and are dependent on preload to maintain cardiac output.

3. **Labetalol** can be administered parenterally (see Table 4-4) in hypertensive crisis, even in patients in the early phase of an acute MI, and is the drug of choice in hypertensive emergencies that occur during pregnancy. When given intravenously, the β-adrenergic antagonist effect is greater than is the α-adrenergic antagonist effect. Nevertheless, symptomatic postural hypotension may occur with IV use; thus, patients should be treated in a supine position. Labetalol may be particularly beneficial during adrenergic excess (e.g., clonidine withdrawal, pheochromocytoma, postcoronary bypass grafting). As the half-life of labetalol is 5–8 hours, intermittent IV bolus dosing may be preferable to IV infusion. IV infusion can be discontinued before oral labetalol is begun. When the supine diastolic BP begins to rise, oral dosing can be initiated at 200 mg PO, followed in 6–12 hours by 200–400 mg PO, depending on the BP response.

4. **Esmolol** is a parenteral, short-acting, cardioselective β-adrenergic antagonist (see Table 4-4) that can be used in the treatment of hypertensive emergencies in patients in whom beta-blocker intolerance is a concern. Esmolol is also useful for the treatment of aortic dissection. β-Adrenergic antagonists may be ineffective when used as monotherapy in the treatment of severe hypertension and frequently are combined with other agents (e.g., with sodium nitroprusside in the treatment of aortic dissection).

5. **Nicardipine** is an effective IV calcium antagonist preparation (see Table 4-4) approved for use in postoperative hypertension. Side effects include headache, flushing, reflex tachycardia, and venous irritation. Nicardipine should be administered via a central venous line. If nicardipine is administered peripherally, the IV site should be changed q12h. Fifty percent of the peak effect is seen within the first 30 minutes, but the full peak effect is not achieved until after 48 hours of administration.

6. **Enalaprilat** is the active de-esterified form of enalapril (see Table 4-4) that results from hepatic conversion after an oral dose. Enalaprilat (as well as other ACE inhibitors) has been used effectively in cases of severe

and malignant hypertension. However, variable and unpredictable results also have been reported. ACE inhibition can cause rapid BP reduction in hypertensive patients with high renin states, such as renovascular hypertension, concomitant use of vasodilators, and sclero-derma renal crisis, but should be used cautiously to avoid precipitating hypotension. Therapy can be changed to an oral preparation when IV therapy no longer is necessary.

7. **Diazoxide, hydralazine, and trimethaphan camsylate** now are used rarely in hypertensive crises and offer little or no advantage to the agents discussed in sec. **III.F.1–6.** It should be noted, however, that hydralazine is a useful agent in pregnancy-related hypertensive emergencies because of its established safety profile.

G. **Oral loading of antihypertensive agents** has been used successfully in patients with hypertensive crisis when urgent but not immediate reduction of BP is indicated.

1. **Oral clonidine loading** is achieved by using an initial dose of 0.2 mg PO followed by 0.1 mg PO q1h to a total dose of 0.7 mg or a reduction in diastolic pressure of 20 mm Hg or more. BP should be checked at 15-minute intervals over the first hour, 30-minute intervals over the second hour, and then hourly. After 6 hours, a diuretic can be added, and an 8-hour clonidine dosing interval can be begun. Sedative side effects are significant.

2. **Sublingual nifedipine** has an onset of action within 30 minutes but can produce wide fluctuations and excessive reductions in blood pressure. **Because of the potential for adverse cardiovascular events (stroke/MI), the use of sublingual nifedipine should be heavily discouraged in the acute management of elevated BP** (*Ann Intern Med* 107:185, 1987). Side effects include facial flushing and postural hypotension.

IV. **Individual patient considerations.** A vast array of effective antihypertensive agents is available. Logical therapeutic choices require consideration of a patient's pathogenic derangement of renin secretion, sympathetic tone, and renal sodium excretion and the attendant changes in cardiac output, peripheral vascular resistance, and volume status.

A. **The elderly hypertensive patient** (>60 years) generally is characterized by increased vascular resistance, decreased plasma renin activity, and greater LVH than in younger patients. Often, elderly hypertensive patients have coexisting medical problems that must be considered in initiating antihypertensive therapy. Drug doses should be increased slowly to avoid adverse effects and hypotension. Diuretics as initial therapy have been shown to decrease the incidence of stroke, fatal MI, and overall mortality in this age group (*JAMA* 283:1967, 2000; *JAMA* 265:3255, 1991; *Lancet* 1:1349, 1985). Calcium channel antagonists decrease vascular resistance, have no adverse effects on lipid levels, and also are good choices for elderly patients. Even though elderly patients tend to have low plasma renin activity, ACE inhibitors and ARBs may be effective agents in this population (*N Engl J Med* 328:914, 1993). Long-term studies have documented the safety and efficacy of β-adrenergic antagonists, especially after acute MI; however, they may increase peripheral resistance, decrease cardiac output, and decrease HDL cholesterol. Agents that produce postural hypotension (i.e., prazosin, guanethidine, guanadrel) should be avoided. Central α-adrenergic agents generally are effective in elderly patients but commonly cause sedation. In elderly patients with isolated systolic hypertension, the same approach to initiating therapy should be used, but smaller doses should be given, and adjustments should be made less frequently.

B. **Black hypertensive patients** generally have a lower plasma renin level, higher plasma volume, and higher vascular resistance than do white patients. Thus, black patients respond well to diuretics, alone or in combination with calcium channel antagonists. ACE inhibitors, ARBs, and labetalol (an α- and β-adrenergic antagonist) are also effective agents in this population.

C. The obese hypertensive patient is characterized by more modest elevations in vascular resistance, higher cardiac output, expanded intravascular volume, and lower plasma renin activity at any given level of arterial pressure. Weight reduction is the primary goal of therapy and is effective in reducing BP and causing regression of LVH. Weight reduction should be part of any therapeutic regimen.

D. The diabetic patient with nephropathy may have significant proteinuria and renal insufficiency, which can complicate management (see Chap. 22). Control of BP is the most important intervention shown to slow loss of renal function. ACE inhibitors should be used as first-line therapy, as they have been shown to decrease proteinuria and to slow progressive loss of renal function independent of their antihypertensive effects (*N Engl J Med* 329:1456, 1993). ACE inhibitors may be beneficial in reducing the rates of death, MI, and stroke in diabetics who have cardiovascular risk factors but lack left ventricular dysfunction (*N Engl J Med* 342:145, 2000). Furthermore, ACE inhibitors may have a lower incidence of MI than the dihydropyridine class of calcium channel antagonists (*N Engl J Med* 338:645, 1998). Hyperkalemia is a common side effect in diabetic patients treated with ACE inhibitors, especially in those with moderate to severe impairment of their glomerular filtration rate. ARBs also are effective antihypertensive agents and have been shown to slow the rate of progression to end-stage renal disease thus supporting a renal protective effect. Calcium channel antagonists are also effective in diabetic patients; diltiazem and verapamil may have a selective beneficial effect in decreasing proteinuria in diabetic patients with renal disease (*Ann Intern Med* 113:987, 1990).

E. The hypertensive patient with chronic renal insufficiency has hypertension that usually is partially volume dependent. Retention of sodium and water exacerbates the existing hypertensive state, and diuretics are important in the management of this problem. With a serum creatinine greater than 2.5 mg/dl, loop diuretics are the most effective class. BP control in this patient group decreases progression to end-stage renal disease (*N Engl J Med* 334:13, 1996).

F. The hypertensive patient with LVH is at increased risk for sudden death, MI, and all-cause mortality. Although there is no direct evidence, regression of LVH could be expected to reduce the risk for subsequent complications. Sodium restriction, weight loss, and all drugs except direct-acting vasodilators can decrease left ventricular mass and wall thickness. ACE inhibitors appear to have the greatest effect on regression (*JAMA* 275:1507, 1996).

G. The hypertensive patient with coronary artery disease is at increased risk for unstable angina and MI. β-Adrenergic antagonists can be used as first-line agents in these patients, as they can decrease cardiac mortality and subsequent reinfarction in the setting of acute MI and can decrease progression to MI in those who present with unstable angina. β-Adrenergic antagonists also have a role in secondary prevention of cardiac events and in increasing long-term survival after MI (*Arch Intern Med* 156:1267, 1996). Care should be exercised in those with cardiac conduction system disease. Calcium channel antagonists should be used with caution in the setting of acute MI, as studies have shown conflicting results from their use. ACE inhibitors are also useful in patients with coronary artery disease and decrease mortality in patients who present with acute MI, especially those with left ventricular dysfunction, and more recently have been shown to decrease mortality in patients without left ventricular dysfunction (*N Engl J Med* 342:145, 2000).

H. The hypertensive patient with HF is at risk for progressive left ventricular dilatation and sudden death. In this population, ACE inhibitors decrease mortality (*N Engl J Med* 327:685, 1992), and in the setting of acute MI, they decrease the risk of recurrent MI, hospitalization for HF, and mortality (*N Engl J Med* 327:669, 1992; *Lancet* 345:669, 1995). It would also be anticipated that, based on this mechanism of action, the angiotensin receptor blockers would have similar beneficial effects, and they appear to be an effective alternative in patients who are unable to tolerate an ACE inhibitor (*Lancet* 355:1582, 2000). Nitrates and hydralazine also decrease mortality in patients with HF irrespective of hypertension, but hydralazine can cause reflex tachycardia and worsening ischemia in patients with unstable coronary syndromes and should be used with caution. Calcium channel antagonists should generally be avoided in patients in whom negative inotropic effects will affect their status adversely.

V. Initial drug therapy. Currently, diuretics, β-adrenergic antagonists, calcium channel antagonists, ACE inhibitors, ARBs, and α-adrenergic antagonists are regarded as first-line agents. Data from long-term trials have shown decreased cardiovascular and cerebrovascular morbidity and mortality with the use of thiazide diuretics and β-adrenergic antagonists; thus, these drugs may be favored as first-line agents in the absence of a contraindication to their use (hyperlipidemia, glucose intolerance, or an elevated uric acid) or if characteristics of a patient's profile (concomitant disease, age, race) mandate institution of a different agent. Calcium channel antagonists and ACE inhibitors have been shown to decrease BP to degrees similar to those observed with diuretics and β-adrenergic antagonists and also are good initial agents because of their low side effect profile. The majority of patients with stage 1 or stage 2 hypertension can attain adequate BP control with single-drug therapy. Initial drug choice may be affected by coexistent factors, such as age, race, angina, HF, renal insufficiency, LVH, obesity, hyperlipidemia, gout, and bronchospasm. Cost and drug interactions also should be considered. The BP response usually is consistent within a given class of agents; therefore, if a drug fails to control BP, another agent from the same class is unlikely to be effective. At times, however, a change within drug class may be useful in reducing adverse effects. The lowest possible effective dosage should be used to control BP, adjusted every 1–3 months as needed.

VI. Additional therapy. When a second drug is needed, it can generally be chosen from among the other first-line agents. A diuretic should be added first, as doing so may enhance effectiveness of the first drug, yielding more than a simple additive effect. Several combination preparations of first-line agents are available.

VII. Adjustments of a therapeutic regimen. In considering a modification of therapy because of inadequate response to the current regimen, the physician should investigate other possible contributing factors. Poor patient compliance, use of antagonistic drugs (i.e., sympathomimetics, antidepressants, steroids, nonsteroidal anti-inflammatory drugs, cyclosporine, caffeine, thyroid hormones, cocaine, erythropoietin), inappropriately high sodium intake, or increased alcohol consumption should be considered before antihypertensive drug therapy is modified. Unacceptable side effects from a particular agent may contribute to poor patient compliance. Excessive fluid retention should be evaluated and treated. Secondary causes of hypertension must be considered when a previously effective regimen becomes inadequate and other confounding factors are absent.

Special Considerations

I. Hypertension associated with withdrawal syndromes. Hypertension may be part of several important syndromes of withdrawal from drugs, including alcohol, cocaine, and opioid analgesics. Rebound increases in BP also may be seen in patients who abruptly discontinue antihypertensive therapy.

  A. Cocaine and other sympathomimetic drugs (e.g., amphetamines, phencyclidine hydrochloride) can produce hypertension in the setting of acute intoxication and when the agents are discontinued abruptly after chronic use. Hypertension often is complicated by other end-organ insults, such as ischemic heart disease, stroke, and seizures. Phentolamine is effective in acute management, and sodium nitroprusside or nitroglycerin can be used as an alternative (see Table 4-3). β-Adrenergic antagonists should be avoided due to the risk of unopposed α-adrenergic activity, which can exacerbate hypertension.

B. **Monoamine oxidase inhibitors** used in association with certain drugs or foods can produce a catecholamine excess state and accelerated hypertension. Interactions are common with tricyclic antidepressants, meperidine, methyldopa, levodopa, sympathomimetic agents, and antihistamines. Tyramine-containing foods that can lead to this syndrome include certain cheeses, red wine, beer, chocolate, chicken liver, processed meat, herring, broad beans, canned figs, and yeast. Nitroprusside, labetalol, and phentolamine have been used effectively in the treatment of accelerated hypertension associated with monoamine oxidase inhibitor use (see Table 4-4).

II. **Withdrawal syndrome associated with discontinuation of antihypertensive therapy.** In substituting therapy in patients with moderate to severe hypertension, it is reasonable to increase doses of the new medication in small increments while tapering the previous medication to avoid excessive BP fluctuations. On occasion, an AWS develops, usually within the first 24–72 hours. Occasionally, BP rises to levels that are much greater than those of baseline values. The most severe complications of AWS include encephalopathy, stroke, MI, and sudden death. The AWS is associated most commonly with centrally acting adrenergic agents (particularly clonidine) and β-adrenergic antagonists but has been reported with other agents as well, including diuretics. Rarely should BP medications be withdrawn, but, in discontinuing therapy, these drugs should be tapered over several days to weeks unless other medications are to substitute in the interim. Discontinuation of antihypertensive medications should be done with caution in patients with pre-existing cerebrovascular or cardiac disease. Management of AWS by reinstitution of the previously administered drug generally is effective. Sodium nitroprusside (see Table 4-3) is the treatment of choice when parenteral administration of an antihypertensive agent is required or when the identity of the previously administered agent is unknown. In the AWS caused by clonidine, β-adrenergic antagonists should not be used because unopposed alpha-adrenergic activity will be augmented and may exacerbate hypertension. However, labetalol (see Table 4-3) may be useful in this situation.

III. **Hypertensive crisis** (see Therapeutic Considerations, sec. **I.D**). In hypertensive emergency, control of acute or ongoing end-organ damage is more important than is the absolute level of BP. BP control with a rapidly acting parenteral agent should be accomplished as soon as possible (within 1 hour) to reduce permanent organ dysfunction and death. A reasonable goal is a 20–25% reduction of mean arterial pressure or a reduction of the diastolic pressure to 100–110 mm Hg over a period of minutes to hours. A precipitous fall in BP may occur in patients who are elderly, volume depleted, or receiving other antihypertensive agents, and caution should be used to avoid cerebral hypoperfusion. BP control in hypertensive urgencies can be accomplished more slowly. The initial goal of therapy in urgency should be to achieve a diastolic BP of 100–110 mm Hg. Excessive or rapid decreases in BP should be avoided to minimize the risk of cerebral hypoperfusion or coronary insufficiency. Normal BP can be attained gradually over several days as tolerated by the individual patient.

IV. **Aortic dissection.** Acute, proximal aortic dissection (type A) is a surgical emergency, whereas uncomplicated, distal aortic dissection (type B) can be treated successfully with medical therapy alone. All patients, including those treated surgically, require acute and chronic antihypertensive therapy to provide initial stabilization and to prevent complications (e.g., aortic rupture, continued dissection). Medical therapy of chronic stable aortic dissection should seek to maintain systolic BP at or below 130–140 mm Hg if tolerated. Antihypertensive agents with negative inotropic properties, including calcium channel antagonists, β-adrenergic antagonists, methyldopa, clonidine, and reserpine, are preferred for management in the postacute phase.

A. Sodium nitroprusside is considered the initial drug of choice because of the predictability of response and absence of tachyphylaxis. The dose should be titrated to achieve a systolic BP of 100–120 mm Hg or the lowest possible BP that permits adequate organ perfusion. Nitroprusside alone causes an increase in left ventricular contractility and subsequent arterial shearing forces, which contribute to ongoing intimal dissection. Thus, in using sodium nitroprusside, adequate simultaneous β-**adrenergic antagonist therapy is essential,** regardless of whether systolic hypertension is present. Traditionally, propranolol has been recommended. **Esmolol,** a cardioselective IV β-adrenergic antagonist with a very short duration of action, may be preferable, especially in patients with relative contraindications to β antagonists. If esmolol is tolerated, a longer-acting β-adrenergic antagonist should be used.

B. IV labetalol has been used successfully as a single agent in the treatment of acute aortic dissection (*JAMA* 258:78, 1987). Labetalol produces a dose-related decrease in BP and lowers contractility. It has the advantage of allowing for oral administration after the acute stage of dissection has been managed successfully.

C. Trimethaphan camsylate, a ganglionic blocking agent, can be used as a single IV agent if sodium nitroprusside or β-adrenergic antagonists cannot be tolerated. Unlike sodium nitroprusside, trimethaphan reduces left ventricular contractility. Because trimethaphan is associated with rapid tachyphylaxis and sympathoplegia (e.g., orthostatic hypotension, blurred vision, and urinary retention), other drugs are preferable.

V. Pregnancy and hypertension. Hypertension in the setting of pregnancy is a special situation because of the potential for maternal and fetal morbidity and mortality associated with elevated BP and the clinical syndromes of pre-eclampsia and eclampsia. The possibility of teratogenic or other adverse effects of antihypertensive medications on fetal development also should be considered.

A. Classification of hypertension during pregnancy has been proposed by the American College of Obstetrics and Gynecology (*N Engl J Med* 335:257, 1996).

    1. Pre-eclampsia or eclampsia. Pre-eclampsia is a condition defined by pregnancy, hypertension, proteinuria, generalized edema, and, occasionally, coagulation and liver function abnormalities at 20 weeks' gestation. Eclampsia encompasses those physical signs in addition to generalized seizures.

    2. Chronic hypertension. This disorder is defined by a BP greater than 140/90 mm Hg before the twentieth week of pregnancy.

    3. Chronic hypertension with superimposed pre-eclampsia or eclampsia

    4. Transient hypertension. This condition results in increases in BP without associated proteinuria or CNS manifestations. BP returns to normal within 10 days of delivery.

B. Therapy. Treatment of hypertension in pregnancy should begin if the diastolic BP is greater than 100 mm Hg. Nonpharmacologic therapy, such as weight reduction and vigorous exercise, is not recommended during pregnancy. Alcohol and tobacco use should be discouraged strongly. Pharmacologic intervention with methyldopa is recommended as first-line therapy because of its proven safety. Hydralazine and labetalol are also safe and can be used as alternative agents; also, both can be used parenterally. Other antihypertensives have theoretical disadvantages, but none except the ACE inhibitors has been proven to increase fetal morbidity or mortality. If a patient is suspected of having pre-eclampsia or eclampsia, urgent referral to an obstetrician who specializes in high-risk pregnancy is recommended.

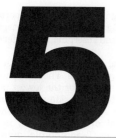

Ischemic Heart Disease

Stacy C. Smith
and Anne C. Goldberg

Ischemic heart disease remains the leading cause of morbidity and mortality in North America. The manifestations of coronary artery disease (CAD) include stable angina, acute coronary syndromes (ACS), heart failure (HF), sudden death, and silent ischemia. **ACS** represent a spectrum of clinical presentations of acute myocardial ischemia, referred to as **unstable angina (UA), non–ST-elevation myocardial infarction (MI), and ST-elevation MI.** Before the reperfusion era, non–ST-elevation MI was referred to as "non–Q-wave MI" and an ST-elevation MI as a "Q-wave MI." However, it is now recognized that Q waves do not develop in all patients with ST elevation on the presenting ECG and that they arise in some patients without ST elevation on the presenting ECG. The most common cause of ACS is erosion of an atherosclerotic plaque, resulting in platelet aggregation and thrombus formation. However, any sudden imbalance between myocardial oxygen supply and demand can result in acute ischemia. In UA and non–ST-elevation MI, the thrombus is platelet rich and usually nonocclusive. In ST-elevation MI, the thrombus is composed of platelets, fibrin, and RBCs, and is usually occlusive. The ECG has a central role in the initial triage of patients who present with suspected ischemic chest pain. Other causes of chest pain should always be considered in the differential diagnosis (see Table 5-3).

Primary Prevention

I. **General considerations.** Approximately 24% of men and 42% of women die in the year after an MI. The timely identification of CAD in women is therefore particularly important. One in 27 women dies of breast cancer, but one in two dies of CAD and stroke. Thus, primary prevention of CAD through risk factor identification and modification remains crucial to the reduction of morbidity and mortality.

II. **Risk factors for CAD** are cigarette smoking, diabetes mellitus, dyslipidemia, and hypertension. Other risk factors include a family history of premature CAD, age, male gender, postmenopausal status, and homocystinemia. The presence of multiple risk factors increases the risk of CAD.

III. **Risk factor identification and modification**

A. **Cigarette smoking** increases the risk of CAD and multiplies the impact of other risk factors. Within 3 years of cessation of smoking, the risk of CAD returns to the level of a nonsmoker (*J Clin Epidemiol* 44:1247, 1991; see Chap. 10).

B. **Diabetes mellitus** is strongly associated with premature CAD, particularly in women (see Chap. 22).

C. **Hyperlipidemia** increases the risk of developing CAD substantially in patients with two or more risk factors and a total cholesterol level in excess of 200 mg/dl, a low-density lipoprotein (LDL)-cholesterol level greater than 130 mg/dl, or a high-density lipoprotein (HDL)-cholesterol level of less than 35 mg/dl. Treatment of hyperlipidemia can reduce the incidence of CAD by 25–60% and the risk of death from CAD by up to 30% (*N Engl J Med* 341:489, 1999; see Hyperlipidemia in Patients with Ischemic Heart Disease).

D. Hypertension should be identified and treated to reduce the risk of CAD and stroke (see Chap. 4).

E. Obesity increases the risk of CAD, and is associated with hypertension, diabetes (insulin resistance), and hyperlipidemia.

F. Aspirin (75–325 mg PO qd) reduces the incidence of cardiac events by 23% (*N Engl J Med* 318:262, 1988) and should be considered for primary prevention, especially in patients with multiple risk factors.

G. Estrogen replacement therapy (ERT) is indicated for women with natural or surgical menopause. Starting ERT is not recommended in postmenopausal women after an MI due to the increased risk of cardiac events after beginning therapy (*JAMA* 280:605, 1998). However, women already receiving ERT who present with an MI can continue their current therapy, although further study is needed (see Secondary Prevention, sec. **II.E**).

Stable Angina

I. Diagnosis

A. Clinical history. Angina typically is described as a retrosternal pain, discomfort, heaviness, or pressure that radiates to the neck, jaw, shoulders, or arms, usually precipitated by exertion or stress and relieved with rest. Women often describe their anginal symptoms differently than men, noting epigastric or back discomfort. Associated symptoms include dyspnea, diaphoresis, nausea, vomiting, and, occasionally, palpitations or lightheadedness. Patients with diabetes may not have classic angina symptoms but may experience the associated symptoms as their "anginal equivalent." Other medical conditions that increase myocardial oxygen demand or that decrease oxygen supply may precipitate or aggravate angina and should be evaluated by history and appropriate laboratory studies. In men and older women, a history of typical angina, especially in the presence of other cardiac risk factors, suggests a 90% probability of CAD. In such patients, the role of invasive and noninvasive cardiac tests is to assess the severity of CAD, guide therapy, and estimate the risk of MI. In patients who experience chest pain that is not likely to be of cardiac origin and who do not demonstrate significant cardiac risk factors, the prevalence of ischemic heart disease is low (<25%), and further cardiac evaluation may be necessary to determine whether CAD is present. Nonetheless, the results of noninvasive tests in patients with these characteristics often are falsely positive. However, noninvasive tests are particularly useful in patients with an intermediate probability of disease.

B. Noninvasive testing

   1. The resting ECG may demonstrate (1) significant Q waves (>40 milliseconds) consistent with a prior MI, (2) resting ST-segment depression or elevation, or (3) T-wave inversion that is suggestive of myocardial ischemia. Frequently, the resting ECG is normal, even in the presence of significant CAD. However, documentation of ST-segment or T-wave abnormalities during an episode of chest discomfort can be useful for confirming the diagnosis of CAD and may limit the need for further noninvasive testing.

   2. Exercise ECG is useful in establishing the diagnosis of CAD and allows risk stratification of patients with angina. Exercise that is sufficient to increase the heart rate to 85% of the predicted maximum for age is necessary for optimal sensitivity (75%). Inability to exercise, resting ECG abnormalities, and medications (e.g., digoxin, β-adrenergic antagonists) adversely affect the accuracy of a stress exercise ECG. A markedly positive test result indicative of severe CAD is defined as the presence of any of the following: (1) new ST-segment depression greater than 1 mm early after the start of exercise, (2) new ST-segment depression greater than 2 mm in multiple leads, (3) inability to exercise for more than 2 minutes, (4) decreased systolic BP with exercise, (5) development of HF or sustained ventricular arrhythmias with exercise, and (6) a prolonged interval after exercise (>5 minutes) before ischemic ST-segment changes return to baseline. Patients who have a markedly positive test result should undergo cardiac catheterization to evaluate the need for coronary revascularization. In patients with known CAD, the ability to complete 7 minutes of a standard Bruce exercise protocol without development of significant ST-segment depression is associated with an excellent prognosis with medical therapy alone.

3. **Stress myocardial perfusion imaging** with thallium 201 or technetium 99m sestamibi has been reported to increase the sensitivity for detection of significant CAD from 70% to 80% and the specificity from 80% to 90% (*Circulation* 83:363, 1991). Stress perfusion imaging also allows the diagnosis of multivessel disease, localizes ischemia, and permits a determination of myocardial viability. However, given the increased cost of perfusion imaging compared with exercise stress testing, these techniques should be reserved for patients with ECG abnormalities at rest [left bundle branch block (LBBB), left ventricular hypertrophy, or baseline ST depression]. In patients who are unable to exercise, pharmacologic stress perfusion imaging can be performed with IV adenosine, dipyridamole, or dobutamine. A markedly positive study may demonstrate multiple areas of ischemia, left ventricular (LV) dilatation, or uptake of tracer in the lungs. Patients with any of these study results should be evaluated via coronary angiography. False-negative tests can occur when there is ischemia in multiple coronary distributions ("balanced ischemia"), such as in some patients with three-vessel CAD.

4. **Exercise and pharmacologic stress echocardiography,** when performed in experienced centers, is useful in the diagnosis of CAD, with a sensitivity and specificity similar to those of nuclear perfusion techniques. Dobutamine, with or without atropine, can be used to induce pharmacologic stress in patients who are unable to exercise. Patients with multiple regions of inducible ischemia should be referred for an invasive study.

5. **Electron beam CT and MRI** are noninvasive techniques that are currently under development for the preclinical detection of CAD.

C. **Coronary angiography with left ventriculography** is the definitive test for the diagnosis of CAD. Significant coronary obstruction is defined as greater than 70% narrowing of the luminal diameter. Coronary angiography can be combined with pharmacologic or exercise stress testing to assess the physiologic significance of observed coronary stenoses. In addition, angiography provides prognostic information about the number of significantly obstructed coronary arteries and the degree of LV dysfunction. Coronary angiography is indicated in high-risk patients, such as those with refractory UA, those with spontaneous or exercise-induced ischemia after MI, and those with markedly abnormal stress tests.

II. **Management**

A. **General principles.** The management of angina should include identification and treatment of cardiac risk factors. Smoking cessation, exercise, and patient education are particularly important. Specific treatment of angina is directed toward improving myocardial oxygen supply, reducing myocardial oxygen demand, and treating precipitating factors or concurrent disorders (e.g., hypertension, anemia) that may exacerbate ischemia (*Circulation* 99:2829, 1999).

B. **Drug therapy.** The selection of an effective regimen is based on the acuity and severity of symptoms, the presence of associated disease (e.g., pulmonary or renal disease), the patient's age and activity level, and the underlying pathophysiologic mechanism that is presumed to be responsible for the ischemia (e.g., arterial spasm, fixed stenosis). Because the etiology of myocardial ischemia is often multifactorial, a combination of agents with different mechanisms of action frequently is more effective than monotherapy. Patients with persistent symptoms despite optimal medical therapy should be referred for coronary angiography and revascularization.

1. **Aspirin.** All patients with CAD should be treated with aspirin (81–325 mg PO qd). In patients who are allergic to aspirin, the adenosine diphosphate receptor antagonist clopidogrel (75 mg PO qd) or ticlopidine (250 mg PO bid) can be used. Ticlopidine has potentially serious side effects, such as a 2.4% incidence of neutropenia; also, there have been several reports of thrombotic thrombocytopenic purpura (TTP), particularly in patients who are receiving long-term therapy. Neutropenia has not been reported with clopidogrel. However, TTP has been rarely associated with clopidogrel administration.

2. β-**Adrenergic antagonists** reduce myocardial oxygen demands by decreasing heart rate, BP, and contractility, and decrease mortality in patients with stable angina and a history of MI. All patients with recurrent episodes of exertional angina should receive a β-adrenergic antagonist as front-line therapy unless contraindications are present.

   a. **Selection** of an appropriate agent begins with a knowledge of the classification of the β-adrenergic antagonists with respect to their selectivity for cardiac β_1-receptors as compared to β_2-receptors (see Chap. 4, Table 4-3). No clear differences have been found among the various β-adrenergic antagonists with respect to their antianginal efficacy. However, lower doses of β_1-selective drugs (metoprolol and atenolol) are less likely to cause bronchospasm or to exacerbate peripheral vascular disease. At higher doses β_1 selectivity is lost. Agents with intrinsic sympathomimetic activity may dilate peripheral vessels and have less effect on resting heart rate.

   b. **Dosage** should be carefully titrated to achieve a resting heart rate of 50–60 beats/minute (bpm) and an exercise heart rate that does not exceed 90–100 bpm. Asymptomatic resting bradycardia does not require a reduction in dosage. Resting heart rate cannot be used to evaluate therapy in patients taking agents with intrinsic sympathomimetic activity. Patients prescribed β-adrenergic antagonists should be evaluated for signs of bronchospasm or HF when therapy is initiated and when the dose is being adjusted.

   c. **Contraindications** to the use of β-adrenergic antagonists include clinical evidence of HF, a history of bronchospasm, atrioventricular (AV) nodal block, severe peripheral vascular disease, and marked resting bradycardia (sick sinus syndrome). In patients with depressed LV function, β-adrenergic antagonist therapy can be attempted but should be initiated at a low dose (see Chap. 6).

   d. **Side effects** of β-adrenergic antagonists include bronchospasm, postural hypotension, claudication, depression, deterioration in intellectual capacity, salt retention, and potential masking of hypoglycemia. Infrequently, abrupt withdrawal of these agents may precipitate UA, arrhythmias, MI, and even sudden death. Therefore, when β-adrenergic antagonists must be stopped abruptly, patients at high risk for these events should be monitored for symptoms of recurrent ischemia.

3. **Nitrates** remain important agents in the treatment of stable angina (Table 5-1). In addition, all patients should be prescribed sublingual or aerosol nitroglycerin to abort episodes of angina. The primary antianginal effect is via an increase in venous capacitance, which reduces ven-

Table 5-1. Dosages and action of commonly used nitrate preparations

Preparation	Dosage[a]	Onset (mins)	Duration
Sublingual nitroglycerin	0.3–0.6 mg prn	2–5	10–30 mins
Aerosol nitroglycerin	0.4 mg prn	2–5	10–30 mins
Oral isosorbide dinitrate	5–40 mg tid	30–60	4–6 hrs
Oral isosorbide mononitrate	10–20 mg bid	30–60	6–8 hrs
Oral isosorbide mononitrate-SR	30–120 mg qd	30–60	12–18 hrs
2% Nitroglycerin ointment	0.5–2.0 in. tid	20–60	3–8 hrs
Transdermal nitroglycerin patches	5–15 mg qd	>60	12 hrs[b]

SR = sustained-release preparation.
[a]Chronic therapy should incorporate asymmetric dosing with 12-hour nitrate-free interval.
[b]Recommended maximum duration of application.

tricular volume and pressure and improves subendocardial perfusion. Coronary vasodilation, improvement in collateral flow, and afterload reduction augment this primary effect.

a. **Sublingual nitroglycerin** is available as 0.3-, 0.4-, and 0.6-mg tablets or as a metered-dose spray (0.4 mg). Usually, 0.4-mg tablets are prescribed, but, occasionally, lower doses are sufficient. Peak pharmacologic action occurs within 2 minutes and continues for approximately 30 minutes. Nitroglycerin dosing can be repeated at 5-minute intervals if symptoms persist. Patients should be informed of possible side effects (e.g., headache, flushing, hypotension), the importance of taking the drug while seated, the need for airtight storage of the drug in the original amber bottle, and replacement of medication every 6 months. The patient should be advised to take nitroglycerin at the first indication of angina and prophylactically before engaging in activities that are known to precipitate angina. Patients should seek prompt medical attention if angina occurs at rest or with increasing frequency or if an anginal episode fails to respond by the third dose.

b. **Long-acting nitrates** are indicated for long-term management of angina pectoris that is refractory to treatment with a β-adrenergic antagonist. Isosorbide-5-mononitrate has high bioavailability, as it does not undergo first-pass hepatic metabolism. If administered twice a day, an eccentric dosing schedule should be used because nitrate tolerance develops with q12h administration. A sustained-release preparation of isosorbide-5-mononitrate permits once-daily dosing. Isosorbide dinitrate should be administered three times a day, with a 12-hour nitrate-free interval to avoid the development of nitrate tolerance.

c. **Topical 2% nitroglycerin** ointment is applied to the skin as a 1- to 2-in. measured dose q4–6h by use of an occlusive dressing. The onset of action is approximately 30 minutes. Nitroglycerin ointment is an acceptable long-acting nitrate for patients who are unable to take oral medications. The absorption of topical nitrates varies. **Sustained-release transdermal nitroglycerin** preparations are limited by the failure of low-dose patches (2.5–5.0 mg/24 hours) to achieve therapeutic drug concentrations and by the tendency of higher-dose patches to produce nitrate tolerance. Patients should be instructed to remove the patch for 12 hours each day to minimize the development of tolerance.

   d. **Nitrate tolerance,** resulting in reduced therapeutic response, may
   occur with all nitrate preparations. The institution of a nitrate-free
   interval of at least 10–12 hours can enhance treatment efficacy. When
   nitrates cannot be discontinued, even for a short time, higher doses
   may be required to compensate for nitrate tolerance.
4. **Calcium channel antagonists** have an antianginal effect due to direct
   coronary vasodilation and reduced peripheral vascular resistance. All calcium channel antagonists have potential negative inotropic effects, but,
   in the absence of significant HF, cardiac performance usually is preserved
   by a reduction in afterload. Calcium channel antagonists are the agents
   of choice for patients who are unable to tolerate β-adrenergic antagonists
   or nitrates and are indicated in the management of stable angina and UA
   (see Chap. 4, Table 4-3). Because these agents are potent coronary vasodilators, they are particularly effective in patients with coronary vasospasm
   (Prinzmetal's angina) (see Coronary Vasospasm and Variant Angina).
   a. **Nifedipine** is a first-generation dihydropyridine with more pro-
      nounced arteriolar vasodilating properties than verapamil or dil-
      tiazem. Although nifedipine has negative inotropic effects in vitro,
      the decrease in peripheral vascular resistance usually results in a
      slight increase in cardiac output and heart rate. Bradycardia and AV
      block are not common problems. In patients with decreased LV func-
      tion, HF may be exacerbated. **Immediate-release preparations of
      nifedipine should be avoided in patients with CAD, UA, or prior MI
      because of concerns about excess cardiovascular morbidity and
      mortality.** Unless it is administered with a β-adrenergic antagonist to
      minimize reflex increases in heart rate, sustained-release nifedipine
      should not be prescribed for those with UA.
   b. **Diltiazem** is an arteriolar vasodilator that also prolongs AV nodal con-
      duction and slows the sinus node rate. It has fewer negative inotropic
      effects than verapamil.
   c. **Verapamil** has arteriolar vasodilating properties and slows AV nodal
      conduction. It has a greater negative inotropic effect than does
      nifedipine or diltiazem, limiting its use in patients with significant LV
      dysfunction. Verapamil is contraindicated in patients with sick sinus
      syndrome, AV nodal disease, and HF, and should be used cautiously
      with β-adrenergic antagonists, which increase the potential for brady-
      cardia or AV block. Verapamil increases serum digoxin levels. The
      most common side effect is constipation.
   d. **Second-generation dihydropyridine calcium channel antagonists**
      include amlodipine, felodipine, isradipine, and nicardipine (see
      Chap. 4, Table 4-3). Like nifedipine, these agents are potent coro-
      nary and peripheral vasodilators, and their side effects are similar to
      those of nifedipine. Bradycardia and AV block have not been
      reported. Amlodipine does not increase mortality in patients with
      CAD and depressed ventricular function, providing that HF is opti-
      mally treated (*N Engl J Med* 335:1107, 1996).
5. **Lipid reduction.** Treatment of hyperlipidemia, especially with 3-
   hydroxy-3-methylglutaryl coenzyme A (HMG-CoA) reductase inhibitors
   (statins), can reduce the incidence of CAD by 25–60% and the risk of
   death from CAD by up to 30% (*N Engl J Med* 341:489, 1999; see Hyperlipidemia in Patients with Ischemic Heart Disease).
C. **Revascularization.** Percutaneous transluminal coronary angioplasty
   (PTCA) and coronary artery bypass grafting (CABG) are invasive procedures designed to improve regional myocardial blood flow by dilating or
   bypassing stenotic coronary vessels.
   1. **Patient selection.** Patients with angina that is refractory to medical man-
      agement or with markedly positive stress tests should be referred for coro-
      nary angiography and assessment of LV function. High-risk patients

include those with left main CAD, multivessel disease with involvement of the proximal left anterior descending coronary artery, and depressed LV function (ejection fraction <40%). Additional clinical indicators of high-risk status include older age, severe angina, diabetes mellitus, hypertension, prior MI, ST-segment depression on the resting ECG, and a markedly positive stress test. Patients at high risk for cardiac mortality should be referred for surgical revascularization. Patients at lower risk can be managed with medical therapy or referred for percutaneous revascularization.

2. **Percutaneous coronary intervention (PCI).** Current percutaneous techniques include balloon angioplasty, intracoronary stenting, and atherectomy devices. In appropriately selected cases, clinical success is achieved in greater than 95% of patients. Risks of elective percutaneous coronary revascularization include a less than 1% mortality, a 2–5% incidence of nonfatal MI, and a less than 1% need for emergency CABG for unsuccessful procedures. Approximately 30–50% of vessels treated with balloon angioplasty alone develop restenosis within 3–6 months. Intracoronary stenting has reduced the incidence of clinical restenosis to less than 10–20% in discrete lesions. Patients who are undergoing PCI should receive aspirin before the procedure and heparin during the procedure, to minimize the risk of coronary thrombosis. Lepirudin, a direct thrombin inhibitor that is not associated with thrombocytopenia, can be used to treat patients with a history of heparin-induced thrombocytopenia (see Unstable Angina and Non–ST-Elevation Myocardial Infarction, sec. **III.A**). The use of platelet glycoprotein (GP) IIb/IIIa receptor antagonists decreases the incidence of abrupt coronary occlusion and nonfatal MI after PCI (*Circulation* 100:2045, 1999). All patients who are receiving intracoronary stents should be given aspirin indefinitely and additional antiplatelet therapy (clopidogrel, 75 mg qd, or ticlopidine, 250 mg bid) for 30 days to reduce the incidence of subacute stent thrombosis to less than 2% (*N Engl J Med* 334:1084, 1996).

3. **CABG.** Improvement of ischemic symptoms is achieved initially in up to 95% of patients with stable angina pectoris who undergo surgical revascularization. The risks of CABG include a 1–3% operative mortality, a 5–10% incidence of perioperative MI, a small risk of perioperative stroke or cognitive dysfunction, and a 10–20% risk of vein graft failure in the first year. Approximately 75% of patients remain free of recurrent angina or adverse cardiac events at 5 years of follow-up. The use of internal mammary artery grafts is associated with 90% graft patency at 10 years, compared with 40–50% for saphenous vein grafts. After 10 years of follow-up, 50% of patients develop recurrent angina or other adverse cardiac events related to late vein graft failure or progression of CAD in native vessels.

4. **PTCA versus CABG.** Randomized trials suggest that PTCA and related techniques are an effective approach to the management of medically refractory angina in patients with one- or two-vessel CAD and normal LV function, with the caveat that more than one procedure will be required in many patients (*Lancet* 346:1184, 1995; *N Engl J Med* 335:217, 1996). Patients with diabetes mellitus and multivessel CAD should be referred for CABG (*Ann Intern Med* 128:216, 1998).

5. **CABG versus medical therapy.** Although medical management can be effective in low-risk patients and carries a low mortality, CABG provides more effective relief of anginal symptoms. A meta-analysis of the 10-year follow-up findings in patients who were randomly assigned to CABG or drug therapy for angina pectoris confirmed improved survival in the following subsets of patients treated with CABG: (1) those with left main artery disease, (2) those with three-vessel disease, (3) those with two-vessel disease involving the proximal left anterior descending coronary artery, and (4) those with multivessel disease and abnormal LV function (*Lancet* 344:563, 1994).

Unstable Angina and Non–ST-Elevation Myocardial Infarction

UA is a clinical syndrome characterized by angina of new onset, angina at rest or with minimal exertion, or a crescendo pattern of angina with episodes of increasing frequency, severity, or duration. UA may develop in a patient with a history of stable exertional angina or may occur in the post-MI setting. A better understanding of the pathophysiologic mechanisms in ACS has led to improved therapies (*N Engl J Med* 342:101, 2000). Occasionally, UA is precipitated by severe anemia, thyrotoxicosis, arrhythmias, hypertension, or HF.

I. **Risk of MI in patients with UA.** The development of UA carries a 10–20% risk of progression to acute MI in the untreated patient; medical treatment reduces the risk of progression to MI to 5–7%. Patients at high risk for progression to acute infarction include those with new onset of angina at rest, those with a sudden change in anginal pattern (particularly when associated with labile ST-T-wave changes on the ECG), and those with recurrent or persistent pain after initiation of treatment. Clinical evidence of LV dysfunction, pulmonary edema, transient mitral regurgitation, or hypotension during episodes of ischemia identifies patients in whom extensive areas of myocardium are at risk or in whom ischemic mitral regurgitation has developed. The development of new ST-segment depression, transient ST elevation, or deep T-wave inversions in the anterior precordial leads in the absence of MI also suggests severe underlying CAD.

II. **Diagnosis.** Patients with UA and those with non–ST-elevation MI cannot be distinguished from one another on the basis of clinical symptoms, ECG findings, or angiographic findings. Approximately 75% of patients with UA or non–ST-elevation MI, or both, have an abnormal ECG with labile ST depression, labile T-wave inversions, or, less frequently, transient ST elevation. **Non–ST-elevation MI,** defined by elevations in creatine kinase isoenzyme (MB-CK) levels or cardiac-specific troponin levels, and the absence of persistent ST elevations, is present in approximately 40% of patients with unstable ischemia (*JAMA* 281:707, 1999). ST-segment depression that persists may be indicative of a non–ST-elevation MI. (see ST-Elevation Myocardial Infarction, sec. I).

III. **Acute management.** Initial medical management includes hospitalization, IV access, continuous ECG monitoring, sedation as needed, and correction of precipitating conditions such as hypertension, arrhythmias, anemia, and hypoxemia. The goals of treatment are to relieve ischemic symptoms aggressively with antianginal drugs and to inhibit thrombosis.

    A. **Aspirin and heparin.** All patients should receive aspirin and an antithrombotic agent in the absence of contraindications. Aspirin and heparin reduce subsequent MI and cardiac death in patients with UA. **Aspirin** has been used in doses as low as 75 mg/day, but current recommendations are for 160–325 mg PO qd. **Unfractionated heparin** can be given as an IV bolus of 60–80 units/kg, followed by an infusion of 14 units/kg/hour. The activated partial thromboplastin time (aPTT) should be measured q6h until a therapeutic level of one and a half to two times the control value is achieved (therapeutic range may vary depending on reagents used). **Low-molecular-weight heparin** (enoxaparin, 1 mg/kg SC bid) is at least as effective as IV unfractionated heparin (*N Engl J Med* 337:447, 1997). Heparin usually is continued for 48 hours or until angiography is performed. In approximately 1–3% of patients who are receiving heparin, heparin-induced thrombocytopenia develops, presenting after 5–7 days of therapy with platelet counts of 30,000–50,000 (*J Am Coll Cardiol* 31:1449, 1998). For patients with heparin-induced thrombocytopenia, **lepirudin** can be used and is administered as a 0.4-mg/kg bolus intravenously (maximum 44 mg) and then continuously infused at 0.15 mg/kg/hour with dose reduction required in renal impairment (see Chap. 19, Table 19-5). The

Table 5-2. Platelet glycoprotein IIb/IIIa receptor inhibitors in acute coronary syndromes

	Abciximab	Eptifibatide	Tirofiban
Drug type	Monoclonal antibody	Cyclic heptapeptide	Nonpeptide small molecule
Dosage	0.25 mg/kg IV bolus, then 10 μg/min × 12 hrs (for UA and planned PCI)	180 μg/kg bolus, then 2 μg/kg/min × 24–48 hrs	0.4 μg/kg/min over 30 mins, then 0.1 μg/kg/min × 24–48 hrs
Metabolism/ excretion	Cellular catabolism	Renal excretion*	Renal excretion*
Recovery of platelet inhibition	48–96 hrs	4–6 hrs	4–6 hrs
Reversibility	Platelet transfusion	None	None

PCI = percutaneous coronary intervention; UA = unstable angina
Notes: Contraindications for glycoprotein IIb/IIIa (GP IIb/IIIa) receptor inhibition include history of bleeding diathesis or active bleeding within the previous 30 days (2 years for abciximab), major surgery within the previous 6 weeks, history of stroke within the previous 30 days (2 years for abciximab), any history of hemorrhagic stroke, severe hypertension, platelet count of less than 100,000, or international normalized ratio greater than 1.2.
All patients should be monitored for the development of thrombocytopenia every 6–8 hours while receiving a GP IIb/IIIa inhibitor.
All patients should receive aspirin and weight-adjusted heparin to achieve an activated partial thromboplastin time of one and a half to two times normal.
*Dosage should be adjusted for patients with a serum creatinine of greater than 2.0.

aPTT is monitored and adjusted as with heparin. **Clopidogrel** and **ticlopidine** are thienopyridine derivatives that inhibit platelet aggregation by affecting the adenosine diphosphate–dependent activation of the glycoprotein IIb/IIIa complex. Clopidogrel, 75 mg/day, is an acceptable alternative for patients who are allergic to aspirin. It is preferred over ticlopidine because it has a lower incidence of side effects (granulocytopenia, GI intolerance, TTP).

B. GP IIb/IIIa receptor antagonists. Activation of platelet GP IIb/IIIa receptors, resulting in fibrinogen binding, is the final common pathway of platelet aggregation and platelet-mediated thrombosis. In patients with UA or non–ST-elevation MI treated with GP IIb/IIIa receptor antagonists, the composite risk of death, MI, and recurrent ischemia is significantly reduced (*Circulation* 100:2045, 1999). All patients with non–ST-elevation MI, indicated by early elevation in cardiac enzymes, or patients with UA and greater than 1 mm ST-segment depression in two contiguous ECG leads derive the most benefit from these drugs. Currently, three GP IIb/IIIa receptor antagonists are available (Table 5-2). Eptifibatide and tirofiban are approved for treatment of patients with UA and non–ST-elevation MI. Abciximab is approved for patients with UA and non–ST-elevation MI and a planned percutaneous revascularization procedure. All agents are administered with aspirin and weight-adjusted IV unfractionated heparin. Because of the additive inhibition of platelet function, all patients should be monitored closely for thrombocytopenia and bleeding complications. The overall rate of significant thrombocytopenia is 0.4–1.0%, and it occurs more often with abciximab. Pseudothrombocytopenia due to platelet clumping should be evaluated by determining platelet counts in ethylenediaminetetra acetic acid and citrate-containing anticoagulants simultaneously. GP IIb/IIIa receptor antagonists are presently not indicated for the treatment of ST-elevation MI, although studies are ongoing to determine the efficacy of these drugs in this patient subset. Contraindications for the use of these drugs include bleeding disorders, active bleeding in the previous 30 days, severe hypertension, major surgery in the last 6 weeks, cerebrovascular accident in the previous 30 days, previous intracranial hemorrhage, or platelet count of less than 100,000. Abciximab is the preferred agent for patients with renal insufficiency.

C. **Antianginal therapy.** In general, IV nitroglycerin is preferred to sublingual, oral, or cutaneous preparations because of the ability to achieve predictable blood levels of drug rapidly (see Appendix D). After 24 hours, the asymptomatic patient should be switched to a long-acting nitrate preparation (see Table 5-1). Patients should also receive a β-adrenergic antagonist when not contraindicated, because this combination reduces the risk of subsequent MI. A calcium channel antagonist, preferably verapamil or diltiazem, is effective in controlling ischemic symptoms but should be considered a second-line agent, as it does not reduce the risk of MI. Nifedipine generally should not be used without concomitant β-adrenergic antagonist therapy in patients with UA. Use of newer dihydropyridines should be avoided until more information is available about their effects in patients with unstable ischemic syndromes. Narcotic analgesics such as morphine sulfate are reserved for treatment of pain that is refractory to aggressive medical therapy.

D. **Fibrinolytic agents** should not be used in patients with UA or non–ST-elevation MI. They are reserved for individuals with ischemic chest pain and persistent ST elevation or new LBBB. These agents increase the incidence of MI in patients with UA and do not reduce mortality in those with non–ST-elevation MI (*Circulation* 89:1545, 1994).

E. **Intra-aortic balloon counterpulsation** is indicated in patients with ischemic symptoms that are refractory to medical therapy. Because this procedure is associated with a 10–15% risk of significant vascular complications, it should be used only to stabilize the patient's condition before CABG or PTCA.

F. **Lipid-lowering therapy** reduces the incidence of subsequent MI and cardiac death in patients with unstable ischemic syndromes (see Hyperlipidemia in Patients with Ischemic Heart Disease).

IV. **Risk stratification and revascularization.** Approximately 80% of patients with unstable ischemic syndromes respond to aggressive pharmacologic treatments. Within the first 6 weeks, the risk of cardiac death is 1% for UA and 5% for non–ST-elevation MI (see Subsequent Management of Myocardial Infarction, sec. **V**). The risk of subsequent MI or recurrent MI is approximately 5% for patients with UA or non–ST-elevation MI, respectively. Patients with refractory ischemia, recurrent symptoms, or elevations of baseline troponin or MB-CK levels despite medical therapy have an increased risk of cardiac death and should be referred for coronary angiography. Patients who are asymptomatic after 48 hours of drug therapy can perform a modified Bruce protocol stress test. Those with a markedly positive stress test should be referred for angiography. An alternative approach in asymptomatic patients is early angiography and revascularization. The early invasive strategy offers the advantage of risk stratification based on coronary anatomy as well as a reduction in the need for rehospitalization and antianginal medications; however, no difference is found in combined rate of death, recurrent MI, and failed symptom-limited stress testing compared with those of conservative medical management (*Circulation* 89:1545, 1994).

ST-Elevation Myocardial Infarction

ST-elevation MI (often referred to as "acute MI" or AMI) is a medical emergency that is most often caused by occlusive coronary thrombus. Approximately

Table 5-3. Selected differential diagnosis of myocardial infarction (MI)

Diagnosis	ECG findings mimicking MI	Diagnostic evaluation
Pericarditis	ST elevation	Echocardiography
Myocarditis	ST elevation, Q waves	cTnI, echocardiography
Acute aortic dissection	ST elevation or depression, nonspecific ST- and T-wave changes	Transesophageal echocardiography, chest CT, aortography, or MRI
Pneumothorax	New poor R-wave progression in leads V_1–V_6, acute QRS axis shift	Chest radiography
Pulmonary embolism	Inferior ST elevation, ST shifts in leads V_1–V_3	Ventilation-perfusion scan
Acute cholecystitis	Inferior ST elevation	Gallbladder ultrasonography or radioisotope scan

cTnI = cardiac-specific troponin I.

33% of patients with ST-elevation MI die, one-half of them within the first hour of symptom onset. Mortality can be significantly reduced by rapid transport to the hospital, institution of prompt pharmacologic or mechanical reperfusion, treatment of ventricular arrhythmias, and recognition and treatment of hemodynamic complications.

I. Diagnosis of MI requires the presence of at least two of the following criteria: (1) a history of prolonged chest discomfort or anginal equivalent, (2) ECG changes consistent with ischemia or necrosis, or (3) elevated cardiac enzymes.

    A. History. Chest pain associated with MI resembles that of angina pectoris but typically is more severe, longer in duration, and not relieved by rest or nitroglycerin. Accompanying symptoms may include dyspnea, nausea, vomiting, fatigue, diaphoresis, and palpitations. MI may occur without chest pain, especially in postoperative patients, the elderly, and patients with diabetes mellitus or hypertension. In these individuals, the symptoms may be isolated dyspnea, exacerbation of HF, or acute confusion. Other causes of chest pain should also be considered (Table 5-3).

    B. Physical examination. The physical examination should be directed at identifying hemodynamic instability and pulmonary congestion. New systolic murmurs are particularly important, suggesting the presence of ischemic mitral regurgitation or an acquired ventricular septal defect.

    C. Clinical stratification on initial presentation. Patients with acute MI are stratified into high- and low-risk subgroups on the basis of the initial physical examination. Those without evidence of pulmonary congestion or shock (Killip class I) have an excellent prognosis (mortality <5%). The prognosis with only mild pulmonary congestion or an isolated S_3 gallop (Killip class II) also is reasonably good. Patients with pulmonary edema (Killip class III) often have extensive LV dysfunction or acute mitral regurgitation and require aggressive management. Patients with hypotension and evidence of shock (Killip class IV) have a mortality that approaches 80% unless the cause of shock is treatable. Cardiogenic shock due to right ventricular infarction usually occurs in patients with inferior wall infarction and often is clinically recognized as the presence of elevated jugular venous pressures without evidence of pulmonary congestion.

D. ECGs. ECGs should be obtained on admission and daily during hospitalization in the cardiac care unit and should be repeated for evaluation of recurrent chest pain or arrhythmias. Although some patients who experience an MI initially have a normal ECG, the majority demonstrate changes on serial ECGs. In patients with inferior MI, right-sided chest leads should be recorded initially to detect right ventricular infarction. ST elevation of 1 mm or more in lead V_4R suggests a right ventricular MI (RVMI).

    1. ST-T-wave changes. Convex ST-segment elevation with either peaked upright or inverted T waves usually is indicative of acute myocardial injury, the early stage of a transmural ST-elevation MI.

    2. Q waves. The development of new Q waves (>40 milliseconds) is generally considered diagnostic of MI but may occur in patients with prolonged ischemia and, occasionally, in patients with myocarditis.

    3. ECG changes that mimic MI (see Table 5-3). ST-segment elevation and evolution of Q waves (transient or permanent) may, on rare occasions, result from pre-excitation syndromes, pericarditis, myocarditis, cardiomyopathy, chronic obstructive pulmonary disease, and pulmonary embolism.

E. Cardiac enzymes. The serum levels of various cardiac enzymes progressively increase as myocardial necrosis evolves.

    1. Cardiac-specific troponins. Assays for cardiac-specific troponin I (cTnI) and troponin T (cTnT) have even greater sensitivity and specificity for myocardial injury than those for MB-CK. In patients with acute ischemic syndromes, the risk of subsequent cardiac death is directly proportional to the increase in cardiac-specific troponin, even when MB-CK levels are not elevated (*N Engl J Med* 335:1333, 1996; *N Engl J Med* 335:1342, 1996). Serum levels of cTnI and cTnT increase 3–12 hours after the onset of MI, peak at 24–48 hours, and return to baseline over 5–14 days. The increased specificity of cTnI and cTnT for myocardial necrosis permits accurate diagnosis of MI in the postoperative setting, in which elevations of MB-CK may be related to skeletal muscle trauma. In addition, the delayed clearance of cardiac troponins is useful in diagnosing MI in patients who seek treatment days after an episode of prolonged chest pain.

    2. Creatine kinase. Increased plasma MB-CK activity has greater than 95% sensitivity and specificity for myocardial injury when measured within 24–36 hours of the onset of chest pain. With MI, serum MB-CK levels increase within 3–12 hours of chest pain, reach a peak in 24 hours, and return to baseline in 48–72 hours. Increased MB-CK not caused by MI occurs infrequently as a result of release from noncardiac sources, delayed clearance of MB-CK, or cross reactivity of some assays for MB-CK with BB-CK. This should be considered when elevations persist without change over serial samples, in contrast to the typical rise and fall that occur with MI (Table 5-4).

    3. Myoglobin is not cardiac specific but is released rapidly from infarcted myocardium, and can be detected as early as 2 hours after MI. For patients who present 2–3 hours after the onset of ischemic chest pain, myoglobin is a useful marker in the diagnosis of AMI.

    4. Use of cardiac enzymes. In patients in whom MI is suspected, determinations of serum CK and MB-CK levels should be made on hospital admission, at 8–12 hours, and at 16–24 hours. Cardiac-specific troponin levels can also be measured on admission and at 12–24 hours afterward, to increase the sensitivity for the diagnosis of MI. Alternatively, cardiac-specific troponin levels only can be obtained at baseline and at 12 hours; if these are elevated, MB-CK levels then can be measured, if necessary, to confirm that MI occurred within the previous 48 hours. An elevated myoglobin level or the presence of CK isoforms within 4–6 hours of the onset of symptoms suggests a diagnosis of MI.

F. Noninvasive cardiac imaging. With the improved cardiac enzyme assays currently available, the routine use of noninvasive cardiac imaging tech-

Table 5-4. Causes of elevated MB–creatine kinase (CK) other than myocardial infarction

Elevated MB-CK and elevated cardiac-specific troponin levels

Myocarditis

Pericarditis

Cardiac contusion

Cardiac surgery

Multiple cardiac defibrillations

Elevated MB-CK and normal cardiac-specific troponin levels

Low percentage of MB-CK relative to total CK

    Extensive skeletal muscle trauma

    Rhabdomyolysis

High percentage of MB-CK relative to total CK

    Polymyositis

    Muscular dystrophy

    Myopathies

    Chronic renal insufficiency (possibly secondary to myopathy)

    Vigorous athletic training (e.g., marathon runners)

Nonmuscle sources of MB-CK or BB-CK

    Intracranial hemorrhage or infarction (BB-CK)

    Prostatic and bronchogenic carcinomas (BB-CK, MB-CK rarely)

    Bowel infarction (BB-CK)

Delayed clearance of MB-CK and total CK

    Hypothyroidism (also possibly secondary to myopathy)

---

niques is not indicated for the initial diagnosis of MI. However, emergency echocardiographic evaluation can be used to detect regional wall motion abnormalities in patients with refractory ischemic chest pain and a nondiagnostic ECG, allowing triage to cardiac catheterization for assessment of coronary occlusion. In addition, Doppler techniques can identify mitral regurgitation and ventricular septal rupture in patients with new or changing systolic murmurs.

  G. Coronary angiography and left ventriculography. These techniques are indicated to evaluate coronary occlusions and to assess whether regional wall motion abnormalities are present in patients with refractory chest pain and nondiagnostic ECG changes.

II. Acute management. The goals of immediate management in patients with ST-elevation MI are to identify candidates for reperfusion therapy, as most patients with ST-elevation MI have occlusive thrombus. Other management priorities are to relieve ischemic pain, provide supplemental oxygen, and recognize and treat potentially life-threatening complications of infarction such as hypotension, pulmonary edema, and arrhythmias (*J Am Coll Cardiol* 34:890, 1999). **Rapid triage to reperfusion therapy** involves a brief screening history and review of the 12-lead ECG within 10 minutes of the patient's arrival in the emergency department. Patients with ST elevation (>1 mm in at least two contiguous leads) or new LBBB who present within 12 hours of the last episode of prolonged chest pain (>30 minutes) should be evaluated for fibrinolytic therapy or primary PTCA. The goal should be initiation of fibrinolytic therapy within 30 minutes or coronary angiography with primary PTCA within 60 minutes of arrival at the hospital. Initial treatment in all patients with chest pain and suspected MI, whether or not they are triaged to reperfusion therapy, includes anticoagulants, antiplatelet therapy, β-adrenergic antagonists, analgesics, nitroglycerin, and oxygen.

A. **General measures** include establishing an IV line and obtaining initial blood samples for cardiac enzyme levels, CBC, electrolytes (including magnesium), and a lipid profile. The cardiac rhythm should be monitored continuously by ECG, and vital signs should be determined frequently. Patients who do not demonstrate ST elevation on the initial ECG should undergo repeat ECGs if chest discomfort is ongoing, as ST elevation may develop. Oxygen saturation should be measured by pulse oximetry, and hypoxemia should be treated promptly. Hypotension is prevented by adequate volume expansion; it may occur in patients with volume depletion or right ventricular infarction and should be treated by elevation of the lower extremities and IV saline. The vagotonic effects of morphine can be treated with 0.5 mg IV atropine.

B. **Antiplatelet therapy** with aspirin reduces mortality in patients with MI. All patients who are not already receiving daily aspirin should immediately be given 160–325 mg non–enteric-coated aspirin PO, preferably chewed to enhance absorption.

C. **Anticoagulation** with heparin should be initiated in all patients with MI as an IV bolus of 60–80 units/kg, followed by an infusion of 14 units/kg/hour to maintain an aPTT of one and a half to two times control (therapeutic range may vary depending on reagents used) unless the patient is receiving streptokinase. In patients who are receiving other fibrinolytic agents, the maximum heparin bolus is 5000 units IV and the maximum initial infusion is 1000 units/hour. The use of anticoagulants in patients who are receiving streptokinase increases the risk of bleeding and has not been clearly shown to be of clinical benefit. Therefore, the current recommendation is for the treating physician to decide on the use of anticoagulants. General guidelines for the use of anticoagulants with streptokinase are to wait 6 hours after completing the infusion before administering anticoagulants and to avoid bolus dosing. The aPTT should be monitored and heparin dosing adjusted to keep the aPTT at one and a half to two times control.

D. **β-Adrenergic antagonists** reduce myocardial ischemia and may limit infarct size. Administration of these drugs should be avoided in patients with any of the following: (1) rales over more than one-third of the lung fields, (2) heart rate of less than 60 bpm, (3) systolic BP of less than 90 mm Hg, (4) PR interval greater than 250 milliseconds, (5) advanced heart block, (6) significant bronchospastic lung disease, and (7) severe peripheral vascular disease. Therapy can be initiated with an IV bolus of metoprolol, 5 mg; this dose can be repeated q5min to a total dose of 15 mg, with monitoring of vital signs. Patients who tolerate IV metoprolol loading can be started on oral metoprolol, 50 mg q6–12h, and then switched to 100 mg PO bid (or atenolol, 100 mg PO qd). Although no evidence exists that esmolol hydrochloride reduces infarct size or decreases mortality, because of its extremely short half-life (10 minutes), it is particularly useful in patients who are at high risk for complications of β-adrenergic antagonists (see Appendix D).

E. **Nitroglycerin.** Sublingual nitroglycerin (0.4 mg) should be administered to most patients with ischemic chest pain except those with hypotension (systolic BP <90 mm Hg), marked sinus tachycardia (heart rate >110 bpm), excessive bradycardia (heart rate <50 bpm), or inferior infarction complicated by right ventricular infarction. Sublingual nitroglycerin can be given q5min in the absence of hypotension. If symptoms persist after three doses, morphine should be given. Hypotension may occur in patients with volume depletion or right ventricular infarction and should be treated by elevation of the lower extremities and IV saline. Patients who respond to sublingual nitroglycerin can be started on IV nitroglycerin at 10 μg/minute for relief of ischemic pain (see Appendix D); dose titration should be guided by careful monitoring of heart rate and BP. In normotensive patients, the IV nitroglycerin dose can be increased q5min until ischemic pain is relieved. Heart rate should not increase, and BP should not decrease by more than 10% from baseline values. A vagotonic response to nitrates occurs on rare occasions, particularly with IV nitroglycerin, and can be treated with 0.5–1.0 mg IV atropine.

F. Morphine. Adequate analgesia decreases levels of circulating catecholamines and reduces myocardial oxygen consumption. Morphine sulfate is the analgesic of choice for the treatment of the pain of MI. Morphine induces modest venodilation, which decreases preload, has a modest arterial vasodilating effect, and has a vagotonic effect that can decrease heart rate. Morphine is given intravenously in doses of 2–4 mg, which can be repeated q5–10min until pain is controlled or side effects develop. Nausea and vomiting can be treated with an antiemetic agent.

G. Oxygen therapy, 2–4 L/minute via nasal cannula, is indicated in most patients with acute MI because mild hypoxemia is common. In stable patients without hypoxemia, nasal oxygen can be discontinued after 6 hours. Arterial blood gas measurements should be obtained on admission only if the patient is in respiratory distress and is not a candidate for fibrinolytic therapy. Increasing oxygen tension to supranormal levels is not indicated because it may produce an increase in BP and systemic vascular resistance. Prompt institution of mechanical ventilation when necessary decreases the work of breathing and reduces myocardial oxygen demand.

H. Glucose-insulin-potassium (GIK). Metabolic modulation in AMI has been evaluated using either high-dose GIK (25% glucose, 50 IU/L insulin, 80 mmol/L KCl at 1.5 ml/kg/hour for 24 hours) or low-dose GIK (10% glucose, 20 IU/L insulin, 50 mmol/L KCl at 1.0 ml/kg/hour for 24 hours). Preliminary data reveal a significant reduction in the combined end point of death, severe HF, and ventricular fibrillation in patients treated with GIK (*Circulation* 98:2227, 1998). This inexpensive therapy may have important implications for the treatment of AMI patients worldwide. A large-scale clinical trial is required to evaluate fully the benefits of this therapy.

III. Acute coronary reperfusion. Approximately 90% of patients with acute MI and ST-segment elevation have complete thrombotic occlusion of the infarct-related coronary artery. Early restoration of perfusion reduces infarct size, preserves LV function, and reduces mortality (*Lancet* 343:311, 1994).

A. Choice of reperfusion therapy. Fibrinolytic therapy and primary PTCA reduce mortality to a similar extent in patients with acute MI (*JAMA* 278:2093, 1997). The American College of Cardiology/American Heart Association revised guidelines for the treatment of AMI recommend primary PTCA as an alternative to fibrinolytic therapy for patients with AMI when performed within 90 minutes of presentation at a center and by an operator skilled in the procedure (*J Am Coll Cardiol* 34:890, 1999). It is critical that prompt coronary reperfusion be considered in all patients who present within 12 hours of a prolonged ischemic episode (>30 minutes) that is associated with new ST-segment elevation of at least 0.1 mV (>1 mm) in at least two contiguous leads. Reperfusion therapy also is indicated in patients with marked ST-segment depression (>2 mm) in the anterior leads that is indicative of posterior wall infarction and in those with prolonged chest pain and presumed new LBBB. Emergency coronary angiography and possible PTCA should also be considered in the following patients: (1) those with chest pain and persistent ST elevation who present more than 12 hours after the onset of acute MI, (2) those with persistent ST depression, (3) those with refractory angina symptoms and nondiagnostic ECG changes, and (4) those in cardiogenic shock. For patients younger than 75 years, an early revascularization strategy in those with shock decreases mortality at 6 months; however, patients who are older than 75 years benefit more from initial medical stabilization than from early revascularization (*N Engl J Med* 341:625, 1999).

Table 5-5. Contraindications to thrombolytic therapy

Absolute contraindications

Active bleeding

Defective hemostasis

Recent major trauma

Surgical procedure <10 days

Invasive procedure <10 days

Neurosurgical procedure <2 mos

GI/GU bleeding <6 mos

Prolonged CPR >10 mins

Stroke/TIA <12 mos

History of CNS tumor, aneurysm, or AVM

Acute pericarditis

Suspected aortic dissection

Active peptic ulcer disease

Active inflammatory bowel disease

Active cavitary lung disease

Pregnancy

Relative contraindications

Systolic BP >180 mm Hg

Diastolic BP >110 mm Hg

Bacterial endocarditis

Hemorrhagic diabetic retinopathy

History of intraocular bleeding

Stroke or TIA ≥ 12 mos ago

Brief CPR <10 mins

Chronic warfarin therapy

Severe renal or liver disease

Severe menstrual bleeding

AVM = arteriovenous malformation; GU = genitourinary; TIA = transient ischemic attack.

B. **Fibrinolytic therapy** offers the advantages of availability and rapid administration. The disadvantage of fibrinolytic therapy is the risk of intracranial hemorrhage (0.7–0.9%) and the uncertainty of whether normal coronary flow has been restored in the infarct-related artery (IRA). Fibrinolytic agents induce clot lysis in 60–90% of patients but normalize coronary blood flow in only 30–60% of IRA by 90 minutes, depending on the agent used. Normal coronary flow in the IRA is directly related to improved LV function (*N Engl J Med* 336:1621, 1997).

1. **Contraindications to fibrinolytic therapy** may be relative or absolute (Table 5-5). The age of the patient should not be an absolute contraindication to fibrinolysis because the prognosis after MI is poorer in the elderly. The overall risk of intracranial hemorrhage with fibrinolytic therapy is approximately 0.7% and is increased by twofold or more in the elderly, in

Table 5-6. Doses of fibrinolytic agents for myocardial infarction

Agents with fibrin specificity

Alteplase (rt-PA): IV bolus of 15 mg, followed by 0.75 mg/kg (up to 50 mg) by IV infusion over 30 mins, then 0.5 mg/kg (up to 35 mg) by IV infusion over 60 mins. Maximum dose: 100 mg IV over 90 mins.

Reteplase (r-PA): IV bolus of 10 units over 2 mins, followed by another IV bolus of 10 units after 30 mins.

Tenecteplase (TNK-tPA): IV bolus of 0.5 mg/kg; ≤60 kg = 30 mg; 61–70 kg = 35 mg; 71–80 kg = 40 mg; 81–90 kg = 45 mg; ≥90 kg = 50 mg.

Agents without fibrin specificity

Streptokinase (SK): IV infusion of 1.5 million units over 60 mins.

patients weighing less than 70 kg, and in patients who present with severe hypertension (BP >180/110 mm Hg). In patients with relative contraindications, the decision to initiate fibrinolytic therapy should be individualized on the basis of an assessment of the risk of severe bleeding compared with the risk of MI complications. Patients with contraindications to fibrinolysis should be considered for primary PTCA.

2. **Specific fibrinolytic agents** (Table 5-6)
   a. **Recombinant tissue-plasminogen activator** (alteplase, rt-PA) is more clot selective than streptokinase and does not cause allergic reactions or hypotension. rt-PA is administered as an IV bolus of 15 mg followed by an IV infusion of 0.75 mg/kg (up to 50 mg) over 30 minutes, then 0.5 mg/kg (up to 35 mg) by IV infusion over 60 minutes. Thus, patients with a body weight of 70 kg or more receive a maximum dose of 100 mg over 90 minutes. Concomitant use of IV heparin reduces the risk of subsequent coronary occlusion (see sec. **III.B.4**)
   b. **Reteplase** (r-PA) has reduced fibrin specificity but a longer half-life than does rt-PA, permitting bolus administration. r-PA resulted in a similar decrease in mortality when compared to streptokinase and rt-PA in randomized trials. The initial dose is 10 units by IV bolus, with a second 10-unit bolus administered 30 minutes later. Guidelines for heparin administration are the same as those for rt-PA (see sec. **III.B.4**).
   c. **Tenecteplase** (TNK-tPA) is a genetically engineered variant of alteplase with slower plasma clearance, better fibrin specificity, and high resistance to plasminogen-activator inhibitor-1, allowing single-bolus administration. When compared to alteplase, TNK-tPA had a similar decrease in mortality in randomized trials (*Lancet* 354:716, 1999). However, the incidence of mild to moderate bleeding was less in patients who received TNK-tPA. Guidelines for heparin administration are the same as those for rt-PA (see sec. **III.B.4**).
   d. **Streptokinase** is a nonselective agent that induces a generalized fibrinolytic state characterized by extensive fibrinogen degradation. Streptokinase is administered as an IV infusion of 1.5 million units over 60 minutes. Allergic reactions (skin rashes and fever) may be seen in 1–2% of patients. Hypotension occurs in 10% of patients and usually responds to volume expansion. Allergic reactions and severe hypotension are treated as anaphylactoid reactions, with IV antihistamines and steroids. Because of the development of antibodies, patients who were previously treated with streptokinase should be given rt-PA, TNK-tPA, or r-PA.

3. **The choice of a fibrinolytic agent** must be guided by considerations of cost, efficacy, and ease of administration. Alteplase, reteplase and tenec-

teplase are more expensive than streptokinase. Compared with streptokinase, alteplase is associated with a slightly greater risk of intracranial hemorrhage but offers the net clinical benefit of an additional 10 lives saved per 1000 patients treated (*N Engl J Med* 329:673, 1993).

4. **Adjuncts to fibrinolytics** include aspirin, IV heparin, and β-adrenergic antagonist therapy (see sec. **II.B–D**). IV heparin (60 units/kg bolus, maximum 4000 units; 12 units/kg/hour infusion, maximum 1000 units/hour; target aPTT of one and a half to two times control; therapeutic range may vary depending on reagents used) reduces the risk of subsequent coronary occlusion in patients given alteplase, reteplase, and tenecteplase, and should be continued for at least 48 hours. aPTT values above 90 seconds are associated with an increased risk of bleeding. The value of IV heparin administered before patients are treated with streptokinase is unproved. In all patients who are not ambulatory, deep vein thrombosis prophylaxis should be considered if they are not already receiving anticoagulation.

5. **Success of fibrinolytic therapy** can be monitored by clinical markers such as improvement in ST-segment elevation and resolution of chest pain. In patients demonstrating at least a 50% reduction of ST-segment elevation and relief of chest pain, it is 80–90% likely that the IRA has TIMI 2 flow. Unfortunately, fewer than one-half of patients demonstrate convincing clinical signs of successful reperfusion. Reperfusion arrhythmias are not a reliable indicator of coronary recanalization. Patients with persistent chest pain and ST elevation at 60–90 minutes after the initiation of fibrinolytic therapy should be considered for urgent coronary angiography and rescue PTCA.

6. **Bleeding complications** are the most common adverse effect of fibrinolytic therapy. Careful monitoring of the aPTT should be performed (see sec. **II.C**) along with daily monitoring of the hematocrit and platelet count. Routine monitoring of fibrinogen and fibrinogen degradation products is not necessary. Venipuncture should be limited and arterial puncture avoided in patients treated with fibrinolytic therapy. Major bleeding complications that require blood transfusions occur in approximately 10% of patients. Intracranial hemorrhage is the most dreaded complication and generally results in death or permanent disability. In patients who experience a sudden change in neurologic status, anticoagulant and fibrinolytic therapies should be reversed, and evaluation with an urgent head CT scan should be undertaken. In patients who hemorrhage, fresh frozen plasma can be given to reverse the lytic state. Cryoprecipitate can also be used to replenish fibrinogen and factor VIII levels. Because platelet dysfunction often accompanies the lytic state, platelet transfusions may be useful in patients with markedly prolonged bleeding times.

C. **Primary PTCA** results in mechanical reperfusion of a thrombotic coronary occlusion with normal arterial flow (TIMI 3) in greater than 95% of patients with ST elevation and acute MI. Other advantages of primary PTCA are immediate assessment of LV function and identification of other diseased vessels. Although it does not carry the risk of intracranial hemorrhage associated with fibrinolytic agents, primary PTCA takes longer to implement and is less widely available.

1. **Indications.** Primary PTCA is indicated for patients with ST-elevation MI or new LBBB in the setting of greater than 30 minutes of ischemic chest pain who present 12 hours or less from the onset of symptoms. Primary PTCA is also indicated for patients who present more than 12 hours from the onset of ischemic chest pain if their symptoms and ECG changes are persistent. Primary PTCA is the preferred reperfusion strategy for patients with contraindications to fibrinolytic therapy and for those in cardiogenic shock. Primary PTCA may also be preferable in patients with increased

risk of intracranial hemorrhage and in patients who have undergone previous CABG. In the absence of facilities for performing primary PTCA, patients with hemodynamic instability still benefit from prompt administration of fibrinolytic therapy. PTCA is not performed routinely during the first 48 hours after successful fibrinolytic therapy, but **rescue (adjuvant) PTCA** is indicated in patients in whom reperfusion has apparently failed, such as those with persistent chest pain and ST-segment elevation.

   2. Adjuncts to PTCA. Adjunctive therapies include antiplatelet agents, anticoagulants, intracoronary stents, and intra-aortic balloon counterpulsation.

   a. Aspirin reduces coronary reocclusion after PTCA. Patients who are not taking chronic aspirin should initially be given 325 mg non-enteric-coated aspirin (see sec. **II.B**).

   b. Heparin is administered during PTCA and can be continued for 24–48 hours after the procedure. If given concurrently with a GP IIb/IIIa inhibitor, the heparin dosing should be reduced to keep the aPTT at one and a half to two times control (therapeutic range may vary depending on reagents used).

   c. Intra-aortic balloon counterpulsation can be combined with PTCA in patients with MI to provide hemodynamic support, to reduce recurrent ischemia, and to decrease the incidence of coronary reocclusion.

   d. Intracoronary stenting can be performed during PTCA. Patients who are receiving intracoronary stents are treated with non–enteric-coated aspirin (325 mg PO qd) and ticlopidine (250 mg PO bid) or clopidogrel (75 mg PO qd) for up to 1 month. Patients on ticlopidine must be monitored for neutropenia. After the first month, they should be maintained on 160–325 mg enteric-coated aspirin/day.

D. Emergency CABG. Delays encountered in preparing for emergency surgery make CABG an unacceptable alternative to fibrinolysis or PTCA. Emergency CABG is indicated in patients with refractory ischemia or cardiogenic shock whose coronary anatomy is not suitable for PTCA, in individuals in whom PTCA has failed, and in patients with mechanical complications of MI (see Complications of Myocardial Infarction, sec. **V**). Insertion of an intra-aortic balloon pump usually is indicated to stabilize these patients before the surgical procedure.

Subsequent Management of Myocardial Infarction

Patients with MI should be admitted to the cardiac care unit for arrhythmia monitoring. Patients who are free from recurrent ischemia, hypotension, arrhythmias, and HF may be candidates for transfer to a telemetry step-down unit after 24–36 hours. Many of the traditional cardiac precautions are not indicated for patients who are revascularized early.

I. Activity level. Stable patients who are free from recurrent chest pain should have bedside commode privileges immediately and may sit in a chair after 12 hours. Within the first day, patients should be allowed to perform low-level activities such as toileting, assisted bathing, and walking in the hospital room. Patients should be cautioned to avoid the Valsalva maneuver, which may predispose to ventricular arrhythmias. After 24–48 hours, stable patients should progressively increase their activity levels.

II. Diet and bowel care. Patients should take no food or drink by mouth until they are pain free; when pain subsides, they should be allowed clear liquids. The diet should be advanced to a 1200- to 1800-calorie diet with low cholesterol and no added salt. Current guidelines do not prohibit ingestion of hot, cold, or caffeinated beverages. Because constipation is a common problem in MI patients, stool softeners or mild laxatives are given routinely.

III. Sedation. No evidence has been found to support the routine administration of anxiolytic drugs. Education and reassurance from the staff may more effectively address patient anxiety. Liberalizing family visiting privileges may also be helpful. Therapy with low doses of benzodiazepines may be necessary in some patients who are experiencing nicotine withdrawal. Patients who are agitated in the ICU can be treated with IV haloperidol, assuming that the QT interval is monitored (see Chap. 1).

IV. Additional pharmacologic therapy. Subsequent therapy for acute MI is aimed at reducing thrombotic and thromboembolic complications, limiting infarct size and recurrent ischemia, favorably affecting ventricular remodeling, and reducing mortality over the short and long term.

    A. Antiplatelet therapy. The minimum daily dose of aspirin is 160 mg. Although not approved by the United States Food and Drug Administration for patients with MI, clopidogrel is an alternative antiplatelet agent for patients who are unable to take aspirin (see Unstable Angina and Non–ST-Elevation Myocardial Infarction, sec. **III.A**).

    B. Anticoagulant therapy. Heparin should be given intravenously to all patients with MI who are treated with fibrinolytic agents, are undergoing PTCA, or are at high risk for development of systemic or venous thromboemboli. However, for patients who are receiving streptokinase, the benefit of subsequent IV heparin has not been proven (see ST-Elevation Myocardial Infarction, sec. **II.C**). Patients at high risk for systemic emboli [e.g., large or anterior MI, atrial fibrillation (AF), previous embolus, documented LV thrombus] should be treated with IV heparin until therapeutic anticoagulation is achieved with warfarin (i.e., international normalized ratio equal to two to three times control). Warfarin should be continued indefinitely in those with AF or severe LV dysfunction and a previous embolic event, and for 3–6 months in patients with an LV mural thrombus. Patients at low risk for systemic emboli who are not candidates for coronary reperfusion can be treated with SC heparin, 5000 units bid, until they are ambulatory.

    C. Angiotensin-converting enzyme (ACE) inhibitors provide a reduction in short-term mortality when initiated within the first 24 hours of acute MI. Patients who receive the greatest benefit are those in high-risk groups, including those with anterior infarctions, HF, and previous MI. However, even high-risk patients without evidence of LV dysfunction or HF have been shown to have a significantly reduced incidence of death, MI, and stroke when treated with ramipril (*N Engl J Med* 342:145, 2000). ACE inhibitors are contraindicated in patients with hypotension and should be used with caution in individuals with renal insufficiency. Therapy can be initiated with captopril, ramipril, trandolapril, or enalapril (see Chap. 4). IV enalaprilat should be avoided as the initial therapeutic agent because of possible increased mortality if BP is reduced excessively. Patients with HF or asymptomatic LV dysfunction (ejection fraction <40%) should receive ACE inhibitors indefinitely.

    D. β-Adrenergic antagonists should be continued for secondary prevention (see Secondary Prevention, sec. **II.B**).

    E. Nitrates. Although a mortality benefit has not been demonstrated, most experts recommend that topical or oral nitrates be continued in patients with large transmural infarcts and in those with MI complicated by HF or recurrent ischemia.

    F. Calcium channel antagonists have not been demonstrated to provide any mortality benefit in patients with acute MI. **Immediate-release nifedipine has been associated with excess mortality and an increased incidence of reinfarction.** Studies of immediate-release verapamil in ST-elevation MI and of diltiazem in non–ST-elevation MI suggest that these agents may reduce the incidence of reinfarction in patients without LV dysfunction who cannot tolerate β-adrenergic antagonists. Diltiazem has been found to increase mortality in patients with LV dysfunction.

G. Prophylactic lidocaine is not indicated in patients with acute MI.

V. Risk stratification and revascularization subsequent to MI. Patients with acute MI (ST elevation or non–ST elevation) can be categorized into low- and high-risk subsets on the basis of initial clinical course, noninvasive assessment of LV function, and stress testing. Ventricular function can be assessed by echocardiography within the first 24–48 hours.

A. High-risk patients have one or more of the following characteristics and therefore higher adverse event rates after acute MI: (1) history of previous MI, (2) sustained hypotension or cardiogenic shock, (3) early ventricular arrhythmias with hemodynamic compromise, (4) HF, (5) advanced heart block, (6) recurrent post-MI angina, and (7) LV ejection fraction of less than 40%. High-risk patients should remain hospitalized for several days after their condition has stabilized and should undergo coronary angiography.

B. Low-risk patients are those without high-risk clinical characteristics who have normal or mildly decreased LV function and may be candidates for transfer from the cardiac care unit to a monitored telemetry floor after 24–36 hours. If these patients are able to ambulate without recurrent ischemia, they can be discharged from the hospital after 3–4 days and undergo outpatient symptom-limited exercise stress testing at 10–14 days. Alternatively, these patients can be referred for submaximal exercise stress testing on day 4 (before hospital discharge) and for maximal stress testing at 2–3 weeks. Those with abnormal resting ECGs (e.g., LBBB, LV hypertrophy, or baseline ST depression) should undergo exercise stress perfusion imaging or exercise stress echocardiography to increase the specificity for detection of ischemia. Patients who can achieve five metabolic equivalents without early ST depression and with a normal increase in systolic BP have a low risk of death or recurrent infarction after acute MI. Those who are unable to exercise can be referred for pharmacologic stress perfusion imaging or dobutamine echocardiography. Patients with inducible ischemia should be considered for surgical or percutaneous revascularization.

VI. Rehabilitation after MI

A. In-hospital phase. Physical activity should be progressively advanced in stable patients (see sec. I). By the third day, such patients can begin ambulation outside of their rooms while being monitored by telemetry. Before discharge from the hospital, patients should receive verbal and written instructions concerning physical activities, medications, diet, and secondary preventive measures, along with a prescription and instructions for use of nitroglycerin tablets or spray.

B. Outpatient phase. Before beginning cardiac rehabilitation, patients may walk two or three times a day for 20–30 minutes as long as their pulse is maintained within 20 bpm of their standing heart rate. Before resuming moderate lifting, driving, working, or sexual activity, patients should successfully complete a symptom-limited stress test (see sec. **V.B**). The majority of patients also benefit from a formal 8- to 12-week cardiac rehabilitation program. In the outpatient phase, it is important to continue to educate the patient about secondary prevention and compliance with medication regimens (see Secondary Prevention).

Complications of Myocardial Infarction

I. Recurrent chest pain after MI may be caused by recurrent ischemia, reinfarction, pericarditis, pulmonary embolism, and subacute cardiac rupture. Initial evaluation should include careful auscultation for a new murmur or pericardial rub and a repeat ECG to document recurrent ST elevation, new ischemic ST- or T-wave changes, or evidence of pericarditis. Myocardial enzyme levels should be repeated to exclude reinfarction. Echocardiography or emergency angiography may be indicated to clarify the cause of recurrent chest pain.

A. Recurrent ischemia. Ischemia recurs in 20–30% of patients after MI, with or without antecedent fibrinolytic therapy. Patients with signs or symptoms of recurrent ischemia in the post-MI period should continue to receive heparin, along with parenteral nitrates and β-adrenergic antagonists. Intraaortic balloon counterpulsation is beneficial in stabilizing patients with ischemia that is refractory to medical therapy. Prompt coronary angiography should be performed to identify those patients who can benefit from PTCA or CABG.

B. Recurrent infarction. Extension or recurrence of infarction occurs in 5–20% of patients after MI and often is preceded by recurrent chest discomfort despite therapy. Patients with recurrent chest pain or ECG changes should be evaluated for new myocardial necrosis by re-elevation of cardiac enzyme levels. Initial therapy is similar to that described for recurrent ischemia. Patients with recurrent ST elevation after fibrinolysis should be considered for immediate rescue PTCA, but, in the absence of facilities for acute intervention, patients can be treated 24 hours after the initial dose with repeat fibrinolysis using rt-PA or r-PA. Because reinfarction increases the probability of death, HF, arrhythmias, and cardiac rupture, these patients should be monitored in-hospital for an extended period and should be evaluated for revascularization.

C. Acute pericarditis. Postinfarction pericarditis develops in approximately 15–25% of patients with large transmural MIs. Pain due to pericarditis is typically substernal with radiation to the back, is unresponsive to nitrates, is exacerbated by deep breathing or movement, and is relieved by sitting up. A pericardial friction rub may be appreciated but often is evanescent. Pericardial effusions that are evident on the echocardiogram are common after transmural infarction and are not, by themselves, diagnostic of pericarditis in the asymptomatic patient. The classic ECG findings associated with pericarditis may be masked by the infarct but include PR depression, J-point elevation, concave upward ST elevation, and initially upright T-wave changes. Aspirin, 650 mg PO q6h, is the preferred treatment. The use of glucocorticoids or non–aspirin-containing nonsteroidal anti-inflammatory drugs (NSAIDs), although efficacious, generally is contraindicated, because these drugs retard myocardial scar formation and may predispose to cardiac rupture. In patients who are being treated with IV heparin, the presence of active pericarditis may increase the risk of hemorrhagic cardiac tamponade. In such individuals, the potential risk should be balanced against the need for continued anticoagulation. In patients with expanding effusions on the echocardiogram or early signs of cardiac tamponade, anticoagulation should be discontinued.

D. Post-MI (Dressler's) syndrome, believed to be an autoimmune phenomenon, is very rare in the reperfusion era. It is characterized by pericarditis, pleuritis, pericardial or pleural effusions, fever, leukocytosis, elevated sedimentation rate, and elevated levels of antimyocardial antibodies. Patients typically have malaise, fever, and chest pain, but the syndrome may be mistaken for angina pectoris or MI, and the ECG may show diffuse, marked ST-segment elevation. Onset of symptoms is usually between the second and tenth weeks after MI, and the course may be lengthy, with frequent remissions and exacerbations. Therapy is aimed at relieving symptoms and consists of NSAIDs such as aspirin (650 mg PO q6–8h) or indomethacin (25–50 mg PO q6–8h). Glucocorticoids such as prednisone (1 mg/kg PO qd) may be required for severe symptoms; when used, the dose should be tapered gradually to minimize exacerbation of symptoms. Anticoagulants should be discontinued if possible, as hemorrhagic pericarditis with tamponade can occur. **Constrictive peri-carditis** may complicate the post-MI syndrome but is rare.

II. **Arrhythmias** are common in patients with acute MI. Although life-threatening arrhythmias such as ventricular tachycardia (VT) and fibrillation (VF) are of most concern, any arrhythmia that results in hemodynamic compromise should be vigorously treated. Sustained arrhythmias that cause hypotension, angina pectoris, or HF should be terminated with electrical cardioversion. Potentially exacerbating conditions should be considered and corrected, including adverse effects of drugs, hypoxemia, acidosis, or electrolyte imbalances (especially disorders of potassium and magnesium). HF, recurrent ischemia, or hypotension also may predispose to arrhythmias and should be managed promptly.

A. **Ventricular arrhythmias** (see Chaps. 7 and 8)

1. **Ventricular premature depolarizations** are common in the acute MI period. Prophylactic suppression of ventricular premature depolarizations no longer is recommended in patients with MI. Patients should be monitored while electrolyte imbalance is corrected and β-adrenergic antagonist therapy for ischemia is initiated.

2. **Accelerated idioventricular rhythm** occurs in up to 20% of patients in the first 2 days after MI, especially in those in whom coronary reperfusion is achieved. It is usually benign, lasting less than 48 hours, and does not require specific therapy. When accelerated idioventricular rhythm is associated with clinical instability, administration of atropine or overdrive atrial pacing is effective treatment (see Chaps. 7 and 8).

3. **Nonsustained monomorphic or polymorphic VT** usually occurs during the first 48 hours after MI. Therapy is not required unless the episode is sustained (>30 seconds) or produces hemodynamic compromise. **Sustained VT** in the first 48 hours after MI is associated with increased in-hospital mortality, whereas late sustained VT increases in-hospital and long-term mortality. Drug therapy generally is continued for at least 24 hours. Patients with recurrent or late sustained VT require further evaluation (see Chap. 7).

4. **The incidence of primary VF** has decreased in the reperfusion era, but it still occurs in up to 5% of hospitalized patients, usually within 4 hours after the onset of MI. VF is treated with immediate unsynchronized defibrillation (see Chap. 8). Patients with late VF (>48 hours after MI) require further evaluation (see Chap. 7).

B. **Supraventricular tachycardias** (see Chap. 7)

1. **Sinus tachycardia** is common in patients with acute MI and frequently is associated with HF, hypoxemia, pain, anxiety, fever, hypovolemia, or adverse drug effects. Persistent sinus tachycardia is indicative of a poor prognosis and often is an indication for invasive hemodynamic evaluation. Treatment is directed at correcting underlying causes. In the absence of HF and after contributing causes have been corrected, judicious use of a β-adrenergic antagonist is indicated, especially when hypertension accompanies sinus tachycardia.

2. **Paroxysmal supraventricular tachycardia** occurs infrequently in patients with MI but should be treated to prevent exacerbation of myocardial ischemia (see Chap. 7).

3. **AF** is deleterious to the ischemic myocardium because the ventricular response usually is rapid and the atrial contribution to ventricular filling is lost. In the acute MI period, AF frequently is transient and does not require anticoagulant or antiarrhythmic treatment beyond 6 weeks if sinus rhythm is maintained.

4. **Junctional rhythms** are most common in patients with inferior MI and may present as a slow AV junctional rhythm (rate, 30–60 bpm) or as an accelerated junctional rhythm (rate, 70–130 bpm). AV junctional rhythm is usually a benign escape rhythm in patients with sinus bradycardia and only rarely requires temporary transvenous AV pacing in

patients with hypotension. Accelerated junctional rhythm (nonparoxysmal junctional tachycardia) is less common and can be related to increased automaticity or to digitalis toxicity (see Chap. 7).

C. Bradycardias and heart blocks

1. **Sinus bradycardia** occurs frequently in patients with acute MI, particularly in those with inferior MI and after reperfusion of the right coronary artery. Treatment is indicated only in patients with hypotension, decreased cardiac output, or ventricular ectopy related to the bradycardia (see Chap. 7).

2. **AV conduction disturbances,** including first-degree, second-degree, or third-degree (complete) AV block, occur commonly in patients with MI.

   a. **First-degree AV block** often is caused by treatment with digoxin or other agents that slow AV node conduction.

   b. **Second-degree AV block** is classified either as **Mobitz type I (Wenckebach),** which usually is associated with an inferior MI, or as **Mobitz type II,** which is located below the bundle of His and usually is associated with a large anterior MI. Mobitz type I AV block rarely necessitates transvenous pacing, but atropine can be administered in the presence of symptomatic bradycardia. Mobitz type II block may progress to complete AV block and requires pacemaker insertion regardless of whether the patient is symptomatic (see sec. **II.F**).

   c. **In third-degree heart block,** there is AV dissociation, often with a slow ventricular escape rhythm. In patients with anterior MI, complete AV block may develop abruptly, often preceded only by first-degree AV block or some form of intraventricular block, and is associated with a large area of infarction and high mortality. In patients with inferior MI, heart block may be preceded by first- or second-degree AV block, and often the junctional or ventricular escape rhythm is not associated with symptoms. Nonetheless, third-degree AV block in the setting of an MI requires emergency transvenous pacing because of the potential for progression to asystole (see Chap. 7).

D. Intraventricular conduction disturbances occur in up to 10% of patients with MI and may involve one or more of the three fascicles of the His-Purkinje system. Patients may present with new or age-indeterminate (1) unifascicular block of the right bundle branch (RBBB), left anterior fascicle (LAFB), or left posterior fascicle (LPFB); (2) bifascicular block that involves either both fascicles of the left bundle branch, or RBBB with LAFB or LPFB; or (3) trifascicular block, which is defined as bifascicular block in the presence of first-degree AV block. Newly acquired bifascicular or trifascicular blocks are more common in large anterior infarcts and carry a high risk of asystole. Treatment of advanced conduction disturbances requires transcutaneous or transvenous pacing (see secs. **II.F** and **G**).

E. Asystole may develop precipitously in patients with MI and advanced AV block or complex fascicular blocks. Asystole is the terminal event in up to 15% of patients with MI. Treatment often includes temporary transcutaneous pacing and insertion of a temporary transvenous pacemaker (see Chap. 8).

F. Indications for temporary transvenous pacing in patients with MI include (1) asystole, (2) third-degree AV block, (3) Mobitz type II second-degree AV block, (4) sinus bradycardia or Mobitz type I second-degree AV block associated with hypotension and refractory to atropine, (5) new or age-indeterminate trifascicular block, (6) alternating bundle branch block (RBBB alternating with LBBB; RBBB alternating with LAFB or LPFB), (7) third-degree AV block in the setting of inferior MI complicated by right ventricular infarction (AV sequential pacing), and (8) incessant VT (overdrive pacing).

G. Transcutaneous pacing systems can be used in active mode as support during emergency placement of a temporary transvenous pacemaker or in standby (demand) mode in lower-risk patients. Patients at lower risk for developing asystole include those with (1) new or age-indeterminate bifascicular block with a normal PR interval, (2) new or age-indeterminate RBBB, (3) new Mobitz type I second-degree AV block in patients with stable hemodynamics, and (4) new or age-indeterminate first-degree AV block with or without unifascicular block (i.e., RBBB, LAFB, or LPFB).

III. **Hypertension** increases afterload and elevates myocardial oxygen demand, which may increase infarct size or produce infarct expansion. In general, patients with hypertension in the setting of acute MI should be treated initially with short-acting, titratable IV agents. Other measures include bed rest, analgesia, and sedation, which frequently are sufficient for controlling mild to moderate elevations in systolic BP.

A. **β-Adrenergic antagonists** are excellent initial therapy, especially in patients with a hyperdynamic state manifested by sinus tachycardia. Therapy should begin with small parenteral doses (see ST-Elevation Myocardial Infarction, sec. **II.D**; and Chap. 4).

B. **ACE inhibitors,** in combination with a β-adrenergic antagonist, should be the preferred approach to moderate hypertension (see Subsequent Management of Myocardial Infarction, sec. **IV.C**; and Chap. 4).

C. **Calcium channel antagonists** may be appropriate if ACE inhibitors or β-adrenergic antagonists are ineffective or contraindicated. Given concerns about the safety of dihydropyridines such as immediate-release nifedipine in patients with MI, verapamil or diltiazem may be preferable. The safety of newer dihydropyridines in patients with MI has not been established (see Subsequent Management of Myocardial Infarction, sec. **IV.F**; and Chap. 4).

D. **Nitroprusside** is indicated in the treatment of moderate to severe hypertension (see Appendix D and Chap. 4).

E. **Nitroglycerin** in doses that are sufficient to decrease modest hypertension can often be given to patients with elevated LV filling pressures but, in the presence of normal LV filling pressures, the antihypertensive effects of nitroglycerin are limited. This drug often is effective in the treatment of hypertension associated with HF or when ischemic symptoms continue (see Appendix D).

IV. **LV failure** in the form of LV systolic and diastolic dysfunction (i.e., stiff ventricle) is associated with acute MI. The severity of pump failure is related to the extent of infarction. Acute mechanical complications of MI, such as acute mitral regurgitation, ventricular septal rupture, or exacerbation of underlying chronic valvular disease, may also result in pulmonary edema or shock. Management and evaluation must be tailored to the severity of ventricular dysfunction (see Chap. 6).

A. **Treatment of mild HF.** Patients with mild pulmonary congestion or an S_3 gallop who are not hypotensive can be treated without invasive monitoring. Ventricular and valvular function should be assessed by echocardiography.

1. **Diuretics** generally are appropriate but must be used cautiously, because most patients with MI are not volume overloaded (see Chap. 6).

2. **Nitrates** reduce pulmonary congestion. Therapy should begin with IV nitroglycerin titrated to reduce systolic BP by 10–15%, but not below 90 mm Hg, while avoiding reflex tachycardia. After 24–48 hours, patients can be changed to oral nitrates (see Table 5-1).

3. **ACE inhibitors** improve symptoms in patients with mild to moderate HF and reduce short-term mortality after acute MI (see Subsequent Management of Myocardial Infarction, sec. **IV.C**).

4. **Digoxin** does not reduce overall mortality, and concerns remain about increased mortality from arrhythmias. Therefore, digoxin should not be used in the acute management of HF in MI patients, with the exception of those in whom acute AF develops.

B. **Pulmonary artery catheterization** should be considered in the following situations: (1) severe or progressive HF; (2) cardiogenic shock or hypotension that is unresponsive to fluid administration; (3) clinical signs suggestive of severe mitral regurgitation, ventricular septal defect, or hemodynamically significant pericardial effusion; (4) unexplained or severe cyanosis, hypoxemia, oliguria, or acidosis; (5) unexplained or refractory sinus tachycardia or other tachyarrhythmias; or (6) the need for vasopressors or high doses of parenteral vasodilators that must be closely monitored to avoid deleterious changes in heart rate or BP (see Chap. 9). In patients with LBBB, consideration should be given to placing a temporary pacemaker because pulmonary artery catheterization may induce complete heart block. Often, patients with an indication for a pulmonary artery catheter also require a radial or femoral arterial catheter to allow frequent and accurate measurement of BP. Urinary output should be closely monitored as well.

C. **Hemodynamic subsets in acute MI.** Patients with MI who require pulmonary artery catheterization can be categorized into several hemodynamic subsets that are useful for defining treatment strategies (*J Am Coll Cardiol* 16:249, 1990). Establishing trends is more important than single absolute values, and therapy must be based on individual responses to initial therapy. All hemodynamic data should be evaluated in terms of the clinical response and viewed critically if they fail to correlate with other physiologic parameters (such as urine output). The duration of catheterization should be minimized (see Chap. 9).

1. **Hypovolemic hypotension.** Decreased LV filling pressure [pulmonary artery occlusive pressure (PAOP) <15–18 mm Hg], when accompanied by hypotension, decreased cardiac index (<2.5 L/minute/m^2), oliguria, or persistent sinus tachycardia, should be treated by rapid infusion of normal saline. Because LV compliance is decreased in patients with anterior MI, a PAOP of 15–18 mm Hg is generally an appropriate end point for volume resuscitation.

2. **Pulmonary congestion.** An elevated LV filling pressure (PAOP >18 mm Hg) with a normal cardiac index (>2.5 L/minute/m^2) is an indication of volume overload or decreased LV compliance. IV nitroglycerin should be initiated to reduce filling pressures, followed by a transition to topical or oral nitrates. Patients with clinical evidence of volume overload benefit from modest diuresis.

3. **Peripheral hypoperfusion.** The combination of an elevated LV filling pressure (PAOP >18 mm Hg), decreased cardiac index (<2.5 L/minute/m^2), and systolic arterial pressure greater than 100 mm Hg is an indication of significant LV systolic dysfunction. Because the BP is maintained, afterload reduction with IV nitroglycerin or nitroprusside is the treatment of choice (see Appendix D). Nitroglycerin is preferred early after the onset of infarction because it may also induce coronary vasodilatation and increase myocardial blood flow to ischemic regions. The hemodynamic goal should be to reduce the systemic vascular resistance below 1000 dynes/second/cm^{-5}. Patients who respond to IV nitroglycerin should be started on oral ACE inhibitor therapy to facilitate weaning from parenteral vasodilator therapy. Nitroprusside has less favorable effects than nitroglycerin in terms of coronary blood flow. Use of nitroprusside should be reserved for patients with marked hypertension that is unresponsive to nitroglycerin. If the BP falls or the cardiac index does not improve with vasodilator therapy, an inotropic agent such as dobutamine should be added.

4. **Cardiogenic shock.** Elevated LV filling pressure (PAOP >18 mm Hg), decreased cardiac index (<2.5 L/minute/m^2), and systolic arterial pressure of less than 100 mm Hg are indications of extensive LV dysfunction. Cardiogenic shock is defined as a systolic BP of less than 90 mm Hg in the presence of organ hypoperfusion (such as oliguria or confusion). Patients with cardiogenic shock have a greater than 50% mortality. All patients should receive initial inotropic support. For patients younger than 75 years, an early revascularization strategy decreases mortality at 6 months; however, patients older than 75 years benefit more from initial medical stabilization than from early revasculariza-

tion (*N Engl J Med* 341:625, 1999). Dopamine is the preferred therapeutic agent in patients with a systolic BP of 70–90 mm Hg, but
norepinephrine may be required in markedly hypotensive patients (systolic BP <70 mm Hg). In patients with a systolic BP near 90 mm Hg,
inotropic support with dobutamine often is sufficient and does not
adversely affect ventricular afterload (see Appendix D). A phosphodiesterase inhibitor, amrinone or milrinone, should be added in patients
who either are not responding to or are developing excessive tachycardia from dobutamine (see Chap. 6). These agents reduce preload in
patients with persistently high filling pressures. Because all inotropes
and vasopressors increase myocardial oxygen demand, patients in
whom contraindications do not exist should be considered for insertion
of an intra-aortic balloon pump. All patients should be evaluated for
surgically treatable mechanical complications of infarction, such as
severe mitral regurgitation or ventricular septal rupture (see sec. **V**).

5. **RVMI.** RVMI is characterized by a decreased cardiac index (<2.5 L/
minute/m^2), with normal or decreased LV filling pressures and elevated right atrial pressure (>10 mm Hg) in patients with inferior MI.
In some patients, elevation of right atrial pressure may not be evident
until IV fluids are administered. Clinical signs may include hypotension, elevation of the jugular venous pulsation, a positive Kussmaul's
sign (increase in jugular venous pressures with inspiration), and
right-sided third and fourth heart sounds with clear lung fields. Right
precordial ECG leads should be obtained and analyzed for ST elevation in lead V_4R, a specific marker of RVMI. Echocardiographic demonstration of decreased right ventricular systolic function often is
useful in confirming the diagnosis of RVMI. Hemodynamic responses
to right ventricular infarction range from asymptomatic elevation of
right-sided pressures to severe shock. Patients with a systolic BP of
90–100 mm Hg and a depressed cardiac index often respond to IV fluids, which should be given until the PAOP is 15–18 mm Hg; excessive
fluid administration should be avoided. If the cardiac index still is
decreased after fluid administration or if the systolic BP is less than
90 mm Hg, dobutamine should be administered. Patients with severe
hypotension that is refractory to dobutamine and volume resuscitation should be supported with intra-aortic balloon counterpulsation.
In patients with heart block that causes AV dyssynchrony, AV sequential pacing may have marked beneficial hemodynamic effects.

V. **Mechanical complications of MI** usually develop within the first week after MI
and are accompanied by abrupt or progressive hemodynamic deterioration.
Rapid diagnosis and emergency surgical repair are essential, but mortality
remains high.

A. **Infarct expansion.** Unlike the other mechanical defects, thinning and expansion of the infarcted myocardial wall develops gradually after MI and may
adversely alter ventricular geometry and function. Agents that decrease afterload, particularly ACE inhibitors, may limit infarct expansion and ventricular
dilatation after MI. Glucocorticoids or NSAIDs should be avoided in patients
with MI because they appear to augment myocardial thinning.

B. **Acute mitral regurgitation** usually occurs with an inferoposterior MI and is
associated with a poor prognosis.

1. **Diagnosis.** Most patients with hemodynamically significant mitral
regurgitation have a typical holosystolic murmur. With moderate to
severe mitral regurgitation, pulmonary edema usually is present. Papillary muscle rupture or severe papillary muscle dysfunction, although
rare, often is associated with severe mitral regurgitation and cardiogenic shock. Two-dimensional echocardiography with Doppler imaging
is the initial diagnostic test of choice. Transesophageal echocardiography is an alternative approach to diagnosing mitral regurgitation.

2. **Management.** Patients with mitral regurgitation should be managed with invasive monitoring and pharmacologic afterload reduction with IV nitroglycerin or nitroprusside. Dobutamine may be of benefit in patients with borderline hypotension. In individuals with severe mitral regurgitation, intra-aortic balloon counterpulsation often is necessary to stabilize their hemodynamic parameters. Emergency surgical repair of a ruptured papillary muscle should be performed, because the mortality with medical management approaches 75% in the first 24 hours.

C. **Rupture of the interventricular septum.** This event complicates 1–3% of MIs and is more common with anterior MI.
   1. **Diagnosis.** Ventricular septal rupture is suggested by the development of a holosystolic murmur, the concomitant onset of pulmonary edema, and, almost always, cardiogenic shock. The murmur is best heard along the lower left sternal border and most often is associated with a systolic thrill. Two-dimensional echocardiography with Doppler imaging should be part of the initial evaluation of patients with a new murmur or cardiogenic shock after MI. The presence of a ventricular septal rupture can be documented by a greater than 5% step-up in hemoglobin oxygen saturation between the right atrium and right ventricle during right heart catheterization.
   2. **Management.** Mortality approaches 90% with medical therapy alone. Initial management is similar to that already outlined for patients with cardiogenic shock and should include invasive hemodynamic monitoring. Vasodilators such as nitroglycerin or nitroprusside are indicated to reduce afterload and left-to-right shunting, but the majority of patients require intra-aortic balloon counterpulsation and inotropic support before surgical repair can be attempted. Patients who are in shock and who experience pulmonary edema require emergent surgical repair. Surgical mortality improves in hemodynamically stable patients when operative repair is deferred for at least 1 week.

D. **LV free wall rupture.** This is a catastrophic complication responsible for 10% of deaths associated with MI. Free wall rupture occurs with equal frequency in anterior and inferior MI but is more common in female patients and in patients with a first large transmural MI, with hypertension, treated late with fibrinolytic agents, and treated with glucocorticoids or NSAIDs. Rupture typically occurs during the first week after MI and is manifested as sudden hemodynamic collapse. Although sudden death from acute cardiac tamponade is usual, some instances of LV rupture may be preceded by recurrent pericardial pain secondary to the accumulation of blood in the pericardial space with or without the signs of pericardial effusion, tamponade, and hypotension. Echocardiography may be useful in identifying patients with thin ventricular walls who are at risk for rupture or those in whom partial rupture has occurred. Prompt recognition at this stage may allow for successful surgical repair. Pericardiocentesis in the event of tamponade and the prompt institution of intra-aortic balloon counterpulsation may prove life sustaining until surgical correction can be accomplished. However, the mortality remains in excess of 90%.

E. **Ventricular pseudoaneurysm.** Incomplete free wall rupture may result in formation of a ventricular pseudoaneurysm in which pericardial extravasation of blood is contained locally by the visceral pericardium. Two-dimensional echocardiography is useful in differentiating pseudoaneurysms from true LV aneurysms. Pseudoaneurysms should be repaired promptly because of the high incidence of rupture.

F. **Ventricular aneurysm.** Formation of a true LV aneurysm is preceded by infarct expansion, thinning of the infarcted wall, dyskinetic wall motion, and mural thrombus formation. Ventricular aneurysm can be diagnosed by angiography or echocardiography and often is associated with persistent ST-segment elevation on the ECG. Patients with ventricular aneurysms should be anticoagulated, especially if associated mural thrombus is present. Ventricular aneurysms may require delayed surgical repair if they produce intractable HF, refractory ventricular arrhythmias, or recurrent systemic embolization.

Silent Ischemia

I. **Definition.** Silent ischemia is defined as objective evidence of myocardial ischemia in the absence of angina or anginal equivalents and may be indicative of increased risk for subsequent cardiac events. It occurs in 2.5% of middle-aged men without signs or symptoms of CAD and in approximately 50% of patients with episodes of symptomatic angina pectoris (*J Am Coll Cardiol* 24:1, 1994). It can be documented by asymptomatic ST depression on an ambulatory ECG or during exercise stress testing. Stress testing is preferred to ambulatory ECG for the detection of silent ischemia in patients with CAD.

II. **Therapy.** In patients with stable angina and silent ischemia, revascularization may be more effective than medical therapy in suppressing silent ischemia, but definitive recommendations for treatment must await further trials (*Circulation* 95:2037, 1997). Revascularization should be considered in those patients with a markedly positive stress test or those with silent ischemia at less than 4 metabolic equivalents during treadmill testing. Surgical revascularization may be preferable in those with multivessel disease and significant LV dysfunction. Percutaneous revascularization should be considered in patients with one- or two-vessel disease and preserved LV function. In patients treated with medical therapy, suppression of increases in heart rate appear critical to decreasing episodes of silent ischemia; therefore, drug therapy should include nitrates and a β-adrenergic antagonist or a calcium channel antagonist with negative chronotropic effects. It is not clear whether drug therapy that is designed to suppress silent ischemia as measured on ambulatory ECG results in a better outcome than that designed to control only symptomatic angina.

Coronary Vasospasm and Variant Angina

I. **Definitions. Prinzmetal's variant angina** is characterized by episodes of chest pain that occur at rest and are associated with transient ST-segment elevations on the ECG due to coronary artery vasospasm. Symptomatic **coronary vasospasm** typically occurs in association with a fixed atherosclerotic lesion but is occasionally seen in normal arteries, in which case it is associated with a better prognosis. Episodes of vasospasm may be accompanied by arrhythmia and may progress to MI or sudden death, although this is rare. Sustained coronary vasospasm is believed to play a role in MI associated with cocaine or amphetamine abuse.

II. **Diagnosis.** Transient ST-segment elevation during chest pain is characteristic of coronary vasospasm. Ambulatory ECG monitoring often is useful in detecting such episodes. Coronary angiography is indicated to evaluate the extent of underlying CAD, and the diagnosis can be confirmed by demonstrating coronary artery narrowing during a spontaneous or provoked episode of characteristic chest pain. Provocative testing (IV ergonovine or intracoronary acetylcholine) carries a small risk of refractory spasm and MI.

III. **Management** of acute episodes of coronary vasospasm includes the use of sublingual nitroglycerin. Nifedipine (10 mg), chewed and then swallowed for more rapid onset of action, can be used for refractory spasm in the absence of hypotension. Long-acting nitrates or calcium channel antagonists reduce the frequency of chest pain when used for long-term treatment of Prinzmetal's angina. Cigarette smoking should be discontinued. CABG or PTCA is of benefit only in the presence of significant fixed obstructions.

Secondary Prevention

Secondary prevention is the aggressive modification of risk factors that contribute to the progression of atherosclerosis in patients with known CAD. This applies to patients with chronic stable angina or those whose conditions have been stabilized after an ACS. Secondary prevention is highly effective in reducing mortality from progression of CAD. For example, treatment of hyperlipidemia in patients with CAD reduced the incidence of death by 30% (*N Engl J Med* 339:1349, 1998).

I. **Modification of cardiac risk factors.** Control of cardiac risk factors improves patient well-being and reduces the likelihood of future cardiac events.
   A. **Dietary therapy.** Patients should be instructed about the American Heart Association step 2 diet for reducing cholesterol and achieving optimal body weight.
   B. **Smoking cessation.** Continued smoking after MI significantly increases the chances of recurrent ischemic events. Patients should be firmly advised to quit smoking and should be provided with information on smoking cessation programs. Bupropion has been shown to improve the rate of sustained smoking cessation. A minimum of 7 weeks of therapy is needed, although many patients require treatment for up to a year. All patients should be slowly tapered off bupropion to reduce the chance of relapse and the risk of seizures. **Bupropion is contraindicated in patients with a known seizure disorder or in those who are taking monoamine oxidase inhibitors.** Nicotine-containing patches and gums should be avoided during acute hospitalization but may be helpful subsequently in a supervised program to reduce nicotine craving (see Chap. 10).
   C. **Exercise program.** Regular aerobic exercise, preferably in a structured setting, is recommended after successful completion of an early submaximal or deferred symptom-limited stress test.
   D. **Coexisting medical conditions.** Treatment of pre-existing or newly diagnosed medical conditions in the post-MI patient is essential. Patients with hypertension should be treated with agents that are beneficial after MI, such as β-adrenergic antagonists and ACE inhibitors. Physicians should be aware that significant depression is common after MI; the rate of rehospitalization for recurrent ischemia and infarction can be reduced by emotional support and psychological therapy.

II. **Medical therapy.** Pharmacologic therapy for secondary prevention should emphasize drugs that have been shown in randomized trials to reduce the incidence of reinfarction and cardiovascular death after MI.
   A. **Antiplatelet and anticoagulant therapy** are recommended after MI. Aspirin (75–325 mg/day) is the preferred antiplatelet agent after MI and should be continued indefinitely to reduce the chances of recurrent infarction, stroke, and cardiac death. The combination of aspirin and low-dose warfarin is not superior to aspirin alone in reducing death and recurrent infarction, but warfarin should be added to low-dose aspirin in patients with AF or severe LV dysfunction. Patients with large anterior MIs, LV aneurysm, or mural thrombus should be treated with low-dose aspirin and warfarin for 3–6 months and then continued on aspirin alone. In patients unable to take aspirin, warfarin targeted to an international normalized ratio of 2.0–3.0 has also been shown to improve outcome after MI. Patients

who are unable to take aspirin and do not require warfarin anticoagulation can be considered for alternative antiplatelet agents such as ticlopidine or clopidogrel.

B. β-Adrenergic antagonists reduce mortality and the rates of reinfarction and sudden death after MI. Therapy with oral cardioselective or noncardioselective agents is acceptable (such as metoprolol, 100 mg bid; atenolol, 100 mg qd; timolol, 10 mg bid; or propranolol, 80 mg tid). β-Adrenergic antagonists with intrinsic sympathomimetic activity do not appear to be effective in secondary prevention (see Chap. 4, Table 4-3). Current recommendations favor treatment for an indefinite period in all but the lowest-risk patients.

C. ACE inhibitors reduce mortality and the incidence of HF and recurrent infarction in asymptomatic patients with LV ejection fractions of less than 40% after MI as well as in high-risk patients without known LV dysfunction. In addition, short-term mortality is improved in all patients treated with ACE inhibitors after MI. Given recent data showing a decrease in mortality, MI, and stroke in high-risk patients without LV dysfunction, it is reasonable to continue ACE inhibitor therapy indefinitely in this population following MI (*N Engl J Med* 342:145, 2000).

D. Lipid-lowering agents should be used in patients with hypercholesterolemia (see Hyperlipidemia in Patients with Ischemic Heart Disease).

E. ERT in postmenopausal women suffering an MI is controversial. Postmenopausal women should not be started on hormone replacement therapy (HRT) for secondary prevention, because of the increased rate of cardiac events in the first year after starting this treatment (*JAMA* 280:605, 1998). Currently, it is thought that postmenopausal women who are already taking HRT can continue without an increased risk of cardiac events; however, further study is needed.

F. Calcium channel antagonists are an alternative in patients who are not candidates for β-adrenergic antagonist therapy. In such patients with preserved LV function, secondary prevention can be initiated with a rate-slowing calcium channel antagonist such as verapamil or diltiazem.

G. Nitrates administered as a long-term therapeutic regimen do not reduce mortality after MI and should be reserved for patients with symptomatic angina pectoris or HF.

H. Antioxidant vitamin therapy after MI has not been shown convincingly in randomized trials to be beneficial.

Hyperlipidemia in Patients with Ischemic Heart Disease

I. Rationale for therapy. Lowering cholesterol levels has been shown to decrease the risk of recurrent coronary events and procedures in patients with CAD as well as reduce the risk of developing CAD in people with hypercholesterolemia. Several randomized, placebo-controlled event trials have shown decreased mortality and cardiovascular event rates in patients with CAD and a broad range of LDL-cholesterol levels at time of entry into the studies (*Lancet* 344:1383, 1994; *N Engl J Med* 335:1001, 1996). Data from the Veterans Administration HDL Intervention Trial (*N Engl J Med* 341:410, 1999) suggest that lowering triglycerides and raising HDL may be beneficial in patients with CAD and low HDL-cholesterol levels.

II. Screening and diagnosis

A. All patients with evidence of coronary disease should have lipid profiles performed. The National Cholesterol Education Program has published guidelines for the diagnosis, evaluation, and treatment of high blood cholesterol levels in adults (*JAMA* 269:3015, 1993). A major feature of the guidelines is an emphasis on secondary prevention.

1. **Lipoprotein analysis** should be performed on serum obtained after a **12-hour fast.** Total cholesterol, triglycerides, and HDL-C are measured, and LDL-C is calculated using the following formula:

   LDL-C = total cholesterol – HDL-C – (triglyceride/5)

   where triglyceride/5 represents the cholesterol contained in very-low-density lipoprotein (VLDL). This formula is not valid when triglyceride levels are greater than 400 mg/dl. In such patients, the most reliable way to ascertain LDL-C is to measure it directly using ultracentrifugation. In patients who have had an acute MI, lipoprotein levels measured within the first 24 hours provide an approximation of their usual levels; otherwise, levels will not be stable for up to 6 weeks.

2. **Desirable LDL** in patients with atherosclerotic cardiovascular disease is less than 100 mg/dl. Patients who have manifestations of atherosclerotic vascular disease should be treated aggressively.

B. **Several primary disorders** of lipoprotein metabolism may lead to increased risk of atherosclerosis. These include familial hypercholesterolemia (FH), familial combined hyperlipidemia (FCHL), dysbetalipoproteinemia, and polygenic hypercholesterolemia.

1. **FH** is an autosomal dominant disorder that involves the LDL receptor.

   a. **Heterozygotes** for FH have 50% of the normal number of LDL receptors, elevated LDL-C levels, and cholesterol levels of 350–550 mg/dl. The incidence is approximately 1 in 500 persons. Affected patients often have premature vascular disease and may have tendinous xanthomas. Treatment usually requires drug as well as diet therapy and may necessitate the combination of two or more medications. Patients with insufficient response to tolerated doses of lipid-lowering medications may be candidates for LDL-apheresis.

   b. **Homozygotes** for FH have few or no LDL receptors and thus have markedly elevated LDL-C levels and blood cholesterol levels of 650–1000 mg/dl. The incidence is 1 in 1 million. Heart disease often begins in early childhood, and many patients die of heart disease in their twenties and thirties. Affected children may have planar and tuberous as well as tendinous xanthomas. They respond poorly to diet and drug therapy, although they may have some response to higher doses of potent HMG-CoA reductase inhibitors. LDL-apheresis is the preferred therapy. Liver transplantation has been done in a few patients.

   c. **Familial defective apolipoprotein B-100** is an autosomal dominant disorder caused by an abnormality in the LDL-receptor binding region of apoprotein B-100, the major protein on the surface of LDL particles. It appears to have frequency, clinical features, and lipoprotein levels similar to those of the FH heterozygous form.

2. **FCHL** is associated with an increased risk of vascular disease. Patients may have elevated cholesterol, triglycerides, or both. The molecular basis of this disorder is unknown; many patients overproduce VLDL. FCHL occurs in 1–2% of the population. The diagnosis is made by the presence of multiple lipoprotein phenotypes within one family. Family members may have elevated VLDL, elevated LDL-C, or increased levels of VLDL and LDL-C. Many patients require drug therapy aimed at correcting specific lipoprotein abnormalities in addition to diet therapy, weight loss, and exercise.

3. **Severe polygenic hypercholesterolemia** is found in adults whose LDL-C is above 220 mg/dl and who do not clearly demonstrate a monogenic inheritance of hypercholesterolemia. These patients are usually at increased risk for premature coronary heart disease.

4. **Hypertriglyceridemia** may be secondary to diet, obesity, excess alcohol intake, diabetes mellitus, hypothyroidism, uremia, dysproteinemias, β-adrenergic antagonists, estrogen, oral contraceptive drugs, and retinoids. Triglyceride levels greater than 400 mg/dl are often associated with an underlying primary disorder. Primary hypertriglyceridemia can be due to FCHL or familial hypertriglyceridemia.

5. **Dysbetalipoproteinemia** (type III hyperlipoproteinemia) is a rare (approximately 1 in 5000) disorder caused by an abnormality of apoprotein E, a protein on the surface of VLDL and other lipoproteins, which is important in the uptake of remnant particles by cell surface receptors. Cholesterol-enriched VLDL (beta-VLDL), an atherogenic particle, accumulates. Cholesterol and triglycerides are elevated. Diagnosis is made by a combination of ultracentrifugation and isoelectric focusing, which shows an abnormal apoprotein E pattern. Patients may have palmar or tuberoeruptive xanthomas, and the risk of vascular disease is increased. Patients with this disorder may respond well to diet and weight loss.

6. **Hyperchylomicronemia** can be seen in patients with primary lipid disorders such as FCHL and secondary disorders such as diabetes. Although chylomicrons are not atherogenic, the underlying etiology may be an atherogenic disorder.

7. **Low HDL-C levels,** less than 35 mg/dl, may be caused by a genetic disorder or secondary causes.

   a. **Primary disorders** include familial hypoalphalipoproteinemia, primary hypertriglyceridemias, and rare disorders such as fish-eye disease, Tangier disease, and lecithin-cholesterol-acyltransferase deficiency.

   b. **Secondary causes** of low HDL-C levels include cigarette smoking, obesity, lack of exercise, androgens, some progestational agents, anabolic steroids, beta-adrenergic antagonists, and hypertriglyceridemia.

C. **Secondary causes of hyperlipidemia** include diet, hypothyroidism, diabetes mellitus, nephrotic syndrome, chronic renal failure, and dysproteinemia. Certain **drugs** can have effects on lipids. Thiazide diuretics, β-adrenergic antagonists (particularly less selective ones), glucocorticoids, estrogens, progestins, retinoids, anabolic steroids, and alcohol have variable effects on cholesterol, triglycerides, and HDL cholesterol. Treatment of diabetes mellitus with good control of blood sugars is particularly important if reasonable control of hypertriglyceridemia is to be achieved.

III. **Treatment**

A. **Patients who already have coronary disease should have LDL-cholesterol levels reduced to 100 mg/dl or less.** Therapy should begin during hospitalization for an acute coronary event if patients are not already being treated. Patients with coronary disease should be treated with a step 2 National Cholesterol Education Program diet, which restricts saturated fat to 7% of total calories and daily cholesterol intake to less than 200 mg. Patients should see a dietitian for assistance in making diet changes. Patients with elevated triglycerides need to restrict simple sugars and alcohol as well.

B. **Drug therapy** should be considered at the time of hospitalization for an acute event or at any point at which atherosclerotic vascular disease is diagnosed.

   1. **LDL cholesterol** can be lowered with the HMG-CoA reductase inhibitors (statins): lovastatin, pravastatin, simvastatin, fluvastatin, atorvastatin, and cerivastatin; the bile acid sequestrant resins cholestyramine and colestipol; and nicotinic acid (also called niacin).

      a. **The HMG-CoA reductase inhibitors** lower LDL cholesterol well in most patients. These are the drugs of choice for lowering LDL for secondary prevention. LDL cholesterol can drop by 20–60%, depending on the drug and dosage. All the statins are similar in mechanism of actions and side effects. Atorvastatin has a longer half-life, approximately 13 hours, than the other reductase inhibitors, which have half-lives of approximately 2–3 hours, and can be given at any time during the day. Lovastatin is best given with food, usually with the evening meal; pravastatin, simvastatin, fluvastatin, and cerivastatin can be administered without food, preferably in the evening. **Side effects** occur infrequently (approximately 5% of patients) and most commonly include bloating, gassiness, nausea, and indigestion.

   (1) Liver function tests should be monitored every 6 weeks for the first 3 months, then every 6 months. Approximately 1% of patients have transaminase elevations to greater than three times the upper limit of normal, and the medication must be discontinued.

   (2) Myopathy is an infrequent side effect but has been reported more often when the reductase inhibitors are combined with cyclosporine, gemfibrozil, niacin, or erythromycin.

b. **Bile acid sequestrant resins** lower LDL by 15–30%. Because the resins can raise triglycerides, they should not be used as monotherapy in patients with triglycerides above 250 mg/dl. Usual dosages are 4–20 g/day cholestyramine or colestipol. Up to 24 g cholestyramine or 30 g colestipol can be used. Cholestyramine and colestipol are available in powder form, in bulk or in single-dose packets. Colestipol is also available in 1-g tablets. Once- or twice-daily dosing close to meals is desirable. A single daily dose of up to 8–12 g may be useful to fit the resin into a medication schedule. Resins can be combined with nicotinic acid or reductase inhibitors in patients with severe elevations of LDL cholesterol when greater reductions of LDL are required. The most common **side effects** of the resins are bloating, hard stools, and constipation. Initiation of therapy with low doses, patient education, and use of stool softeners or psyllium can increase compliance. Patients with severe constipation and very complicated drug regimens are not usually good candidates for resin therapy. **Other medications must be taken 1 hour before or 4 hours after the resins. Colesevelam** is a bile acid–binding drug. It is available in 625-mg tablets with a recommended dose of 6 tablets/day and a maximum dose of 7 tablets/day. LDL-cholesterol reduction is 15–18%. Interactions with other drugs may be less frequent due to the structure of this compound.

c. **Nicotinic acid** can lower triglycerides, raise HDL, and lower LDL in higher doses. It is particularly useful in combined hyperlipidemia and in patients with low levels of HDL. Niacin requires extensive patient education because of the flushing and other side effects that can occur.

   (1) To initiate therapy with nicotinic acid, patients should begin taking 100 mg/day for 1 day, then increase to 100 mg tid for 1 week, then 200 mg tid the second week, and 300 mg tid the third week, and repeat lipids and serum chemistries should be obtained after another 3 weeks while patients remain on 300 mg tid. The dose can be gradually increased to the highest dose the patient can tolerate that produces desired results, up to 3000 mg/day. Patients should report any nausea or increased fatigue, as these may be signs of toxicity; liver function tests should be measured and the dose decreased if these are elevated. A prescription-only, extended-release formulation can be given once a day at bedtime; significant liver toxicity was not reported at doses up to 2000 mg/day in clinical trials. Thus, the maximum recommended dose is 2000 mg/day.

   (2) Adverse effects. Some over-the-counter sustained-release preparations have been associated with severe liver toxicity; crystalline or non–time-release preparations should be used. Flushing may be decreased by starting with low doses, use of aspirin before the first few doses, and having the patient take nicotinic acid with meals. Uric acid, blood glucose, and serum transaminases should be monitored every 6–8 weeks during a titration phase. Nicotinic acid should be avoided in patients with a history of gout, active peptic ulcer disease, liver disease, and diabetes.

2. **Hypertriglyceridemia** can be treated with nicotinic acid or a fibric acid derivative. Statins may be effective in patients with mild to moderate hypertriglyceridemia in addition to elevated LDL cholesterol.

   a. **Gemfibrozil and fenofibrate** are the fibric acid derivatives that are available in the United States. The usual dose of gemfibrozil is 600 mg bid before meals. Triglyceride levels are reduced by 30–50%. The drug should not be used in patients with very low creatinine clearances. Abdominal pain and nausea are the most common side effects. The incidence of gallstones is increased in patients who are receiving the fibric acid derivatives due to the increased cholesterol content of bile. Patients on warfarin need to have their prothrombin time monitored closely after they start taking gemfibrozil. The use of fenofibrate is similar to that of gemfibrozil. Fenofibrate is available in 67-, 134-, and 200-mg capsules, with a usual starting dose of 67 mg/day. Many patients require the full dose of 200 mg/day; however, a lower dose should be used in patients with renal insufficiency. It can be given once a day with a meal. Side effects, which occur in 5–10% of patients, are primarily mild GI discomfort and, less frequently, rash and pruritus. Increased transaminases occur in approximately 5% of patients and return to normal when the drug is discontinued. Infrequently, myalgias and increased CK have been reported. In addition to its use for lowering triglycerides, fenofibrate may be helpful in some patients with combined hyperlipidemia who have moderately elevated LDL-cholesterol levels and high triglycerides.

   b. **Nonpharmacologic approaches** to the therapy of hypertriglyceridemia should be combined with medication to achieve the best results. In particular, patients need to decrease intake of alcohol and simple sugars, and they should exercise regularly. Modest amounts of weight loss can be extremely helpful. In addition, patients with diabetes, especially those with very high triglyceride levels, should have good glycemic control. Drugs such as estrogen, retinoids, and thiazides may contribute to hypertriglyceridemia. The use of transdermal estrogen instead of oral estrogen preparations may lead to significant decreases in triglyceride levels in women who are receiving postmenopausal HRT. **Oral estrogen preparations should be avoided in women with triglyceride levels above 500 mg/dl.**

   c. **Patients with triglycerides of 400 mg/dl or less** and elevated LDL-cholesterol levels may respond adequately to a statin added to nonpharmacologic measures. **If the triglycerides are above 400 mg/dl** despite adequate dietary modifications and exercise, the choice of medication could include a statin at higher doses, gemfibrozil, fenofibrate, or niacin. For patients with **triglycerides over 1000 mg/dl,** fibrates and niacin are the drugs of choice. If LDL-cholesterol levels remain high after the triglycerides are lowered, combination therapy should be considered.

3. **Low HDL-cholesterol levels** are associated with an increased risk of cardiovascular disease. Attention should be given to factors that lower HDL, such as cigarette smoking and certain medications, including β-adrenergic antagonists, androgenic compounds, and progestins. Nonpharmacologic therapy, such as exercise, weight loss, and smoking cessation, should be stressed. Niacin is the most effective agent for increasing HDL. Some increase (approximately 10–20%) can occur with fibrates.

Heart Failure, Cardiomyopathy, and Valvular Heart Disease

Gregory A. Ewald and
Joseph G. Rogers

Heart Failure

I. **Clinical diagnosis**
   A. **Definition. Heart failure (HF)** is the inability of the heart to maintain an output adequate to meet the metabolic demands of the body. It is an increasingly common condition associated with extremely high morbidity and mortality.
   B. **Etiology.** HF may be secondary to abnormalities in myocardial contraction (systolic dysfunction), ventricular relaxation and filling with normal contractile function (diastolic dysfunction), or systolic and diastolic dysfunction (Table 6-1). Hypertension and coronary artery disease are the most frequent causes of HF in the United States. Additional etiologies include primary diseases of myocardial muscle, abnormalities of valvular function, and pericardial disease. High-output HF may occur with severe anemia, arteriovenous shunts, thyrotoxicosis, or beriberi.
   C. **Pathophysiology.** HF is manifested as organ hypoperfusion and inadequate tissue oxygen delivery due to a low cardiac output and decreased cardiac reserve, as well as pulmonary and systemic venous congestion. A variety of "compensatory adaptations" occur, including (1) increased left ventricular (LV) volume (dilatation) and mass (hypertrophy), (2) increased systemic vascular resistance (SVR) secondary to enhanced activity of the sympathetic nervous system and elevated levels of circulating catecholamines, and (3) activation of the renin-angiotensin and vasopressin (antidiuretic hormone) systems. These secondary mechanisms, in conjunction with pump failure, play a role in the pathophysiology of HF.
   D. **Clinical manifestations** of HF vary depending on the rapidity of cardiac decompensation, underlying etiology, and age and comorbidities of the patient. **Signs and symptoms** of low cardiac output include fatigue, exercise intolerance, and decreased peripheral perfusion. Extreme deterioration in cardiac output and elevated SVR result in hypoperfusion of vital organs such as the kidney (decreased urine output) and brain (confusion and lethargy) and, ultimately, in cardiogenic shock. Elevations in LV diastolic pressure and pulmonary venous pressure result in pulmonary edema. Chronic pulmonary and systemic venous congestion results in orthopnea, dyspnea on exertion, paroxysmal nocturnal dyspnea, peripheral edema, elevated jugular venous pressure, pleural and pericardial effusions, hepatic congestion, and ascites. Associated laboratory abnormalities include elevated levels of BUN and creatinine, hyponatremia, and elevated serum levels of hepatic enzymes.
   E. **The diagnosis of HF** should be suspected by clinical presentation. Radiographic evidence of cardiomegaly and pulmonary vascular redistribution is common. Depressed ventricular function should be confirmed by echocardiography, radionuclide ventriculography, or cardiac catheterization with left ventriculography. Abnormalities in the ECG are common and include supraventricular and ventricular arrhythmias, conduction delays, and nonspecific ST-T changes.

Table 6-1. Common causes of heart failure

Predominant systolic failure

Coronary artery disease

Hypertension

Dilated cardiomyopathy

    Idiopathic

    Toxic (alcohol, doxorubicin)

    Infection (viral, parasitic, and others)

Predominant diastolic failure

Hypertension

Hypertrophic cardiomyopathy

Restrictive cardiomyopathy

    Amyloidosis

    Sarcoidosis

    Hemachromatosis

Constrictive pericarditis

High-output failure

    Chronic anemia

    Atrioventricular shunts

    Thyrotoxicosis

    F. Precipitants of HF may include myocardial ischemia or infarction, hypertension, arrhythmias, infection, anemia, pregnancy, thyroid disease, volume overload, toxins (alcohol, doxorubicin), drugs (β-adrenergic antagonists, nonsteroidal anti-inflammatory drugs, calcium channel antagonists), pulmonary embolism, and dietary or medical noncompliance.

II. General principles in the management of HF

    A. The initial approach to the patient with HF must be individualized according to severity, acuity of presentation, etiology, presence of coexisting illness, and precipitating factors. Identification of the underlying etiology and precipitating factors is essential, as the beneficial effect of one type of treatment (e.g., nitrates for ischemia) may be deleterious when applied to another situation [e.g., severe aortic stenosis (AS)]. After a careful history has been obtained and a physical examination and directed diagnostic evaluation have been undertaken, treatment should be based on the degree of myocardial dysfunction, total body and intravascular volume status, and extent of peripheral vasoconstriction. General principles of treatment include correction of precipitating processes, control of fluid and sodium retention, optimization of myocardial contractile function, minimization of cardiac workload, and reduction of pulmonary and systemic venous congestion. Close attention to clinical parameters, such as weight, vital signs, fluid intake, and urine output, is critical to guiding HF therapy.

    B. Nonpharmacologic therapeutic measures generally are used in conjunction with specific pharmacologic treatment.

        1. Restriction of physical activity may be useful in acute HF to reduce myocardial workload and oxygen consumption in patients with symptomatic HF. After stabilization, carefully guided cardiac rehabilitation and aerobic exercise may improve functional capacity in selected patients with HF (*Circulation* 85:2119, 1992).

2. **Weight loss** in obese patients reduces SVR as well as myocardial oxygen demand. However, maintenance of adequate caloric intake in patients with severe HF is necessary to prevent or correct cardiac cachexia.

3. **Dietary sodium restriction** (Na^+, <2 g/day) facilitates control of signs and symptoms of HF and minimizes diuretic requirements.

4. **Fluid and free water restriction** (<1.5 L/day) is especially important in the setting of hyponatremia (serum sodium <130 mEq/L) and volume overload (see Chap. 3).

5. **Minimization of medications with negative inotropic effects** (e.g., verapamil, diltiazem, disopyramide, and flecainide), if possible, may acutely improve signs and symptoms of HF in patients with impaired ventricular contractility.

6. **Administration of oxygen** may relieve dyspnea, improve oxygen delivery, reduce the work of breathing, and limit pulmonary vasoconstriction in patients with hypoxemia.

7. **Dialysis or ultrafiltration** may be necessary in patients with severe HF and renal dysfunction who cannot respond adequately to fluid and sodium restriction or diuretics. Other mechanical methods of fluid removal such as therapeutic thoracentesis and paracentesis may provide temporary symptomatic relief of dyspnea. Care must be taken to avoid excessively rapid fluid removal and subsequent hypotension.

C. **Pharmacologic therapy of HF. General principles** of pharmacologic therapy include vasodilatation, control of sodium and fluid retention, β-adrenergic receptor blockade, and inotropic support of depressed LV function. Vasodilators are the cornerstone of therapy for patients with HF. Diuretics are reserved for individuals with volume overload. Most patients require a multidrug regimen to control symptoms and prolong survival.

1. **Vasodilator therapy** is the mainstay of treatment in HF. Arterial and venous vasoconstriction occurs in patients with HF due to activation of the adrenergic and renin-angiotensin systems, as well as increased secretion of arginine vasopressin. Arterial vasoconstriction impairs myocardial performance by increasing the impedance (afterload) against which the ventricle ejects blood, which raises intracardiac filling pressures, increases myocardial wall stress and oxygen demand, and predisposes to subendocardial ischemia. In patients with severe HF, reflexive arteriolar vasoconstriction in renal, hepatic, mesenteric, cerebral, and myocardial vascular beds results in further hypoperfusion and end-organ dysfunction. Venous vasoconstriction limits venous capacitance, resulting in venous congestion and elevated diastolic ventricular filling pressures (preload). Pulmonary arterial vasoconstriction may occur as a result of hypoxia, in response to chronically elevated pulmonary blood flow (e.g., left-to-right intracardiac shunts) or in response to chronically elevated left atrial pressure [e.g., mitral stenosis (MS), mitral regurgitation (MR), or LV failure]. Vasodilators can selectively reduce afterload, preload, or both. Agents with predominantly venodilatory properties decrease preload and ventricular filling pressures. In the absence of LV outflow tract obstruction, arterial vasodilators reduce afterload by decreasing SVR, resulting in increased cardiac output, decreased ventricular filling pressure, and decreased myocardial wall stress. Patients with valvular regurgitation, severe HF with elevated SVR, or HF with associated hypertension will most likely benefit from afterload reduction with arterial vasodilators. The efficacy and toxicity of vasodilator therapy depend on intravascular volume status and preload. Hypotension, orthostasis, and prerenal azotemia may result from treatment with venous or arterial dilators in the setting of low or normal ventricular filling pressures. Vasodilators should be used with caution in patients with a fixed cardiac output [e.g., AS or hypertrophic cardiomyopathy (HCM)] or with predominantly diastolic dysfunction (restrictive cardiomyopathy or HCM).

Table 6-2. Angiotensin-converting enzyme inhibitors in heart failure*

Drug	Initial dose	Half-life (hrs)	Recommended daily dosage (mg)
Benazepril	5–10 mg qd; can use q12h	10	40–80
Captopril	6.25–12.5 mg q6–8h	<2	150–400
Enalapril	2.5–10.0 mg qd; can use q12h	11	40–80
Fosinopril	5–10 mg qd; can use q12h	12	40–80
Lisinopril	2.5–5.0 mg qd; can use q12h	12	40–80
Moexipril	5.0–7.5 mg qd; can use q12h	12	30–60
Quinapril	5 mg × 1 day; then 5 mg q12h	25	40–80
Ramipril	1.25–2.5 mg q12h	13–24	20–40
Trandolapril	1–2 mg qd	6–10	2–8

*Captopril, enalapril, and ramipril have U.S. Food and Drug Administration (FDA) approval for symptomatic improvement and mortality reduction. Fosinopril, lisinopril, and quinapril have FDA approval for adjunctive treatment in heart failure (i.e., symptomatic improvement). Moexipril, benazepril, and trandolapril are approved for the treatment of hypertension.

    a. Oral vasodilators should be the initial therapy in patients with symptomatic chronic HF and in patients in whom parenteral vasodilators are being discontinued. When treatment with oral vasodilators is being initiated, it is prudent to use agents with a short half-life.

    (1) Angiotensin-converting enzyme (ACE) inhibitors (Table 6-2) attenuate vasoconstriction, vital organ hypoperfusion, hyponatremia, hypokalemia, and fluid retention attributable to compensatory activation of the renin-angiotensin system. Treatment with ACE inhibitors decreases ventricular filling pressures and SVR while increasing cardiac output, with little or no change in BP or heart rate. Large clinical trials have clearly demonstrated that ACE inhibitors improve symptoms and survival in patients with mild to severe HF. ACE inhibitors may also prevent the development of HF in patients with asymptomatic LV dysfunction. Hypotension and renal insufficiency may develop on ACE inhibitor therapy in the setting of reduced preload and may respond to a reduction in the dose of diuretics or venodilating agents or to cautious volume expansion. Absence of an initial beneficial response to treatment with an ACE inhibitor does not preclude long-term benefit. Acute renal insufficiency may occur in patients with bilateral renal artery stenosis. Additional adverse effects include rash, angioedema, dysgeusia, increases in serum creatinine, proteinuria, hyperkalemia, leukopenia, and cough. Levels of serum creatinine and electrolytes, urinalysis, and blood counts should be monitored periodically during treatment. Oral potassium supplements, potassium salt substitutes, and potassium-sparing diuretics should be used with caution during treatment with ACE inhibitors. Most ACE inhibitors are excreted by the kidneys, necessitating careful dose titration in patients with renal insufficiency. Captopril contains a sulfhydryl group; agranulocytosis and angioedema may be more common than with other ACE inhibitors, particularly in patients with associated collagen vascular disease or serum creatinine greater than 1.5 mg/dl.

    (2) Angiotensin II receptor blockers (ARB) (Table 6-3) inhibit the renin-angiotensin system via specific blockade of the angiotensin

Table 6-3. Angiotensin receptor blockers in heart failure*

Medication	Initial dose	Half-life (hrs)	Recommended daily dosage (mg)
Candesartan cilexetil	8–16 mg qd	5–9	2–32
Eprosartan	200–400 mg qd; can use q12h	5–9	400–800
Irbesartan	75–150 mg qd	11–15	75–300
Losartan	25 mg qd; can use q12h	6–9	25–100
Telmisartan	20–40 mg qd	24	40–80
Valsartan	80 mg qd	6–9	80–320

*Angiotensin receptor blockers have U.S. Food and Drug Administration approval for the treatment of hypertension. They are recommended in patients with heart failure who are intolerant to angiotensin-converting enzyme inhibitors (see text).

II receptor. In contrast to ACE inhibitors, they do not increase bradykinin levels, which may be responsible for adverse effects such as cough. They currently are approved for the treatment of hypertension but also produce favorable hemodynamic effects in patients with HF (*Circulation* 91:691, 1995) and may reduce mortality in patients with symptomatic HF (*Lancet* 349:747, 1997). Preliminary data suggest that patients treated with ARBs do not have a survival benefit when compared to those treated with ACE inhibitors (*Lancet* 355:1582, 2000). ARBs should be considered in those patients who are unable to tolerate ACE inhibitors due to side effects. (*Lancet* 355:1582, 2000)

(3) **Nitrates** are predominantly venodilators and help relieve symptoms of venous and pulmonary congestion. Nitrates reduce myocardial ischemia by decreasing ventricular filling pressures and by directly dilating coronary arteries. In combination with hydralazine, nitrates have been demonstrated to decrease mortality in patients with HF (*N Engl J Med* 314:1547, 1986). Nitrate therapy may precipitate hypotension in patients with reduced preload. Improved hemodynamics and symptomatic relief may be seen after the first dose in the majority of patients but may be transient due to development of nitrate tolerance (see Chap. 5).

(4) **Hydralazine** acts directly on arterial smooth muscle to produce vasodilation and to reduce afterload. This agent is particularly useful in the treatment of regurgitant valvular lesions. In combination with nitrates, hydralazine improves survival in patients with HF. Dosage requirements vary widely, but most patients benefit from 25–100 mg PO three or four times a day. Hemodynamic tolerance has been reported and may be reduced by concomitant diuretic use. Reflex tachycardia and increased myocardial oxygen consumption may occur, requiring cautious use in patients with ischemic heart disease. Other adverse effects are described in Chap. 4.

(5) **Vasopeptidase inhibitors** are potent vasodilators. They are synthetic molecules that inhibit ACE and neutral endopeptidase, which results in inhibition of the renin-angiotensin system and increased levels of vasodilatory peptides such as bradykinin and atrial natriuretic factor, and appear to be effective in systolic hypertension; studies of efficacy in HF are ongoing.

(6) α-**Adrenergic receptor antagonists** such as prazosin and doxazosin have vasodilatory properties and are effective antihypertensive medications (see Chap. 4). α-Adrenergic blockade reduces
vasoconstriction, SVR, and afterload by antagonizing the effects
of norepinephrine. These agents have not been shown to improve
survival in HF patients, and doxazosin has been demonstrated to
contribute to a higher incidence of HF in hypertensive patients
treated with doxazosin as first-line therapy (*JAMA* 283:1967,
2000).

**b. Parenteral vasodilators should be reserved for patients with
severe HF** or those who are unable to take oral medications. Frequently, IV vasodilator therapy is guided by central hemodynamic
monitoring (pulmonary artery catheterization) to assess efficacy and
avoid hemodynamic instability. Parenteral agents should be started
at low doses, titrated to the desired hemodynamic effect, and discontinued slowly to avoid rebound vasoconstriction.

(1) Nitroglycerin is a potent vasodilator, with effects on venous and,
to a lesser extent, arterial vascular beds. It relieves pulmonary
and systemic venous congestion and is an effective coronary
vasodilator. Nitroglycerin is the preferred vasodilator for treatment of HF in the setting of acute myocardial infarction (MI) or
unstable angina (for dosing, see Chap. 5).

(2) Sodium nitroprusside is a direct arterial vasodilator with less
potent venodilatory properties. Its predominant effect is to
reduce afterload, and it is particularly effective in patients with
HF who are hypertensive or who have severe aortic or mitral valvular regurgitation. Nitroprusside should be used cautiously in
patients with myocardial ischemia because of a potential reduction in regional myocardial blood flow (coronary steal). The initial dose of 10 μg/minute can be titrated (maximum dose of 300–
400 μg/minute) to the desired hemodynamic effect or until
hypotension develops. The half-life of nitroprusside is 1–3 minutes, and its metabolism results in the release of cyanide, which
is metabolized hepatically to thiocyanate and then is excreted
renally. Toxic levels of thiocyanate (>10 mg/dl) may develop in
patients with renal insufficiency, necessitating close monitoring
of serum levels. Thiocyanate toxicity is manifested as nausea,
paresthesias, mental status changes, abdominal pain, and seizures (see Chap. 4). Methemoglobinemia is a rare complication of
treatment with nitroprusside.

(3) Enalaprilat is an active metabolite of enalapril that is available
for IV administration. Its onset of action is more rapid and its
pharmacologic half-life shorter than that of enalapril. The initial
dose is 1.25 mg IV q6h, which can be titrated to a maximum dosage of 5 mg IV q6h. Patients who take diuretics or those with
impaired renal function serum creatinine >3 mg/dl, creatinine
clearance <30 ml/minute) initially should receive 0.625 mg IV
q6h. When dosing is being converted from IV to PO administration, enalaprilat, 0.625 mg IV q6h, is approximately equivalent to
enalapril, 2.5 mg PO daily.

2. β-**Adrenergic receptor antagonists** (see Chap. 4) are useful in the
treatment of HF by blocking the cardiac effects of chronic adrenergic
stimulation, which include direct myocyte toxicity and down-regulation
of cardiac β-receptors. Large randomized trials have documented the
beneficial effects on functional status and survival of β-adrenergic
antagonists. β-Adrenergic antagonists should be added to vasodilator
and diuretic therapy for HF patients with stable heart failure symptoms. Many HF patients experience improvement in ejection fraction,

exercise tolerance, and functional class after the institution of a β-adrenergic antagonist. Typically, 2–3 months of therapy are required to observe significant hemodynamic improvement, but the effect appears to be long-lasting (*JAMA* 283:1295, 2000). β-Adrenergic antagonists should be instituted at a low dose and titrated with careful attention to BP and heart rate, as some patients experience increased volume retention and worsening HF symptoms that usually respond to transient increases in diuretic therapy.

a. Bisoprolol is a β_1-selective agent that improves survival in patients with New York Heart Association class III or IV HF. It also decreases the need for hospitalization in patients with HF (*Lancet* 353:9, 1999). It is initiated at a dose of 1.25 mg/day PO and gradually increased to 10 mg/day.

b. Carvedilol is a nonselective antagonist of β_1- and β_2-adrenoreceptors as well as α_1-adrenergic receptors that also has antioxidant properties. It improves the functional status, ameliorates symptoms, and decreases mortality in patients with HF (*Circulation* 94:2793, 1996; *Circulation* 94:2817, 1996). Carvedilol is initiated at a dosage of 3.125–6.250 mg PO bid and is titrated to 25–50 mg PO bid.

c. Metoprolol is a β_1-selective agent that improves survival and functional status of patients with HF due to ischemic and nonischemic cardiomyopathy and reduces the need for hospital admission due to worsening HF (*JAMA* 283:1295, 2000). It is initiated at a dose of 12.5–25.0 mg/day PO in divided doses or as a single dose of the extended-release preparation and is titrated gradually to a target dose of 100–200 mg/day.

3. Calcium channel antagonists directly relax vascular smooth muscle and inhibit calcium entry into myocardial cells. These agents have a beneficial effect on diastolic relaxation and are useful in the treatment of ischemic heart disease. However, the vasodilatory effects of some of the first-generation calcium channel antagonists (diltiazem and verapamil) are counterbalanced by their negative inotropic properties and may have detrimental effects in patients with LV dysfunction. The addition of amlodipine to diuretics, digoxin, and an ACE inhibitor does not have a beneficial effect on the incidence of hospitalization for worsening HF, MI, arrhythmias, or survival (*N Engl J Med* 335:1107, 1996).

4. Digitalis glycosides increase myocardial contractility and may attenuate the neurohormonal activation that occurs in patients with HF. Digoxin appears to decrease the number of hospitalizations in patients with HF, without an impact on overall mortality (*N Engl J Med* 336:525, 1997). Discontinuation of digoxin in patients who are stable on a regimen of digoxin, diuretics, and an ACE inhibitor may result in clinical deterioration (*N Engl J Med* 329:1, 1993). **The toxic:therapeutic ratio is narrow,** and serum levels should be followed closely, particularly in patients with unstable renal function. Hypokalemia and hypoxemia may exacerbate toxicity and should be corrected before initiation of and during digoxin therapy.

a. Dosage and route of administration should be dictated by the underlying condition and the severity of illness. Digoxin loading is accomplished by giving 0.25–0.50 mg PO or IV initially, followed by 0.25 mg q6h to a total dose of 1.0–1.5 mg. Maintenance therapy is affected by the patient's age, lean body weight, and renal function. The usual daily dose is 0.125–0.375 mg and should be decreased in patients with renal insufficiency. The serum half-life is 33–44 hours with normal renal function. Assessment of serum digoxin levels ultimately should determine optimum dosing. Digoxin levels of 0.8–2.0 ng/ml generally are considered therapeutic, but toxicity can occur in this range.

b. Drug interactions with digoxin are frequent and include impaired absorption of digoxin by cholestyramine, kaolin-pectin, and antacids, which may decrease bioavailability by 25%. Oral antibiotics such as erythromycin and tetracycline may increase digoxin levels by 10–40%. Quinidine, verapamil, flecainide, and amiodarone increase digoxin levels significantly.

c. Contraindications to digoxin use are rare. Atrioventricular (AV) conduction disturbances may be exacerbated by digoxin; conversely, conduction through accessory AV pathways may be potentiated. Electrolyte abnormalities, especially hypokalemia and hypomagnesemia, increase the likelihood of digoxin toxicity and should be corrected. Cardioversion in the presence of digoxin toxicity is relatively contraindicated, as potentially fatal ventricular arrhythmias may be precipitated; however, with serum levels in the therapeutic range, cardioversion can be attempted with little increased risk.

d. Digoxin toxicity remains an important clinical problem. Toxicity may develop despite serum levels within the usual therapeutic range. Factors that contribute to the development of toxicity include drug interactions, electrolyte abnormalities (particularly hypokalemia), hypoxemia, hypothyroidism, renal insufficiency, and volume depletion.

(1) Clinical manifestations of digoxin toxicity include virtually all forms of cardiac arrhythmias. Ventricular premature depolarizations, junctional tachycardia, and varying degrees of second-degree AV block are frequently present. Bidirectional ventricular tachycardia, paroxysmal atrial tachycardia with AV block, and a regular accelerated junctional rhythm in the presence of atrial fibrillation occur almost exclusively as a result of digoxin toxicity. Noncardiac manifestations of toxicity include GI and neuropsychiatric symptoms. Anorexia, nausea, vomiting, and diarrhea may compound toxic effects by worsening hypokalemia. Altered mental status, agitation, lethargy, and visual disturbances (scotomas and color perception changes) can occur.

(2) Treatment of digoxin toxicity includes discontinuation of the drug, correction of precipitating factors, and continuous ECG monitoring. The serum potassium level should be maintained in the high-normal range but should be replenished cautiously because rapid increases can precipitate complete heart block. Symptomatic bradycardia can be controlled with atropine or temporary pacing; sympathomimetics should be avoided, as they may precipitate or worsen ventricular arrhythmias. Lidocaine or phenytoin should be used to control ventricular and atrial arrhythmias; quinidine should not be used, because it may elevate serum levels further (see Chap. 7). Cardioversion is contraindicated unless all other measures of controlling hemodynamically significant arrhythmias have been exhausted.

(3) Digoxin-specific Fab antibody fragments are effective in rapidly reversing life-threatening digoxin intoxication and should be considered when other modes of therapy are inadequate. Digoxin-specific Fab fragment complexes are cleared from the circulation via renal excretion. **Total serum digoxin levels are no longer meaningful after administration of Fab fragments;** free (unbound) digoxin can be measured when serum level monitoring is required. Significant adverse effects have not been reported with the use of these antibody fragments. Each 40-mg vial of Fab fragments neutralizes approximately 0.6 mg digoxin. Dosage is based on the estimated amount of drug ingested or the steady-state serum level (see Table 26-2 for calculation).

Table 6-4. Diuretics in heart failure

Drug	Dose/frequency
Thiazide diuretics	
Chlorthalidone	25–50 mg qd
Hydrochlorothiazide	25–50 mg qd
Metolazone	5–10 mg qd or bid
Loop diuretics	
Bumetanide	0.5–5.0 mg qd; can use q6h PO or IV
Ethacrynic acid	25–100 mg qd; can use q6h PO or IV
Furosemide	10–240 mg qd; can use q6h PO or IV
Indapamide	2.5–5.0 mg qd
Torsemide	5–100 mg qd; can use q6h PO or IV
Potassium sparing	
Amiloride	5–10 mg qd
Spironolactone	25–100 mg qd or bid
Triamterene	50–100 mg bid

5. **Diuretics** (Table 6-4), in conjunction with restriction of dietary sodium and fluids, often lead to clinical improvement in patients with mild to moderate HF. The potassium-sparing diuretic spironolactone has been shown to improve survival and decrease hospitalizations in patients with New York Heart Association class III and IV HF (*N Engl J Med* 341:753, 1999). Frequent assessment of the patient's weight along with careful observation of fluid intake and output is essential during initiation and maintenance of therapy. When diuretics are initiated for an acute exacerbation of HF, the goal of therapy should be a maximum net loss of 0.5–1.0 L of fluid/day (0.5–1.0 kg body weight) to prevent intravascular volume depletion. Frequent complications of therapy include hypokalemia, hyponatremia, hypomagnesemia, volume contraction alkalosis, intravascular volume depletion, and hypotension. Serum electrolytes, BUN, and creatinine levels should be followed after institution of diuretic therapy. Hypokalemia may be life-threatening in patients who are receiving digoxin or in those who have severe LV dysfunction that predisposes them to ventricular arrhythmias. Potassium supplementation or a potassium-sparing diuretic should be considered in addition to careful monitoring of serum potassium levels.

   a. **Thiazide diuretics** (hydrochlorothiazide, chlorthalidone) can be used as initial agents in patients with normal renal function in whom only a mild diuresis is desired. Metolazone, unlike other thiazides, exerts its action at the proximal as well as the distal tubule and may be useful in combination with a loop diuretic in patients with a low glomerular filtration rate.

   b. **Loop diuretics** should be used in patients who require significant diuresis and in those with markedly decreased renal function. Furosemide reduces preload acutely by causing direct venodilation when administered intravenously. This property renders furosemide particularly useful for managing severe HF or acute pulmonary edema. Chronic HF may become refractory to oral diuretics as a result of diminished GI absorption secondary to bowel edema but may respond readily when an equivalent dose of IV diuretic is given. Use of loop diuretics may be complicated by hyperuricemia, hypocalcemia, ototoxicity, rash, and vasculitis. Furosemide and bumetanide are sulfa derivatives and may cause drug reactions in sulfa-sensitive patients. Ethacrynic acid can generally be used safely in such patients.

   c. **Potassium-sparing diuretics** do not exert a potent diuretic effect when used alone. Spironolactone has been shown to improve survival and decrease hospitalizations in symptomatic patients. The potential for development of life-threatening hyperkalemia exists with the use of these agents. Serum potassium must be monitored closely after their administration; concomitant use of ACE inhibitors and nonsteroidal anti-inflammatory drugs and the presence of renal insufficiency (creatinine >2.5 mg/dl) increase the risk of hyperkalemia.

6. **Inotropic agents**

   a. **Sympathomimetic agents** (see Appendix D) are potent inotropes primarily used to treat severe HF. Beneficial and adverse effects are mediated by stimulation of myocardial β-adrenergic receptors. The most important adverse effects are related to the arrhythmogenic nature of these agents and the potential for exacerbation of myocardial ischemia. Drug-related tachycardia and ventricular arrhythmias may be decreased by lower dosage. Treatment should be guided by careful hemodynamic and ECG monitoring.

      (1) **Dopamine** is an endogenous catecholamine that exerts selective renal and mesenteric vasodilatation at doses of 1–3 µg/kg/minute via dopaminergic-receptor stimulation, resulting in improved renal blood flow and urine output. Positive inotropic effects are produced with dosages of 2–8 µg/kg/minute and are secondary to β_1-adrenergic receptor stimulation. At dosages of 7–10 µg/kg/minute, α-adrenergic receptor stimulation predominates; the resulting peripheral vasoconstriction increases SVR and may be deleterious in patients with low cardiac output and HF. Dopamine should be used primarily for stabilization of the hypotensive patient.

      (2) **Dobutamine** is a synthetic analog of dopamine that selectively stimulates β_1-adrenergic receptors; β_2- and α-receptors are activated to a much lesser degree. Its predominant hemodynamic effect is direct inotropic stimulation with reflex arterial vasodilatation, resulting in afterload reduction and augmentation of cardiac output. BP generally remains constant, and heart rate may increase minimally. Tachycardia may result from excessive doses or if LV filling pressure falls in response to improved ventricular performance. Dobutamine is administered as a constant infusion that is initiated at a rate of 1–2 µg/kg/minute and is titrated to obtain the desired hemodynamic effect or until excessive tachycardia or ventricular arrhythmias occur. In the absence of tachycardia, dobutamine does not increase myocardial oxygen requirements excessively. Patients with refractory chronic HF may benefit symptomatically from intermittent dobutamine infusion or from continuous ambulatory administration. Dobutamine tolerance has been described, and some studies have indicated an increased mortality for patients treated with continuous dobutamine. Patients who are undergoing continuous therapy should be closely monitored, and infusion rates of 10 µg/kg/minute or less should be used. Dobutamine has no significant role in the treatment of HF resulting from diastolic dysfunction (e.g., HCM) or a high-output state.

   b. **Phosphodiesterase inhibitors** (see Appendix D) increase myocardial contractility and produce vasodilation by increasing intracellular cyclic adenosine monophosphate. **Amrinone** and **milrinone** are currently available for clinical use and are indicated for treatment of refractory HF. Amrinone has hemodynamic effects similar to those of dobutamine but with more vasodilatory properties. Thus, hypotension may develop in patients who receive vasodilator therapy or who have intravascular volume contraction. Amrinone may improve hemodynamics in patients treated concurrently with digoxin, dobutamine, or dopamine. Administration of a 750-μg/kg bolus IV over 2–3 minutes, followed by a continuous infusion of 2.5–10.0 μg/kg/minute, is recommended. Milrinone is structurally similar to amrinone and has comparable hemodynamic effects. A loading dose of 50 μg/kg is administered over 10 minutes, followed by a continuous infusion of 0.375–0.750 μg/kg/minute to achieve the desired clinical response. Lower doses are required in patients with renal dysfunction. The principal side effects of the phosphodiesterase inhibitors include atrial and ventricular arrhythmias and thrombocytopenia (more common with amrinone).

D. Mechanical circulatory support can be considered for patients in whom other therapeutic modalities have failed, who have transient myocardial dysfunction, or in whom a more definitive procedure is planned.

    1. The intra-aortic balloon pump is positioned in the aorta with its tip distal to the left subclavian artery. Balloon inflation is synchronous with the cardiac cycle and occurs during diastole. The hemodynamic consequences of balloon counterpulsation are decreased myocardial oxygen demand and improved coronary blood flow. Additionally, significant preload and afterload reduction occurs, resulting in improved cardiac output. Severe aortoiliac atherosclerosis and aortic valve insufficiency are relative contraindications to intra-aortic balloon pump placement.

    2. Ventricular assist devices require surgical implantation and are indicated for patients with severe HF after cardiac surgery, for individuals who have intractable cardiogenic shock after acute MI, and for patients whose conditions deteriorate while they await cardiac transplantation. Currently available devices vary with regard to degree of mechanical hemolysis, intensity of anticoagulation required, and difficulty of implantation. Therefore, the decision to institute ventricular assist device circulatory support must be made in consultation with a cardiac surgeon who is experienced in this procedure.

E. Cardiac transplantation is an option for selected patients with severe end-stage heart disease that has become refractory to aggressive medical therapy and for whom no other conventional treatment options are available.

    1. Candidates considered for transplantation should be younger than 65 years (although selected older patients may also benefit), have advanced HF (New York Heart Association functional class III–IV), have a strong psychosocial support system, have exhausted all other therapeutic options, and be free of irreversible extracardiac organ dysfunction that would limit functional recovery or predispose them to posttransplantation complications (*J Am Coll Cardiol* 22:1, 1993).

    2. Survival rates of 90% at 1 year and 70% at 5 years have been reported since the introduction of cyclosporine-based immunosuppression. In general, functional capacity and quality of life improve significantly after transplantation.

    3. Immunosuppressive therapy typically includes glucocorticoids, cyclosporine, and azathioprine.

    4. Posttransplantation complications include acute rejection, infection caused by immunosuppression, and adverse effects of immunosuppressive agents (see Chap. 16). Aggressive posttransplantation coronary artery disease is the leading cause of death after the first year.

III. Acute HF and cardiogenic pulmonary edema (CPE)

A. Pathophysiology. CPE occurs when the pulmonary capillary pressure exceeds the forces (serum oncotic pressure and interstitial hydrostatic pressure) that maintain fluid within the vascular space. Accumulation of fluid in the pulmonary interstitium is followed by alveolar flooding and disturbance of gas exchange. Increased pulmonary capillary pressure may be caused by LV failure of any cause, obstruction to transmitral flow (e.g., MS, atrial myxoma), or, rarely, by pulmonary veno-occlusive disease.

B. Diagnosis

1. **Clinical manifestations** of CPE usually occur rapidly and include dyspnea, anxiety, and restlessness. Physical signs of decreased peripheral perfusion, pulmonary congestion, use of accessory respiratory muscles, and wheezing often are present. The patient may expectorate pink frothy fluid.

2. **Radiographic abnormalities** include cardiomegaly, interstitial and perihilar vascular engorgement, Kerley B lines, and pleural effusions. The radiographic abnormalities may follow the development of symptoms by several hours, and their resolution may be out of phase with clinical improvement.

C. Management

1. **Initial supportive treatment** of CPE includes administration of oxygen to raise the arterial oxygen tension to greater than 60 mm Hg. Mechanical ventilation is indicated if hypercapnia coexists or if oxygenation is inadequate by other means. A sitting position improves pulmonary function and assists in venous pooling. Cardiac workload should be decreased by placing the patient on strict bed rest and by reducing pain and anxiety.

2. **Pharmacologic treatment**

   a. **Morphine sulfate** reduces anxiety and dilates pulmonary and systemic veins. Morphine, 2–5 mg IV, can be given over several minutes and can be repeated every 10–25 minutes until an effect is seen.

   b. **Furosemide** is a potent venodilator and decreases pulmonary congestion within minutes of IV administration, well before its diuretic action begins. An initial dose of 20–40 mg IV should be given over several minutes and can be increased based on response, to a maximum of 200 mg in subsequent doses.

   c. **Nitroglycerin** is a venodilator that can potentiate the effect of furosemide. Administration IV is preferable to oral and transdermal forms because it may be rapidly titrated.

   d. **Nitroprusside** [see sec. **II.C.2.b.(2)**] is an effective adjunct in the treatment of acute CPE. It is useful in CPE that results from acute valvular regurgitation or hypertension (see Valvular Heart Disease, sec. **III.B.2.a**). Pulmonary and systemic arterial catheterization should be considered to guide titration of nitroprusside therapy.

   e. **Inotropic agents** such as dobutamine or phosphodiesterase inhibitors may be helpful after initial treatment of CPE in patients with concomitant hypotension or shock (see sec. **II.C.6**).

3. **Acute hemodialysis and ultrafiltration** may be effective, especially in the patient with significant renal dysfunction and diuretic resistance.

4. **Right heart catheterization** (e.g., Swan-Ganz catheter) may be helpful in cases in which a prompt response to therapy does not occur. The pulmonary artery catheter allows differentiation between cardiogenic and noncardiogenic causes of pulmonary edema via measurement of central hemodynamics and cardiac output and helps to guide subsequent therapy (see Chap. 5, Myocardial Infarction, sec. **V.C,** and Chap. 9).

5. **Precipitating factors should be corrected.** Common precipitants of pulmonary edema include severe hypertension, MI or myocardial ischemia (particularly if associated with MR), acute valvular regurgitation, new-onset tachyarrhythmias or bradyarrhythmias, and volume overload in the

setting of severe LV dysfunction. Successful resolution of pulmonary edema can often be accomplished only by correction of the underlying process.

Cardiomyopathy

I. **Dilated cardiomyopathy** is a disease of heart muscle characterized by dilatation of the cardiac chambers and reduction in ventricular contractile function. Dilatation may be secondary to progression of any process that causes HF, although certain etiologies appear primarily to cause an isolated myopathic process (see Table 6-1). The majority of cases are idiopathic.
   A. **Pathophysiology and clinical features.** Dilatation of the cardiac chambers and varying degrees of hypertrophy are anatomic hallmarks. Symptomatic HF often is present. Tricuspid and MR are common due to the effect of chamber dilatation on the valvular apparatus. Atrial and ventricular arrhythmias are seen in as many as one-half of these patients and probably are responsible for the high incidence of sudden death in this population.
   B. **Diagnosis.** The diagnosis can be confirmed with echocardiography or radio-nuclide ventriculography. Two-dimensional and Doppler echocardiography is helpful in differentiating this condition from hypertrophic or restrictive cardiomyopathy, pericardial disease, and valvular disorders. The ECG is usually abnormal, but changes are typically nonspecific. Endomyocardial biopsy provides little information that affects treatment of patients with dilated cardiomyopathies and is not routinely recommended (*Am Heart J* 124:1251, 1992).
   C. **The medical management** of symptomatic patients is similar to that for HF from any cause. The therapeutic strategies include control of total body sodium and volume as well as appropriate preload and afterload reduction using vasodilator therapy. β-Adrenergic antagonists should be used unless a contraindication exists or they are poorly tolerated. Immunizations against influenza and pneumococcal pneumonia are recommended. Additional therapeutic considerations are as follows.
      1. **Complex ventricular ectopy,** including nonsustained ventricular tachycardia (NSVT), is often seen during ambulatory monitoring of these patients. Patients with complex ventricular ectopy and HF experience a high incidence of sudden death. However, the empiric use of antiarrhythmic agents for NSVT has not been shown to improve survival and could result in drug-induced depression of ventricular function, proarrhythmic effects, or both (*N Engl J Med* 321:406, 1989). The value of signal-averaged ECGs and electrophysiologic studies for the prediction of sudden death in patients with dilated cardiomyopathy is controversial (see Chap. 7). Patients with dilated cardiomyopathy and asymptomatic NSVT should be treated with aggressive medical therapy to improve HF symptoms and myocardial ischemia (if present). Electrolyte imbalances should be corrected, and proarrhythmic drugs should be discontinued. Patients in high-risk groups, including those with (1) a history of sudden cardiac death, (2) sustained VT, (3) ischemic cardiomyopathy (ejection fraction <35%) and NSVT or inducible VT, and (4) nonischemic cardiomyopathy (ejection fraction <35%) with inducible VT should be considered for an implantable cardioverter-defibrillator (see Chap. 7) because of a documented survival advantage (*N Engl J Med* 337:1576, 1997; *N Engl J Med* 335:1933, 1996; *N Engl J Med* 341:1882, 1999).
      2. **Chronic oral anticoagulation** has not been shown to decrease the risk of thromboembolism in patients with LV dysfunction. Anticoagulation should be strongly considered in patients with a history of thromboembolic events, atrial fibrillation, or evidence of a LV thrombus. The level

of anticoagulation recommended varies but is generally an international normalized ratio of 2.0–3.0 (see Chap. 19).

3. **Immunosuppressive therapy** with agents such as prednisone, azathioprine, and cyclosporine for biopsy-proven active myocarditis has been advocated by some, but efficacy has not been established (*N Engl J Med* 333:269, 1995).

D. **Surgical management.** Primary valvular disease and coronary disease should be evaluated and surgically corrected as indicated (see Valvular Heart Disease and Chap. 5). Coronary revascularization reduces ischemia and may improve systolic function in some patients with coronary artery disease. Intra-aortic balloon counterpulsation or placement of a ventricular assist device may be necessary for stabilization of patients in whom cardiac transplantation is an option or before other definitive surgical therapies.

II. **HCM** is a myocardial disorder characterized by ventricular hypertrophy, diminished LV cavity dimensions, normal or enhanced contractile function, and impaired ventricular relaxation. The idiopathic form of HCM has an early onset (as early as the first decade of life) without associated hypertension. Many cases have a genetic component, with mutations in the myosin heavy-chain gene that follow an autosomal dominant transmission with variable phenotypic expressivity and penetrance. An acquired form also occurs in elderly patients with chronic hypertension.

A. **The pathophysiologic changes** in HCM are myocardial hypertrophy that is typically predominant in the ventricular septum (asymmetric hypertrophy) but may involve all ventricular segments equally. The disease can be classified according to the presence or absence of LV outflow tract obstruction. LV outflow obstruction may occur at rest but is enhanced by factors that increase LV contractility or decrease ventricular volume. Delayed ventricular diastolic relaxation and decreased compliance are common and may lead to pulmonary congestion. Myocardial ischemia occurs and is likely secondary to a myocardial oxygen supply-demand mismatch. Systolic anterior motion of the anterior leaflet of the mitral valve often is associated with MR and may contribute to LV outflow tract obstruction.

B. **The clinical presentation** varies but may include dyspnea, angina, arrhythmias, syncope, cardiac failure, or sudden death. Patients of all ages may be affected, but sudden death is most common in children and young adults between the ages of 10 and 35 years and often occurs during periods of strenuous exertion. Physical findings include a bisferious carotid pulse (in the presence of obstruction), a forceful double or triple apical impulse, and a coarse systolic outflow murmur localized along the left sternal border that is accentuated by maneuvers that decrease preload (e.g., Valsalva maneuver).

C. **The diagnosis** is suspected on the basis of clinical presentation or a family history suggestive of familial HCM and is confirmed by two-dimensional echocardiography. Doppler flow studies may be useful in establishing the presence of a significant LV outflow gradient at rest or with provocation.

D. **Management** is directed toward relief of symptoms and prevention of endocarditis, arrhythmias, and sudden death. Treatment in asymptomatic individuals is controversial, and no conclusive evidence has been found that medical therapy is beneficial. **All individuals with HCM should avoid strenuous physical activity,** including most competitive sports.

1. **Medical therapy**

a. **β-Adrenergic antagonists** may reduce symptoms of HCM by reducing myocardial contractility and heart rate. Unfortunately, symptoms may recur during long-term therapy. Many patients show improvement with oral doses of propranolol in the range of 160–320 mg/day (or an equivalent dose of another β-adrenergic antagonist). Higher doses of β-adrenergic antagonist therapy may be necessary in patients with refractory or recurrent symptoms, although dosages in excess of 480 mg/day are associated with a higher incidence of side effects.

   b. **Calcium channel antagonists,** particularly **verapamil** and **diltiazem,** often improve the symptoms of HCM, primarily by augmentation of diastolic ventricular filling. Because of their vasodilatory properties, the dihydropyridines should be avoided in patients with LV outflow tract obstruction. Therapy should be initiated at low doses, with careful hemodynamic monitoring in patients with outflow obstruction. The dose should be increased gradually over several days to weeks if symptoms persist.

   c. **Diuretics** may improve pulmonary congestive symptoms in patients with elevated pulmonary venous pressures (particularly in the small subset of patients in whom a congestive form of cardiomyopathy develops). These agents should be used cautiously in patients with severe LV outflow obstruction because excessive preload reduction will worsen the obstruction.

   d. **Nitrates and vasodilators should be avoided** because of the risk of increasing the LV outflow gradient.

2. **Atrial and ventricular arrhythmias occur commonly** in patients with HCM. Supraventricular tachyarrhythmias are tolerated poorly and should be treated aggressively; direct current cardioversion is indicated if hemodynamic compromise develops. **Digoxin is relatively contraindicated** because of its positive inotropic properties and potential for exacerbating ventricular outflow obstruction. Atrial fibrillation should be converted to sinus rhythm when possible. Diltiazem, verapamil, or β-adrenergic antagonists can be used to control the ventricular response before cardioversion. Procainamide, disopyramide, or amiodarone (see Chap. 7) may be effective in the chronic suppression of atrial fibrillation. Patients with NSVT detected on ambulatory monitoring are at increased risk for sudden death. However, the benefit of suppressing these arrhythmias with medical therapy has not been established, and the risk of a proarrhythmic effect of antiarrhythmic therapy exists. Invasive electrophysiologic testing or implantable cardioverter-defibrillator placement should be considered in high-risk patients (*N Engl J Med* 342:365, 2000). Symptomatic ventricular arrhythmias should be treated as outlined in Chap. 7.

3. **Dual-chamber pacing** (see Chap. 7) has been used successfully in treating patients with HCM (*Circulation* 85:2149, 1992). Alteration of the ventricular activation sequence via right ventricular (RV) pacing is a useful way to minimize LV outflow tract obstruction secondary to asymmetric septal hypertrophy. The effect of dual-chamber pacing on patient morbidity and mortality is not known.

4. **Prophylaxis for endocarditis** is indicated (see Chap. 14).

5. **Anticoagulation** is recommended if paroxysmal or chronic atrial fibrillation develops.

6. **Surgical therapy** is useful in the treatment of symptoms but has not been shown to alter the natural history of HCM. The most frequently used operative procedure involves septal myotomy or myectomy or mitral valve replacement (MVR).

III. **Restrictive cardiomyopathy** results from pathologic infiltration of the myocardium by a variety of processes such as amyloidosis and sarcoidosis. Less common causes include glycogen storage diseases, hemochromatosis, endomyocardial fibrosis, and hypereosinophilic syndromes.

   A. **Pathophysiology and diagnosis.** Myocardial infiltration results in abnormal diastolic ventricular filling and varying degrees of systolic dysfunction, depending on the duration and nature of the underlying disease. Echocardiography may reveal thickening of the myocardium and varying degrees of systolic ventricular dysfunction. Doppler echocardiographic analysis may demonstrate evidence of abnormal diastolic filling patterns and elevated venous pressure. The ECG may show conduction system disease or low voltage, in contrast to the increased voltage seen with ventricular hypertrophy. Cardiac catheterization reveals elevated RV and LV filling pressures and a classic dip-and-plateau pattern in the RV and LV pressure tracing. RV endomyocardial biopsy may be diagnostic and should be considered in patients in whom a diagnosis is not established. **It is often difficult to differentiate between restrictive cardiomyopathy and constrictive pericarditis** because of similar clinical presentations and hemodynamics, but this distinction is critical, as surgical therapy may be effective for constrictive pericarditis.

B. Management
   1. **General measures** include judicious use of diuretics for pulmonary and systemic congestion and digoxin if LV systolic dysfunction is present. **Digoxin should be avoided in patients with cardiac amyloidosis** because of these patients' enhanced susceptibility to digoxin toxicity. In some cases, vasodilator therapy may be beneficial, but these agents should be used with caution to avoid excessive reduction in preload; elevated filling pressures may be required to maintain adequate cardiac output.
   2. **Specific therapy aimed at amelioration of the underlying cause should be instituted.** Cardiac hemochromatosis may respond to reduction of total body iron stores via phlebotomy or chelation therapy with deferoxamine. Cardiac sarcoidosis may respond to glucocorticoid therapy, but prolongation of survival with this approach has not been established. No therapy is known to be effective in reversing the progression of cardiac amyloidosis.

Pericardial Disease

 I. **Constrictive pericarditis** may develop as a late complication of pericardial inflammation. Most cases are idiopathic, but postpericardiotomy syndrome following cardiac surgery and mediastinal irradiation are important identifiable causes. Tuberculous pericarditis is a leading cause of constrictive pericarditis in some underdeveloped countries.
   A. **Pathophysiology and diagnosis.** The noncompliant pericardium causes impairment of ventricular filling and progressive elevation of venous pressure. In contrast to cardiac tamponade, the clinical presentation is characteristically insidious, with gradual development of fatigue, exercise intolerance, and venous congestion. Physical findings include jugular venous distention with prominent X and Y descents, inspiratory elevation of the jugular venous pressure (Kussmaul's sign), peripheral edema, ascites, and a pericardial knock during diastole. Echocardiography may reveal pericardial thickening and diminished diastolic filling. In addition, a chest CT scan or MRI may detect pericardial thickening. Cardiac catheterization usually is necessary to demonstrate elevated and equalized diastolic pressures in all four cardiac chambers. Constrictive pericarditis often is difficult to distinguish from restrictive cardiomyopathy (see Cardiomyopathy, sec. **III.A**).
   B. **Definitive treatment requires complete pericardiectomy,** which is accompanied by significant perioperative mortality (5–10%) but results in clinical improvement in 90% of patients. Patients who are minimally symptomatic can be managed with judicious sodium and fluid restriction and diuretic therapy but must be followed closely to detect hemodynamic deterioration.
II. **Cardiac tamponade** results from increased intrapericardial pressure secondary to fluid accumulation within the pericardial space. Pericarditis of any cause may lead to cardiac tamponade. Idiopathic (or viral) and neoplastic forms are the most frequent etiologies.
   A. **The diagnosis** should be suspected in patients with elevated jugular venous pressure, hypotension, pulsus paradoxus, tachycardia, evidence of poor

peripheral perfusion, and distant heart sounds. The ECG often reveals a tachycardia with low-voltage and electrical alternans. Echocardiography can confirm the diagnosis of pericardial effusion and demonstrate hemodynamic significance by right atrial and RV diastolic collapse, increased right-sided flows during inspiration, and respiratory variation of the transmitral flow. Right heart catheterization also is helpful in determining the hemodynamic significance of a pericardial effusion, especially in patients with a subacute or chronic presentation. Hemodynamic findings of elevated, equalized diastolic pressures are present in the patient with cardiac tamponade.

B. **Treatment consists of drainage of the pericardial space** via pericardiocentesis or surgical pericardiotomy. Urgent pericardiocentesis should be performed with echocardiographic guidance, if possible. If pericardial drainage cannot be performed, stabilization with parenteral inotropic support and aggressive administration of IV saline to maintain adequate ventricular filling are indicated. **Diuretics, nitrates, or any other preload-reducing agents are absolutely contraindicated.**

Valvular Heart Disease

I. **MS** impedes blood flow from the lungs and left atrium into the left ventricle. Rheumatic heart disease is the most common etiology; much less commonly, MS may result from calcium deposition in the mitral annulus and leaflets, from a congenital valvular malformation, or in association with connective tissue disorders. Left atrial myxoma and cor triatriatum may mimic MS clinically. Prosthetic mitral valves (particularly bioprosthetic valves) may become stenotic late after implantation.

A. **Pathophysiology.** Significant MS results in elevation of left atrial, pulmonary venous, and pulmonary capillary pressures, with consequent pulmonary congestion. The degree of pressure elevation depends on the severity of obstruction, flow across the valve, time allowed for diastolic filling, and presence of effective atrial contraction. Therefore, factors that augment flow across the mitral valve, such as tachycardia, exercise, fever, and pregnancy, result in a marked increase in left atrial pressure and may exacerbate HF symptoms. Left atrial enlargement and fibrillation may result in atrial thrombus formation, which is primarily responsible for the high incidence (20%) of systemic embolization in patients with MS who are not anticoagulated.

B. **Diagnosis.** Symptoms of pulmonary congestion, such as dyspnea, cough, and, occasionally, hemoptysis, are prominent. Physical signs of pulmonary venous congestion and right heart volume and pressure overload often are present. A loud first heart sound, early diastolic opening snap, and rumbling diastolic murmur are present on auscultation. The diagnosis and severity of MS can be confirmed by two-dimensional and Doppler echocardiography. Transesophageal echocardiography (TEE) can also be used to confirm the diagnosis, define the anatomy more fully, and provide diagnostic information in patients in whom transthoracic echocardiography is suboptimal. Cardiac catheterization is indicated in patients in whom there is a likelihood of concomitant coronary artery disease and in whom echocardiographic studies are either technically suboptimal or nondiagnostic.

C. **Medical management**
   1. **Factors that increase left atrial pressure,** including tachycardia and fever, should be identified and alleviated. Vigorous physical activity should be avoided in patients with moderate to severe MS.
   2. **Diuretics** (see Heart Failure, sec. **II.C.6,** and Table 6-4) are the mainstay of therapy for pulmonary congestion and edema.
   3. **Anticoagulant therapy** is indicated for patients with MS and atrial fibrillation, because they are at high risk for thromboembolic events. Heparin

therapy should be instituted at the onset of atrial fibrillation, followed by long-term warfarin therapy (see Chap. 19). In the absence of prior embolic events, marked left atrial enlargement, or demonstrable atrial thrombi, patients with sinus rhythm do not require anticoagulation.

4. **Atrial fibrillation may not be well tolerated.** Synchronized direct current cardioversion should be performed if hemodynamic compromise (hypotension, pulmonary edema, and angina) accompanies the onset of atrial fibrillation. In less urgent situations, the ventricular response rate to atrial fibrillation can be controlled without cardioversion (see Chap. 7). Ultimately, an attempt to restore and maintain sinus rhythm is indicated except in the presence of marked left atrial enlargement (i.e., >6 cm). After institution of rate control measures, elective chemical or electrical cardioversion should be attempted (see Chap. 7) but should be preceded by anticoagulation therapy for at least 3 weeks to minimize the risk of systemic embolization on resumption of normal sinus rhythm. After conversion to sinus rhythm has been accomplished, antiarrhythmics can be continued in an effort to maintain sinus rhythm.

5. **Infective endocarditis prophylaxis is indicated** (see Chap. 14).

6. **Continuous prophylaxis against recurrent rheumatic fever** is indicated in young patients, patients at high risk for streptococcal infection (parents of young children, schoolteachers, medical and military personnel, and those in crowded living conditions), and those who have had acute rheumatic fever within the previous 5 years (see Chap. 14).

D. **Surgical considerations**

1. **Patients with severe symptoms** or pulmonary hypertension and significant MS (mitral valve area <1 cm^2/m^2 body surface area) should undergo commissurotomy or MVR.

2. **Patients with mild to moderate symptoms** generally show improvement with diuretic therapy and can be followed with serial echocardiograms.

3. **A single systemic thromboembolic event** does not necessarily mandate MVR. However, the recurrence rate of systemic thromboembolism in patients with MS is high, even with systemic anticoagulation, and MVR should be strongly considered.

4. **Percutaneous balloon mitral valvuloplasty** can reduce the mitral valve pressure gradient and improve cardiac output in patients with MS. This procedure can be considered an alternative to surgery and carries acceptable morbidity and mortality in select patients without significant MR or severe valvular calcification.

II. **AS** in the adult population may result from (1) calcification and degeneration of a normal valve, (2) calcification and fibrosis of a congenitally bicuspid aortic valve, or (3) rheumatic valvular disease.

A. **Pathophysiology.** AS produces a pressure gradient between the left ventricle and the aorta, causing pressure overload of the left ventricle that leads to concentric hypertrophy. As a result, LV compliance is reduced, LV end-diastolic pressure (LVEDP) rises, and myocardial oxygen demand is increased. Elevated LVEDP decreases the perfusion pressure across the myocardium, leading to subendocardial ischemia.

B. **Diagnosis.** The diagnosis of significant AS may be difficult, as the condition may be asymptomatic for a number of years. Clinical suspicion often is raised by the presence of one or more of the classic symptoms in the triad of angina, syncope, and HF. Physical findings include a slowly rising carotid pulse that is sustained (pulsus parvus et tardus) and a mid- to late-peaking systolic murmur that is typically harsh in quality. The pressure gradient across the stenotic aortic valve is directly related to the severity of obstruction and cardiac output. Therefore, the intensity of the systolic murmur may diminish as the cardiac output decreases with increasingly severe AS. In general, murmurs of long duration that peak late in systole indicate severe AS. Doppler echocardiography provides a noninvasive estimation of the aortic valve gradient and aortic valve area, which correlates well with the findings at cardiac catheterization. Most patients being considered for aortic valve replacement (AVR) require preoperative cardiac catheterization to determine the extent of concomitant coronary artery disease.

C. **Medical management**

1. **Infective endocarditis** occurs with increased frequency, and prophylaxis is indicated (see Chap. 14).

2. **Vigorous exercise and physical activity** should be avoided in patients with moderate to severe AS.

3. **Atrial (and ventricular) arrhythmias are poorly tolerated** and should be treated aggressively (see Chap. 7).

4. **Digoxin may be useful** in patients with HF in the presence of LV dilatation and impaired systolic function. However, in severe AS caused by the fixed obstruction of LV outflow, inotropic therapy is of little benefit.

5. **Diuretics may be useful** in treating congestive symptoms but must be used with extreme caution. Reduction of LV filling pressure in patients with AS may decrease cardiac output and systemic BP.

6. **Nitrates and other vasodilators should be avoided** in patients with severe AS, if possible. These agents reduce LV filling pressure and may lower systemic BP, resulting in hemodynamic collapse. Patients with AS in whom angina develops occasionally require treatment with nitroglycerin. Such therapy should be initiated only under strict supervision by a physician at the bedside. Volume expansion with saline may be necessary to avoid excessive preload reduction. If nitroglycerin results in hypotension that does not respond to aggressive volume expansion, parenteral inotropic agents (e.g., dobutamine), vasopressors, or both should be given.

7. **Asymptomatic patients with mild to moderate AS** can be followed closely with clinical assessment and Doppler echocardiography performed at 6- to 12-month intervals.

D. **Surgical considerations**

1. Symptomatic patients should undergo evaluation for AVR, including two-dimensional and Doppler echocardiography. In patients with suboptimal transthoracic echocardiograms, TEE may be helpful. Coronary arteriography should be performed in men older than 40 years and women older than 50 years, as well as in all patients with anginal symptoms; left ventriculography is indicated in patients with coexistent MR (although a high-quality transthoracic echocardiogram or a TEE may provide adequate information and limit the total amount of contrast material administered). **Patients with severe AS (aortic valve area <0.75 cm^2) should undergo AVR** unless comorbid conditions preclude surgery. Asymptomatic patients with severe AS are rare and should be considered for AVR if LV dilatation or decreased systolic function is present. Patients with significant concomitant coronary artery disease should undergo surgical revascularization at the time of AVR, because current surgical techniques have limited the morbidity and mortality of the combined procedure to nearly that of AVR alone.

2. **Intra-aortic balloon counterpulsation** may stabilize patients with critical AS and hemodynamic decompensation until AVR can be accomplished. It should not be used when significant aortic insufficiency (AI) coexists with AS.

3. **Percutaneous balloon aortic valvuloplasty** can reduce the aortic valve gradient and improve symptoms and LV function with relatively low morbidity and mortality in selected patients. Unfortunately, restenosis occurs in approximately 50% of patients within 6 months. At present, use of this therapeutic modality should **be limited to patients who are poor surgical candidates.**

III. MR

A. Chronic MR, as an isolated lesion, is caused most commonly by myxomatous degeneration of the mitral valve. Other etiologies include rheumatic heart disease, calcification of the mitral valve annulus, coronary artery disease with associated papillary muscle dysfunction, infective endocarditis, and connective tissue diseases (e.g., Marfan's syndrome, Ehlers-Danlos syndrome). MR may occur as a secondary phenomenon in patients with LV dilatation.

1. **Pathophysiology.** Chronic MR imposes volume overload on the left ventricle as a result of regurgitation of a fraction of the LV blood flow into the left atrium. Normal forward cardiac output is maintained early in the course of the disease, but, with progressive MR, compensatory mechanisms no longer accommodate increasing LV end-diastolic volume. Accordingly, ejection fraction falls, and symptoms of right and left HF develop.

2. **Diagnosis.** The diagnosis is suggested by characteristic physical findings of well-preserved carotid pulsations, an enlarged point of maximal impulse, and an apical holosystolic murmur. Doppler and two-dimensional echocardiography may confirm the diagnosis, estimate the severity of MR, and provide clues to its etiology. TEE is particularly useful for the evaluation of the mitral valve and is used instead of left ventriculography in some institutions.

3. **Medical management**

   a. **Infective endocarditis prophylaxis** should be given (see Chap. 14).

   b. **Anticoagulant therapy** should be considered, particularly in the presence of atrial fibrillation, an enlarged left atrium, or a previous embolic event. However, the incidence of thromboembolic events is lower than in MS.

   c. **Atrial fibrillation should be anticipated** in the later stages of MR as the left atrium dilates, and it should be treated as outlined in sec. **I.C.3–4.**

   d. **Vasodilators provide hemodynamic improvement** in MR by reducing SVR, thus decreasing the mitral regurgitant fraction and augmenting forward cardiac output. Beneficial effects have been demonstrated with nitroprusside, captopril, enalapril, and hydralazine.

   e. **Digoxin may be useful** in the presence of impaired LV systolic function.

   f. **Diuretics** are useful for treating congestive symptoms.

   g. **Nitrates** can also be used to reduce preload and ventricular size, which may decrease the severity of MR.

4. **Surgical considerations**

   a. **Patients with moderate to severe symptoms** despite medical therapy should be considered for mitral valve repair or replacement, if the LV ejection fraction is greater than 40%.

   b. **Patients with severe MR** secondary to LV dilatation associated with depressed LV systolic function (ejection fraction <25%) may experience decreased symptoms and demonstrate improved cardiac output after mitral valve repair (*Am Heart J* 129:1165, 1995).

   c. **Patients with minimal or no symptoms** should be followed closely with assessment of LV size and systolic function (by echocardiography or radionuclide ventriculography) every 6–12 months. Patients should be considered for mitral valve repair (or replacement) when the echocardiographic end-systolic dimension exceeds 45 mm or an angiographic end-systolic volume exceeds 55 ml/m² (*Chest* 108:842, 1995). Generally, by the time that a decrease in ejection fraction is noted, marked LV dysfunction has occurred and MVR with its attendant increase in LV afterload may be poorly tolerated or may fail to improve the patient's symptoms.

B. Acute MR can result from papillary muscle dysfunction or rupture caused by myocardial ischemia or infarction, infective endocarditis with flail or perforated leaflets, severe myxomatous disease with rupture of a chorda that results in a flail leaflet, or trauma.

1. **Pathophysiology.** The pathophysiologic features of acute MR differ from those of chronic MR in that compensatory increases in left atrial and LV compliance do not occur. The result is a sudden increase in pulmonary venous pressure that leads to acute pulmonary edema. Acute MR frequently results in cardiogenic shock.

2. **Medical management**
   a. **Afterload reduction** should be initiated urgently with sodium nitroprusside [see Heart Failure, sec. **II.C.1.b.(2)**] and should be guided by systemic BP and central hemodynamic monitoring. Approximately 50% of patients with acute MR can be stabilized in this manner, allowing MVR to proceed under more controlled conditions.
   b. **Diuretics** (see Heart Failure, sec. **II.C.6**), with or without nitrates, can be used (as the systemic BP tolerates) to relieve pulmonary congestion. However, the direct venodilatory effect of nitroprusside may render other preload-reducing maneuvers unnecessary.
   c. **Intra-aortic balloon counterpulsation** is indicated in cases of severe hemodynamic instability to reduce SVR and improve forward cardiac output.

3. **Surgical therapy.** Surgery is indicated urgently in patients with acute MR and hemodynamic compromise whose condition cannot be stabilized medically. In those with infective endocarditis who are hemodynamically stable, MVR should be delayed for several days while antibiotic therapy is initiated. If refractory hemodynamic deterioration develops, surgery should not be delayed.

IV. **AI** may result from an abnormality of the aortic valve itself, dilatation and distortion of the aortic root, or both. Causes of valvular AI include rheumatic fever, endocarditis, trauma, connective tissue diseases, and congenital bicuspid aortic valve. Dilatation or distortion of the aortic root may be due to systemic hypertension, ascending aortic dissection, syphilis, cystic medionecrosis, Marfan's syndrome, or ankylosing spondylitis. Chronic AI typically presents insidiously, whereas acute AI usually manifests as severe HF and impending cardiogenic shock.

A. **Pathophysiology.** The diastolic regurgitant flow from the aorta into the left ventricle causes increased LV end-diastolic volume and pressure. In turn, the LV becomes dilated and hypertrophied, which maintains stroke volume and prevents further increase in LVEDP. In acute AI, the chronic compensatory mechanisms are not active, and, therefore, the increase in LVEDP is marked. In chronic AI, increases in peripheral resistance (e.g., hypertension) lead to increased regurgitant flow and raise diastolic filling pressure and volume.

B. **Diagnosis.** AI may be suspected on the basis of clinical findings, including a wide pulse pressure, bounding pulses, and an aortic diastolic murmur. The presence of AI can be confirmed by two-dimensional and Doppler echocardiography or cardiac catheterization with ascending aortography.

C. **Medical management.** Medical therapy is reserved for patients with chronic stable AI or for stabilization of patients with severe or acute AI before definitive surgical treatment.

1. **Treatment of underlying or precipitating causes,** such as endocarditis, syphilis, and connective tissue diseases, should occur concomitantly with treatment of HF.

2. **Patients should receive prophylaxis for endocarditis** (see Chap. 14).

3. **Strenuous physical activity should be restricted** in patients with AI and associated LV dysfunction. Activities that involve increases in isometric work (lifting heavy objects) are more detrimental than are activities such as walking or swimming.

4. **Fluid and salt restriction, diuretics, digoxin, and vasodilators** are the cornerstones of therapy for patients with chronic AI who have evidence of

LV dysfunction. Nifedipine may reduce the need for AVR in patients with symptomatic AI and normal LV function (*N Engl J Med* 331:689, 1994).

5. **Sodium nitroprusside or positive inotropes** (see Heart Failure, sec. **II.C**) should be used in a patient with acute AI to stabilize the patient's condition before AVR.

D. Surgical treatment

1. **AVR and repair of associated aortic root abnormalities** should be performed urgently in individuals with acute AI. In patients with infective endocarditis who are hemodynamically stable with medical therapy, AVR can be deferred for several days while treatment with antibiotics is initiated. Patients in whom hemodynamic instability develops require urgent surgery.

2. **AVR should be recommended in patients with severe chronic AI** in whom signs or symptoms of moderate HF (New York Heart Association functional class II–III) or LV dysfunction develop. Echocardiography should be performed serially and AVR considered when LV dilatation or LV systolic dysfunction becomes significant. The clinical outcome and extent of reversibility of LV dysfunction after AVR depend on the duration of dysfunction, dilatation of the left ventricle (end-systolic diameter and volume), and degree of systolic dysfunction.

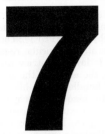

Cardiac Arrhythmias

Mitchell N. Faddis

Recognition and Diagnosis

I. **Clinical history and physical examination.** The treatment of cardiac arrhythmias begins with a thorough understanding of the range of symptoms that can be attributed to an arrhythmia and the manifestations of arrhythmias on physical examination. Clinically significant tachyarrhythmias may produce symptoms of palpitations, lightheadedness, dyspnea, angina, or syncope. Most patients who have an episode of a sustained tachyarrhythmia report the sensation of a rapid pulse or palpitations provided that they do not have syncope. A sudden onset and termination of the palpitations are highly suggestive of a tachyarrhythmia. Patients may report that a particular maneuver, such as Valsalva or breath-holding, may terminate the episode. Many forms of supraventricular tachycardia (SVT) can be terminated by vagal stimulation. Patients with a significant bradyarrhythmia may report exercise intolerance, fatigue, lightheadedness, or syncope. A history of familial or congenital causes of arrhythmias [e.g., hypertrophic cardiomyopathy, Wolff-Parkinson-White syndrome (WPW), congenital long QT syndrome, congenital structural heart disease, or maternal systemic lupus erythematosus], organic heart disease (e.g., ischemic, cardiomyopathic, valvular, etc.), or endocrinopathies (e.g., thyroid disease, pheochromocytoma, etc.) should be sought. A history of a toxic ingestion should be investigated. Physical examination should emphasize pulse rate and regularity. Blood pressure should be measured supine and standing with orthostatic changes recorded. A thorough cardiovascular examination should be performed as well as a search for signs of systemic disease. Serum electrolytes, CBC, and a toxicology screen should be considered for all patients under evaluation for a suspected arrhythmia.

II. **Clinical syndromes associated with arrhythmias.** The diagnosis of an arrhythmia may also be aided by the recognition of a particular clinical syndrome in which the arrhythmia participates.

A. **Sick sinus syndrome (SSS)** is usually a disorder of the elderly presumed to arise from intrinsic disease of the sinoatrial node caused by aging, or in association with structural heart disease. Extrinsic causes of sinus node dysfunction that should be excluded are hypothyroidism, hypothermia, or drugs that produce sinus node dysfunction, such as digoxin, antiarrhythmic agents (particularly amiodarone), beta-blockers, diltiazem, verapamil, or clonidine. The manifestations of SSS are often nonspecific and include palpitations, fatigue, confusion, and syncope. Symptoms arise from inappropriate sinus bradycardia or prolonged sinus pauses caused by sinus arrest, exit block, or both. Bradyarrhythmias may alternate with tachyarrhythmias, especially atrial fibrillation (AF), to create the tachycardia-bradycardia syndrome. The diagnosis of SSS is established by ECG or ambulatory monitoring in the majority of cases. Permanent pacemaker implantation is indicated for symptomatic bradycardia associated with SSS in the absence of a treatable or reversible medical condition.

B. **WPW** is characterized by pre-excitation on 12-lead ECG, defined as a short PR interval together with a delta wave slurring the upstroke of the QRS complex, and paroxysmal supraventricular tachycardia (PSVT). The most common form of associated PSVT is orthodromic atrioventricular re-entrant tachycardia (AVRT), in which excitation proceeds down the atrioventricular (AV) node with retrograde excitation, reaching the atria via the accessory pathway. The resultant SVT, in the absence of bundle branch block, has a normal QRS (not pre-excited). Less commonly, the associated tachyarrhythmia may be antidromic-AVRT in which conduction down the accessory pathway produces a fully pre-excited (wide) QRS complex. The retrograde limb of antidromic-AVRT proceeds through the His-Purkinje system and the AV node to the atria (see Mechanisms of Arrhythmia, sec. **III.E.2**). The most common wide-complex tachycardia seen in patients with WPW is orthodromic-AVRT with rate-related, bundle branch block, with antidromic-AVRT being less common. AF in patients with pre-excitation is of special concern, as the accessory pathway may facilitate a very rapid ventricular response to AF that can initiate ventricular fibrillation (VF).

C. **Syncope,** defined as the transient loss of consciousness and postural tone, is common in the general population. Of an unselected population, 40% report at least one lifetime syncopal event. Syncope accounts for approximately 6% of all hospital admissions. Because a syncopal event may herald an otherwise unsuspected, potentially lethal cardiac condition, a careful evaluation of the patient with syncope is warranted. The etiologies of syncope are myriad and can be divided into primary cardiac and noncardiac mechanisms. Primary cardiac syncope is caused either by mechanical obstruction of cardiac output (e.g., hypertrophic cardiomyopathy, valvular stenosis, aortic dissection, myxomas, pulmonary embolism) or by arrhythmias, including bradyarrhythmias (e.g., sinus node disease, AV node disease, conduction system disease, pacemaker malfunction) or tachyarrhythmias, including either SVTs or ventricular tachycardia (VT). Neurocardiogenic syncope is a common cause of syncope, particularly in those without underlying heart disease or other comorbidities. A variety of afferent neural pathways may participate in neurocardiogenic syncope, including mechanoreceptors and chemoreceptors in the heart, carotid body, and viscera. Efferent neural pathways result in peripheral vasodilatation and/or bradycardia leading to hypotension and syncope. Specific stimuli may evoke a neurocardiogenic mechanism leading to a situational syncope (e.g., associated with micturition, defecation, coughing, swallowing). Other noncardiac causes of syncope include orthostatic hypotension, toxic or metabolic influences (e.g., drug toxicities, hypoglycemia, hypoxia, etc.), neurologic etiologies (e.g., seizures or cerebrovascular events), and psychiatric etiologies (e.g., conversion disorders and anxiety disorders).

1. **History and physical examination.** The clinical history and physical examination have the highest utility for identification of a potential mechanism of a syncopal event. In addition to a careful interview of the patient, historical details should be sought from witnesses and emergency medical services personnel. Special attention should be focused on the events or symptoms that precede and follow the syncopal event, the time course of loss and resumption of consciousness (abrupt vs. gradual), and any description of vital signs before, during, and after the event. A characteristic prodrome of nausea, diaphoresis, or flushing preceding loss of consciousness suggests neurocardiogenic syncope, as does the identification of a particular emotional or situational trigger or a postsyncopal sensation of fatigue that lasts for many minutes to hours. Alternatively, an unusual sensory prodrome, incontinence, or a decreased level of consciousness that gradually clears suggests a seizure as a likely etiology. With transient ventricular arrhythmias, an abrupt loss of consciousness may occur with a rapid recovery. A clear history of palpitations is elicited infrequently. Physical examination should include

assessment of orthostatic vital signs and careful neurologic, pulmonary, and cardiovascular assessment. Bedside manipulations may be useful, including Valsalva maneuvers and squatting, with attention to cardiac auscultatory findings to detect valvular and subvalvular lesions. The diagnostic utility of carotid sinus massage is highest in patients with syncope and no structural cardiovascular disease. Carotid sinus massage should be performed in a monitored setting by trained personnel. Carotid sinus massage is contraindicated in patients with a carotid bruit.

2. **Diagnostic testing.** An initial 12-lead ECG and ECG monitoring (24- to 72-hour Holter recordings, patient-activated event recorders, implantable loop recorders) may lead to a diagnosis in only about 10% of cases. Routine laboratory tests typically are unhelpful; however, for patients with comorbid conditions or those who take electrophysiologically active drugs, such screening should be performed. Toxicology screening should be performed for suspected illicit drug use or inadvertent drug exposure. Two-dimensional echocardiography with Doppler flow studies should be performed in patients whose history or physical examination suggests the presence of structural heart disease. In the presence of a structurally normal heart, malignant ventricular arrhythmias are an uncommon cause of syncope. Invasive electrophysiologic studies (EPS) are most useful in patients with syncope and structural heart disease or a documented tachyarrhythmia. EPS in this setting is useful to identify an arrhythmic mechanism of syncope. Head-up tilt-table testing may be helpful in establishing a neurocardiogenic mechanism for syncope, although the test suffers from a low predictive value in unselected populations. Generally, it is performed in those with a structurally normal heart (or a negative EPS) and a clinical history suggestive of a neurocardiogenic mechanism. Neurologic or psychiatric testing is reserved for those with a suggestive clinical history. Routine CT scans, EEGs, or both in unselected patients with syncope are not supported by available data.

3. **Therapy.** Appropriate therapy for patients with syncope is determined by the underlying etiology. When the clinical history or diagnostic testing is suggestive of a neurocardiogenic mechanism, empiric therapy targeted at various aspects of the physiologic response may be initiated. Treatment can be targeted at minimizing the impact of peripheral vasodilatation by the use of support stockings, α agonists, or volume expansion with fludrocortisone. β-Adrenergic blockers may be useful to block peripheral adrenergic-mediated vasodilatation and to decrease cardiac inotropy. Disopyramide may have utility, probably through its strong negative inotropic action in reducing stimulation of ventricular mechanoreceptors, to prevent neurocardiogenic syncope. Centrally acting agents such as serotonin-reuptake inhibitors (SRI) or yohimbine may be useful to attenuate central reflex centers involved in neurocardiogenic mechanisms. Permanent dual-chamber pacemakers with a hysteresis function (high-rate pacing in response to a detected sudden drop in heart rate) have been shown to be useful in highly selected patients with recurrent neurocardiogenic syncope with a prominent cardioinhibitory component (*J Am Coll Cardiol* 33:16, 1999).

D. **Sudden cardiac death (SCD).** SCD is defined as a sudden death that occurs within 1 hour of the onset of symptoms. It accounts for 80–90% of all sudden nontraumatic deaths. In the United States, 350,000 cases of SCD occur annually. Among patients with aborted SCD, ischemic heart disease is the most common associated cardiac structural abnormality. Most cardiac arrest survivors do not evolve evidence of an acute myocardial infarction (MI); however, more than 75% have evidence of previous infarcts. In the absence of an acute MI, an underlying pathophysiologic cause should always be corrected if possible (e.g., aortic valve replacement in critical aortic

Table 7-1. Drugs associated with torsades de pointes

Amiodarone	Erythromycin	Perhexiline
Amitriptyline	FK506	Prenylamine
Astemizole	Flecainide	Probucol
Bepridil	Haloperidol	Procainamide
Bretylium	Ibutilide	Propafenone
Chlorpromazine	Imipramine	Quinidine
Cisapride	Indapamide	Quinine
Cocaine	Itraconazole	Sotalol
Disopyramide	Ketanserin	Sparfloxacin
Dofetilide	Ketoconazole	Sultopride
Doxepin	Maprotiline	Terfenadine
Droperidol	Moricizine	Terodiline
Encainide	Pentamidine	Thioridazine

stenosis, revascularization of critical multivessel coronary artery disease) (see Treatment, sec. **II.C**).

E. Congenital long QT syndrome. A familial history of SCD and a prolonged QT interval on a 12-lead ECG is suggestive of the congenital long QT syndrome. Considerable genetic and phenotypic heterogeneity has been identified in this syndrome. At present, the affected gene in approximately 50% of cases has been shown to be a cardiac ion channel. Beta-blocker therapy or unilateral sympathectomy has been shown retrospectively to decrease the mortality in this syndrome. Consideration of an implantable cardioverter-defibrillator (ICD) should be given for patients with a malignant family history (see Treatment, sec. **II.C.1**).

F. Acquired long QT syndrome. A variety of influences can prolong the QT interval in patients who do not have the congenital long QT syndrome and, thereby, promote torsades de pointes (TDP). Factors that have been associated with the acquired long QT syndrome include electrolyte abnormalities (hypokalemia, hypomagnesemia, and, rarely, hypocalcemia), drugs (Table 7-1), cardiac disease (ischemia or myocarditis), bradycardia, CNS disease (intracranial trauma, subarachnoid hemorrhage, or cerebrovascular accident), and toxic exposures (organophosphate poisoning, cesium). Therapy for sustained TDP is immediate direct current (DC) cardioversion. Reversal or treatment of the underlying condition should be undertaken, if possible, in patients who have had an episode of TDP or in whom the QT_c is greater than 500 milliseconds. Magnesium sulfate, 1–2 g administered by IV bolus up to 4–6 g, is highly effective in the treatment and prevention of drug-induced TDP. Elimination of long-short triggering sequences and shortening of the QT interval can be achieved by increasing the heart rate to the range of 90 to 120 beats/minute (bpm) by either IV isoproterenol infusion (initial rate at 2 µg/minute) or temporary transvenous pacing.

III. ECG data. For hemodynamically stable arrhythmias or arrhythmias that are transient in nature, ECG data should be used initially to identify the relationship between atrial and ventricular activation.

A. 12-lead ECG. Initial data should consist of a standard 12-lead ECG and a continuous rhythm strip with leads that best demonstrate atrial activation (e.g., V1, II, III, aVF). Comparison of a 12-lead ECG at baseline with that obtained during an arrhythmia can highlight subtle features of the QRS deflection that indicate the superposition of atrial and ventricular depolarization. The continuous rhythm strip (of at least 3 leads) documents (1) the effect of spontaneous atrial or ventricular depolarizations; (2) changes in rate, morphology, or regularity; and (3) the response to interventions (e.g., vagal maneuvers, antiarrhythmic drug therapy, electrical cardioversion). If atrial activity is not discernible in the available ECG leads, other recording methods that enhance detection of atrial activity can be considered, such as transesophageal or transvenous recordings.

B. **Continuous ambulatory ECG monitoring** for 24–72 hours may be useful for documentation of symptomatic transient arrhythmias that occur with sufficient frequency, such as sinus node dysfunction, or symptomatic ectopic beats. This recording mode is also useful for assessment of a patient's heart rate response to daily activities or response to an antiarrhythmic drug treatment. The correlation between patient-reported symptoms in a time-marked diary and heart rhythm recordings is helpful for diagnostic purposes. Clinically significant paroxysmal tachyarrhythmias may be missed by this recording method because of the finite recording period.

C. **Event recordings.** Patient-actuated ECG recording is useful for diagnosis of transient arrhythmias that occur infrequently. Three types of this recording mode are available. The first is a "loop" memory unit worn by the patient that continuously records the ECG. When the patient is symptomatic, the monitor is triggered and the ECG recording is saved with the preceding time period. A second type of ECG recording system is connected only when the patient experiences symptoms. A third type is an implantable loop memory unit, placed surgically, to provide automated or patient-actuated recording of significant arrhythmic events that occur infrequently over several months.

D. **Exercise ECG.** The 12-lead ECG recording during a standard exercise tolerance test is useful for studying exercise-induced arrhythmias or to assess the sinus response to exercise.

Mechanisms of Arrhythmia

I. **Premature complexes** represent the most common interruption of normal sinus rhythm (NSR), most frequently arising from the ventricles and less often from the atria and the AV node.

A. **Premature atrial complexes (PACs)** often occur in the absence of structural heart disease and are commonly seen in the clinical settings of infection, inflammation, myocardial ischemia, drug toxicity, catecholamine excess, electrolyte imbalance, or excessive use of tobacco, alcohol, or caffeine. Symptoms range from none to the sensation of "skipped" beats. PACs typically require no therapy. If they are symptomatic, therapy should be directed toward correction or removal of provocative stimuli. β-Adrenergic antagonists or calcium channel antagonists may be useful.

B. **Premature junctional complexes (PJCs)** often occur in the absence of structural heart disease. PJCs typically result in a premature, normally conducted QRS. With intact retrograde AV nodal conduction, an inverted P wave will occur on the ECG during or just after the inscription of the QRS. The next, normally timed sinus P wave may experience delay or block in the AV node, owing to retrograde conduction of the PJC. Symptoms and therapy are similar to those pertinent to PACs.

C. **Premature ventricular complexes (PVCs)** often occur in the absence of structural heart disease and are increasingly frequent with age. Potential triggers are similar to those for PACs. The frequency, the number of morphologies, and the occurrence of complex forms have limited prognostic significance. The ECG reveals a premature QRS complex with a bizarre morphology, typically greater than 120 milliseconds in duration, with a T-wave polarity opposite to that of the QRS complex. The patient may be asymptomatic or feel skipped beats. PVCs typically require no therapy. When patients are symptomatic, therapy should be directed toward correction of underlying abnormalities. β-Adrenergic antagonists may be useful to reduce PVC occurrence in symptomatic patients. Other antiarrhythmic agents may be effective in suppressing PVCs, but adverse effects (e.g., arrhythmia aggravation, proarrhythmia, death) preclude their widespread use (*N Engl J Med* 321:406, 1989). In the setting of acute myocardial ischemia or infarction, IV lidocaine may suppress PVCs but does not decrease mortality, and toxic effects (e.g., increased risk of asystole and CNS effects) appear to outweigh potential benefits in most cases.

II. **Bradyarrhythmias.** A bradyarrhythmia is any rhythm that results in a ventricular rate of less than 60 bpm. Mechanisms of bradyarrhythmias include the following.

   A. **A sinus pause or sinus arrest** occurs when the sinus node intermittently fails to produce an impulse or when sinus node inactivity is prolonged, respectively. Sinus pauses or sinus arrest are manifestations of sinus node dysfunction that result from intrinsic sinus node disease or extrinsic factors, particularly vagal stimulation. In the case of intrinsic sinus node disease, sinus pauses often occur after termination of a PSVT, particularly AF. Sinus pauses or arrest may produce lightheadedness or syncope. Sinus pauses that result in ventricular asystole of greater than 3 seconds in the awake patient are an indication for permanent pacemaker therapy in the absence of reversible causes.

   B. **Sinus bradycardia** is defined as a sinus rate of less than 60 bpm with a normal P-wave configuration consistent with an origin in the sinus node area. Increased vagal tone, drug effects, ischemia, and primary sinus node disease are typical etiologies. Affected patients may be asymptomatic or may complain of fatigue, exercise intolerance, dyspnea or angina with exertion, or confusion in elderly patients. Asymptomatic patients require no therapy. In symptomatic patients, therapy is directed toward the underlying etiology, and treatment includes atropine, 0.5 mg IV every 2 minutes to a maximum of 0.04 mg/kg, or cardiac pacing (see Treatment, sec. **I.B**).

   C. **AV block** occurs when an atrial impulse is conducted with delay or fails to conduct to the ventricle at a time when the AV node should not be refractory.

      1. **First-degree AV block** usually results from conduction delay within the AV node, but, rarely, intra-atrial delay or delay within the His-Purkinje system (often seen in conjunction with bundle branch block) may be responsible. The **ECG** reveals a PR interval greater than 200 milliseconds. **Etiologies** include increased vagal tone, a drug effect, electrolyte abnormalities, ischemia, and conduction system disease. First-degree block is usually asymptomatic but may exacerbate heart failure (HF) from loss of AV synchrony caused by an excessively prolonged PR interval. Asymptomatic patients require no therapy. In symptomatic patients, dual-chamber pacemaker therapy can be considered in the absence of treatable causes (see Treatment, sec. **I.B**).

      2. **Second-degree AV block** is present when some atrial impulses are not conducted to the ventricle when the AV node should not be refractory. Two types of second-degree AV block are recognized based on the pattern of impulse conduction, and distinctions between type I and type II are important, as they carry different prognostic implications.

         a. **Mobitz type I (Wenckebach) block** demonstrates progressive delay in AV conduction with successive atrial impulses, as evidenced by **progressive PR interval prolongation,** before the block of an atrial impulse. The characteristic ECG pattern is of QRS complexes occurring in regular groupings (grouped beating) separated by the blocked beat. The RR interval progressively shortens before a blocked P wave. The site of conduction block almost always is within the AV node. **Etiologies** include increased vagal tone, antiarrhythmic drug effects, electrolyte abnormalities, myocardial ischemia (typically in an inferior or posterior distribution), and conduction system disease. Mobitz type I block, especially with a normal QRS, is benign and usually does not portend development of complete heart block. Symptomatic type I AV block is managed initially with atropine, 0.5. mg IV every 2 minutes to a maximum of 0.04 mg/kg. For persistent symptoms, permanent pacemaker therapy should be instituted (see Treatment, sec. **I.B**).

  b. **Mobitz type II block** is characterized by abrupt AV conduction block without evidence of conduction delay in preceding conducted impulses. The **ECG** demonstrates no change in PR intervals preceding a nonconducted P wave. The site of block is localized most often to the His-Purkinje system. **Etiologies** include conduction system disease, antiarrhythmic drug effects, myocardial ischemia (typically in an anterior distribution), and increased vagal tone. Type II block, especially in the setting of a bundle branch block (BBB), often antedates the development of complete heart block. Symptoms may include fatigue, palpitations, lightheadedness, and syncope. Hemodynamically unstable patients should be treated initially with temporary transvenous pacemaker insertion followed by permanent pacemaker implantation. Because of the propensity for progression to complete heart block, asymptomatic patients can also be treated with permanent pacemaker implantation (see Treatment, sec. **I.B**). **Atropine should not be used to treat Mobitz type II block associated with BBB,** as this can exacerbate the degree of block by accelerating the sinus rate.

  c. **2:1 AV block** may be caused by either type I or type II mechanisms. The concomitant presence of bundle branch block or fascicular block suggests the presence of type II second-degree AV block.

3. **Third-degree (complete) AV block** is present when all atrial impulses fail to conduct to the ventricle and the prevailing ventricular escape rhythm is slower than the atrial rate. This pattern is distinct from **AV dissociation,** typically a benign condition, which is present when the ventricular rate exceeds the atrial rate. The site of block in complete AV block may be the AV node (as occurs in congenital heart block) or within the His-Purkinje system (typical for acquired heart block). **Etiologies** of acquired complete AV block include ischemia or infarction, drug toxicity, idiopathic degeneration of the conduction system, infiltrative diseases (amyloidosis, sarcoidosis, metastatic disease), rheumatologic disorders (polymyositis, scleroderma, rheumatoid nodules), infectious diseases (Chagas' disease, Lyme disease), calcific aortic stenosis, or endocarditis. Symptoms depend on the degree of bradycardia of the underlying escape rhythm and include lightheadedness, dyspnea, CHF, angina, and syncope. In the absence of reversible causes of complete heart block, permanent pacemaker therapy is indicated for acquired complete heart block. Congenital complete heart block with significant bradycardia (<45 bpm) can be treated with permanent pacemaker implantation to prevent a malignant ventricular arrhythmia.

III. **Tachyarrhythmias** are defined as heart rhythms with a rate in excess of 100 bpm and are further distinguished as being SVT or VT, depending on the mechanism and site of origin. Although the underlying mechanism of the tachycardia critically determines prognosis and therapy, initial investigation may allow only for characterization of the tachycardia as either narrow complex (QRS duration <120 milliseconds) or wide complex (QRS duration >120 milliseconds).

  A. **Narrow-complex tachycardias** that have an apparent 1:1 association between atrial and ventricular activation, visible on 12-lead ECG or rhythm strip, are almost exclusively supraventricular in origin. A differential diagnosis of tachycardia mechanisms can be generated on the basis of the **R-P**

interval, the time interval between the peak of an R wave and the subsequent P wave, during the tachycardia.

1. **Short R-P tachycardias** have an R-P interval that is less than 50% of the R-R interval. Arrhythmia mechanisms in this classification include the following.

   a. **"Typical" AV nodal re-entrant tachycardia (AVNRT).** This re-entrant rhythm occurs in patients who have functional dissociation of two discrete conduction pathways around the AV nodal region, so-called dual AV nodal physiology. The two pathways, which differ in conduction velocity and refractory period, are referred to as the "slow" and "fast" AV nodal pathways in reference to the relative conduction velocity. Conduction proceeds antegrade down the slow pathway with retrograde conduction up the fast pathway. Atrial and ventricular excitation occur concurrently with every tachycardia circuit.

   b. **Orthodromic AV re-entrant tachycardia (O-AVRT).** This accessory pathway–mediated re-entrant rhythm occurs when anterograde conduction to the ventricle takes place through the AV node and retrograde conduction to the atrium occurs through the accessory pathway.

   c. **Sinus tachycardia or ectopic atrial tachycardia (EAT)** associated with first-degree AV block sometimes occurs as a short R-P tachycardia. The two rhythms differ with respect to the P-wave axis and morphology. EAT may be due to either a triggered or automatic mechanism. Sinus tachycardia is usually secondary to a physiologic stimulus, although a syndrome of inappropriate sinus tachycardia has been described.

2. **Long R-P tachycardias** have an R-P interval that is greater than 50% of the RR interval. Arrhythmia mechanisms in this classification include the following.

   a. **Sinus tachycardia** (see sec. **III.A.1.c**)

   b. **EAT** (see sec. **III.A.1.c**)

   c. **"Atypical" AVNRT.** Less common than the "typical" form of AVNRT, this arrhythmia mechanism occurs when anterograde conduction proceeds over the fast AV nodal pathway with retrograde conduction over the slow AV nodal pathway in patients with dual AV nodal physiology (see sec. **III.A.1.a**).

   d. **O-AVRT mediated by an accessory bypass tract with slow or decremental conduction properties.** In this less common form of O-AVRT, retrograde conduction over the accessory pathway to the atrium proceeds slowly enough for atrial activation to occur in the second half of the RP interval (see sec. **III.A.1.b**). The associated tachycardia is often incessant and may be associated with a tachycardia-mediated cardiomyopathy.

B. **AF** is the most common sustained tachyarrhythmia for which patients seek treatment. It is typically a disease of the elderly, affecting as many as 10% of those older than 75 years. Thromboembolism as a result of AF may account for as many as 50% of all cerebrovascular accidents. Significant structural heart disease is often associated with AF, particularly valvular, hypertensive, and ischemic heart disease. Disease processes that increase atrial size or disrupt atrial conduction may increase the susceptibility to AF. Transient or reversible etiologies include cardiac surgery, hypertension, acute alcohol ingestion, theophylline or other stimulant toxicity, endocrinopathies (hypothyroidism, hyperthyroidism, pheochromocytoma), pericarditis, and MI. AF that occurs in the absence of structural heart disease is termed "lone" AF. An irregularly fluctuating baseline on the 12-lead ECG with an irregular and frequently rapid ventricular response (>100 bpm in the untreated patient) is a hallmark of the 12-lead ECG that is typical of AF. Symptoms include palpitations, skipped beats, lightheadedness, breathlessness, CHF, angina, and syncope. Therapies are discussed in Treatment, sec. **II.A.**

C. **Atrial flutter (AFL)** results from a single re-entrant circuit around functional or structural barriers to conduction within the atria. It may occur in structurally normal hearts but is seen more commonly in association with structural heart disease that predisposes to the development of AF. Prior cardiac surgery that involved an atriotomy incision may promote AFL by providing a nonconductive scar around which re-entry can occur. In typical or type I flutter (most common), the 12-lead ECG baseline has a characteristic "sawtooth" pattern that is apparent in the inferior leads (II, III, aVF), with an effective atrial rate of 280 to 350 bpm. The RR intervals may be regular, reflecting a fixed-ratio AV block (2:1, 3:1), or variable, reflecting a Wenckebach periodicity. In the presence of class Ia or class Ic antiarrhythmic drugs, AFL rates may be slowed substantially. Atypical or type II flutter lacks the characteristic sawtooth pattern of type I and may have atrial rates up to 420 bpm. Treatments are considered later in this chapter (see Treatment, sec. **II.A**).

D. **Multifocal atrial tachycardia** is an irregular SVT distinguished by at least three P-wave morphologies apparent on a 12-lead ECG. It often is associated with chronic obstructive pulmonary disease and HF and may be potentiated by concomitant therapy with theophylline. Therapy is targeted at treatment of the underlying pathophysiologic process.

E. **Wide-complex tachycardias** may be either supraventricular or ventricular in origin, and correct identification of the origin and mechanism of the tachycardia is critical to the selection of appropriate treatment. Demographic and ECG criteria are helpful in distinguishing between SVT and VT (see sec. **II.E.4.b**).

   1. **SVT with aberration** can present as a wide-complex tachycardia as a result of rate-dependent conduction block within one of the two major divisions of the His-Purkinje system **[right bundle branch block (RBBB), left bundle branch block (LBBB)]** or to the presence of a fixed intraventricular conduction defect.

   2. **Wide-complex tachycardias associated with WPW syndrome.** In the setting of WPW, three different wide-complex tachycardias are possible: orthodromic-AVRT with aberrant conduction, antidromic-AVRT, and pre-excited AF as described previously (see Recognition and Diagnosis, sec. **II.B**). Pre-excited AF deserves special consideration because of a propensity to initiate VF. The ECG is characterized by an irregularly undulating baseline without recognizable P waves, an irregular and typically rapid ventricular rate (180–300 bpm), and QRS complexes that demonstrate variable fusion between normal complexes and fully pre-excited (wide, bizarre) complexes. **For hemodynamically stable pre-excited AF, IV procainamide may be used, but AV nodal blocking agents (adenosine, calcium channel antagonists, digoxin) must be avoided,** as they may increase the ventricular rate paradoxically initiating VF. Hemodynamic compromise or clinical instability should be treated with prompt DC cardioversion.

   3. **Accelerated idioventricular rhythm (AIVR)** is a ventricular rhythm that arises from abnormal automaticity of the terminal Purkinje system or from the ventricular myocardium. It may occur with acute MI (particularly after reperfusion of an infarct-related coronary), drug toxicity (e.g., digitalis), or inflammatory processes. The ECG reveals a ventricular rate of 60–110 bpm, usually exceeding the spontaneous atrial rate. The QRS complex is wide (typically >120 milliseconds) and bizarre. Retrograde P waves can be seen in patients with retrograde AV conduction, whereas in those with retrograde AV block, narrow-complex or fusion beats (atrial capture) occasionally may be seen. AIVR is suppressed when the atrial rate exceeds the ventricular rate. AIVR usually is transient and asymptomatic but may be a cause of hemodynamic deterioration in patients who require AV synchrony. In symptomatic patients, therapy is directed at increasing the sinus rate (e.g., with atropine, isoproterenol, overdrive atrial pacing).

4. **VT** is the most frequently encountered life-threatening arrhythmia. It is defined as a series of three or more ventricular complexes that occur at a rate of 100–250 bpm, where the origin of activation is within the ventricle. Typically, the QRS is wide (usually >120 milliseconds), with T-wave polarity opposite to that of the major QRS deflection. Monomorphic VT, usually associated with significant structural heart disease, has a single QRS morphology throughout the arrhythmia, whereas polymorphic VT is characterized by an ever-changing QRS morphology. In the setting of significant structural heart disease, sustained VT (defined as an episode longer than 30 seconds) predicts a poor long-term prognosis. **Prompt recognition and acute treatment of an episode of VT are critical to prevent morbidity and cardiac arrest.** Coronary artery disease is the most common structural heart disease that predisposes to VT. Nonischemic cardiomyopathies, infiltrative diseases, infectious diseases (viral myocarditis, Chagas' disease, Lyme disease), congenital myocardial defects, inflammatory diseases that affect the myocardium (systemic lupus erythematosus, rheumatoid arthritis), surgical repairs for congenital heart disease, and primary and metastatic malignancies that involve the heart also may provide the substrate for VT. Finally, various distinct forms of VT have been described in otherwise normal patients without evidence of structural heart disease.

   a. **Symptoms** associated with an episode of sustained VT depend on the rate of the tachycardia. VT may be asymptomatic, particularly when the rate of the tachycardia is relatively slow, the patient is supine, and cardiac function is preserved. For faster tachycardias, symptoms include palpitations, breathlessness, lightheadedness, angina, and syncope. Untreated, VT may degenerate to VF, resulting in hemodynamic collapse and death.

   b. **Differentiation of SVT with aberrancy from VT** on the basis of analysis of the surface ECG may be critical in determining appropriate acute and chronic therapy. Features that favor VT include (1) absence of an RS complex in all precordial leads, (2) onset of R wave to nadir of S wave longer than 100 milliseconds in any precordial lead, (3) AV dissociation, (4) the presence of capture or fusion beats, and (5) QRS morphology criteria present in precordial leads $V_{1(2)}$ and V_6. One of two sets of QRS morphology criteria is applied, depending on whether the QRS in the tachycardia resembles an RBBB or an LBBB morphology. Features characteristic of RBBB morphology VT are, in $V_{1(2)}$, a monophasic R, QR, or RS morphology, and, in V_6, any Q wave, R-S ratio less than 1, or a monophasic R morphology. Features characteristic of LBBB morphology VT are, in $V_{1(2)}$, an R-wave duration greater than 30 milliseconds, a duration of greater than 60 milliseconds from onset of R to nadir of S wave, or notching in downstroke of S wave, and, in lead V_6, a QR or QS morphology (*Circulation* 83:1649, 1991).

   c. **Repetitive monomorphic VT** is a form of VT usually noted in the absence of structural heart disease. Episodes of VT are typically paroxysmal and nonsustained, with an LBBB morphology and an inferior axis. Intracardiac mapping in patients with this disorder usually demonstrates a single focus in the right ventricular outflow tract, although sites in the left ventricle have been described. The prognosis of this form of VT is benign; however, patients may suffer from symptoms of lightheadedness, palpitations, dyspnea, and angina.

5. **VF** is the result of rapid, repetitive activation of the ventricles from multiple coalescing and fractionating wave fronts of depolarization. It is associated with disorganized mechanical contraction, hemodynamic collapse, and sudden death. Any structural, toxic, or metabolic derangement that adversely affects the homogeneity of ventricular repolarization can pre-

dispose to VF. The ECG reveals irregular and rapid oscillations (250–400 bpm) of highly variable amplitude without uniquely identifiable QRS complexes or T waves. VF without an identifiable and reversible cause requires chronic therapy in the form of either prophylactic antiarrhythmic drug therapy (e.g., amiodarone, sotalol) or implantation of an ICD (see Treatment, sec. **II.C.1**).

Treatment

I. **Treatment of bradyarrhythmias.** Identification of reversible causes of symptomatic bradycardia should be undertaken immediately following diagnosis. Symptomatic sinus bradycardia, first-degree AV block, or Mobitz I second-degree AV block may respond acutely to atropine treatment, 0.5–2.0 mg IV. For irreversible causes and other mechanisms of symptomatic bradycardia, pacemaker therapy should be considered.

A. **Temporary pacemakers.** Temporary pacing can be achieved by either placement of an external transthoracic unit (external pacemaker-defibrillator combination) or insertion of a temporary transvenous pacemaker. Temporary pacing is indicated for symptomatic second- or third-degree heart block caused by transient drug intoxication or electrolyte imbalance. In the setting of an acute MI, complete heart block, or Mobitz II second-degree AV block, temporary pacing is required. In addition, a temporary pacemaker is indicated for Mobitz I second-degree AV block if the arrhythmia causes hemodynamic compromise or angina (see Chap. 5). Symptomatic sinus bradycardia, AF with a slow ventricular response, or other bradycardic manifestations of conduction system disease may necessitate temporary pacing until a permanent pacemaker can be inserted.

B. **Permanent pacemaker implantation.** Contemporary pacemakers can maintain AV synchrony and adapt the rate of pacing to mimic the normal physiologic heart rate response to exertion. Before the decision is made to implant a pacemaker, the indications, appropriate mode of pacing, and arrangements for follow-up should be considered.

1. **Pacing modalities.** A four-letter alphabetic code is used to identify pacing modalities. The first initial defines the chamber that is paced (**V**entricle, **A**trium, **D**ual chamber), the second identifies the chamber in which electrograms are sensed (**V**entricle, **A**trium, **D**ual chamber), the third indicates the response to a sensed event (**I**nhibited, **T**riggered, and **D**ual function), and the fourth, when present, denotes **R**ate response mode. The VVI and DDD modes are used most commonly. VVI units pace and sense in the ventricle; a sensed (native) event inhibits the ventricular stimulus. DDD units pace and sense in both chambers. Events sensed in the atrium inhibit the atrial stimulus and trigger a ventricular response after an appointed interval, whereas ventricle-sensed events inhibit ventricular and atrial outputs. Other pacing modalities, particularly DDI and DVI, are useful in patients with PSVT. Modern pacemakers have supraventricular tachyarrhythmia detection protocols that allow automatic switching of pacing modes to prevent rapid ventricular pacing in response to a PSVT.

2. **Permanent pacemaker indications** are discussed fully in joint recommendations from the American Heart Association and the American College of Cardiology (*J Am Coll Cardiol* 31:1175, 1998). Indications for permanent pacing are grouped into three classifications. Class I indications are conditions in which permanent pacing is considered to be acceptable and necessary for adequate treatment. Class II indications are conditions for which permanent pacing is considered acceptable as a therapy but some controversy exists. Class III indications are conditions for which permanent pacemaker therapy is considered inappropriate.

Symptomatic bradycardia, due to either sinus node dysfunction or AV nodal block, in the absence of a reversible cause, constitutes a class I indication for permanent pacing. Asymptomatic conditions that are also considered class I indications for permanent pacemaker implantation in adults include (1) AV block in the setting of myotonic dystrophy, (2) persistent advanced second-degree or third-degree AV block after acute MI with demonstrated block in the His-Purkinje system (BBB), (3) chronic bifascicular or trifascicular block with intermittent type II second- or third-degree AV block, and (4) third-degree AV block with an escape rate <40 bpm.

II. **Treatment of tachyarrhythmias.** The acute treatment of symptomatic tachyarrhythmias should follow the protocols of advanced cardiac life support outlined in Chap. 8. Chronic treatment for tachyarrhythmias is aimed at either prevention of recurrence or prevention of the complications associated with the specific tachyarrhythmia.

A. **AF and AFL**

1. **Indications for anticoagulation.** Chronic warfarin anticoagulation is the most effective therapy for attenuating the risk of stroke associated with AF and AFL (see Chap. 19). Clinical characteristics identifying those at increased risk for thromboembolic events include a previous transient ischemic attack, valvular heart disease, CHF, hypertension, diabetes, age older than 75 years, and coronary artery disease *(Arch Intern Med* 154:1449, 1994). Left atrial spontaneous echo contrast also appears to identify those at increased risk, although large clinical studies are lacking *(J Am Coll Cardiol* 24:755, 1994). Patients with thromboembolic risk factors and contraindications to anticoagulation should be given daily aspirin or, if aspirin intolerant, ticlopidine or clopidogrel. The need for anticoagulation and the role of aspirin are controversial in patients younger than 65 years with no risk factors for thromboembolic events because of the low rate of strokes in this population.

2. **Rate control** of the ventricular response to AF or AFL can be achieved with agents that prolong conduction through the AV node. These include diltiazem, verapamil, β-adrenergic blockers, and digoxin. In patients with severe LV systolic dysfunction, digoxin may be the only agent tolerated because of the negative inotropic effect of calcium channel blockers and β-adrenergic blockers.

3. **Electrical cardioversion.** Therapy for acute AF or AFL with a rapid ventricular response in the setting of ongoing myocardial ischemia, MI, hypotension, or marked CHF should receive prompt electrical (DC) cardioversion. Before attempting to restore sinus rhythm, whether through antiarrhythmic agents (chemical cardioversion) or DC cardioversion, one must consider the potential for a thromboembolic event. In general, if AF has persisted for longer than 48 hours (or for an unknown duration), patients should be anticoagulated, with an international normalized ratio of 2–3, for at least 3 weeks before cardioversion, and anticoagulation should be continued for at least 3 weeks, in the same therapeutic range, following successful cardioversion for full atrial contractility to return. *(Circulation* 89:1469, 1994).

a. **Technique.** Before cardioversion, all antiarrhythmic drug levels should be titrated to their therapeutic ranges, and digoxin levels should be determined to exclude digoxin toxicity. Concerns about the duration of therapeutic anticoagulation, particularly for AF and AFL, should be addressed. Informed consent should be obtained, reliable IV access should be established, and continuous monitoring of the ECG should be initiated. Supplemental oxygen and equipment that is necessary for intubation and manual ventilation should be available. Adhesive defibrillation pads or hand-held paddles then should be positioned, with consideration given to the arrhythmia being treated. For ventricular arrhythmias, the anterior electrode should be placed just right of the sternum at the level of the third or fourth intercostal space, with the second electrode being positioned lateral to the cardiac apex or more posteriorly in the left infrascapular region. For atrial arrhythmias, the anterior electrode should be positioned just right or left of the sternum at the level of the third or fourth intercostal space, with the second electrode positioned just below the left scapula. In all cases, care should be taken to position electrodes at least 6 cm from permanent pacemaker or defibrillator generators. When practical, amnesia should be induced with midazolam (1–2 mg IV q2min to a maximum of 5 mg), methohexital (25–75 mg IV), etomidate (0.2–0.6 mg/kg IV), or propofol (initial dose, 5 mg/kg/minute IV). Proper synchronization by the cardioverter-defibrillator should be confirmed by noting the presence of a synchronization marker superimposed on the QRS complex. If electrode paddles are being used, firm pressure should be applied to minimize contact impedance. Direct contact with the patient or the bed should be avoided.

   b. **Adverse effects.** DC cardioversion rarely produces adverse effects. Sinus pauses and atrial, junctional, or ventricular ectopic beats may occur transiently after restoration of sinus rhythm, especially in patients with long-standing AF and a slow ventricular response. Reports of serious arrhythmias, such as VT, VF, or asystole, are rare and are more likely in the setting of improperly synchronized cardioversion, digitalis toxicity, or concomitant antiarrhythmic drug therapy. Systemic or pulmonary embolic events are uncommon if appropriate anticoagulation has been achieved (see sec. **II.A.1**). Muscle pain, with a concomitant rise in lactate dehydrogenase, SGOT, and creatine kinase, and irritation of the skin at the paddle site may occur. Although creatine kinase–MB is elevated in 12% of patients after cardioversion, troponin I, a more cardiospecific marker of myocardial necrosis, was found not to increase after cardioversion with up to 400 joules in this same group of patients (*Am J Cardiol* 78:825, 1996).

   c. **Contraindications.** DC cardioversion is relatively contraindicated in certain circumstances. If **digitalis toxicity** is known or suspected, elective cardioversion for AF or AFL should be deferred. Cardioversion is generally ineffective in **multifocal atrial tachycardia** or paroxysmal arrhythmias without an antiarrhythmic agent to prevent the recurrence of the arrhythmia. Patients with **hyperthyroidism** should be functionally euthyroid before elective cardioversion to limit the likelihood of recurrence.

4. **Overdrive atrial pace-termination** of AFL can be attempted, particularly in patients with temporary pacemaker leads or with some models of permanent pacemakers that allow temporary programming of high atrial rates. Similar considerations regarding anticoagulation for electrical cardioversion should be observed before an attempt is made at overdrive pace-termination of AFL of longer than 48 hours in duration.

5. **Pharmacologic cardioversion** of AF or AFL to NSR requires similar considerations regarding anticoagulation for electrical cardioversion of an episode of AF or AFL greater than 48 hours in duration. Class Ia, Ic, and III agents have some efficacy at converting AF to NSR. The efficacy of a particular antiarrhythmic drug to convert AF or AFL to NSR pharmacologically is typically lower than the efficacy of the drug to prevent a recurrence of the arrhythmia.

6. **Antiarrhythmic therapy for maintenance of NSR.** Long-term antiarrhythmic therapy to prevent the recurrence of AF is controversial. Antiarrhythmic agents (classes Ia, Ic, and III) are modestly effective but have not been shown to reduce stroke risk or to reduce overall mortality and are associated with a small risk for life-threatening proarrhythmia

(*Circulation* 82:1106, 1990). As a result, antiarrhythmic therapy should be reserved for patients who have highly symptomatic AF or AFL.

7. **Catheter ablation of the AV node with pacemaker implantation.** This strategy can be considered (1) when adequate control of the ventricular response to AF or AFL is accompanied by symptomatic ventricular pauses or (2) for CHF exacerbation in patients for whom LV dysfunction limits pharmacologic doses of agents for control of the ventricular response to AF or AFL.

8. **Catheter ablation of typical (and atypical) forms of AFL** can replace antiarrhythmic drug therapy as a means to restore and maintain sinus rhythm (*Circulation* 86:1233, 1992). Chronic therapy for preventing recurrences of AFL has been limited by the lack of efficacy of drug therapy.

B. **Treatment of SVT with 1:1 AV association.** Initial therapy of acute episodes of narrow-complex tachycardias, particularly AVNRT, includes vagal maneuvers (e.g., carotid massage, Valsalva maneuver) and, if unsuccessful, bolus administration of short-acting agents that slow or block AV nodal conduction, such as adenosine (initially 6 mg IV), verapamil (5 mg IV q5min for a maximum of 3 doses), or diltiazem (15- to 20-mg bolus over 2 minutes). Bolus administration of adenosine infrequently causes transient AF; therefore, it is prudent to have a DC cardioverter present when administering adenosine to patients with WPW. Chronic drug therapy can include calcium channel antagonists, β-adrenergic antagonists, or digoxin. Chronic therapy with nodal-blocking agents in WPW carries a small risk of promoting a rapid ventricular response to AF and subsequent VF. Pharmacologic therapy for WPW patients is targeted at slowing conduction and prolonging refractoriness of the accessory bypass tract with an antiarrhythmic agent (class Ia, Ic, and III agents). Radiofrequency catheter ablation now can obviate the need for such therapy in most patients (*N Engl J Med* 324:1605, 1991). Radiofrequency catheter ablation for all forms of SVT with 1:1 AV association typically makes long-term drug therapy unnecessary.

C. **Treatment of VT and VF.** Immediate unsynchronized DC cardioversion is the primary therapy for pulseless VT and VF (see Chap. 8). After successful cardioversion, continuous IV infusion of effective antiarrhythmic therapy should be maintained until any reversible causes have been corrected. The choice of chronic antiarrhythmic therapy depends on the nature of the conditions responsible for the initial VT or VF episode. In the case of TDP associated with acquired long QT syndrome, bolus administration of magnesium sulfate in 1- to 2-g increments up to 4–6 g IV is highly effective. Primary VF that occurs within the first 72 hours of an acute MI is not associated with an elevated risk of recurrence and does not require antiarrhythmic therapy. VF without an identifiable and reversible cause requires chronic therapy in the form of either prophylactic antiarrhythmic drug therapy (e.g., amiodarone, sotalol) or implantation ICD. ICD implantation has been demonstrated to provide a survival benefit for SCD survivors when compared to antiarrhythmic drug therapy (*N Engl J Med* 337:1576, 1997). Patients with significant anoxic brain injury or intractable CHF were excluded from this analysis.

1. **ICD implantation.** ICDs provide automatic recognition and treatment of ventricular arrhythmias. These devices include tiered therapy providing (1) high-energy defibrillation for VF or rapid VT, (2) low-energy cardioversion for stable VT, (3) antitachycardia pacing algorithms to terminate VT, and (4) ventricular or dual-chamber bradycardia pacing. ICD implantation improves survival in (1) patients resuscitated from near-fatal ventricular arrhythmias and (2) patients with a history of nonsustained VT, coronary artery disease, and depressed LV function [ejection fraction (EF) <35%] who have VT induced during an EPS that is not suppressed with IV procainamide (*N Engl J Med* 335:1933, 1996). Complications associated with ICDs are similar to those described for pacemakers. In addition, inappropriate therapy initiated by SVTs or

spurious sensing (e.g., myopotential sensing, sensing electrical artifacts caused by lead fracture) remains a common problem despite refinements in device technology.

2. **Antiarrhythmic drug therapy.** Chronic antiarrhythmic drug therapy is indicated for the treatment of recurrent symptomatic ventricular arrhythmias. In the setting of hemodynamically unstable ventricular arrhythmias treated with an ICD, antiarrhythmic drug therapy is often necessary to suppress frequent device therapy. Antiarrhythmic drugs differ in mechanism of action, efficacy, and side effect profiles, as described below. Prospective, randomized, placebo-controlled trials have shown that class I or class III antiarrhythmic drugs either increase mortality (*N Engl J Med* 321:406, 1989) or have no benefit (e.g., *Lancet* 349:675, 1997; *N Engl J Med* 341:857, 1999) in patients with asymptomatic nonsustained VT (NSVT) and left ventricular dysfunction caused by ischemic heart disease. In contrast, chronic beta-adrenoreceptor blocker therapy has been shown to reduce mortality significantly in patients without a contraindication after MI or with chronic HF (*Circulation* 98:1184, 1998).

3. **Radiofrequency catheter ablation of VT** can be considered for hemodynamically stable forms of VT. Repetitive monomorphic VT from the right ventricular outflow tract is particularly amenable to catheter ablation, with long-term cure rates similar to those achieved for catheter ablation of SVT. Bundle branch re-entry VT has also been treated by catheter ablation, with similarly high success rates. VT associated with ischemic heart disease can also be treated by catheter ablation; however, success rates are lower. Catheter ablation of ischemic VT in patients with antiarrhythmic drug–refractory VT and an implanted ICD has been successful in reducing frequent ICD shocks (*Circulation* 96:1525, 1997).

4. **Primary prevention of VT/VF episodes.** Primary prevention of SCD is indicated for all patients after MI with beta-blocker treatment in whom this therapy is not contraindicated. Large, randomized, placebo-controlled clinical trials with beta-blocker treatment have demonstrated an approximately 50% reduction in the rate of SCD and total mortality in the first year after MI (e.g., the Beta-Blocker Heart Attack trial: *JAMA* 246:2073, 1981). In patients with significant LV dysfunction (EF <35%) and asymptomatic NSVT, risk stratification by invasive EPS is indicated to identify patients at high risk of SCD as described previously (see sec. **II.C.1**).

Antiarrhythmic Drug Therapy

I. **General principles.** Antiarrhythmic agents are classified according to the Vaughan-Williams classification (*J Clin Pharmacol* 24:129, 1984). Class I agents inhibit the fast sodium channel, class II agents are β-adrenergic antagonists, class III agents primarily block potassium channels, and class IV agents are calcium channel antagonists. Specific antiarrhythmic agents may have actions that span multiple classes. In addition, active metabolites of a given antiarrhythmic agent may have electrophysiologic (EP) actions that are substantially different from those of the parent compound. (See Table 7-2 and Appendix D for further dosing details.) Class I agents possess local anesthetic and membrane-stabilizing effects, and their predominant action is to bind to sodium channels and to impede sodium influx during phase 0 of the action potential, resulting in depression of intracardiac conduction. Class I drugs can be further classified into Ia, Ib, and Ic. Class Ia agents prolong ventricular refractoriness and QT interval through their potassium channel–blocking action. Class Ib agents are less potent sodium channel blockers and, at high

Table 7-2. Commonly used antiarrhythmic drugs

Drug	Normal half-life (hrs)	Half-life in ESRD (hrs)	Elimination (R or H)	Oral dosage	IV dosage
Ia					
Procaina-mide	3–6	6–59	R 76–93% H 7–24%	1–6 g/day in divided doses	Load: 17 mg/kg up to 50 mg/min in divided doses Maint: 2–5 mg/min
Quinidine	5–7	5–14	H 80–90% R 10–20%	Sulfate, 200–400 mg q6h Pg, 275–550 mg q8–12h Glc, 324–648 mg q8–12h	—
Ib					
Lidocaine	1–2	1–3	H 90% R 10%	—	Load: 1 mg/kg; repeat 0.5 mg/kg q8–10min up to 3 mg/kg total Maint: 1–4 mg/min
Ic					
Flecainide	12–27	26	H 65% R 35%	100–200 mg q12h	—
Propafenone	2–10	—	H	150–300 mg q8h	—
III					
Amiodarone	18–60 days	—	H	Load: 600–1600 mg/day Maint: 200–400 mg/day	Load: 150-mg bolus, then 1 mg/min for 6 hrs, then 0.5 mg/min
Bretylium	4–17	24–36	R 80% H 20%	—	Load: 5–10 mg/kg over 10 mins up to 30 mg/kg in 24 hrs Maint: 1–3 mg/min

(continued)

Table 7-2. (continued)

Drug	Normal half-life (hrs)	Half-life in ESRD (hrs)	Elimination (R or H)	Oral dosage	IV dosage
Dofetilide	10	NA	R 70% H 30%	125–500 µg q12h	—
Ibutilide	2–12	NA	R <10%	—	1 mg (0.01 mg/kg if weight <60 kg) over 10 mins; can repeat once after 10 mins
Sotalol	12	36	R 90% H 10%	80–240 mg q12h	—

ESRD = end-stage renal disease; Glc = gluconate; H = hepatic; Maint = maintenance; NA = not applicable; Pg = polygalacturonate; R = renal.

tissue concentrations, shorten action potential duration and refractoriness. Class Ic agents are potent sodium channel–blocking agents, markedly slowing conduction with little effect on repolarization. Although class Ia and class Ic drugs have been commonly used empirically to treat non–life-threatening arrhythmias (AF, AFL, atrial and ventricular ectopy), these agents have been associated with increased mortality, presumably due to proarrhythmia (*N Engl J Med* 324:781, 1991; *Circulation* 82:1106, 1990).

II. **ECG monitoring when antiarrhythmic agents are initiated** fulfills the following two roles.

    A. **The efficacy** of an antiarrhythmic agent in reduction or elimination of the tachyarrhythmia can be measured directly with continuous ECG monitoring. For patients whose arrhythmias are nonsustained and well tolerated, Holter monitoring or event recorders are useful in establishing efficacy. However, day-to-day variability in arrhythmia frequency limits the utility of this strategy. For assessing the efficacy of antiarrhythmic therapy in preventing recurrence of sustained VT or VF, the frequency and duration of nonsustained VT are of limited value (*N Engl J Med* 329:445, 1993). In post-MI patients, the ability to reduce the frequency of ventricular ectopy has been associated with increased overall mortality (*N Engl J Med* 321:406, 1989). Exercise testing may be useful in the evaluation of antiarrhythmic drug efficacy, particularly in the small subset of patients with arrhythmias triggered by exertion or changes in sympathetic tone. In a minority of patients with sustained ventricular arrhythmias and frequent ventricular ectopy, exercise testing in combination with ambulatory monitoring may be useful in identifying antiarrhythmic therapy that prevents recurrence of sustained ventricular arrhythmias (*N Engl J Med* 329:445, 1993).

    B. **The risk of proarrhythmia,** defined as the exacerbation of a rhythm disturbance or the initiation of a potentially life-threatening arrhythmia, associated with antiarrhythmic drugs is a primary concern. Proarrhythmia can occur at doses or plasma concentrations below those considered to be toxic. In general, class Ia, Ic, and III agents have a propensity for proarrhythmia, with the likelihood being highest in the setting of ischemic heart disease and left ventricular dysfunction. The initiation and titration of antiarrhythmic drug therapy should be performed with ECG monitoring. In most patients, particularly those with significant structural heart disease, inpatient ECG monitoring is preferable. For patients without significant structural heart disease or coronary artery disease, outpatient ECG monitoring can be considered.

III. Antiarrhythmic agents

A. Class Ia agents

1. **Quinidine** is moderately effective in suppressing symptomatic atrial premature depolarizations and complex ventricular ectopy, converting AF to sinus rhythm and preventing its recurrence, and terminating and preventing paroxysmal SVTs. In a minority of patients, quinidine may be useful in preventing recurrence of sustained VT or VF.

   a. **Loading** regimens of quinidine sulfate range from 600–1000 mg in divided doses over 6–10 hours, with a typical initial maintenance regimen of 200 mg quinidine sulfate PO q6h and a maximum dosage of 2.4 g/day. Extended-release quinidine gluconate tablets are given every 8–12 hours. Quinidine polygalacturonate may reduce gastric irritation and, like quinidine gluconate, can be administered every 8–12 hours.

   b. **IV administration** of quinidine preparations has been associated with marked hypotension and should be avoided.

   c. **Pharmacokinetics.** Absorption of an oral dose of quinidine sulfate or gluconate is virtually complete; serum levels peak 90 minutes after a dose of quinidine sulfate and 3–4 hours after a dose of quinidine gluconate. The serum half-life is 5–8 hours. It increases significantly with age and hepatic dysfunction and modestly with HF and renal failure. Serum levels of 1.3–5.0 mg/L correlate with clinical efficacy.

   d. **Drug toxicity** frequently limits the use of quinidine. GI side effects are common and include nausea, vomiting, diarrhea, abdominal pain, and anorexia. CNS toxicity, referred to as *cinchonism*, includes tinnitus, hearing loss, visual disturbances, confusion, delirium, and psychosis. Adverse reactions include rash, fever, immune-mediated thrombocytopenia, and hemolytic anemia. Proarrhythmia, often manifested as recurrent episodes of TDP, is seen in 1–3% of cases. Quinidine and all class Ia agents should be avoided in patients with a history of TDP and discontinued if the QT_c exceeds 500 milliseconds or is prolonged by more than 25%. Hypokalemia, hypomagnesemia, and severe left ventricular dysfunction identify patients at increased risk for development of quinidine-induced TDP. New or increased cardiac conduction abnormalities may occur; therefore, quinidine should be avoided in patients with high-degree AV block or evidence of extensive conduction system disease. Ventricular rate control during AF and flutter must be achieved with AV nodal blocking agents before initiation of quinidine, owing to its vagolytic effects, which may enhance AV nodal conduction. Serum digoxin levels increase approximately twofold with therapeutic doses of quinidine. Warfarin effects may be potentiated by quinidine. Phenobarbital and phenytoin reduce the serum half-life significantly. Other agents that prolong the QT interval (see Table 7-1) should be avoided in patients who are taking quinidine.

2. **Procainamide** shares quinidine's effects on automaticity, conduction, and refractoriness. Its major metabolite, *N*-acetylprocainamide (NAPA), exerts an action typical of class III agents. The clinical utility of procainamide parallels that of quinidine. Additionally, IV procainamide can be as effective as lidocaine in the acute termination of sustained VT (*Circulation* 80:652, 1989).

   a. **Oral loading** can be achieved rapidly with an oral loading dose of 750–1000 mg. Sustained-release tablets are available for dosing qid and in a new formulation for dosing bid. Typical maintenance dosing is 2000–4000 mg/day in divided doses.

    b. IV administration should be given at a rate that does not exceed 50 mg/minute (to avoid hypotension) until the arrhythmia is suppressed, the QRS widens by 50%, or a maximum loading dose of 17 mg/kg has been administered. Vital signs should be observed continuously during the initial infusion. A maintenance infusion of 2–4 mg/minute then can be used (see Appendix D).

    c. Pharmacokinetics. The peak serum concentration is reached 1 hour after an oral dose and almost immediately with IV administration. Elimination is by hepatic metabolism and renal excretion. The major metabolic pathway is hepatic acetylation to NAPA. In some patients (i.e., slow acetylators), this process is slowed, and significant drug accumulation can result. The serum half-life of procainamide is approximately 3 hours and may be prolonged significantly by HF or renal dysfunction. NAPA has a serum half-life of 6–8 hours, but it may be as long as 70 hours in patients with severe renal dysfunction. Serum procainamide levels of 4–12 mg/L correlate with clinical efficacy. Combined procainamide and NAPA levels greater than 30 mg/L are associated with increased toxicity.

    d. Toxicity and side effects of procainamide include a lupus-like syndrome (fever, pleuropericarditis, hepatomegaly, arthralgias), which may be seen in up to one-third of patients during chronic therapy and may be more likely in the slow acetylator phenotype. This syndrome usually spares the kidneys and resolves when the drug is discontinued. Antinuclear antibodies, frequently in high titers, develop in 75% of patients during chronic administration; however, this abnormality does not mandate discontinuation of the drug in the absence of other symptoms. Agranulocytosis may result from a hypersensitivity reaction to procainamide. Proarrhythmia and ECG changes are similar to those associated with quinidine (see sec. **II.A.1.d**).

3. Disopyramide's EP effects in slowing conduction and prolonging refractoriness are similar to those of procainamide and quinidine. Additionally, disopyramide is potentially effective for preventing inducible and spontaneous neurally mediated syncope (*Am J Cardiol* 65:1339, 1990).

    a. The usual maintenance dosage is 100–300 mg PO q6–8h. In patients with hepatic dysfunction, HF, or moderate renal insufficiency (creatinine clearance >40 ml/minute), the dosage should not exceed 100 mg q6h. In patients with marked renal impairment, a 200-mg loading dose, followed by 100 mg q12h for creatinine clearances of 15–40 ml/minute or 100 mg q24h for creatinine clearances less than 15 ml/minute, is recommended. A sustained-release preparation is available, permitting q12h dosing interval.

    b. Pharmacokinetics. Peak plasma concentration is reached in approximately 2 hours. The serum half-life ranges from 4–10 hours. Serum levels of 2–4 mg/L correlate with clinical efficacy.

    c. Toxicity and side effects include precipitation or worsening of CHF (caused by negative inotropy), dry mouth, urinary retention, constipation, blurred vision, abdominal pain, exacerbation of glaucoma, and drying of bronchial secretions (caused by anticholinergic effects). Disopyramide can provoke a myasthenic crisis in patients with that disease. Proarrhythmia risk and ECG changes are similar to those observed with quinidine (see sec. **III.A.1.d**). Hypoglycemia and masking of hypoglycemic symptoms may occur, particularly in patients with renal dysfunction.

B. Class Ib agents (see Table 7-2) are similar to type Ia agents with regard to their effect on fast sodium channels and intracardiac conduction but cause shortening of the action potential and thus shorten repolarization.

    1. Lidocaine is effective in the management of ventricular tachyarrhythmias, particularly in the setting of acute MI; however, the routine prophylactic administration of lidocaine in patients with acute MI is not indicated (*Arch Intern Med* 149:2694, 1989).

a. **Initial therapy** should consist of an IV bolus of 1 mg/kg, with subsequent bolus injections of 0.5 mg/kg q8–10min, if necessary, to a total of 3 mg/kg. Maintenance therapy IV at 2–4 mg/minute should follow the bolus immediately (see Appendix D). Maintenance dosages are reduced by 50% in patients with CHF, shock, or hepatic dysfunction and in those older than 70 years. Endotracheal or IM administration can be used when IV administration is not possible. The recommended dose is 300 mg when these alternative routes are used, although higher doses may be necessary.

b. **Pharmacokinetics.** Therapeutic serum levels are 2–6 mg/L, but adverse reactions have been observed at even lower levels. Plasma levels should be monitored during prolonged infusions. Serum half-life is prolonged in patients with hepatic dysfunction or HF, in the elderly, with prolonged administration, and with propranolol or cimetidine use.

c. **Toxicities** of lidocaine include CNS effects (convulsions, confusion, stupor, and, rarely, respiratory arrest), all of which resolve with discontinuation of therapy. Negative inotropic effects are seen only at high drug levels. Induction of arrhythmias may occur occasionally, including sinus arrest, AV block, and asystole. Rapid ventricular rate, caused by augmentation in AV conduction, can be seen with AFL or AF.

2. **Mexiletine** is similar to lidocaine in its chemical structure and EP properties but, in general, has a less potent antiarrhythmic activity. Mexiletine can be used alone or in combination with a class Ia drug for treatment of ventricular arrhythmias in selected patients, although it has not been shown effective in preventing recurrence of sustained life-threatening ventricular arrhythmias when used alone. It may have a limited role in the treatment of some patients with congenital long QT syndromes.

a. **A loading dose** of 400 mg can be administered, and the usual maintenance dosage is 200 mg PO q8h. A minimum of 2–3 days between dosage adjustments is recommended. When the drug is used in combination with type Ia or type III agents, a synergistic interaction may allow a lower dose of each agent to be used.

b. **Pharmacokinetics.** Peak plasma concentrations are observed within 2–4 hours. Mexiletine is eliminated primarily by the liver, but 10% is excreted unchanged by the kidneys. Hepatic dysfunction and MI may prolong elimination half-life (>20 hours). The margin between therapeutic (0.75–2.00 mg/L) and toxic (>2 mg/L) concentrations is narrow.

c. **Toxicities.** CNS toxicity includes tremor, dizziness, and blurred vision. Higher levels may result in dysarthria, diplopia, nystagmus, and an impaired level of consciousness. Nausea and vomiting are common. Proarrhythmic effects, particularly TDP, are less common than those with type Ia and type III agents. Drug interactions may be observed with concomitant use of mexiletine and lidocaine. Rifampin and phenytoin reduce plasma levels of mexiletine by enhancing hepatic metabolism. Mexiletine increases theophylline plasma levels.

3. **Tocainide** has been used alone or in combination with class Ia drugs for treatment of ventricular arrhythmias. It has not been shown to be effective in preventing recurrences of sustained life-threatening ventricular arrhythmias.

a. **The usual daily dose** is 1200–1800 mg PO in divided doses q8–12h.

b. **Pharmacokinetics.** Peak plasma concentrations occur within 2 hours. The half-life ranges from 10–14 hours and may be prolonged in patients with acute MI. Therapeutic serum levels are 4–10 mg/L, with increased toxicity at levels that exceed 10 mg/L.

c. **Toxicities** and side effects include neurologic symptoms and GI side effects similar to those associated with mexiletine. Pulmonary complications include pulmonary fibrosis, interstitial pneumonitis, and fibrosing alveolitis. Agranulocytosis, leukopenia, hypoplastic anemia, and thrombocytopenia have been reported in 0.1–0.2% of those who take tocainide. CBCs should be monitored weekly for the first 3 months and then at least monthly.

4. **Phenytoin** is used primarily in the treatment of digitalis-induced ventricular and supraventricular arrhythmias. It may have a limited role in the treatment of ventricular arrhythmias associated with congenital long QT syndromes. The IV loading dose is 250 mg given over 10 minutes (maximum rate of 50 mg/minute). Subsequent doses of 100 mg can be given q5min as necessary and as blood pressure tolerates, to a total of 1000 mg. Frequent monitoring of the ECG, BP, and neurologic status is required. Continuous infusion is not recommended (see Chap. 25).

5. **Moricizine** is structurally similar to the phenothiazines and has EP effects that represent a combination of class Ia and Ib actions. Moricizine can be used to treat ventricular arrhythmias; however, it has not been shown to be effective in preventing recurrences of sustained life-threatening ventricular arrhythmias.

   a. **The initial dosage** is 200 mg PO q8h, with a maximum dose of 900 mg/day.

   b. **Toxicities** of moricizine include proarrhythmia, nausea, vomiting, diarrhea, tremor, mood changes, headache, vertigo, dizziness, and nystagmus. Moricizine may decrease serum levels of theophylline.

C. **Class Ic agents** (see Table 7-2) profoundly depress the slope of phase 0 of the cardiac action potential and markedly slow conduction throughout the specialized conduction system and myocardium, with less prolongation of refractoriness than that with class Ia agents. Automaticity also is decreased throughout. The ECG characteristically shows a widening of the QRS and lengthening of the QT_c interval (largely attributable to QRS prolongation).

1. **Flecainide** generally is more effective than are other class I agents in the management of a variety of supraventricular arrhythmias, including AF, AFL, and the PSVTs. It may be effective in suppressing complex ventricular ectopy and nonsustained VT; however, its routine use in this setting is not recommended because of the risk of proarrhythmia and sudden death (*N Engl J Med* 324:781, 1991).

   a. **The initial dosage** is 50–100 mg PO bid and can be increased by an increment of 50 mg bid every fourth day until clinical efficacy is obtained or a total dose of 400 mg/day is reached. Dosages that exceed 400 mg/day should be avoided in patients with CHF or renal failure.

   b. **Pharmacokinetics.** Therapeutic serum levels range from 0.4–0.9 mg/L. The mean plasma elimination half-life is approximately 20 hours and is prolonged in the setting of renal impairment or HF.

   c. **Toxicities** of flecainide include conduction abnormalities, with 20% increases in the PR and QRS intervals commonly being observed. Patients who have an increase of more than 50% in the PR interval or QRS duration should be monitored closely. The dose should be reduced or the drug should be discontinued if the PR interval exceeds 0.3 seconds, the QRS duration exceeds 0.2 seconds, or bifascicular block, second-degree AV block, or third-degree AV block occurs. Proarrhythmic effects have been reported in up to 5% of patients and may be higher in patients with underlying heart disease or ventricular arrhythmias. Flecainide serum levels above 1 mg/L appear to be associated with a higher risk of proarrhythmia. When used in the treatment of AF (particularly in the absence of AV nodal blocking agents), flecainide may result in conversion to AFL with 1:1 AV conduction. Negative inotropic effects may precipitate or exacerbate CHF. Atrial and ventricular pacing thresholds may increase by as much as 200%; therefore, threshold testing of pacemakers and

ICDs must be performed after drug initiation. Noncardiac effects include confusion, irritability, blurred vision, dizziness, nausea, and headache. Flecainide causes modest increases in plasma digoxin levels. Plasma levels of flecainide and propranolol increase when they are used concurrently. Amiodarone increases flecainide levels, requiring a one-third reduction in dose.

   2. **Propafenone** is related structurally to flecainide. At therapeutic levels, it has type Ic actions and moderate beta-adrenergic antagonism. Its clinical utility is similar to that of flecainide (see sec. **III.C.1**).

      a. **The initial dosage** is 150 mg PO tid, which can be increased at 3- to 4-day intervals up to 300 mg tid. The dosage should be increased cautiously in patients with hepatic or renal insufficiency.

      b. **Pharmacokinetics.** Peak plasma concentration is reached in 2–3 hours, and metabolism occurs in the liver. However, the relationship between serum level and therapeutic efficacy is poor. Bioavailability increases with dose, such that a threefold increase in dose may result in a tenfold increase in plasma concentration. Caution is advised in patients with renal insufficiency, as the parent drug and the metabolites are eliminated in the urine. Therapeutic serum concentrations range from 0.2–1.5 mg/L. The dose in patients with hepatic insufficiency is reduced by 20–30%.

      c. **Toxicities** and proarrhythmia risk of propafenone are similar to those seen with flecainide (see sec. **III.C.1**). Bronchospasm may occur as a result of its beta-adrenergic antagonistic actions. Negative inotropic effects may precipitate or worsen CHF. Noncardiac effects include dizziness, disturbances in taste, blurred vision, and nausea. Drugs that inhibit the cytochrome P450 system in the liver may inhibit propafenone metabolism. Plasma digoxin concentration, effects of β-adrenergic antagonists, and effects of warfarin are increased by propafenone.

D. **Class II agents** are β-adrenergic antagonists that exert their antiarrhythmic actions by attenuating the binding at catecholamine receptor sites (see Chap. 4). They are effective in decreasing automaticity and in preventing re-entrant arrhythmias involving the AV node. β-Adrenergic antagonists appear to influence ventricular arrhythmogenesis favorably by altering myocardial oxygen supply versus demand and by blunting tissue response to circulating catecholamines. Toxicities and side effects of beta-adrenergic antagonist agents include negative inotropic effects that can precipitate or exacerbate CHF in patients with severe left ventricular dysfunction. Negative chronotropic effects may cause symptomatic sinus bradycardia and may exacerbate AV nodal conduction abnormalities. Coronary artery spasm may be potentiated by β-adrenergic antagonists, owing to unopposed α-adrenergic stimulation. Abrupt withdrawal of β-adrenergic antagonists may precipitate cardiac arrhythmias or angina. Discontinuation of drug therapy should be tapered over several days. Potential noncardiac effects are numerous (see Chap. 4). Class II agents are clinically useful in certain situations.

   1. **After MI,** β-adrenergic antagonists reduce overall death rate and sudden death rate (*Circulation* 85:1107, 1992).

   2. **In thyrotoxicosis, pheochromocytoma,** and states of catecholamine excess (exercise, postoperative state, extreme emotional stress), the associated arrhythmias often respond to therapy.

   3. **In AF and AFL,** β-adrenergic antagonists reduce the ventricular response rate and reduce the incidence of postoperative AF in cardiac surgery patients (*Circulation* 84:236, 1991).

   4. **PSVTs** may respond to therapy with β-adrenergic antagonists with a reduction in the recurrence rate.

   5. **Sinus tachycardia,** although rarely requiring specific treatment, responds to β-adrenergic blockade.

6. **In congenital long QT syndromes** complicated by recurrent episodes of TDP, β-adrenergic antagonists may be effective in preventing recurrent episodes of TDP (*Ann N Y Acad Sci* 644:112, 1992).

7. **Neurocardiogenic syncope** can be managed effectively with β-adrenergic antagonists (see Recognition and Diagnosis, sec. **II.C.3**)

E. **Class III agents** (see Table 7-2) prolong action potential duration and repolarization to a greater extent than they depress conduction velocity.

1. **Amiodarone** prolongs repolarization and refractoriness in atrial and ventricular tissue. It slows the sinus rate and prolongs AV nodal conduction. It is also a noncompetitive α- and β-adrenergic antagonist. It can reduce systemic vascular resistance and mean arterial BP, particularly with IV loading. Hemodynamic deterioration has been reported in patients with severe underlying left ventricular dysfunction. Amiodarone is a potent antiarrhythmic agent that is effective for a variety of arrhythmias but, in high doses, is associated with significant toxicities (*Am Heart J* 125:109, 1993). After oral loading, amiodarone prevents the recurrence of sustained VT or VF in up to 60% of patients. A therapeutic latency of >5 days exists before beneficial antiarrhythmic effects are observed with oral dosing, and full suppression of arrhythmias may not occur for 4–6 weeks after therapy is initiated.

a. **For VT or VF,** amiodarone has efficacy similar to that of bretylium, with less hypotension (*Circulation* 92:3255, 1995). In the setting of ventricular arrhythmias with hemodynamic collapse, beneficial response to amiodarone can be seen even after failures with other agents (*JACC* 27:67, 1996). **Supraventricular arrhythmias** also can be treated effectively with amiodarone, but the potential toxicities of this drug limit its use. It prevents recurrences of AF and AFL and can effect chemical conversion of AF to NSR. In chronic AF, it slows the ventricular response, but the onset of this effect is slow in comparison to that of conventional agents (calcium channel antagonists, β-adrenergic antagonists, and digoxin).

b. **Oral dosage loading** schedules are empiric and vary between 800 and 1600 mg PO qd for 1–2 weeks. The usual maintenance dose rarely exceeds 400 mg qd, and the minimum effective dose should be used to avoid the potential toxicities. Approximately 50% of an oral dose is absorbed, and a peak plasma concentration occurs 3–8 hours after ingestion.

c. **Loading IV** is 150 mg over 10 minutes followed by infusion at 1 mg/minute for 6 hours, then 0.5 mg/minute. A more rapid bolus may cause hypotension. Repeat 150-mg boluses can be given if arrhythmias recur. The maintenance infusion is equivalent to an oral loading dose of 1000–1200 mg/day.

d. **Pharmacokinetics.** Elimination is via hepatic excretion into bile. The slow uptake and release from reservoir tissues contribute to a multiphasic elimination half-life in which plasma levels fall to 50% within the first 3–5 days after discontinuation of therapy, with a subsequent half-life of 26–107 days. Therapeutic serum levels range from 1.0–2.5 mg/L. Measurements of serum concentrations are of limited value but may assist in documenting compliance and absorption.

e. **Toxicity.** Adverse effects are partially dose dependent and may occur in up to 75% of patients treated with amiodarone at high doses for 5 years. However, at lower dosages (200–300 mg/day), adverse effects that require discontinuation occur in approximately 5–10% of patients per year. Specific toxicity syndromes include the following: (1) Pulmonary toxicity occurs in 1–15% of treated patients but appears less likely in patients who receive less than 300 mg/day (*Circulation* 82:51, 1990). Patients characteristically have a dry cough and dyspnea associated with pulmonary infiltrates and rales. The process appears to be reversible if detected early, but undetected cases may result in a mortality of up to 10% of those affected. A chest radiograph and pulmonary function tests should be obtained every 6 months. The presence of interstitial changes on the chest radiograph and decreased diffusing capacity raise concern of amiodarone pulmonary toxicity. (2) Photosensitivity is a common adverse reaction, and, in some patients, a violaceous skin discoloration develops in sun-exposed areas. The blue-gray discoloration may not resolve completely with discontinuation of therapy. (3) Thyroid dysfunction is a common adverse effect. Hypothyroidism and hyperthyroidism have been reported, with an incidence of 2–5% per year. Thyroid function should be monitored annually. If hypothyroidism develops, concurrent treatment with levothyroxine may allow continued amiodarone use. (4) Corneal microdeposits, detectable on slit-lamp examination, develop in virtually all patients. Their occurrence is dose dependent and reversible with discontinuation of the drug. These deposits rarely interfere with vision, although some patients notice halos around lights. Optic neuritis, leading to blindness, has also been reported in association with amiodarone. (5) Cardiovascular effects include asymptomatic sinus bradycardia and prolonged AV node conduction; however, severe bradycardia or high-grade AV block may occur in patients who have pre-existing conduction abnormalities. Exacerbation of ventricular arrhythmias is rare, as is TDP. The ECG effects include a lengthened PR interval, QRS duration, and QT interval. Other agents that prolong the QT interval (see Table 7-1) should be avoided in patients who are taking amiodarone. (6) Other side effects, including nausea and anorexia, may occur, especially during the high-dose loading phase. A transient rise in hepatic transaminases commonly is observed early in the course of therapy but usually is asymptomatic. If the increase exceeds three times normal or doubles in a patient with an elevated baseline level, amiodarone should be discontinued or the dose should be reduced. Maintenance doses of warfarin and digoxin should be reduced routinely by one-half when amiodarone is started, and levels should be followed closely.

2. **Sotalol** decreases the frequency and duration of nonsustained VT in up to 40% of patients, prevents inducibility of sustained VT via programmed electrical stimulation in 35% of patients, and prevents recurrence of sustained VT and VF in 70% of patients (*N Engl J Med* 329:452, 1993). Sotalol is also useful as an agent to prevent recurrences of symptomatic AF and AFL.

   a. **Initial dosage** is 80 mg bid, with dosage increments every 2–3 days until the desired dose is attained. The usual therapeutic dose is 160–320 mg/day.

   b. **Pharmacokinetics.** Peak plasma concentrations occur in 2.5–4.0 hours, with an elimination half-life of approximately 12 hours. Sotalol is excreted predominantly unchanged in the urine. The dosing interval should be increased to 24 hours for a creatinine clearance of 30–60 ml/minute, with extension to 36–48 hours for a creatinine clearance of 10–30 ml/minute.

   c. **Toxicities** of sotalol include proarrhythmic effects, typically TDP, the risk of which appears to be dose dependent and related to the QT interval. Prolongation of the QT_c to greater than 500 milliseconds is associated with a 5% incidence of TDP. Concomitant use of other agents that prolong the QT interval (see Table 7-1) should be avoided. Due to sotalol's β-antagonist activity, multiple cardiac and noncardiac side effects are possible (see sec. **III.D**). Bradyarrhythmias are common, particularly when used in combination with other agents that suppress sinus node function or AV nodal conduction. Sotalol is contraindicated in patients with sinus bradycardia or second- or third-degree AV block. Bronchospasm and HF may be precipitated or exacerbated by sotalol, with new-onset HF occurring in approximately 3% of patients.

3. **Bretylium** tosylate is a quaternary ammonium compound that has direct EP effects and interactions with the autonomic nervous system. Bretylium markedly prolongs action potential duration and refractoriness in Purkinje fibers and ventricular muscle. It also affects peripheral adrenergic nerve terminals, initially causing an abrupt release of norepinephrine; subsequently, it prevents further release and blocks norepinephrine reuptake. Automaticity may increase transiently, owing to the initial norepinephrine release. Bretylium's efficacy is thought to be related to alterations in refractoriness and effects on the autonomic nervous system. Bretylium's chief clinical utility is in the treatment of VT and VF. It may be effective in cardiac arrest, even after protracted episodes of VF that is refractory to conventional maneuvers (see Chap. 8).

   a. **For VF** or hemodynamically unstable VT, the **initial dose** is 5 mg/kg, with repeat boluses as needed to a maximum of 35 mg/kg total (see Chap. 8). For patients with hemodynamically stable refractory or recurrent VT, rapid injections of bretylium should be avoided, as they may cause hypotension, nausea, and vomiting. In those patients who do not require immediate cardioversion, 5–10 mg/kg bretylium should be injected over 10 minutes, followed by a maintenance infusion of 2 mg/minute.

   b. **Pharmacokinetics.** The onset of action is prompt with IV administration, although maximum efficacy may require 15–20 minutes. The serum half-life varies from 4–17 hours. Bretylium is cleared by the kidneys.

   c. **Toxicities** include proarrhythmia, transient hypertension, and increased sinus rate, which may accompany initiation of therapy, owing to initial elaboration of catecholamines. Common side effects with sustained infusion include hypotension, nausea, and vomiting. Bretylium may potentiate the response to infused catecholamines. The hypotensive effects of diuretics or vasodilator drugs also may be augmented during chronic bretylium administration.

4. **Ibutilide** is a class III agent available in IV form for chemical cardioversion of AF and AFL. It prolongs the atrial and ventricular refractory period, with minimal effect on conduction. The mechanism appears to be increasing the slow inward sodium plateau current while decreasing the outward potassium current. Initial experience with ibutilide demonstrates a 45% conversion rate for AF and a 60% conversion rate for AFL at 4 hours after infusion.

   a. **For patients who weigh** less than 60 kg, the recommended dosage is 0.01 mg/kg IV over 10 minutes. For patients who weigh more than 60 kg, the dose is 1 mg IV over 10 minutes. After 10 minutes, the dose can be repeated once if indicated.

   b. **Pharmacokinetics.** The onset of action is nearly immediate, with approximately half of responders converting to sinus rhythm during the initial infusion. Remaining responders convert over the next 1–2 hours. Ibutilide is metabolized in the liver and excreted in the kidneys, with a mean half-life of 6 hours.

   c. **Initial toxicity** studies suggest that ibutilide is associated with a 4–8% risk of serious proarrhythmia (principally TDP). It is recommended that, during administration of ibutilide, DC cardioversion and other resuscitative equipment be in close proximity and that patients be observed closely for at least 4 hours after the infusion. Experience with the drug is limited, particularly in patients with serious comorbid conditions.

5. **Dofetilide** is indicated for the chronic treatment of patients with AF and AFL. The antiarrhythmic action of dofetilide is through blockade of the rapid component of the delayed rectifier potassium current, I_{Kr}. As a result of this effect, the myocyte action potential is prolonged because of the inhibition of repolarization. At clinically effective doses, the QT interval on the 12-lead ECG is usually prolonged. Dofetilide is contraindicated in patients with a QT_c greater than 440 milliseconds (500 milliseconds in patients with BBB or interventricular conduction delay). Dofetilide is hemodynamically neutral and has no effect on AV node conduction or sinus node function.

   a. **Oral dosing.** Initial oral dosing of 500 µg bid is recommended for patients with normal creatinine clearance. Dofetilide is contraindicated for patients with a creatinine clearance of less than 20 ml/minute. A dosage reduction to 250 µg bid is indicated for patients with a creatinine clearance of 40–60 ml/minute and 125 µg bid for patients with a creatinine clearance of 20–40 ml/minute. A 12-lead ECG should be obtained before the first dose of dofetilide and 2–3 hours later. If the QT_c interval after the first dose prolongs by 15% of the baseline or exceeds 500 milliseconds, a 50% dosage reduction is indicated. Daily 12-lead ECGs and continuous inpatient ECG monitoring are indicated for the first 3 days of therapy. If the QT_c prolongs to greater than 500 milliseconds (>550 milliseconds for patients with BBB or intraventricular conduction delay) after a dose reduction, dofetilide should be discontinued.

   b. **Pharmacokinetics.** Oral bioavailability of dofetilide is greater than 90%, with peak plasma concentrations at 2–3 hours in the fasted state. The terminal half-life of dofetilide is about 10 hours. Approximately 80% of each dose is renally cleared by active secretion. Several medications block this secretion (cimetidine, prochlorperazine, trimethoprim, megestrol, ketoconazole) and are, therefore, contraindicated with dofetilide.

   c. **Toxicity.** The risk of TDP from dofetilide treatment is less than 3% when the dosage is adjusted for renal function and QT_c interval (*N Engl J Med* 341:857, 1999).

F. **Class IV agents** are calcium channel antagonists (see Table 4-3). These agents selectively block the slow inward current carried primarily by calcium ions. In tissues dependent on slow channel activity (sinoatrial and AV nodes and some areas of diseased atrial and ventricular tissue), verapamil and diltiazem induce a concentration-dependent depression in phase 4 depolarization and a prolongation in refractoriness, resulting in depressed automaticity and slowed conduction.

   1. **Verapamil** is effective in slowing the ventricular response rate of AF and flutter and in slowing or abolishing the SVTs that use the AV node in their re-entrant circuit. Although IV formulations are useful for termination of re-entrant SVTs, bolus administration of adenosine appears equally effective and avoids the possibility of prolonged hypotension that can result from IV verapamil.

      a. **For IV administration,** an initial dose of 5–10 mg should be given as an IV bolus over 2–3 minutes. It can be repeated after 15–30 minutes if necessary. A continuous infusion seldom is used. The cardiac rhythm and vital signs should be monitored closely during administration.

      b. **Pharmacokinetics.** The onset of action is within 1–2 minutes after IV administration, with a peak effect occurring in 10–15 minutes. Depression of AV node conduction is detectable for up to 6 hours. Hemodynamic effects occur 3–5 minutes after bolus injection and usually dissipate within 20 minutes. After oral ingestion, peak plasma concentrations are reached in 1–2 hours. The half-life is 4–12 hours, with extensive first-pass metabolism in the liver and 70% of metabolites excreted by the kidneys.

c. **Toxicities** include bradycardia, high-degree AV block, and asystole. Verapamil should not be used in patients with pre-existing second- or third-degree AV block or in those with sinus node dysfunction. Pretreatment with IV calcium salts (1 g calcium gluconate IV) may blunt verapamil-induced hypotension. Verapamil should be used with extreme caution in patients with mild to moderate HF, and it is contraindicated in severe HF and hypotension. Verapamil is contraindicated also in patients with WPW syndrome and AF (see Mechanisms of Arrhythmia, sec. **III.E.2**). In hepatic dysfunction, toxic levels may be reached quickly. Concomitant use with β-adrenergic antagonists may produce significant negative inotropy or conduction blockade.

2. **Diltiazem** has EP properties similar to those of verapamil, but its shorter half-life allows easier titration of effect in critical care settings. An IV bolus of diltiazem is effective in terminating nearly 90% of PSVTs within 3 minutes of a first or second bolus.

a. **The recommended dosage** for IV bolus administration is 0.25 mg/kg body weight over 2 minutes, with a repeat bolus of 0.35 mg/kg if the desired effect is not obtained. After bolus administration, a continuous infusion can be initiated at 10 mg/hour, with the infusion rate titrated to the desired effect. Oral preparations include 30-, 60-, 90-, and 120-mg tablets for tid or qid dosing, with longer-acting preparations available for qd or bid dosing. Oral administration should begin at 120–240 mg/day, initially in divided doses.

b. **Pharmacokinetics.** The plasma half-life is 3–4 hours after a single IV injection and is prolonged by as much as 50% with continuous IV administration. For conversion from IV to PO dosing, the approximate PO daily dose is 150% of the 24-hour cumulative IV infusion.

c. **Toxicity** and side effects of diltiazem are essentially the same as those of verapamil (see sec. **III.F.1.c**), reflecting negative chronotropic and inotropic effects. Symptomatic hypotension occurs in up to 3% of patients after IV bolus infusion. Hepatic dysfunction may allow for accumulation to toxic levels. Diltiazem has been shown to increase propranolol levels, increasing the possibility of bradycardia and AV block.

G. **Other antiarrhythmic agents**

1. **Adenosine** is an endogenous nucleoside with significant EP effects, including inhibition of sinus node automaticity, shortening of atrial refractory period duration, depression of AV node conduction, and prolongation of AV nodal refractoriness. Adenosine is indicated for the treatment of re-entrant PSVTs that can be terminated by blocking AV node conduction transiently. Adenosine and verapamil have comparable efficacy for termination of AV nodal re-entry and orthodromic AVRT (*Ann Intern Med* 113:104, 1990). Adenosine is not effective in converting AFL, AF, or VT to sinus rhythm, but adenosine-induced AV nodal blockade may facilitate the diagnosis of these arrhythmias by causing transient AV dissociation. In a small number of patients, adenosine induces AF, likely secondary to its transient shortening of the atrial refractory period.

a. **The recommended initial dose** is 6 mg given IV as a rapid bolus via an antecubital vein, followed by a 10- to 30-ml saline flush. If within 1–2 minutes SVT is not terminated and AV block is not seen, 12 mg followed by 18 mg can be given. A lower initial dose (3 mg) should be used if the drug is injected through a central venous line.

b. **Pharmacokinetics.** The serum half-life of adenosine, approximately 4–8 seconds, is not affected by hepatic or renal failure. A continuous infusion of adenosine is not effective and should not be used for control of supraventricular arrhythmias.

    c. Toxicities of adenosine include precipitation of prolonged asystole in patients with SSS or second- or third-degree AV block. Adenosine effects are antagonized by methylxanthines (caffeine or theophylline), and larger doses may be required. Effects are potentiated by dipyridamole and carbamazepine and in heart transplant recipients, such that a smaller initial dosage should be used. Common adverse side effects—facial flushing, dyspnea, and chest pressure—usually are of brief duration. Adenosine also rarely may exacerbate bronchoconstriction. It should not be used in pre-excited tachycardias unless equipment for immediate defibrillation is present, in light of risk of inducing AF with rapid conduction over the accessory pathway (see Mechanisms of Arrhythmia, sec. **III.D.2**).

2. Digitalis glycosides are useful in the control of the resting ventricular rate in AF or AFL in the setting of left ventricular dysfunction and CHF. They may be useful also as adjunctive therapy in combination with calcium channel antagonists or beta-adrenergic antagonists for optimum rate control of chronic AF (*Am J Cardiol* 69:78G, 1992).

    a. Digoxin, the most commonly used digitalis glycoside, is available in capsules, tablets, as a solution for injection, and as an elixir, with bioavailability that varies with preparation. Loading regimens for digoxin vary widely, with as much as 0.5 mg given as a single IV dose and loading accomplished after 1.0–1.5 mg has been administered in divided doses over 8–24 hours. Usual maintenance doses range between 0.125 and 0.5 mg PO qd, with decreased doses in patients with renal dysfunction.

    b. Pharmacokinetics. Therapeutic digoxin levels are not well defined, but a range of 0.8–2.0 µg/L correlates with effect in most patients. Levels greater than 2 µg/L should raise concern of digitalis toxicity. Digoxin levels should not be measured within 6 hours after an IV dose or 8 hours after a PO dose because of incomplete distribution. Most of an oral dose is absorbed, with peak effect occurring in 90 minutes to 5 hours. After IV injection, peak effect is observed in 1–4 hours. The average serum half-life is 36–48 hours. Excretion is predominantly renal, and serum half-life is prolonged with renal insufficiency (see Chap. 6).

    c. Digitalis toxicity. A wide range of brady- and tachyarrhythmias have been associated with digitalis toxicity. Paroxysmal atrial tachycardia with varying degrees of AV block and bidirectional VT are seen almost exclusively in association with digitalis toxicity. Treatment of digoxin toxicity is discussed in Chap. 6.

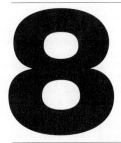

Cardiopulmonary Resuscitation and Advanced Cardiac Life Support

Michael Lippmann

Health care providers should be experienced in the practices and procedures of **basic life support (BLS) and advanced cardiac life support (ACLS)**. The ultimate goals of resuscitation are to maintain cerebral perfusion until cardiopulmonary function is restored and to return the patient to baseline neurologic function. Availability of early defibrillation is critical, as the majority of adult arrests are secondary to ventricular arrhythmias. **Adult resuscitation** should expeditiously follow this sequence: assessment of unresponsiveness, activation of emergency medical services, BLS until defibrillation is available, defibrillation if indicated, intubation, and administration of appropriate medications. The specific clinical circumstances regarding any particular patient may require deviation from these guidelines [*JAMA* 268:2171, 1992; *Circulation* 102(Suppl I):I-86, 2000].

Basic Life Support

Airway, breathing, and circulation are the essentials of BLS. When encountering an unconscious patient, the following are recommended.

I. **Determine unresponsiveness** by gently shaking the patient. Avoid shaking the patient's head or neck if trauma to this area is suspected.

II. **Activate the emergency medical services system**

III. **Position the patient** on a firm, flat surface. If the victim must be moved from the face-down position, roll the patient as a unit so that the head, neck, and torso move simultaneously.

IV. **Open the patient's airway.** The patient's mouth needs to be open, and dentures should be left in place. If neck injury is not suspected, the head tilt–chin lift should be performed. If a cervical spine injury is suspected, use the jaw-thrust maneuver to limit the potential for spinal cord injury.

V. **Assess for the presence of respiration** once the airway is open. An open airway may be all that is necessary for spontaneous respiration to resume and continue.

VI. **If spontaneous respiration is not present, give two slow breaths** (1.5–2.0 seconds per breath), taking a breath after each ventilation. Each ventilation should be performed with sufficient volume to make the patient's chest rise. Rapid or high-pressure breaths may result in gastric distention. If the chest does not rise, the patient's head should be repositioned and ventilation attempted again. If ventilation is unsuccessful after a second attempt, obstructed airway maneuvers should be used (see sec. **X**).

VII. **Assess circulation** by palpating for pulses and checking for signs of perfusion, including swallowing or breathing for more than occasional gasps.

VIII. **Chest compressions** should be initiated at a rate of 80–100/minute in the absence of a carotid pulse. The patient should be lying on a firm surface. Chest compressions are performed with the heel of one hand on the back of the other hand. Hand position should be 1 in. cephalad to the patient's xiphoid process. With shoulders directly above the hands and elbows in a locked position, the rescuer compresses the patient's sternum 1.5–2.0 in. The adequacy of compressions should be assessed periodically by having another rescuer palpate the carotid pulse. Fifteen chest compressions should be performed followed by two ventilations. Once the patient is intubated, ventilations can be performed at a rate of 12–15/minute without pausing for compressions.

IX. **Stop BLS for 5 seconds** at the end of the first minute and every 1–2 minutes thereafter to determine whether the patient has resumed spontaneous breathing or circulation. If a spontaneous pulse has returned, check the BP and continue ventilation as needed. BLS should otherwise not be withheld for more than 5 seconds except to intubate or defibrillate the patient. Attempts at intubation should not exceed 30 seconds before CPR is resumed.

X. **If an unconscious patient cannot be ventilated** after two attempts at positioning the head and chin and a laryngoscope is unavailable (see Chap. 26), 6–10 abdominal thrusts (the Heimlich maneuver) should be performed. Careful technique should be used to avoid improper hand position, which may cause damage to the internal organs. After this maneuver is performed, debris should be swept from the patient's mouth with a finger, and then one should attempt to ventilate the patient. This sequence should continue to be repeated until ventilation is successful. Cricothyrotomy and transtracheal ventilation rarely are necessary for ventilating the patient (see Chap. 9).

XI. **Active compression and decompression and interposed abdominal compression** are experimental techniques that hold promise for increasing cerebral and cardiac blood flow.

General Considerations of Advanced Cardiac Life Support

ACLS is an extension of BLS and usually is implemented by a team. Early designation of a team leader facilitates coordination of the effort. The team leader is responsible for ensuring proper implementation of ACLS. The leader should ascertain that BLS is being properly performed and that defibrillation occurs early when indicated. After this, the leader should ensure that proper endotracheal intubation and ventilation, placement of a functioning IV catheter, administration of appropriate cardiovascular medicines, and diagnosis and treatment of the cause of the arrest are performed correctly. The team leader should examine the patient and determine the events preceding the arrest, obtain a relevant history including current medications and treatments, and obtain appropriate tests (electrolytes, hematocrit, arterial blood gases, ECG, radiographs, etc.) to determine and treat the cause of the arrest. The patient's rhythm and pulse should be assessed after every intervention. The team leader also should determine when termination of resuscitative efforts is warranted.

I. **Arrhythmia recognition and defibrillation** should be performed as quickly as possible. Use of quick-look paddles on defibrillators avoids delay before the establishment of ECG monitoring.

A. **Pulseless ventricular tachycardia (VT) or ventricular fibrillation (VF)** should be defibrillated immediately.

1. **Proper technique** is essential for successful defibrillation. One paddle should be placed along the upper right sternal border below the clavicle and the other paddle positioned lateral to the left nipple centered in the midaxillary line. Conductive gel or pads and firm pressure reduce transthoracic impedance. Before defibrillation, the operator must ensure that no one is touching the bed or the patient.

2. **A solitary precordial "thump"** is delivered only when the onset of VT or VF is witnessed on a monitor. Although the precordial thump may convert VT or VF to a more stable rhythm if delivered quickly, it **should not delay**

defibrillation attempts. Use of a precordial thump in unmonitored situations may induce VT or VF in patients with organized electrical activity.

3. Patients with an **automatic implantable cardioverter-defibrillator** or a **pacemaker** can be externally defibrillated without damage to the device, provided that a defibrillation paddle is not placed over the device. In these patients, especially those with an epicardial patch, higher energy levels (>200 joules) and anterior-posterior paddle positions may be necessary.

4. **Blind defibrillation** in the absence of a rhythm diagnosis rarely is necessary because of the monitoring capabilities on most modern defibrillators.

B. A **"flat line" on the monitor** might indicate loose leads, a lack of connection between the patient and monitor, isoelectrical VF, or true asystole. Operator mistakes are the most frequent cause of misdiagnosed asystole. **Asystole should always be confirmed in two leads** that are perpendicular to each other.

II. **Ventilation and airway management** are essential to any resuscitative effort. Oxygen (100%) should be administered, and a qualified individual should accomplish endotracheal intubation (see Chap. 9) as soon as possible. BLS should not be interrupted for more than 30 seconds for intubation. Ventilation with a well-fitting pocket mask and protection of the airway by suctioning are preferable to making repeated unsuccessful attempts at intubation. Because of the difficulty in maintaining a seal, only experienced personnel should use a bag-valve device with a mask. Bag-valve-mask ventilation is best accomplished by two practitioners to assure that an adequate seal is achieved and sufficient tidal volume is delivered. Initial airway management following endotracheal tube placement consists of excluding esophageal intubation by auscultation over the stomach upon delivering the first breath. If esophageal intubation is suspected by the presence of stomach gurgling and the absence of chest wall expansions the endotracheal tube should be removed immediatly. In the absence of stomach gurgling and in the presence of chest wall expansion, proper endotracheal positioning is assessed by checking for equal bilateral breath sounds during ventilation. Endotrachael placement should also be confirmed using nonphysical examination techniques including esophageal detector devices, qualitative end-tidal CO_2 indicators, and capnographic and capnometric devices. If airway obstruction is present and cannot be relieved, (see Basic Life Support, sec. **X**), transtracheal catheter ventilation or cricothyrotomy is indicated (see Chap. 9).

III. **Route of drug administration**

A. A **peripheral IV line,** especially in the antecubital vein, should be placed if no venous access is available. Using a long IV catheter, elevating the extremity, and flushing with a 20- to 30-ml bolus of IV fluid can facilitate rapid entry of drugs into the central circulation. The agents take up to 1 minute to reach the central circulation.

B. An **internal jugular or subclavian central venous line,** in place before the arrest, should be used for drug administration. There is no advantage to placing a central line if a functioning peripheral line is present. If adequate peripheral IV access cannot be established quickly, a central vein should be cannulated with minimal interruption of CPR. If the femoral vein is used, a long catheter that reaches above the diaphragm should be used to avoid a delay in the transit of drugs into the central circulation.

C. **Endotracheal administration** of atropine, lidocaine, and epinephrine can be given if there is a delay in obtaining IV access. The dose for drugs used in this manner should be two to two and a half times the recommended IV dose, and the agents should be diluted in 10 ml saline. Once injected into the endotracheal tube, the medicine is distributed into the bronchi by several forceful lung inflations while chest compressions are held.

D. **Intracardiac injections** are not recommended.

IV. **Fluids given intravenously** (normal saline is preferred) are indicated for volume expansion in patients with cardiac arrest and evidence of acute blood loss, hypovolemia, or hypotension. Patients with acute myocardial infarction (MI), especially right ventricular infarction, also might benefit from volume expansion. Routine IV fluid administration in patients with cardiac arrest and no evidence of volume depletion does not increase cardiac output and dilutes hemoglobin, decreasing tissue oxygen delivery to the cerebral and cardiac circulations.

V. **Internal cardiac compression** along with defibrillation rarely is practical but can be considered in the following situations: (1) penetrating chest trauma, (2) chest deformity that precludes adequate chest compressions, (3) severe hypothermia, (4) ruptured aortic aneurysm or pericardial tamponade that is unresponsive to pericardiocentesis, (5) during or shortly after procedures that require open thoracotomy, and (6) penetrating abdominal trauma. This procedure is successful only if implemented early during the arrest sequence by experienced personnel, rather than as a last resort.

VI. **Initiation and discontinuation**

A. **Resuscitation should be initiated in all patients who have had an arrest** unless those efforts would be futile or are against the patient's known wishes. The primary physician should have previously discussed with the patient or his or her surrogate the degree of intervention that the patient would wish permitted and should have communicated those desires in the chart (e.g., no CPR, no intubation, no defibrillation, no vasopressors).

B. **The decision to terminate ACLS should be individualized and influenced by the prearrest condition** (sepsis, metastatic cancer, stroke, cirrhosis, left ventricular dysfunction, etc.), **the intra-arrest condition, the response to resuscitative efforts, and the patient's wishes.** Only 16% of patients who have had cardiac arrest in the hospital survive to discharge (*Chest* 108:1009, 1995). Asystole, unwitnessed arrest, pulseless electrical activity (PEA), VF or VT refractory to more than three defibrillations, delay in initiating CPR, delay in defibrillation, resuscitative efforts of longer than 15 minutes' duration, or end-tidal carbon dioxide of less than 10 mm Hg all are associated with a poor outcome. The following conditions should be met before resuscitative efforts are discontinued: (1) countershocks for VF (if present) have been delivered, (2) the patient has been oxygenated and ventilated via a properly placed endotracheal tube, (3) IV access has been achieved and appropriate medications have been administered according to ACLS protocols, and (4) asystole or an agonal rhythm persists despite continued resuscitative efforts and an appropriate search for reversible causes. The duration of the resuscitative effort should be considered, as studies have shown that resuscitation attempts that persist for 30 minutes usually are unsuccessful. Neither the presence nor absence of neurologic signs, short of regained consciousness, provides a reliable end point for resuscitative efforts.

Specific Arrest Sequences in Advanced Cardiac Life Support

The following sequences and the figures in this chapter are useful in treating a broad range of patients with cardiac arrhythmias but should be modified as the clinical situation warrants. The decision to use specific interventions is guided by the overall condition of the patient, not only the arrhythmia displayed on the cardiac monitor. Figs. 8-1 through 8-5 outline the algorithms recommended by the American Heart Association; however, some patients may require care that is not specified in these algorithms.

I. **VF and pulseless VT** are the most common causes of nontraumatic adult cardiac arrests. Early defibrillation improves the chance of survival. Diagnosing and treating the underlying cause of arrest (e.g., hypokalemia, MI, hypoxia) should be performed promptly after successful defibrillation (Fig. 8-1).

A. **Early defibrillation** is critical and should be performed without delay before intubating or obtaining IV access. **Initial** defibrillation in a stacked sequence

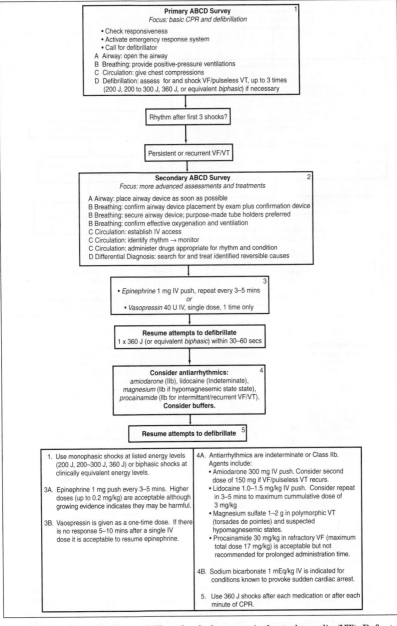

Fig. 8-1. Ventricular fibrillation (VF) and pulseless ventricular tachycardia (VT). Refer to the text for further details. [Adapted from Guidelines 2000 for Cardiopulmonary Resuscitation and Emergency Cardiovascular Care. Part 6: advanced cardiovascular life support: section 1: Introduction to ACLS 2000: overview of recommended changes in ACLS from the guidelines 2000 conference. The American Heart Association in collaboration with the International Liaison Committee on Resuscitation. *Circulation* 102(Suppl I):I86, 2000.]

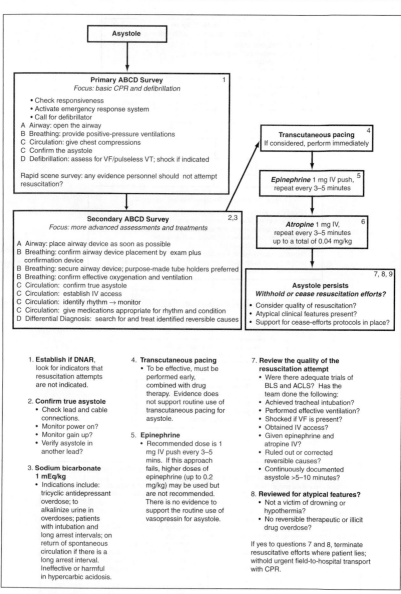

Fig. 8-2. Asystole algorithm. Refer to the text for further details. (ACLS = advanced cardiac life support; BLS = basic life support; DNAR = do not attempt resuscitation; VF = ventricular fibrillation; VT = ventricular tachycardia.) [Adapted from Guidelines 2000 for Cardiopulmonary Resuscitation and Emergency Cardiovascular Care. Part 6: advanced cardiovascular life support: section 1: Introduction to ACLS 2000: overview of recommended changes in ACLS from the guidelines 2000 conference. The American Heart Association in collaboration with the International Liaison Committee on Resuscitation. *Circulation* 102(Suppl I):I86, 2000.]

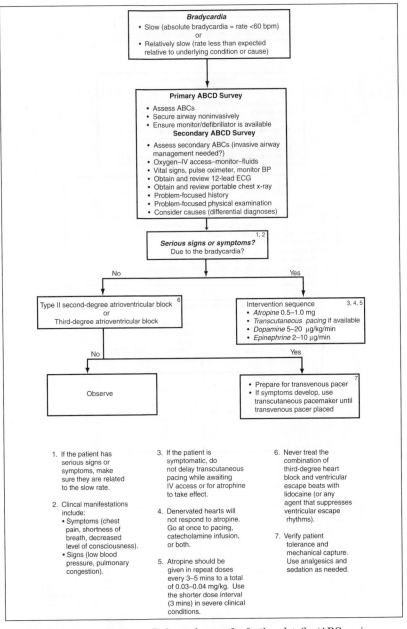

Fig. 8-3. Bradycardia algorithm. Refer to the text for further details. (ABC = airway, breathing, circulation; AV = atrioventricular; bpm = beats/min.) [Adapted from Guidelines 2000 for Cardiopulmonary Resuscitation and Emergency Cardiovascular Care. Part 6: advanced cardiovascular life support: section 1: Introduction to ACLS 2000: overview of recommended changes in ACLS from the guidelines 2000 conference. The American Heart Association in collaboration with the International Liaison Committee on Resuscitation. *Circulation* 102(Suppl I):I86, 2000.]

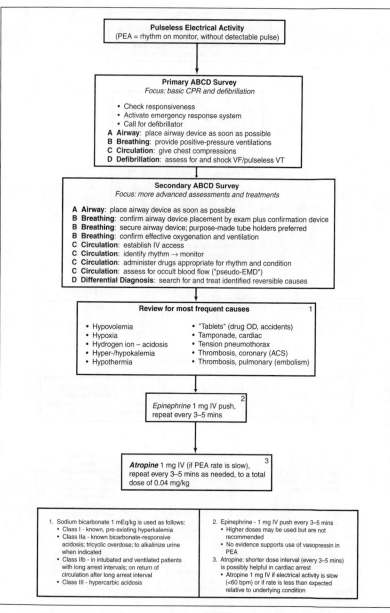

Fig. 8-4. Pulseless electrical activity algorithm. Refer to the text for further details. (ACS = acute coronary syndrome; EMD = electromechanical dissociation; OD = overdose; VF = ventricular fibrillation; VT = ventricular tachycardia.) [Adapted from Guidelines 2000 for Cardiopulmonary Resuscitation and Emergency Cardiovascular Care. Part 6: advanced cardiovascular life support: section 1: Introduction to ACLS 2000: overview of recommended changes in ACLS from the guidelines 2000 conference. The American Heart Association in collaboration with the International Liaison Committee on Resuscitation. *Circulation* 102(Suppl I):I86, 2000.]

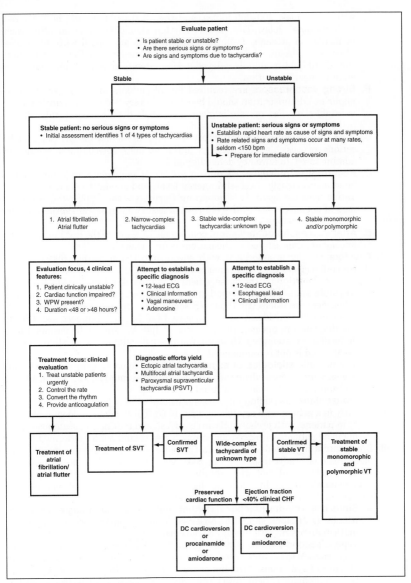

Fig. 8-5. Tachycardia overview algorithm. Algorithm assumes patient has a pulse. If patient becomes unstable at any point, move to immediate cardioversion. If delays in synchronization occur and the patient is unstable, proceed to immediate unsynchronized cardioversion. Refer to the text for further details. (bpm = beats/min; CHF = congestive heart failure; DC = direct current; SVT = supraventricular tachycardia; VT = ventricular tachycardia; WPW = Wolff-Parkinson-White.) [Adapted from Guidelines 2000 for Cardiopulmonary Resuscitation and Emergency Cardiovascular Care. Part 6: advanced cardiovascular life support: section 1: Introduction to ACLS 2000: overview of recommended changes in ACLS from the guidelines 2000 conference. The American Heart Association in collaboration with the International Liaison Committee on Resuscitation. *Circulation* 102(Suppl I):I86, 2000.]

with 200 joules, 200–300 joules, and then 360 joules should be delivered with minimal delay. The cardiac rhythm should be assessed after each defibrillation attempt. Defibrillation should be attempted with 360 joules after each subsequent dose of antiarrhythmic medication. Repeat defibrillation should not be unduly delayed during attemts at venous cannulation or endotracheal intubation.

B. **Strong vasopressors** are required for all patients in cariac arrest. Epinephrine administration should be repeated every 3–5 minutes until a pulse is established. Vasopressin is given as a single dose, one time only. Epineprine is continued 10-20 minutes after the dose of vasopressin.

C. If **VF or pulseless VT is refractory** to defibrillation and vasopressors, medications of possible benefit (e.g., antiarrythmics and buffers) should be administered, followed by defibrillation.

D. **Recurrent or pulseless VT** during the arrest sequence should be defibrillated at previously successful energy levels and should be treated with an antiarrhythmic agent. It is important to reassess continually the effectiveness of ongoing resuscitative efforts and assure adequacy of ventilation and chest compressions.

E. **After successful defibrillation,** continuous infusion of the last antiarrhythmic agent administered to the patient is undertaken.

II. **Asystole** usually is associated with severe underlying cardiac disease. This rhythm often constitutes a terminal condition, and the likelihood of resuscitation is poor. An algorithm for the management of asystole is outlined in Fig. 8-2.

A. **Asystole should be confirmed in two leads** that are perpendicular to each other, because isoelectric (fine) VF sometimes can masquerade as asystole (see General Considerations of Advanced Cardiac Life Support, sec. **I.B**). If the diagnosis is unclear, the presence of fine VF should be assumed and defibrillation attempted. However, routine defibrillation for asystole is detrimental and is not recommended.

B. The possible **etiologies of asystole** (hypoxia, hyperkalemia, hypokalemia, pre-existing acidosis, drug overdose, and hypothermia) should be considered and appropriate therapy instituted if identified.

C. **Transcutaneous pacing** may, in some instances, be of benefit if it is instituted early in a patient with asystole (see sec. **III.C**). This modality seldom is of benefit in patients with prehospital cardiac arrest, and routine transcutaneous pacing in all patients with asystolic cardiac arrest should not be performed.

III. **Bradycardia** is treated according to the patient's hemodynamic stability and mechanism of bradycardia (see Fig. 8-3). The focus should be on the patient's clinical status and not the absolute heart rate. The manifestations of hemodynamic instability include hypotension, pulmonary edema, altered mentation, ischemic chest pain, or acute MI.

A. **Sinus bradycardia, junctional rhythm, and type I second-degree atrioventricular (AV) block** should be observed in asymptomatic patients. Symptomatic patients require therapy as outlined below.

B. **Type II second-degree and complete AV block** are unstable rhythms and may progress to asystole or VF. A pacemaker should be considered even in the absence of symptoms. Atropine or transcutaneous pacing should be used in the symptomatic patient until a transvenous pacemaker can be placed. Pacing should be used preferentially for AV block at or below the His-Purkinje level (manifesting as a widened QRS complex). Atropine may exacerbate ischemia or induce VT and VF when used to treat bradycardia associated with acute MI (see Chap. 5).

C. **Transcutaneous pacing** results in improved survival in patients with hemodynamically unstable bradycardia and should be considered early in the resuscitative effort. Transvenous pacing should follow transcutaneous pacing. Signs of adequate circulation indicate effective cardiac pacing.

D. **Transvenous pacing** should be considered if transcutaneous pacing is not immediately available or is ineffective. In the postresuscitation period, transvenous pacing is more effective and can be placed more safely than during active resuscitation.

E. **If the bradycardia is a ventricular escape rhythm, the use of lidocaine may be lethal.** Additionally, lidocaine is not indicated for suppression of ventricular escape beats induced by the bradycardia.

IV. **PEA** includes idioventricular, ventricular escape, postdefibrillation idioventricular, and bradyasystolic rhythms and electromechanical dissociation, all of which are characterized by electrical activity (other than VT and VF) in the absence of a pulse. These arrhythmias are associated with a very poor outcome, especially in the prehospital setting. Rapid identification and treatment of an underlying cause increase the chance of survival. An algorithm for management of PEA is outlined in Fig. 8-4.

A. **Reversible causes** of PEA include hypovolemia, hypoxia, cardiac tamponade, tension pneumothorax, hypothermia, massive pulmonary embolism, drug overdose, hyperkalemia, severe acidosis, and massive MI.

B. **Doppler ultrasound** may reveal blood flow not detected by arterial palpation. Patients in whom these findings are made should be treated aggressively for severe hypotension (see Chap. 9).

V. **Tachycardias,** like bradycardias, are treated according to the patient's hemodynamic stability and the type of arrhythmia. Manifestations of hemodynamic instability (hypotension, pulmonary edema, altered mentation, ischemic chest pain, or acute MI) should be sought before appropriate therapy is determined. An algorithm for the approach to patients with a tachyarrhythmia is outlined in Fig. 8-5.

A. A **hemodynamically unstable patient** with a nonsinus rhythm that is greater than 150 beats/minute requires cardioversion. A brief trial of appropriate medication can be used while preparations for cardioversion are under way, but the delay should be minimal.

1. **IV access and supplemental oxygen** should be in place. The equipment and personnel that are necessary to support the airway should also be readily available. If possible, a short-acting sedative should be administered. Assistance from trained anesthesia personnel is optimal if these specialists are available and if the patient's condition permits.

2. **Synchronized cardioversion** should be performed starting at 100 joules and then increasing to 200, 300, and 360 joules if the tachycardia does not respond. Atrial flutter and supraventricular tachycardia (SVT) often respond to an initial shock of 50 joules. Polymorphic VT should initially be cardioverted with 200 joules. If delays in synchronization occur and the patient's condition is critical, unsynchronized cardioversion should be performed immediately.

3. **For heart rates of less than 150 beats/minute,** immediate cardioversion seldom is necessary. In the case of sinus tachycardia, cardioversion is not appropriate, and a search for the underlying cause should be performed.

B. **If the patient's condition is stable,** treatment is based on the determination of the underlying cardiac rhythm and function.

1. **Hemodynamically stable, monomorphic VT with normal cardiac function** is treated with one of the following agents: procainamide, sotalol, amiodarone, or lidocaine.

2. **Patients with underlying impaired cardiac function and stable monomorphic VT** should receive an amiodarone or lidocaine bolus. If there is no response to pharmacologic therapy, synchronized cardioversion is indicated.

3. **Torsades de pointes** is a characteristic form of VT that displays a gradual alteration in the amplitude and direction of electrical activity and commonly occurs with a prolonged QT interval. It should be considered when VT is refractory to the treatment outlined previously. Defibrillation should always be attempted if the arrhythmia is sustained or asso-

ciated with hemodynamic instability. See Chap. 7 for further details of management.

4. **Treatment of stable wide-complex tachycardias whose diagnosis remains unclear** despite careful evaluation is based on the patient's cardiac functional status. Cardioversion and amiodarone are recommended for patients with clinical heart failure. Cardioversion or procainamide or amiodarone are used in patients with preserved function.

5. **Paroxysmal SVTs** can initially be treated with vagal stimulation if this is not contraindicated. Various maneuvers are possible, but the most commonly used is unilateral carotid sinus massage, which should be performed carefully and avoided in elderly patients or those with carotid bruits. If maneuvers that cause vagal stimulation are contraindicated or are unsuccessful, IV adenosine should be given. Verapamil or diltiazem is an acceptable alternative but might cause hypotension. If patients do not respond to adenosine or verapamil, other drugs (digoxin, β-adrenergic antagonist, diltiazem) or elective synchronized cardioversion can be used.

6. Treatment of atrial fibrillation and flutter is outlined in Chap. 7.

Postresuscitation Management

The management of successfully resuscitated patients should focus on the treatment of the underlying disease process and the maintenance of electrical, hemodynamic, and respiratory stability. All patients require careful and repeated assessment and should be initially monitored in an intensive care unit. Evaluation and management of serum electrolytes, volume status, and previously initiated therapies (e.g., antiarrhythmic agents or pacing) are essential to successful long-term survival. Hypotension frequently is encountered in the postresuscitation period, and successful management depends on rapid determination of its etiology. Hypotension after cardiac arrest frequently is caused by derangements in a patient's intravascular volume, heart rate, cardiac performance, or a combination of these etiologies, and often requires invasive hemodynamic monitoring (see Chap. 9).

Common Medications Used in Advanced Cardiac Life Support

I. **Epinephrine** produces beneficial effects during CPR by increasing myocardial and cerebral blood flow. The recommended dose is 1 mg (10 ml of a 1:10,000 solution) repeated at 3- to 5-minute intervals. Higher doses of epinephrine (5.0 mg or 0.1 mg/kg) do not seem to be more effective (*N Engl J Med* 339:1595, 1998) and may be associated with worse neurologic outcomes (*Ann Intern Med* 129:450, 1998).

II. **Vasopressin** in high doses acts as a nonadrenergic peripheral vasoconstrictor and may be more effective than epinephrine in promoting the return of spontaneous circulation in cardiac arrest. It is administered once with a single dose of 40 units intravenously.

III. **Atropine** sulfate is used for symptomatic bradycardia and asystole. It may be beneficial for treatment of AV block at the nodal level and slow PEA. The recommended dose for symptomatic bradycardia is 0.5–1.0 mg IV, repeated every 3–5 minutes (q3–5min) if necessary. For asystole or PEA, the dose is 1 mg repeated q3–5min. The maximum dose is 0.04 mg/kg, which results in full vagal blockade. Atropine should be used cautiously in the setting of acute myocardial ischemia or MI, as excessive increases in heart rate may worsen ischemia.

IV. **Amiodarone** is recommended after defibrillation and vasopressors in cardiac arrest with persistent VT or VF. IV amiodarone is administered as a 300-mg rapid infusion diluted in a volume of 20–30 ml normal saline or dextrose in water. Supplementary doses of 150 mg by rapid infusion are administered for recurrent or refractory VT/VF, followed by an infusion of 1 mg/minute for 6 hours, then 0.5 mg/minute to a maximum daily dose of 2 g. Amiodarone is the preferred agent for the treatment of atrial and ventricular arrhythmias in patients with severely impaired heart function. It is effective for control of hemodynamically stable VT and wide-complex tachycardia of uncertain origin. It can control rapid ventricular rate due to accessory pathway conduction in pre-excited atrial arrhythmias. Amiodarone-induced hypotension and bradycardia are avoided by slowing the infusion rate or treated by fluids, pressors, chronotropic agents or temporary pacing.

V. **Lidocaine** can be used to treat VT or VF that persists after defibrillation and administration of epinephrine. Lidocaine is also beneficial in stable VT. An initial bolus of 1.0–1.5 mg/kg is required to achieve therapeutic levels rapidly. Additional boluses of 0.5–1.5 mg/kg can be administered q5–10min as needed to a total of 3 mg/kg. Only bolus dosing should be used in cardiac arrest. With the return of perfusion, a maintenance infusion of 2–4 mg/minute is recommended. Lidocaine levels should be monitored. Toxicity is more likely in patients with decreased cardiac output (i.e., acute MI, shock, and congestive heart failure), those who are older than 70 years, or patients with hepatic dysfunction. In these situations, the bolus dose remains unchanged, but the maintenance infusion should be decreased by half.

VI. **Procainamide hydrochloride** is recommended for treatment in patients with recurrent VT when lidocaine is contraindicated or has failed. Procainamide is more effective than lidocaine for hemodynamically stable monomorphic VT that is not associated with acute MI (*Am J Cardiol* 78:43, 1996). Procainamide is acceptable for treatment of wide-complex tachycardias associated with a pulse that cannot be distinguished from VT. Procainamide is administered by infusing 20–50 mg/minute until one of the following end points is reached: The arrhythmia is suppressed, hypotension ensues, the QRS complex is widened by 50%, or a total dose of 17 mg/kg is reached. The maintenance infusion rate is 1 to 4 mg per minute and is halved in patients with renal or cardiac dysfunction. The maintenance dose is adjusted according to subsequent drug levels. This drug should be avoided in patients with pre-existing QT prolongation, hypokalemia, hypomagnesemia, or torsades de pointes. Hypotension frequently occurs if procainamide is injected too rapidly.

VII. **Magnesium sulfate** might be beneficial in the treatment of torsades de pointes, VT, or VF associated with a hypomagnesemic state. The dose is 1–2 g IV administered over 1–2 minutes up to 4–6 g.

VIII. **Adenosine** is the first-line drug for SVT. The initial dose is 6 mg delivered as a rapid IV bolus over 1–3 seconds, followed immediately by a 20-ml saline flush. If no response occurs in 1–2 minutes, the dose should be increased to 12 mg followed by 18 mg delivered in the same fashion. The dose should be halved if a central line is used and can be repeated if necessary. Theophylline antagonizes the actions of adenosine, and therefore patients who take this drug might require larger doses of adenosine. Dipyridamole and carbamazepine prolong adenosine's effects. Adenosine should be used with caution in patients who are taking these medications or in heart transplant recipients.

IX. **Diltiazem or verapamil** is useful in the management of atrial fibrillation or flutter and multifocal atrial tachycardia. These agents can also be administered for treatment of SVT if adenosine has failed, the patient is hemodynamically stable, and the patient has a narrow QRS complex. The initial IV diltiazem bolus is 0.25 mg/kg. If necessary, a second dose of diltiazem (0.35 mg/kg) can be administered after 15 minutes. The maintenance infusion of diltiazem is 5–15 mg/hour, which is titrated to control the ventricular rate. Verapamil initially is given at a dose of 2.5–5.0 mg IV, followed by IV doses of 5–10 mg up to a maximum dose of 20 mg. The administration of IV calcium might prevent the hypotensive effects of these agents.

X. Isoproterenol (2–10 μg/minute) might be useful for refractory torsades de pointes (after magnesium and overdrive electrical pacing have failed). Isoproterenol is useful also for hemodynamically significant bradycardia in the denervated heart of a transplant patient until a pacemaker is available. Isoproterenol should rarely be used because it decreases cerebral and cardiac perfusion pressure. Epinephrine or dopamine is preferred for refractory bradycardia.

XI. Sodium bicarbonate is not recommended for routine use during the resuscitative effort. Use of this agent should be based on a clearly defined diagnosis. Bicarbonate administration is indicated for hyperkalemia and might also be beneficial for a known pre-existing acidosis, in the event of overdose with tricyclic antidepressants, and to alkalinize the urine in patients with a drug overdose. The initial dose is 1.0 mEq/kg given intravenously, followed by 0.5 mEq/kg given q10min. In most patients who experience cardiac arrest, acidosis is uncommon if BLS is performed adequately. Acidosis, if present, usually is due to inadequate ventilation; therefore, treatment should be directed at increasing the minute ventilation. No convincing evidence exists that acidosis adversely affects the ability to defibrillate the patient, the effectiveness of adrenergic agents, or survival. The utility of bicarbonate is poorly defined for patients with a prolonged arrest interval. The agent is not useful in patients with hypoxic lactic acidosis.

XII. Calcium has not been shown to improve survival in patients who experience cardiac arrest. Use of IV calcium should be limited to situations in which definite indications exist, including hyperkalemia, hypocalcemia, and calcium channel antagonist toxicity. When indicated, 10% calcium chloride is the preferred preparation, given as an IV bolus of 5–10 ml (500–1000 mg). Caution should be exercised in patients who are also taking digitalis because the toxic effects of digitalis may be potentiated by calcium.

9

Critical Care

Marin H. Kollef

The goals of critical care medicine are to save the lives of patients with life-threatening but reversible medical or surgical conditions and to offer the dying a peaceful and dignified death. Open discussions between physicians and patients and their family members ensure that critical care is provided in a manner that is most consistent with the patient's wishes.

Respiratory Failure

I. **General considerations.** Hypercapnic respiratory failure occurs with acute carbon dioxide retention [arterial carbon dioxide tension ($PaCO_2$) >45–55 mm Hg], producing a respiratory acidosis (pH <7.35). Hypoxic respiratory failure occurs when normal gas exchange is seriously impaired, resulting in hypoxemia [arterial oxygen tension (PaO_2) <60 mm Hg or arterial oxygen saturation (SaO_2) <90%]. Usually, this type of respiratory failure is associated with tachypnea and hypocapnia; however, its progression can lead to hypercapnia as well. Hypoxic respiratory failure can result from a variety of insults, as shown in Table 9-1. The acute respiratory distress syndrome (ARDS) is a form of hypoxic respiratory failure caused by acute lung injury. The common end result is disruption of the alveolar capillary membrane, leading to increased vascular permeability and accumulation of inflammatory cells and protein-rich edema fluid within the alveolar space. The American-European Consensus Conference has defined ARDS as follows: (1) acute bilateral pulmonary infiltrates, (2) ratio of PaO_2 to inspired oxygen concentration (FIO_2) less than 200, and (3) no evidence for heart failure or volume overload as the principal cause of the pulmonary infiltrates (*Am J Respir Crit Care Med* 149:818, 1994).

II. **Pathophysiology**

   A. **Hypoxic respiratory failure** usually is the result of the lung's reduced ability to deliver oxygen into the bloodstream, owing to one of the following six processes.

   1. **Shunt.** This term refers to the fraction of mixed venous blood that passes into the systemic arterial circulation after bypassing functioning lung units. Congenital shunts are due to developmental anomalies of the heart and great vessels. Acquired shunts usually result from diseases that affect lung units, although acquired cardiac and peripheral vascular shunts also can occur. Table 9-1 lists some of the more common disease processes that produce clinically significant pulmonary shunts. Shunts are associated with a widened alveolar-arterial oxygen tension [$P(A-a)O_2$] gradient, and the resultant hypoxemia is resistant to correction with supplemental oxygen alone when the shunt fraction of the cardiac output (CO) is greater than 30%.

   2. **Ventilation-perfusion mismatch.** Diseases associated with airflow obstruction [e.g., chronic obstructive pulmonary disease (COPD),

Table 9-1. Causes of shunts and hypoxic respiratory failure

Symptoms	Causes
Cardiogenic pulmonary edema (low permeability, high hydrostatic pressure)	Acute myocardial infarction
	Left ventricular failure
	Mitral regurgitation
	Mitral stenosis
	Diastolic dysfunction
Noncardiogenic pulmonary edema/ ARDS (high permeability, low hydrostatic pressure)	Aspiration
	Sepsis
	Multiple trauma
	Pancreatitis
	Near-drowning
	Pneumonia
	Reperfusion injury
	Inhalational injury
	Drug reaction (aspirin, narcotics, interleukin-2)
Mixed pulmonary edema (high permeability, high hydrostatic pressure)	Myocardial ischemia or volume overload associated with sepsis, aspiration, etc.
	High-altitude exposure
Pulmonary edema of unclear etiology	Upper airway obstruction
	Neurogenic cause
	Lung re-expansion

ARDS = acute respiratory distress syndrome.

asthma], interstitial inflammation (e.g., pneumonia, sarcoidosis), or vascular obstruction (e.g., pulmonary embolism) often produce lung regions with abnormal ventilation-to-perfusion relationships. In ventilation-perfusion mismatch, unlike shunt physiology, increases in FIO_2 result in increases in PaO_2.

3. **Low inspired oxygen.** Usually, FIO_2 is reduced at high altitudes or when toxic gases are inhaled. In patients with other cardiopulmonary disease processes, an inappropriately low FIO_2 can contribute to hypoxic respiratory failure.

4. **Hypoventilation.** This condition is associated with elevated $PaCO_2$ values, and the resultant hypoxemia is due to increased alveolar carbon dioxide, which displaces oxygen. Usually, oxygen therapy improves hypoxemia due to hypoventilation but may worsen the overall degree of hypoventilation, especially in patients with chronic airflow obstruction. Primary treatment is directed at correcting the cause of the hypoventilation.

5. **Diffusion impairment.** Hypoxemia due to diffusion impairments usually responds to supplemental oxygen therapy, as is seen in patients with interstitial lung diseases.

6. **Low mixed venous oxygenation.** Normally, the lungs fully oxygenate pulmonary arterial blood, and mixed venous oxygen tension ($P\overline{v}O_2$) does not affect PaO_2 significantly. However, a decreased $P\overline{v}O_2$ can lower the

PaO_2 significantly when either intrapulmonary shunting or ventilation-perfusion mismatch is present. Factors that can contribute to low mixed venous oxygenation include anemia, hypoxemia, inadequate CO, and increased oxygen consumption. Improving oxygen delivery to tissues by increasing hemoglobin or CO usually decreases oxygen extraction and improves mixed venous oxygen saturation ($S\bar{v}O_2$) and PaO_2.

B. Hypercapnic respiratory failure usually involves some combination of the following three processes.

1. **Increased carbon dioxide production** (i.e., respiratory acidosis) can be precipitated by fever, sepsis, seizures, and excessive carbohydrate loads in patients with underlying lung disease. The oxidation of carbohydrate fuels is associated with more carbon dioxide production per molecule of oxygen consumed as compared to the oxidation of fat fuels.

2. **Increased dead space** occurs when areas of the lung are ventilated but not perfused or when decreases in regional perfusion exceed decreases in ventilation. Examples include intrinsic lung diseases (e.g., COPD, asthma, cystic fibrosis, pulmonary fibrosis) and chest wall disorders associated with parenchymal abnormalities (e.g., scoliosis). Usually, these disorders are associated with widened $P(A-a)O_2$ gradients.

3. **Decreased minute ventilation** can result from CNS disorders (e.g., spinal cord lesions), peripheral nerve diseases (e.g., Guillain-Barré syndrome, botulism, myasthenia gravis, amyotrophic lateral sclerosis), muscle disorders (e.g., polymyositis, muscular dystrophy), chest wall abnormalities (e.g., thoracoplasty, scoliosis), drug overdoses, metabolic abnormalities (e.g., myxedema, hypokalemia), and upper airway obstruction. These disorders normally are associated with a normal $P(A-a)O_2$ gradient unless accompanying lung disease is also present.

C. Mixed respiratory failure is seen most commonly after surgery, particularly in patients with underlying lung disease who are undergoing upper abdominal procedures. Abnormalities in oxygenation usually occur on the basis of atelectasis, which often is multifactorial in origin (decreased lung volumes and cough due to the effects of anesthesia, abnormal diaphragmatic function resulting from the surgery or associated pain, and interstitial edema causing small airways to close). Hypoventilation can also result from abnormal diaphragmatic function, particularly when complete paralysis occurs, as with phrenic nerve injury.

III. Blood gas analysis (see Chap. 3, Acid-Base Disturbances)

Oxygen Therapy

The goal of oxygen administration is to facilitate adequate uptake of oxygen into the blood to meet the needs of peripheral tissues. When this goal cannot be accomplished with the methods outlined in secs. **I–IV**, endotracheal intubation may be necessary.

I. Nasal prongs allow patients to eat, drink, and speak during oxygen administration. Their disadvantage is that the exact FIO_2 delivered is not known, as it is influenced by the patient's peak inspiratory flow demand. As an approximation, the following guide can be used: 1 L/minute of nasal prong oxygen flow is approximately equivalent to an FIO_2 of 24%, with each additional liter of flow increasing the FIO_2 by approximately 4%. Flow rates should be limited to less than 5 L/minute.

II. Venturi masks allow the precise administration of oxygen. Usual FIO_2 values delivered with these masks are 24%, 28%, 31%, 35%, 40%, and 50%. Often,

Venturi masks are useful in patients with COPD and hypercapnia because one can titrate the PaO_2 to minimize carbon dioxide retention.

III. **Nonrebreathing masks** achieve higher oxygen concentrations (approximately 80–90%) compared to partial rebreathing systems. A one-way valve prevents exhaled gases from entering the reservoir bag in a nonrebreathing system, thereby maximizing the FIO_2.

IV. **A continuous positive airway pressure (CPAP) mask** can be used if the PaO_2 is less than 60–65 mm Hg during use of a nonrebreathing mask and the patient is conscious and cooperative, able to protect the lower airway, and hemodynamically stable (*N Engl J Med* 339:429, 1998). CPAP is delivered by a tight-fitting mask equipped with pressure-limiting valves. Many patients cannot tolerate a CPAP mask because of persistent hypoxemia, hemodynamic instability, or feelings of claustrophobia or aerophagia. In these patients, endotracheal intubation should be performed. Initially, 3–5 cm H_2O of CPAP should be applied while monitoring the PaO_2 or SaO_2. If the PaO_2 is still less than 60 mm Hg (SaO_2 <90%), the level of CPAP should be increased in steps of 3–5 cm H_2O up to a level of 10–15 cm H_2O.

V. **Bilevel positive airway pressure (BiPAP)** is a method of noninvasive ventilation whereby inspiratory and expiratory pressure can be applied by a mask during the patient's respiratory cycle. The inspiratory support decreases the patient's work of breathing. The expiratory support (CPAP) improves gas exchange by preventing alveolar collapse. Noninvasive ventilation using face or nasal masks has been successfully performed in patients with neuromuscular disease, COPD, and postoperative respiratory insufficiency as a means of decreasing the need for endotracheal intubation and mechanical ventilation (*Ann Intern Med* 128:721, 1998). In using BiPAP, a pressure-support ventilation (PSV) level of 5–10 cm H_2O and a CPAP level of 3–5 cm H_2O are reasonable starting points. The PSV level can be increased in increments of 3–5 cm H_2O, using the patient's respiratory rate as a guide of effectiveness.

Airway Management and Tracheal Intubation

Establishment of a patent airway and ventilatory support are required by many ICU patients. Specific indications for airway support in the form of endotracheal intubation include (1) initiation of mechanical ventilation, (2) airway protection, (3) inadequate oxygenation using less invasive methods, (4) prevention of aspiration and allowing for the suctioning of pulmonary secretions, and (5) hyperventilation for the treatment of increased intracranial pressure. In an emergency situation, such simple maneuvers as a jaw thrust with mask-to-face ventilation may assist the patient in clearing an obstructed airway and in maintaining adequate ventilation until endotracheal intubation can be performed.

I. **Airway management**

A. **Head and jaw positioning.** The oropharynx should be inspected, and all foreign bodies should be removed. For patients with inadequate respirations, the jaw thrust or head tilt–chin lift maneuvers should be performed (see Chap. 8, Basic Life Support, sec. **IV**, and Chap. 26, Acute Upper Airway Obstruction).

B. **Oral and nasopharyngeal airways.** When head and jaw positioning fail to establish a patent airway or when more permanent airway maintenance is desired, an oral or nasopharyngeal airway can be used. Initially, oral airways are positioned with the concave curve of the airway facing up into the roof of the mouth. The oral airway then is turned 180 degrees so that the concave curve of the airway follows the natural curve of the tongue. A tongue depressor can also be used to displace the tongue inferiorly and laterally to allow direct positioning of the oral airway. Careful monitoring of airway patency is required, as malpositioning of oral airways can push the tongue posteriorly and can result in obstruction of the oropharynx. Nasopharyngeal airways are made of soft plastic. These airways are passed easily down one of the nasal passages to the posterior pharynx after topical nasal lubrication and anesthesia with viscous lidocaine jelly.

C. **Laryngeal mask airway (LMA).** The LMA is an endotracheal tube with a small mask on one end that can be passed orally over the larynx to provide ventilatory assistance and prevent aspiration. Placement of the LMA is more easily performed than endotracheal intubation. However, it should be considered a temporary airway for patients who require prolonged ventilatory support.

D. **Mask-to-face ventilation.** After an airway is established, respiratory efforts should be evaluated and monitored closely. Ineffective respiratory efforts can be augmented with simple mask-to-face ventilation. Proper fitting and positioning of the mask ensure a tight seal around the mouth and nose, optimizing ventilation. Additionally, proper head positioning (see sec. **II.A**) and the use of airway adjuncts (e.g., oral or nasopharyngeal airways) optimize ventilation with a mask-to-face system.

II. **Endotracheal intubation** (*Respir Care* 44:615, 1999)

A. **Technique.** Depending on the skill of the operator and the urgency of the situation, one of several techniques can be selected for intubation of the trachea. Such techniques include (1) direct laryngoscopic orotracheal intubation, (2) blind nasotracheal intubation, and (3) flexible fiberoptically guided orotracheal or nasotracheal intubation. In emergency situations, the direct laryngoscopic technique allows for the most rapid intubation of the trachea with the largest endotracheal tube. Nasotracheal intubation often requires smaller endotracheal tubes that are more susceptible to kinking and obstruction and is associated with a higher incidence of otitis media and sinusitis. Before endotracheal intubation is attempted, a systematic evaluation of the patient's head and neck positioning must be performed. The oral, pharyngeal, and tracheal axes should be aligned before any intubation attempts. This "sniffing" position is achieved by flexing the patient's neck and extending the head. A small pillow or several towels placed under the occiput can assist in maintaining this position. Table 9-2 offers a step-by-step approach to performing successful orotracheal intubation. After successful intubation of the trachea, the tracheal tube cuff pressures should be monitored at regular intervals and should be maintained below capillary filling pressure (i.e., <25 mm Hg) to prevent ischemic mucosal injury.

B. **Verification of correct endotracheal tube positioning.** Proper tube positioning must be ensured by (1) direct view of the endotracheal tube entering the trachea through the vocal cords, (2) fiberoptic inspection of the airways through the endotracheal tube, or (3) use of an end-tidal carbon dioxide monitor. Clinical evaluation of the patient (i.e., listening for bilateral breath sounds over the chest and the absence of ventilation over the stomach) and radiographic evaluation (e.g., standard portable chest radiograph) can be unreliable for establishing correct endotracheal tube positioning. If uncertainty exists regarding the positioning of the endotracheal tube, it should be withdrawn and the patient reintubated.

C. **Complications.** Improper endotracheal tube positioning is the most important immediate complication to be recognized and corrected. Ideally, the tip of the endotracheal tube should be 3–7 cm above the carina, depending on head and neck positioning. Esophageal or right main-stem intubation should be suspected if hypoxemia, hypoventilation, barotrauma, or cardiac decompensation occurs. Abdominal distension, lack of breath sounds over the thorax, and regurgitation of stomach contents through the endotracheal tube indicate an esophageal intubation. Any uncertainty regarding the possibility of an esophageal intubation calls for immediate verification of tube

Table 9-2. Procedure for direct orotracheal intubation

1. Administer oxygen by face mask.
2. Ensure that basic equipment is present and easily accessible [oxygen source, bag-valve device, suctioning device, endotracheal (ET) tube, blunt stylet, laryngoscope, 20-ml syringe].
3. Place patient on nonmobile rigid surface.
4. If patient is in hospital bed, remove backboard and adjust bed height.
5. Depress patient's tongue with tongue depressor and administer topical anesthesia to patient's pharynx.
6. Position patient's head in sniffing position (see sec. **II.A**).
7. Administer intravenous sedation and neuromuscular blocker if necessary.*
8. Have assistant apply Sellick maneuver (compressing cricothyroid cartilage posteriorly against vertebral bodies) to prevent regurgitation and aspiration of stomach contents from esophagus.
9. Grasp laryngoscope handle in left hand while opening patient's mouth with gloved right hand.
10. Insert laryngoscope blade on right side of patient's mouth and advance to base of tongue, displacing tongue to the left.
11. Lift laryngoscope away from patient at a 45-degree angle using arm and shoulder strength. Do not use patient's teeth as a fulcrum.
12. Suction oropharynx and hypopharynx if necessary.
13. Grasp ET tube with inserted stylet in right hand and insert it into right corner of patient's mouth, avoiding obscuration of epiglottis and vocal cords.
14. Advance ET tube through vocal cords until cuff is no longer visible and remove stylet.
15. Inflate cuff with enough air to prevent significant air leakage.
16. Verify correct ET tube positioning by auscultation of both lungs and the abdomen.
17. Obtain a chest radiograph to verify correct position of the ET tube.

---

*Neuromuscular blockade can result in complete airway collapse and airway obstruction. Personnel who are skillful in establishment of an emergency surgical airway should be available if paralysis is used.

positioning or reintubation of the patient, with direct confirmation of endotracheal tube positioning. Other complications associated with endotracheal intubation include dislodgment of teeth, trauma to the upper airway, and increased intracranial pressure.

III. Surgical airways

A. Tracheostomy. The main indications for surgical tracheostomy are (1) the need for prolonged respiratory support, (2) potentially life-threatening upper airway obstruction (due to epiglottitis, facial burns, or worsening laryngeal edema), (3) obstructive sleep apnea that is unresponsive to less invasive therapies, and (4) congenital abnormalities (e.g., Pierre-Robin syndrome). Tracheostomy sites usually require at least 72 hours to mature. Tube dislodgment before site maturation, followed by blind attempts at tube reinsertion, can lead to tube malpositioning within a false channel in the pretracheal space; this misplacement can result in complete loss of the airway followed by progressive hypoxemia and hypotension. If a tracheostomy tube cannot be reinserted easily, standard direct orotracheal intubation should be performed (see Table 9-2). Optimal timing of surgical tracheostomy is controversial but should be considered after 10–14 days of mechanical ventilation if prolonged ventilation is anticipated (*Chest* 114:605, 1998).

B. **Cricothyrotomy.** This procedure is indicated for the establishment of an emergency airway when direct tracheal intubation cannot be performed owing to upper airway obstruction. A pillow or towel roll should be placed under the patient's shoulders to extend the neck. The thyroid cartilage superiorly and the cricoid cartilage inferiorly should be located where they border the cricothyroid membrane. The thumb and second finger of the surgeon's nondominant hand should grasp and stabilize the lateral aspects of the cricothyroid membrane. With a scalpel, a transverse skin incision is made over the entire distance of the membrane. The incision then is deepened to the cricothyroid membrane, avoiding injury to surrounding structures. Standard tracheostomy tubes or endotracheal tubes can be inserted into the stoma to ventilate the patient. Alternatively, prepackaged kits using the Seldinger technique with progressive dilatation of the stoma can be used.

C. **Cricothyroid needle cannulation.** In emergency settings when standard endotracheal intubation cannot be performed and placement of a surgical airway is not immediately possible, needle cannulation of the cricothyroid membrane can be performed as an intermediate procedure until a more definitive airway can be established. The ends of the cricothyroid membrane are grasped with the nondominant hand and a 22-gauge needle is inserted into the airway, aspirating air to confirm positioning. Lidocaine then is injected into the trachea to blunt the patient's cough reflex before the needle is withdrawn. By the same technique, a 14-gauge (or larger) needle-through-cannula device can be passed through the cricothyroid membrane at a 45-degree angle to the skin. When air is aspirated freely, the outer cannula is passed into the airway caudally, and the needle is removed. A 3-ml syringe barrel then can be attached to the catheter and a 7-mm inner-diameter endotracheal tube adapter attached to the syringe to allow bag-valve ventilation. Alternatively, the cannula can be attached directly to high-flow oxygen (i.e., 10–15 L/minute).

Mechanical Ventilation

I. **Indications.** The decision to begin mechanical ventilation is a clinical judgment that should take into account the reversibility of the underlying disease process as well as the patient's overall medical condition. Usual indications include severely impaired gas exchange, rapid onset of respiratory failure, an inadequate response to less invasive medical treatments, and increased work of breathing with evidence of respiratory muscle fatigue. Parameters that can help to guide the decision as to whether mechanical ventilation is needed include respiratory rate (>35), inspiratory force (≤25 cm H_2O), vital capacity (<10–15 ml/kg), PaO_2 (<60 mm Hg with FIO_2 >60%), $PaCO_2$ (>50 mm Hg, with pH <7.35), and an absent gag or cough reflex.

II. **Initiation of mechanical ventilation.** Certain variables should be considered when initiating mechanical ventilation.

A. **Ventilator type.** Often, ventilator selection is dictated by what is available at a particular hospital. A volume-cycled ventilator is used in most clinical circumstances.

B. **Mode of ventilation.** Several modes of mechanical ventilation are available. General guidelines for the use of the more commonly administered or referred to modes are provided.

1. **Assist-control ventilation (ACV)** should be the initial mode of ventilation used in most patients with respiratory failure. It produces a venti-

lator-delivered breath for every patient-initiated inspiratory effort. Controlled ventilator-initiated breaths are delivered automatically when the patient's spontaneous rate falls below the selected backup rate. Respiratory alkalosis is a potential concern when using ACV for patients with tachypnea.

2. **Intermittent mandatory ventilation (IMV)** allows patients to breathe at a spontaneous rate and tidal volume without triggering the ventilator, while the ventilator adds additional mechanical breaths at a preset rate and tidal volume. **Synchronized IMV (SIMV)** allows the ventilator to become sensitized to the patient's respiratory efforts at intervals determined by the frequency setting. This capability allows coordination of the delivery of the ventilator-driven breath with the respiratory cycle of the patient to prevent inadvertent stacking of a mechanical breath on top of a spontaneous inspiration. Potential advantages of SIMV include less respiratory alkalosis, fewer adverse cardiovascular effects due to lower intrathoracic pressures, less requirement for sedation and paralysis, maintenance of respiratory muscle function, and facilitation of long-term weaning. However, considerable patient-initiated respiratory muscle work may contribute to respiratory muscle fatigue and failure to wean from mechanical ventilation in some patients. This nonphysiologic work of spontaneous breathing can be alleviated by the addition of low levels of PSV (4–8 cm H_2O) or the addition of flow-by, or both (see sec. **II.C.6**).

3. **PSV** augments each patient-triggered respiratory effort by an operator-specified amount of pressure that is usually between 5 and 50 cm H_2O. PSV is used primarily to augment spontaneous respiratory efforts during IMV modes of ventilation or during weaning trials (see sec. **IV**). PSV can also be used as a primary form of ventilation in patients who can trigger the ventilator spontaneously. Increased airway resistance, decreased lung compliance, and decreased patient effort result in diminished tidal volumes and, frequently, in decreased minute ventilation. PSV is not recommended as a primary ventilatory mode in patients in whom any of the aforementioned parameters are expected to fluctuate widely.

4. **Inverse ratio ventilation (IRV)** uses an inspiratory-to-expiratory ratio that is greater than the standard 1:2–1:3 ratio (i.e., ≥1:1) to stabilize terminal respiratory units (i.e., alveolar recruitment) and to improve gas exchange primarily for patients with ARDS (*Crit Care Clin* 14:707, 1998). The goals of IRV are to decrease peak airway pressures, to maintain adequate alveolar ventilation, and to improve oxygenation. The use of IRV can be considered in patients with a PaO_2 of less than 60 mm Hg despite an FIO_2 of greater than 60%, peak airway pressures greater than 40–45 cm H_2O, or the need for positive end-expiratory pressure (PEEP) of greater than 15 cm H_2O. Most patients need heavy sedation and often muscle paralysis during the implementation of IRV.

5. **Lung-protective, pressure-targeted ventilation** (i.e., permissive hypercapnia) is a method whereby controlled hypoventilation is allowed to occur with elevation of the $PaCO_2$ to minimize the detrimental effects of excessive airway pressures. This form of ventilation has been used in patients with respiratory failure due to asthma and ARDS. For patients with ARDS it has been shown to improve survival (*N Engl J Med* 338:347, 1998).

6. **Independent lung ventilation** uses two independent ventilators and a double-lumen endotracheal tube. Usually, this modality is used for severe unilateral lung disease, such as unilateral pneumonia, respiratory failure associated with hemoptysis, or a bronchopleural fistula.

7. **High-frequency ventilation** uses rates substantially faster [60–3000 breaths/minute (bpm)] than conventional ventilation with small tidal volumes (2–4 ml/kg). The use of high-frequency ventilation is controversial except during upper airway surgery.

8. **Partial liquid ventilation** involves the partial filling of the lung with a perfluorocarbon solution. This type of ventilation has been demonstrated to improve pulmonary mechanics, oxygenation, and ventilation and perfusion matching in patients with ARDS. Partial liquid ventilation appears to improve gas exchange by recruiting previously atelectatic lung regions and by facilitating the transport of oxygen to all lung regions.

9. **Mechanical ventilation with inhaled nitric oxide (NO)** has been demonstrated to improve gas exchange in adults and children with respiratory failure, including patients with ARDS, primary pulmonary hypertension, or cor pulmonale secondary to congenital heart disease, and after cardiac surgery or heart or lung transplantation. Inhaled NO acts as a selective pulmonary artery (PA) vasodilator, decreasing PA pressures (without decreasing systemic BP or CO) and improving oxygenation by reducing intrapulmonary shunt (*Crit Care Med* 26:15, 1998). Generally, 5–20 parts/million of NO is administered, and the level of methemoglobin is monitored periodically.

C. **Ventilator management**

1. **FIO_2.** Hypoxemia is more dangerous than is brief exposure to high inspired levels of oxygen. The initial FIO_2 should be 100%. Adjustments in the FIO_2 can be made to achieve a PaO_2 of greater than 60 mm Hg or an SaO_2 greater than 90%.

2. **Minute ventilation.** Minute ventilation is determined by the respiratory rate and the tidal volume. In general, a respiratory rate of 10–15 bpm is an appropriate rate with which to begin. Close monitoring of minute ventilation is especially important in ventilating patients with COPD and carbon dioxide retention. In these individuals, the minute ventilation should be adjusted to achieve the patient's baseline $PaCO_2$ and not necessarily a normal $PaCO_2$. Inadvertent hyperventilation with resultant metabolic alkalosis in these patients may be associated with serious serum electrolyte shifts and arrhythmias. Initial tidal volumes usually can be set at 10–12 ml/kg. Patients with decreased lung compliance (e.g., ARDS) often need smaller tidal volumes (6–8 ml/kg) to minimize peak airway pressures and iatrogenic morbidity.

3. **PEEP** is defined as the maintenance of positive airway pressure at the end of expiration. It can be applied to the spontaneously breathing patient in the form of CPAP or to the patient who is receiving mechanical ventilation. The appropriate application of PEEP usually increases lung compliance and oxygenation while decreasing the shunt fraction and the work of breathing. PEEP increases peak and mean airway pressures, which can increase the likelihood of barotrauma and cardiovascular compromise. PEEP is used primarily in patients with hypoxic respiratory failure (e.g., ARDS, cardiogenic pulmonary edema). Low levels of PEEP (3–5 cm H_2O) may also be useful in patients with COPD, to prevent dynamic airway collapse from occurring during expiration. The main goal of PEEP is to achieve a PaO_2 of greater than 55–60 mm Hg with an FIO_2 of less than or equal to 60% while avoiding significant cardiovascular sequelae. Usually, PEEP is applied in 3- to 5-cm H_2O increments during monitoring of oxygenation, organ perfusion, and hemodynamic parameters. Patients who receive significant levels of PEEP (i.e., >10 cm H_2O) should not have their PEEP removed abruptly, because removal can result in collapse of distal lung units, the worsening of shunt, and potentially life-threatening hypoxemia. PEEP should

be weaned in 3- to 5-cm H_2O increments while oxygenation is monitored closely.

4. **Inspiratory flow rate.** Flow rates set inappropriately low can be associated with prolonged inspiratory times that can lead to the development of auto-PEEP. The resultant lung hyperinflation (i.e., auto-PEEP) can affect patient hemodynamics adversely by impairing venous return to the heart. Patients with severe airflow obstruction are at the greatest risk for development of lung hyperinflation when improper flow rates are used. Increasing the inspiratory flow rate usually allows for longer expiratory times that help to reverse this process.

5. **Trigger sensitivity.** Most mechanical ventilators use pressure triggering to initiate either a machine-assisted breath or to permit spontaneous breathing between IMV breaths, or during trials of CPAP. The patient must generate a decrease in the airway circuit pressure equal to the selected pressure sensitivity. Most patients do not tolerate a trigger sensitivity less than -1 or -2 cm H_2O due to autocycling of the ventilator. Alternatively, excessive trigger sensitivity can increase the patient's work of breathing, contributing to failure to wean from mechanical ventilation. In general, the smallest trigger sensitivity should be selected, allowing the patient to initiate mechanical or spontaneous breaths without causing the ventilator to autocycle.

6. **Flow-by.** To decrease the patient work of breathing, flow-by can be used as an adjunct to conventional modes of mechanical ventilation. Flow-by refers to triggering of the ventilator by changes in airflow as opposed to changes in airway pressures. A continuous base flow of gas is provided through the ventilator circuit at a preselected flow rate (5–20 L/minute). A flow sensitivity (i.e., patient rate of inhaled flow that triggers the ventilator to switch from base flow to either a machine-delivered or a spontaneous breath) is selected (usually 2 L/minute). Flow-triggered systems are more responsive than are pressure-triggered systems and result in a decreased work of breathing.

III. **Management of problems and complications**

A. **Airway malpositioning and occlusion** (see Airway Management and Tracheal Intubation, sec. **II.C**).

B. **Worsening respiratory distress or arterial oxygen desaturation** may develop suddenly as a result of changes in the patient's cardiopulmonary status or secondary to a mechanical malfunction. The first priority is to ensure patency and correct positioning of the patient's airway so that adequate oxygenation and ventilation can be administered during the ensuing evaluation.

1. **Briefly note ventilator alarms, airway pressures, and tidal volume.** Low-pressure alarms with decreased exhaled tidal volumes may suggest a leak in the ventilator circuit.

2. **Disconnect the patient from the ventilator and manually ventilate with an anesthesia bag using 100% oxygen.** For patients receiving PEEP, manual ventilation with a PEEP valve should be used to prevent atelectasis and hypoxemia.

3. **If manual ventilation is difficult, check airway patency by passing a suction catheter through the endotracheal tube or tracheostomy.** Additionally, listen for prolonged expiration continuing up to the point of the next manual breath. This suggests the presence of gas trapping and auto-PEEP.

4. **Check vital signs and perform a rapid physical examination with attention to the patient's cardiopulmonary status.** Be attentive to asymmetry in breath sounds or tracheal deviation suggesting tension PTX. Note other parameters, including cardiac rhythm and hemodynamics.

5. **Treat appropriately on the basis of the foregoing evaluation.** Treatment should be specific to the identified problems. If the presence of gas trapping and auto-PEEP is suspected, a reduction in the minute venti-

lation is appropriate. In some circumstances, periods of hypoventilation (4–6 bpm) or even apnea for 30–60 seconds may be necessary to reverse the hemodynamic sequelae of auto-PEEP (e.g., shock, electromechanical dissociation).

6. Return the patient to the ventilator only after checking its function. Increase the level of support provided by the ventilator to the patient after an episode of respiratory distress or arterial oxygen desaturation. Usually, this adjustment means increasing the FIO_2 and the delivered minute ventilation unless significant auto-PEEP is present.

C. An **acute increase** in the **peak airway pressure** usually implies either a decrease in lung compliance or an increase in airway resistance. At a minimum, considerations that should be entertained as causes of increased airway pressure include (1) pneumothorax (PTX), hemothorax, or hydropneumothorax; (2) occlusion of the patient's airway; (3) bronchospasm; (4) increased accumulation of condensate in the ventilator circuit tubing; (5) main-stem intubation; (6) worsening pulmonary edema; or (7) the development of gas trapping with auto-PEEP.

D. Loss of tidal volume, as evidenced by a difference between the tidal volume setting and the delivered tidal volume, implies a leak in either the ventilator or the inspiratory limb of the circuit tubing. A difference between the delivered tidal volume and the expired tidal volume implies the presence of a leak at the patient's airway due either to cuff malfunction or to malpositioning of the airway (e.g., positioning of the cuff at or above the level of the glottis) or a leak within the patient (e.g., presence of a bronchopleural fistula in a patient with a chest tube).

E. Asynchronous breathing ("fighting" or "bucking" the ventilator) occurs when a patient's breathing coordinates poorly with the ventilator. This difficulty may indicate unmet respiratory demands. A careful evaluation is mandated, with attention focused at the identification of leaks in the ventilator system or airway, inadequate FIO_2, or inadequate ventilatory support. The problem can be alleviated by adjustments in the mode of mechanical ventilation, rate, tidal volume, inspiratory flow rate, and level of PEEP. The identification of gas trapping with auto-PEEP may require changing multiple settings to allow adequate time for exhalation (e.g., decreasing rate and tidal volume, increasing inspiratory flow rate, switching from assist-control to SIMV in selected cases). Additionally, measures aimed at reducing the work of breathing with mechanical ventilation also may resolve the problem (addition of flow-by triggering or low levels of PSV to patients taking spontaneous breaths). If these adjustments are unsuccessful, sedation should be attempted. Muscle paralysis should be reserved for patients in whom effective gas exchange and ventilation cannot be achieved with other measures.

F. Organ hypoperfusion or hypotension can occur. Positive pressure ventilation can result in decreased CO and BP by decreasing venous return to the right ventricle, increasing pulmonary vascular resistance, and impairing diastolic filling of the left ventricle because of increased right-sided heart pressures. Increasing the preload to the left ventricle with fluid administration should increase stroke volume and CO in most cases. Occasionally, the administration of dobutamine (after appropriate preload replacement) or vasopressors becomes necessary. Under these circumstances, consideration should be given to reducing airway pressures (peak airway pressures <40 cm H_2O) at the expense of relative hypoventilation (i.e., pressure-targeted ventilation).

G. Auto-PEEP is the development of end-expiratory pressure caused by airflow limitation in patients with airway disease (emphysema, asthma), excessive minute ventilation, or an inadequate expiratory time. Graphic tracings on modern ventilators can suggest the presence of gas trapping by demonstrating persistent airflow at end expiration. The level of auto-PEEP can be estimated in the spontaneously breathing patient by occluding the expiratory port of the ventilator briefly just before inspiration and measuring the end-expiratory pressure reading on the ventilator's manometer. The presence of auto-PEEP can increase the work of breathing, contribute to barotrauma, and result in organ hypoperfusion by impairing CO. Appropriate adjustments to the ventilator can reduce or eliminate the presence of auto-PEEP (see sec. **II.C**).

H. Barotrauma or volutrauma in the form of subcutaneous emphysema, pneumoperitoneum, pneumomediastinum, pneumopericardium, air embolism, and PTX is associated with high peak airway pressures, PEEP, and auto-PEEP. Subcutaneous emphysema, pneumomediastinum, and pneumoperitoneum seldom threaten the patient's well-being. However, the occurrence of these disorders usually indicates a need to reduce peak airway pressures and the total level of PEEP. The occurrence of a PTX is a potentially life-threatening complication and should be considered whenever airway pressure rises acutely, breath sounds are diminished unilaterally, or BP falls abruptly (see Chap. 26, Pneumothorax). In most cases, acute tension PTX should be treated as an emergency by inserting a 14-gauge catheter-over-needle device into the pleural space at the xiphoid level in the midaxillary line or anteriorly into the second or third intercostal space in the midclavicular line. Chest tube insertion should follow.

I. Positive fluid balance and hyponatremia in mechanically ventilated patients often develop from several factors, including applied PEEP, humidification of inspired gases, administration of hypotonic fluids and diuretics, and increased levels of circulating antidiuretic hormone.

J. Cardiac arrhythmias, particularly multifocal atrial tachycardia and atrial fibrillation, are common in respiratory failure and should be treated as outlined in Chap. 7.

K. Aspiration commonly occurs despite the use of a cuffed endotracheal tube, especially in patients who are receiving enteral nutrition. Elevating the head of the bed and avoiding excessive gastric distension help to minimize the occurrence of aspiration. Additionally, pooling of secretions around the cuff of the endotracheal tube requires suctioning of these secretions before deflation or manipulation of the cuff.

L. Ventilator-associated pneumonia is a frequent complication associated with increased patient morbidity and mortality. Prevention of ventilator-associated pneumonia is aimed at avoiding colonization in the patient by pathogenic bacteria and their subsequent aspiration into the lower airway (*N Engl J Med* 340:627, 1999).

M. Upper GI hemorrhage may develop secondary to gastritis or ulceration. The prevention of stress bleeding requires ensuring hemodynamic stability and, in high-risk patients [e.g., those receiving prolonged mechanical ventilation (>48–72 hours) or with a coagulopathy], the administration of H_2-receptor antagonists, antacids, or sucralfate.

N. Thromboembolism (deep venous thrombosis and pulmonary embolism) may complicate the clinical course of patients who require mechanical ventilation. This disorder can be prevented in most patients by the prophylactic administration of SC heparin, 5000 units q8–12h, or the use of intermittent pneumatic compression devices.

O. Acid-base complications are common in the critically ill patient (see also Chap. 3).

    1. Nonanion gap metabolic acidosis may render weaning difficult, as minute ventilation must increase to normalize pH.

    2. Metabolic alkalosis may compromise weaning by blunting ventilatory drive to maintain a normal pH. In patients with chronic ventilatory insufficiency (e.g., emphysema, cystic fibrosis), correction of metabolic alkalosis usually is inappropriate and can cause an unsustainable minute ventilation requirement. Under these circumstances, a patient should be allowed to slow minute ventilation gradually to a more appropriate level. This change may be facilitated by switching from ACV to SIMV or PSV.

3. **Respiratory alkalosis** may develop rapidly during mechanical ventilation. When severe, it can lead to arrhythmias, CNS disturbances (including seizures), and a decrease in CO. Changing the ventilator settings to reduce the minute ventilation or changing the mode of ventilation (ACV to SIMV) usually corrects the alkalosis. However, some patients (such as those with ARDS, interstitial lung disease, pulmonary embolism, asthma) are driven to high respiratory rates by local pulmonary stimuli. In such patients, sedation with or without paralysis may be indicated briefly during the acute phase of the respiratory compromise.

P. **Oxygen toxicity** commonly is accepted to occur when an FIO_2 of greater than 0.6 is administered, particularly for more than 48 hours. However, the highest FIO_2 necessary should be used initially to maintain the SaO_2 at more than 0.9. The application of PEEP or other maneuvers that increase mean airway pressure (e.g., IRV) can be used to reduce FIO_2 requirements. However, an FIO_2 of 0.6 to 0.8 should be accepted before a plateau pressure above 35 cm H_2O is accepted. This cautionary note is due to the greater risk of morbidity associated with plateau pressures above this level (*N Engl J Med* 338:347, 1998).

IV. **Weaning from mechanical ventilation.** Weaning is the gradual withdrawal of mechanical ventilatory support (*Chest* 114:886, 1998). Successful weaning depends on the condition of the patient and on the status of the cardiovascular and respiratory systems. In patients who have had brief periods of mechanical ventilation, the manner in which ventilatory support is discontinued often is not crucial. In patients with marginal respiratory function, chronic underlying lung disease, or incompletely resolved respiratory impairment, the approach to weaning may be critical to obtaining a favorable outcome.

A. **Weaning strategies.** In general, the level of supported ventilation (minute ventilation) is decreased gradually, and the patient assumes more of the work of ventilation with each of the techniques described. However, it is important during the weaning process not to fatigue the patient excessively, which can prolong the duration of mechanical ventilation.

1. **IMV** allows a progressive change from mechanical ventilation to spontaneous breathing by decreasing the ventilator rate gradually. However, the weaning process may be prolonged if ventilator changes are not made often enough. Prolonged periods at low rates (<6 bpm) may promote a state of respiratory muscle fatigue because of the imposed work of breathing through a high-resistance ventilator circuit. The addition of PSV (see sec. **II.B.3**) may alleviate this fatigue but can prolong the weaning process if not titrated appropriately. Very often, tachypnea occurring during weaning of the IMV rate may represent a problem related to the imposed work from the ventilator circuit and the endotracheal tube rather than a diagnosis of persistent respiratory failure. In circumstances in which this problem is suspected, a trial of extubation may be appropriate.

2. **T-tube technique** intersperses periods of unassisted spontaneous breathing through a T tube (or other continuous-flow circuit) with periods of ventilator support (*N Engl J Med* 332:345, 1995). Short daytime periods (5–15 minutes 2–4 times/day) are used initially and then are increased progressively in duration. Small amounts of CPAP (3–5 cm H_2O) during these periods may prevent distal airway closure and atelectasis, although its effects on weaning success appear to be negligible (*Chest* 100:1655, 1991). Similar to IMV weaning, small amounts of pressure support (4–8 cm H_2O) can be used to decrease inspiratory resistance imposed by the ventilator circuit and the endotracheal tube. Extubation may be appropriate when the patient can comfortably tolerate more than 30–90 minutes of T-tube ventilation. More prolonged periods of T-tube breathing may produce fatigue, especially when small endotracheal tubes (i.e., <8-mm internal diameter) are used.

Table 9-3. Factors to be considered in the weaning process

Weaning parameters

   See Appendix H

Endotracheal tube

   Use largest tube possible

   Consider use of supplemental pressure-support ventilation

   Suction secretions

Arterial blood gases

   Avoid or treat metabolic alkalosis

   Maintain PaO_2 at 60–65 mm Hg to avoid blunting of respiratory drive

   For patients with carbon dioxide retention, keep carbon dioxide at or above the baseline level

Nutrition

   Ensure adequate nutritional support

   Avoid electrolyte deficiencies

   Avoid excessive calories

Secretions

   Clear regularly

   Avoid excessive dehydration

Neuromuscular factors

   Avoid neuromuscular-depressing drugs

   Avoid unnecessary corticosteroids

Obstruction of airways

   Use bronchodilators when appropriate

   Exclude foreign bodies within the airway

Wakefulness

   Avoid oversedation

   Wean in morning or when patient is most awake

---

      3. PSV is preferred by some practitioners when respiratory muscle weakness appears to be compromising weaning success (*Am J Respir Crit Care Med* 150:896, 1994). PSV can reduce the patient's work of breathing through the endotracheal tube and the ventilator circuit. The optimal level of PSV (PSV_{max}) is selected by increasing the PSV level from a baseline of 15–20 cm H_2O in increments of 3–5 cm H_2O. A decrease in respiratory rate with achieved tidal volumes of 10–12 ml/kg signals that the optimal PSV level has been reached. When the patient is ready to begin weaning, the level of PSV is reduced gradually by 3- to 5-cm H_2O increments. Once a PSV level of 5–8 cm H_2O is reached, the patient can be extubated without further decreases in PSV.

      4. Protocol-guided weaning of mechanical ventilation has been safely and successfully used by nonphysicians (*Crit Care Med* 25:567, 1997). The use of protocols or guidelines can reduce the duration of mechanical ventilation by expediting the weaning process.

   B. Failure to wean. Patients who do not wean from mechanical ventilation after 48–72 hours of the resolution of their underlying disease process need further investigation. Table 9-3 lists the factors that should be considered

Table 9-4. Guidelines for assessing withdrawal of mechanical ventilation

1. Patient's mental status: awake, alert, cooperative
2. PaO_2 >60 mm Hg with an FIO_2 <50%
3. PEEP ≤5 cm H_2O
4. $PaCO_2$ and pH acceptable
5. Spontaneous tidal volume >5 ml/kg
6. Vital capacity >10 ml/kg
7. Minute ventilation (MV) <10 L/min
8. Maximum voluntary ventilation double of MV
9. Maximum negative inspiratory pressure (MIP) ≥25 cm H_2O
10. Respiratory rate <30 breaths/min
11. Static compliance (Cst, rs) >30 ml/cm H_2O
12. Rapid shallow breathing index <100
13. Stable vital signs following a 1- to 2-hr spontaneous breathing trial

PEEP = positive end-expiratory pressure.
Source: From KL Yang, MJ Tobin. A prospective study of indexes predicting the outcome of trials of weaning from mechanical ventilation. *N Engl J Med* 324:1445, 1991; and EW Ely, AM Baker, DP Dunagan, et al. Effect on the duration of mechanical ventilation of identifying patients capable of breathing spontaneously. *N Engl J Med* 335:1864, 1996.

when weaning failure occurs. The acronym WEANS NOW has been developed to aid in addressing each of these factors (*J Respir Dis* 6:80, 1985). Commonly used parameters that can be assessed in predicting weaning success are listed in Table 9-4.

   C. Extubation. Usually, extubation should be performed early in the day, when full ancillary staff are available. The patient should be clearly educated about the procedure, the need to cough, and the possible need for reintubation. Elevation of the head and trunk to more than 30–45 degrees improves diaphragmatic function. Equipment for reintubation should be available, and a high-humidity, oxygen-enriched gas source with a higher-than-current FIO_2 setting should be available at the bedside. The patient's airway and the oropharynx above the cuff should be suctioned. The cuff of the endotracheal tube should be deflated partially, and airflow around the outside of the tube—indicating the absence of airway obstruction—should be detected. After the cuff is deflated completely, the patient should be extubated, and high-humidity oxygen should be administered by a face mask. Coughing and deep breathing should be encouraged while the examiner monitors the patient's vital signs and upper airway for stridor. Inspiratory stridor may result from glottic and subglottic edema. If clinical status permits, treatment with nebulized 2.5% racemic epinephrine (0.5 ml in 3 ml normal saline) should be administered. If upper airway obstruction persists or worsens, reintubation should be performed. Extubation should not be reattempted for 24–72 hours after reintubation for upper airway obstruction. Otolaryngology consultation may be beneficial to exclude other causes of upper airway obstruction and to perform tracheostomy if upper airway obstruction persists.

V. Drugs are commonly used in the ICU to facilitate tracheal intubation and mechanical ventilation (Table 9-5). Nondepolarizing muscle relaxants have been implicated in muscle dysfunction and prolonged weakness after their use in ICU patients (*Am Rev Respir Dis* 147:234, 1993). Some reports suggest a drug interaction between muscle relaxants and glucocorticoids, potentiating this effect. To minimize the chances of this complication, the continuous use of muscle relaxants should be limited to as brief a period as possible. Peripheral

Table 9-5. ICU drugs to facilitate endotracheal intubation and mechanical ventilation

Drug	Bolus dosages (IV)	Continuous-infusion dosages[a]	Onset	Duration after single dose
Succinylcholine	1.0–1.5 mg/kg	—	45–60 secs	2–10 mins
Pancuronium	0.05–0.08 mg/kg	0.2–0.6 µg/kg/min	2–4 mins	40–60 mins
Vecuronium	0.08–0.10 mg/kg	0.3–1.0 µg/kg/min	2–4 mins	30–45 mins
Atracurium	0.4–0.5 mg/kg	5–10 µg/kg/min	2–4 mins	20–45 mins
Diazepam	2.5–5.0 mg up to 20–30 mg	1–10 mg/hr or titrate to effect	1–5 mins	30–90 mins[b]
Midazolam	1–4 mg	1–10 mg/hr or titrate to effect	1–5 mins	30–60 mins[b]
Morphine	2–5 mg	1–10 mg/hr or titrate to effect	2–10 mins	2–4 hrs[b]
Fentanyl	0.5–1.0 µg/kg	1–2 µg/kg/hr or titrate to effect	30–60 secs	30–60 mins[b]
Thiopental	50–100 mg; repeat up to 20 mg/kg	—	20 secs	10–20 mins[b]
Methohexital	1–2 mg/kg	—	15–45 secs	5–20 mins[b]
Etomidate	0.3–0.4 mg/kg	—	10–20 secs	4–10 mins
Propofol	0.25–1.00 mg/kg	50–100 µg/kg/min	15–60 secs	3–10 mins[b]

[a]A continuous infusion should be started or titrated upward only after the desired level of sedation is achieved with bolus administration.
[b]Duration is prolonged with continued use either as repeated boluses or continuous IV administration. Frequent titration to the minimum effective dose is required to prevent accumulation of drug.

nerve stimulators should be used to titrate the dose of the muscle relaxant to the lowest effective dose. Finally, glucocorticoids should be avoided in patients who are receiving muscle relaxants unless their use is clearly indicated (e.g., for status asthmaticus, anaphylactic shock).

Shock

Circulatory shock is a process in which blood flow and oxygen delivery to tissues are disturbed; this event leads to tissue hypoxia, with resultant compromise of cellular metabolic activity and organ function. Oliguria, decreased mental status, decreased peripheral pulses, and diaphoresis represent the major clinical manifestations of circulatory shock. Survival from shock is related to the adequacy of the initial resuscitation and the degree of subsequent organ system dysfunction. The main goal of therapy is rapid cardiovascular resuscitation with the re-establishment of tissue perfusion using fluid therapy and vasoactive drugs. The definitive treatment of shock requires reversal of the underlying etiologic process.

I. **Resuscitative principles**
   A. **Fluid resuscitation** usually is the first treatment used. All patients in shock should receive an initial IV fluid challenge. The amount of fluid necessary is unpredictable but should be based on changes in clinical parameters, including arterial BP, urine output, cardiac filling pressures, and CO. Crystalloid fluid solutions (0.9% sodium chloride or Ringer's lactate) usually are administered, owing to their lower cost and comparable efficacy compared to colloid solutions (5% and 25% albumin, 6% hetastarch, dextran 40, and dextran 70). Blood products should be administered to patients with significant anemia or active hemorrhage. Young, adequately resuscitated patients usually tolerate hematocrits of 20–25%. In older patients, individuals with atherosclerosis, and patients who exhibit ongoing anaerobic metabolism, hematocrits of 30% or greater may be required to optimize oxygen transport to tissues.
   B. **Vasopressors and inotropes** play a crucial role in the management of shock states. Their use usually requires monitoring with intra-arterial and PA catheters. **Dopamine** is capable of stimulating cardiac β_1-receptors, peripheral α-receptors, and dopaminergic receptors in renal, splanchnic, and other vascular beds. The effects of dopamine are dose dependent. At dosages of 2–3 µg/kg/minute, dopamine primarily acts as a vasodilator, increasing renal and splanchnic blood flow. At dosages of 4–8 µg/kg/minute, dopamine increases cardiac contractility and CO via the activation of cardiac β_1-receptors. At higher dosages (>10 µg/kg/minute), dopamine increases BP by activation of peripheral α-receptors. **Dobutamine** is an inotropic agent that activates the α_1-, β_1-, and β_2-receptors. It exerts powerful inotropic effects, reduces afterload by indirect (reflex) peripheral vasodilation, and is a relatively weak chronotropic agent, accounting for its favorable hemodynamic response (increased stroke volume with modest increases in heart rate unless used in high dose or in the setting of hypovolemia). **Epinephrine** has α- and β-adrenergic activity. It is the agent of choice for anaphylactic shock. Like dopamine, its relative effects are dose dependent. **Norepinephrine** also has α- and β-adrenergic activity but primarily is a potent vasoconstricting agent. **Dopexamine** stimulates dopaminergic and β_2-adrenergic receptors without stimulating β_1- and α-adrenergic receptors, but this drug is not currently available in the United States. **Amrinone and milrinone** are noncatecholamine inhibitors of phosphodiesterase III that act as inotropes and as direct peripheral vasodilators to increase CO.

II. **Individual shock states** usually can be classified into four broad categories. These categories include hypovolemic shock (e.g., hemorrhage, dehydration), cardiogenic shock (e.g., acute myocardial infarction, cardiac tamponade), obstructive shock (e.g., acute pulmonary embolism), and distributive shock (septic shock and anaphylactic shock). Table 9-6 gives the main hemodynamic patterns seen with each of these shock states.
   A. **Hypovolemic shock** results from a decrease in effective intravascular volume that decreases venous return to the right ventricle. Significant hypovolemic shock (i.e., >40% loss of intravascular volume) that lasts more than several hours is often associated with a fatal outcome despite resuscitative efforts. Therapy of hypovolemic shock usually is aimed at re-establishing the adequacy of the intravascular volume. At the same time, ongoing sources of volume loss, such as a bleeding vessel, may require surgical intervention. Crystalloid solutions are used initially for the resuscitation of patients in hypovolemic shock. Fluid resuscitation must be prompt and should be given through large-bore catheters placed in large peripheral veins. **Rapid infusers or pumps** are available to increase the rate of fluid resuscitation. In the absence of overt signs of congestive heart failure, the patient should receive a 500- to 1000-ml initial bolus of normal saline or Ringer's lactate, with further infusions adjusted to achieve adequate BP and tissue perfusion. When shock is due to hemorrhage, packed RBCs should be given as soon as feasi-

Table 9-6. Hemodynamic patterns associated with specific shock states

Type of shock	CI	SVR	PVR	$S\bar{v}O_2$	RAP	RVP	PAP	PAOP
Cardiogenic (e.g., MI, cardiac tamponade*)	↓	↑	N	↓	↑	↑	↑	↑
Hypovolemic (e.g., hemorrhage)	↓	↑	N	↓	↓	↓	↓	↓
Distributive (e.g., septic)	—	↓	N	N–↑	N–↓	N–↓	N–↓	N–↓
Obstructive (e.g., massive pulmonary embolism)	↓	↑–N	↓	↑	↑	↑	↑	N–↓

CI = cardiac index; MI = myocardial infarction; N = normal; PAOP = pulmonary artery occlusion pressure; PAP = pulmonary artery pressure; PVR = pulmonary vascular resistance; RAP = right atrial pressure; RVP = right ventricular pressure; $S\bar{v}O_2$ = mixed venous oxygen saturation; SVR = systemic vascular resistance.
*Equalization of RAP, PAOP, diastolic PAP, and diastolic RVP establishes a diagnosis of cardiac tamponade.

ble. When hemorrhage is massive, type-specific unmatched blood can be given safely. Rarely, type O-negative blood may be needed.

B. Cardiogenic shock is seen most commonly after acute myocardial infarction (see Chap. 5) and usually is the result of pump failure. Other causes of cardiogenic shock include septal wall rupture, acute mitral regurgitation, myocarditis, dilated cardiomyopathy, arrhythmias, pericardial tamponade, and right ventricular failure due to pulmonary embolism. Cardiogenic shock secondary to acute myocardial infarction usually is associated with hypotension (mean arterial BP <60 mm Hg), decreased cardiac index (<2.0 L/minute/m²), elevated intracardiac pressures [PA occlusive pressure (PAOP) >18 mm Hg], increased peripheral vascular resistance, and organ hypoperfusion (e.g., decreased urine output, altered mentation; see Table 9-6).

1. Certain **general measures** should be undertaken. A PaO_2 of greater than 60 mm Hg should be achieved, and the hematocrit should be maintained at equal to or greater than 30%. Endotracheal intubation and mechanical ventilation should be considered to reduce the work of breathing (and therefore oxygen requirements) and to increase juxtacardiac pressures (P_{JC}), which may improve cardiac function. Similarly, noninvasive mechanical ventilation with BiPAP can be used to accomplish similar end points in patients who are able to sustain spontaneous breathing. Careful attention to fluid management is necessary to ensure that an adequate preload is present to optimize ventricular function (especially in the presence of right ventricular infarction) and to avoid excessive volume administration with resultant pulmonary edema.

2. **Pharmacologic treatment** usually involves two classes of drugs: inotropes and vasopressors. Vasodilators generally are not used in patients with cardiogenic shock due to severe hypotension. The use of vasodilators can be considered after the patient's hemodynamics have stabilized as a means of improving left ventricular function. Dopamine usually is administered first in patients with cardiogenic shock because it has both inotropic and vasopressor properties. Typically, the dose is titrated to maintain a mean arterial BP equal to or greater than 60 mm Hg. Subsequent guidance using a PA catheter helps to define what further

measures are required, including inotropic support (dobutamine, amrinone), afterload reduction (nitroprusside), and changes in intravascular volume (fluid administration vs. diuresis).

   3. **Mechanical circulatory assist devices** are required in patients who do not respond to medical therapy or who have specific conditions identified as the cause of shock (e.g., acute mitral valve insufficiency, ventricular septal defect). Intra-aortic balloon counterpulsation usually is performed with the device inserted percutaneously. The balloon filling is controlled electronically so that it is synchronized with the patient's ECG. The balloon inflates during diastole and deflates during systole, thus reducing afterload and improving CO. Additionally, coronary artery blood flow is improved during diastolic inflation. Intra-aortic balloon pumps should be considered only as an interim step to more definitive therapy.

   4. **Definitive treatment** must be considered for any patient with cardiogenic shock. This treatment can take the form of relatively noninvasive procedures (e.g., angioplasty) or more invasive surgical procedures (e.g., coronary artery bypass surgery, valve replacement, heart transplantation).

C. **Obstructive shock** usually is caused by massive pulmonary embolism. Occasionally, air embolism, amniotic fluid embolism, or tumor embolism also may cause obstructive shock. When shock complicates pulmonary embolism, therapy is directed toward preserving peripheral organ perfusion and removing the vascular obstruction. Fluid administration and the use of vasoconstrictors (e.g., norepinephrine, dopamine) may preserve BP while more definitive measures, such as thrombolytic therapy (e.g., streptokinase, alteplase, reteplase) or surgical embolectomy, are considered.

D. **Distributive shock** occurs primarily as septic shock or anaphylactic shock. These two forms are associated with significant decreases in vascular tone.

   1. **Septic shock** is caused by the systemic release of mediators that usually are triggered by circulating bacteria or their products, although the systemic inflammatory response syndrome can be seen without evidence of infection (e.g., pancreatitis, crush injuries, and certain drug ingestions such as salicylates) (*Chest* 101:1644, 1992). Septic shock is characterized primarily by hypotension due to decreased vascular tone. CO also is increased, owing to increased heart rate and end-diastolic volumes despite overall myocardial depression (*N Engl J Med* 328:1471, 1993). The main goals of treatment of septic shock include initial fluid resuscitation, adequate treatment of the underlying infection, and interruption of the mediator-associated systemic inflammatory response. Initial resuscitation includes appropriate large-volume fluid administration, to compensate for the decrease in vascular tone and dilated ventricular capacity. PA catheter-directed therapy may be important in such patients to determine the adequacy of preload and the need for inotropic or vasoconstrictor agents.

   2. **Anaphylactic shock** is discussed further in Chap. 11, Anaphylaxis.

Hemodynamic Monitoring and Pulmonary Artery Catheterization

I. **Indications.** A PA catheter can be placed to differentiate between cardiogenic and noncardiogenic forms of pulmonary edema, to identify the etiology of shock (see Table 9-6), for the evaluation of acute renal failure or unexplained acidosis, for the evaluation of cardiac disorders, or to monitor high-risk surgical patients in the perioperative setting. The PA catheter allows measurement of intravascular and intracardiac pressures, CO, and $P\overline{v}O_2$ and $S\overline{v}O_2$.

II. **Obtaining a PAOP "wedge pressure" tracing.** The PA catheter is advanced through a central vein after the distal balloon is inflated. Bedside waveform analysis is used to determine successful passage of the catheter through the right atrium, right ventricle, and PA into a PAOP position. Fluoroscopy should be used when difficulty is encountered in positioning the PA catheter. If, at any time after passage into the PA, the tracing is found to move off the scale of the graph, overwedging of the catheter has occurred. An overwedged catheter should be withdrawn immediately 2–3 cm after balloon deflation, and catheter positioning should then be rechecked with reinflation of the balloon. Overwedging of a PA catheter increases the likelihood of serious complications (e.g., PA rupture).

III. **Acceptance of PAOP readings.** Respiratory variation on the waveform, atrial pressure characteristics (including "a" and "v" waves), mean value of the PAOP tracing obtained at end expiration at less than the mean value of the PA pressure measurement, and the aspiration of highly oxygenated blood with the catheter in the PAOP position all indicate an accurate reading.

IV. **Transmural pressure.** When PEEP is present (applied or auto-PEEP), the positive intra-alveolar pressure at end expiration is transmitted through the lung to the pleural space. In these circumstances, the measured PAOP reflects the sum of the hydrostatic pressure within the vessel and the juxtacardiac pressure (P_{JC}). When significant levels of total PEEP are present (>10 cm H_2O), it is more appropriate to use the transmural pressure as a measure of left ventricular filling (transmural pressure = PAOP – P_{JC}). For patients with normal lung compliance, one-half of the total PEEP can be used as an estimate of P_{JC}. When lung compliance is depressed significantly (e.g., in ARDS), one-third of the total PEEP can be used as an estimate for P_{JC}.

V. **CO.** PA catheters are equipped with a thermistor to measure CO. At least two measurements that differ by less than 10–15% should be obtained. Injections should be synchronized with the respiratory cycle to minimize variability between results. Often, thermodilution measurements of CO are inaccurate at an extremely low CO (e.g., <1.5 L/minute) or an extremely high CO (e.g., >7.0 L/minute), in the presence of significant valvular disease (e.g., severe tricuspid insufficiency), and when large intracardiac shunts are present. Calculation of the CO using the Fick formula (see Appendix H) may be more accurate in these circumstances.

VI. **Interpretation of hemodynamic readings.** PAOP can be used as an index of left ventricular filling (preload) and as an index of the patient's propensity for developing pulmonary edema.

A. **Optimizing cardiac function.** Improving cardiac function by optimizing preload is more efficient in terms of myocardial oxygen consumption in comparison to similar improvements in cardiac function by use of inotropes when preload is inadequate. As a general rule, preload should be optimized before inotropic agents (which can increase myocardial oxygen consumption) or vasodilators (which can cause hypotension when preload is inadequate) are used. Fluid boluses should be administered in patients who are suspected of having inadequate cardiac filling pressures (i.e., inadequate preload) and should be followed by repeat measurements of PAOP, CO, heart rate, and stroke volume. In low CO states, if the PAOP increases by less than 5 mm Hg without significant changes in heart rate, CO, and stroke volume, additional fluid boluses may have to be given. An increase in the PAOP by more than 5 mm Hg usually signals that adequate ventricular filling is being achieved. Once the patient's preload has been optimized, cardiac performance can be reassessed and, if necessary, further therapy with inotropes (e.g., dobutamine, amrinone) or with vasodilators (e.g., nitroprusside, hydralazine, angiotensin-converting enzyme inhibitors) can be initiated to achieve further improvements in cardiac performance and tissue perfusion.

B. Reducing unnecessary lung water. PAOP is a reflection of the lung's tendency to develop pulmonary edema. Decreased left ventricular compliance results in a "critical pressure" being reached sooner for similar volume changes as compared to a normally compliant left ventricle. This difference is due to the increased stiffness of the noncompliant ventricle that causes higher pressures to be achieved for similar changes in volume. To optimize cardiac performance and to minimize the tendency for pulmonary edema formation, PAOP should be kept at the lowest point at which cardiac performance is acceptable.

C. Differentiating hydrostatic from nonhydrostatic pulmonary edema. The management of pulmonary edema depends in large part on whether the excessive accumulation of lung water is due to increased hydrostatic pressures (e.g., left ventricular failure, mitral stenosis, acute volume overload), increased permeability of the alveolocapillary barrier (e.g., ARDS due to sepsis, aspiration, or trauma), or a combination of these factors. Clinical and radiographic criteria alone often are insufficient to determine the underlying mechanisms of pulmonary edema. Therefore, less than optimal management of the patient's underlying disease process may occur. In general, a PAOP of less than 18 mm Hg suggests that the primary mechanism of pulmonary edema is nonhydrostatic. Values above 18 mm Hg support a hydrostatic cause for the increased lung water.

D. Adequacy of organ perfusion. Oxygen delivery to tissues depends on (1) an intact respiratory system to provide oxygen for hemoglobin saturation, (2) the concentration of hemoglobin, (3) CO, (4) tissue microcirculation, and (5) the unloading of oxygen from hemoglobin for diffusion into the tissue beds. Oxygen delivery can be measured as the product of CO and arterial oxygen content (CaO_2). CaO_2 is the sum of hemoglobin-bound and dissolved oxygen (see Appendix H). Inadequate organ perfusion generally is associated with elevated blood lactate levels and decreased $S\overline{v}O_2$ (usually <0.6). Factors that contribute to a low $S\overline{v}O_2$ include anemia, hypoxemia, inadequate CO, and increased oxygen consumption. Factors that may elevate measured $S\overline{v}O_2$ despite tissue hypoxia include peripheral arteriovenous shunting, the blood flow maldistribution of sepsis or cirrhosis, and cellular poisoning, such as that associated with cyanide toxicity. In general, optimization of gas exchange and CO along with an adequate hemoglobin (usually ≥10 g/dl) results in improved oxygen delivery to tissues.

Pulmonary Diseases

10

Subramanian Paranjothi
and Dan Schuller

Pulmonary Symptoms

I. **Cough** is a normal reflex that protects the lung from injury by inhaled or aspirated foreign material. Cough also can be a pathologic symptom signaling the presence of abnormal conditions within the respiratory tract or anywhere along the cough reflex afferent component. A chronic cough is one that has been persistent for at least 3 weeks.

A. **The diagnostic evaluation** of chronic cough is simplified by following a systematic approach based on the anatomic location of the cough receptors (nose, sinuses, pharynx, larynx, tracheobronchial tree, pleura, pericardium, diaphragm, and stomach). Cigarette smoking is associated with the highest prevalence of cough. Among smokers of one pack/day, 25% report a chronic cough. After smoking cessation, the cough resolves within 1 month in half of the patients. In patients with a normal chest radiograph, more than 90% of cases of cough are attributable to the isolated or combined presence of postnasal drip (allergic or nonallergic sinusitis or vasomotor rhinitis), asthma, gastroesophageal reflux, and chronic bronchitis. Chronic cough may be the sole presenting manifestation of bronchial asthma or gastroesophageal reflux disease (GERD). *Bordetella pertussis* infection has been postulated as a common cause of persistent cough in adults (*JAMA* 273:1044, 1995). Drugs associated with cough include angiotensin-converting enzyme inhibitors, β-adrenergic blockers (oral or ophthalmic), aspirin, nonsteroidal anti-inflammatory medications, cholinesterase inhibitors, tryptophan, nitrofurantoin, amiodarone, inhaled medications (corticosteroids, pentamidine, ipratropium), and sulfites. A detailed history and physical examination usually provide cardinal clues to the diagnosis.

B. **Specific therapy** directed at the cause of cough is successful in eliminating chronic cough in most patients. However, the average length of time for resolution can be approximately 2 months for postnasal drip syndrome or asthma and as long as 6 months for GERD (*Am Rev Respir Dis* 141:640, 1990). (For treatment of GERD, see Chap. 17.) Often, cough due to asthma is refractory to bronchodilators alone and improves with anti-inflammatory therapy, such as inhaled corticosteroids, cromolyn, or nedocromil (*Chest* 96:583, 1989). GERD is treated initially with physical measures, dietary modification, and pharmacologic intervention with H_2 receptor antagonists or omeprazole. Often, prolonged treatment is necessary (*JAMA* 276:983, 1996; see Chap. 17). If the patient is a smoker and has a negative chest radiograph, an aggressive strategy for smoking cessation should be instituted, with re-evaluation in 4–6 weeks before embarking on an extensive evaluation. For nonsmokers without clues from the history and a normal chest radiograph, pulmonary function testing with bronchoprovocation should be considered. Paranasal sinus imaging and 24-hour esophageal pH monitoring can be obtained when the diagnosis still is in question or the patient has failed an empiric therapeutic trial.

C. Nonspecific therapy consists of agents that suppress the cough reflex centrally or peripherally. Antitussive agents are not particularly effective and are associated with potential side effects. They are appropriate only when the underlying abnormality is not responsive to specific therapy and the deleterious effects from coughing (e.g., fatigue, insomnia, bronchoconstriction, hemodynamic complication, musculoskeletal consequences, bladder or bowel incontinence) outweigh the side effects. All narcotics are effective antitussive agents; however, their use is limited by the potential for addiction and abuse. Among the narcotic medications, codeine (15–30 mg PO q4–6h) is the drug of choice. Hydrocodone (5–10 mg PO q4–6h) or hydromorphone (1 mg PO q3–4h) are more potent alternatives with a higher potential for abuse. Dextromethorphan (10–20 mg PO q4–6h) is a nonnarcotic agent derived from levorphanol; it has no analgesic effect and thus no significant abuse potential. It is contraindicated in patients receiving monoamine oxidase inhibitors. Benzonatate (100 mg PO tid) is thought to act on peripheral and central receptors. Cough productive of copious bronchial secretions that need to be cleared is a relative contraindication for antitussive agents.

II. Hemoptysis is a nonspecific sign associated with many pulmonary diseases, including infection (e.g., bronchitis, lung abscess, tuberculosis, aspergilloma, pneumonia, bronchiectasis), neoplasm, cardiovascular disease (e.g., mitral stenosis, pulmonary embolus, pulmonary vascular malformations, aortic aneurysm), iatrogenic causes, autoimmune disorders (e.g., Wegener's granulomatosis, Goodpasture's syndrome, systemic lupus erythematosus), and drugs or toxins (e.g., cocaine, anticoagulants, thrombolytic agents, penicillamine, solvents, amiodarone, dextran 70). Often, the specific etiology of hemoptysis never is determined.

A. Diagnosis

1. **History and physical examination** should confirm that the source of bleeding is located in the lower respiratory tract and not in the GI tract or nasopharynx. An attempt should be made to estimate the amount of bleeding. The remainder of the clinical evaluation should focus on obtaining clues to the cause of hemoptysis.

2. **Laboratory studies** include a chest radiograph, sputum cytology, appropriate sputum stains and cultures, arterial blood gas levels (ABGs), tests of hemostasis, and urinalysis to detect RBCs or RBC casts that may be associated with Wegener's granulomatosis or Goodpasture's syndrome.

3. **Bronchoscopy** is indicated in patients who have hemoptysis and have a risk factor for carcinoma, even if hemoptysis is minor and the radiograph is normal. Risk factors for carcinoma include (1) age greater than 40 years, (2) significant smoking history, (3) hemoptysis of more than 1 week's duration, and (4) unexplained abnormality on chest radiograph. If bleeding is brisk, rigid bronchoscopy is required.

B. Therapy is tailored to the severity of the episode and to the underlying cause. Minor hemoptysis. Therapy for minor bleeding or blood-streaked sputum should be directed at the specific etiology. **Massive hemoptysis** is defined as more than 600 ml blood over 48 hours or quantities that are sufficient to impair gas exchange. The primary goals of therapy are to maintain the airway, optimize oxygenation, and stabilize the hemodynamic status.

1. **Supportive care.** While awaiting surgical consultation, clinically stable patients should be positioned with the bleeding side in a dependent position to reduce aspiration of blood into the contralateral lung. Supplemental oxygen should be supplied. Sedatives aid patient cooperation, but excessive sedation may suppress airway protection and mask signs of respiratory decompensation. Bed rest, mild cough suppression, and avoidance of excessive thoracic manipulation (e.g., chest percussion, incentive spirometry) are helpful.

2. **Definitive therapy.** Once stabilization is accomplished, diagnostic and therapeutic interventions should be performed promptly, because recurrent bleeding occurs unpredictably.

a. **Early bronchoscopy,** preferably during active bleeding, helps to localize the specific site and to identify the cause of the bleeding. In those patients with lateralized or localized persistent bleeding, immediate control of the airway can be obtained during the procedure with topical therapy, endobronchial tamponade, or unilateral intubation of the nonbleeding lung.

b. **If bleeding continues** but the site of origin is uncertain, lung isolation or use of a double-lumen tube is reasonable, provided that the staff is skilled in this procedure. If the bleeding cannot be localized because the rate of hemorrhage renders visualization of the airway impossible, emergency rigid bronchoscopy or arteriography and embolization are indicated.

c. **Urgent surgical intervention** should be considered in operative candidates with unilateral bleeding when embolization is unavailable or unfeasible, when bleeding continues despite embolization, or when bleeding is associated with persistent hemodynamic and respiratory compromise. Contraindications to surgical resection include inoperable lung cancer and previous pulmonary function studies precluding pulmonary resection [e.g., predicted postoperative forced expiratory volume in 1 second (FEV_1) of <800 ml].

Pleural Effusion

Transudative pleural effusions are formed when the normal hydrostatic or oncotic pressures are perturbed [e.g., increased mean capillary pressure (heart failure) or decreased oncotic pressure (cirrhosis or nephrotic syndrome)]. **Exudative pleural effusions** occur when damage or disruption of the normal pleural membranes or vasculature occurs and leads to increased capillary permeability or decreased lymphatic drainage (e.g., tumor involvement of the pleural space, infection, inflammatory conditions, or trauma).

I. **Diagnosis.** Most pleural effusions require further evaluation unless their origin is clear (e.g., heart failure) and the patient is responding well to therapy (*Am Rev Respir Dis* 140:257, 1989).

A. **Thoracentesis** can be performed safely in the absence of disorders of hemostasis on effusions that demonstrate a thickness of greater than 10 mm on lateral decubitus films. Loculated effusions can be localized with ultrasonography or CT scan. Proper technique and sonographic guidance minimize the risk of pneumothorax and other complications.

1. **The etiology** of an effusion frequently can be deduced from the clinical circumstances (e.g., CHF or hepatic failure with ascites). Exudates have at least one (and transudates none) of the following: (1) a pleural fluid protein–serum protein ratio of greater than 0.5, (2) a pleural fluid–serum lactate dehydrogenase (LDH) ratio of greater than 0.6, or (3) a pleural fluid LDH of more than two-thirds of the upper limit of normal for serum LDH. Proposed additional criteria for an exudative pleural effusion include (1) a cholesterol level of greater than 45 mg/dl, (2) a serum–pleural albumin gradient of less than 1.2 g/dl, or (3) a pleural–serum bilirubin ratio of greater than 0.6 (*Chest* 111:970, 1997). Parapneumonic effusions are exudates that develop secondary to pulmonary infections. An empyema is pus in the pleural space. The pleural fluid glucose, pH, and LDH are helpful in differentiating complicated parapneumonic effusions (Table 10-1) and are useful to identify the patients who usually will require chest tube drainage.

2. **Other studies** involving pleural fluid that may be useful in specific clinical settings include cell count and differential, amylase, triglycerides, microbiologic stains, cultures, and cytology. Some useful observations have been obtained from the results of studies on pleural fluid.

Table 10-1. Parapneumonic effusions and empyema

Type	Pleural fluid chemistry	Pleural fluid bacteriology	Management
Typical parapneumonic effusion	pH >7.20, LDH <1000 IU/L, glucose >40 mg/dl	Negative Gram stain	Antibiotics alone
Complicated parapneumonic effusion—borderline	pH 7.00–7.20, LDH >1000 IU/L, glucose >40 mg/dl	Negative Gram stain	May require drainage; repeat thoracentesis within 24 hrs is recommended
Complicated parapneumonic effusion—simple	pH <7.00, LDH >1000 IU/L, glucose <40 mg/dl	Gram stain–positive or culture-positive fluid but not frank pus or loculated	Tube thoracostomy plus antibiotics
Complicated parapneumonic effusion—complex	pH <7.00, LDH >1000 IU/L, glucose <40 mg/dl	Gram stain–positive or culture-positive loculated fluid but not frank pus	Tube thoracostomy, antibiotics, and (if unsuccessful) consideration for use of intrapleural thrombolytic agents or thoracoscopy
Empyema—simple	—	Free-flowing frank pus in a single loculus	Large-tube thoracostomy, antibiotics, and consideration for decortication if an empyema cavity remains after 1 wk of drainage
Empyema—complex	—	Multiloculated frank pus	Large-tube thoracostomy, antibiotics, and consideration for intrapleural thrombolytic therapy; most require thoracoscopy or decortication

Source: Adapted from RW Light. *Pleural Diseases*. Baltimore: Williams & Wilkins, 1995.

  a. The diagnosis of a **hemothorax** is established by the demonstration of a pleural fluid–blood hematocrit ratio of more than 0.5. Gross blood is seen with tumor, pulmonary infarction, or trauma.
  b. A **pH of less than 7.3** is seen with empyema, tuberculosis, malignancy, collagen vascular disease, or esophageal rupture.
  c. **Glucose** concentration of less than 40 mg/dl is associated with an empyema, rheumatoid arthritis, tuberculosis, or malignancy.
  d. An **elevation of eosinophil count** (>10% of total nucleated cell count) may occur with bloody effusions, pneumothorax (or previous thoracentesis), fungal and parasitic infection, drug-induced disease, and malignancy.

    e. An **elevation of amylase** may occur with pancreatitis, pancreatic pseudocyst, renal failure, malignancy, esophageal rupture, or ruptured ectopic pregnancy.

    f. **Elevation of triglycerides** (>110 mg/dl) indicates chylous effusions, which are caused by thoracic duct rupture from trauma, surgery, or malignancy (usually lymphoma).

    g. **Cytology** is positive in approximately 60% of malignant effusions. Priming the fluid collection bag with 300–1000 IU heparin and submitting a large pleural fluid volume maximize the diagnostic yield for cytologic diagnosis.

B. **Closed pleural biopsy** should be performed when the cause of an exudative pleural effusion cannot be determined by thoracentesis. For tuberculous effusions, pleural fluid cultures alone are positive in only 20–25% of cases; however, the combination of pleural fluid studies and pleural biopsy (demonstrating granulomas or organisms) is 90% sensitive in establishing tuberculosis as the etiology of the effusion. For malignant effusions, pleural biopsies add a small but significant diagnostic yield to fluid cytology alone.

C. **Other diagnostic procedures** that are useful in establishing the etiology of a pleural effusion when the foregoing tests are normal include biopsy of other abnormal sites (e.g., a mediastinal or lung mass), diagnostic thoracoscopy, and evaluation for pulmonary emboli.

II. Treatment

A. **Symptomatic pleural effusions** may require removal of large amounts of pleural fluid. The rapid removal of more than 1 L of pleural fluid may result (rarely) in re-expansion pulmonary edema. When frequent or repeated thoracentesis is required for effusions that reaccumulate, early consideration should be given to tube drainage and pleurodesis.

B. **Parapneumonic effusions and empyema.** Appropriate management is instituted according to a classification based on the size of the effusions, the gross characteristics of the pleural fluid, the biochemical analysis, and the presence of loculations (*Chest* 108:299, 1995). Insignificant parapneumonic effusions (small, <10 mm thick on decubitus film) almost always resolve with antibiotic therapy alone. Performing a thoracentesis is unnecessary unless the effusion becomes symptomatic or increases in size. Pleural effusions greater than 10 mm thick require a thoracentesis, and management depends on the pleural fluid characteristics (see Table 10-1).

C. **Malignant pleural effusions** arise from tumor involvement of the pleura or mediastinum. Patients with malignancy are also at increased risk for pleural effusions from postobstructive pneumonia, pulmonary emboli, chylothorax, and drug or radiation reactions. If pleural tissue or cytology is positive for malignancy or if other causes of effusion are reasonably excluded in a patient with malignancy, several therapeutic options exist (*Clin Chest Med* 14:189, 1993).

    1. **Therapeutic thoracentesis** may improve patient comfort and relieve dyspnea. The subjective response to drainage and the rate of fluid reaccumulation should be monitored. Repeated thoracenteses are reasonable if they achieve symptomatic relief and if fluid reaccumulation is slow.

    2. **Chemical pleurodesis** is an effective therapy for recurrent effusions. This treatment is recommended in patients whose symptoms are relieved with initial drainage but who have rapid reaccumulation of fluid. Talc pleurodesis appears to be the most effective and least expensive agent, particularly in malignant pleural effusions with a pH of less than 7.30 (*Chest* 113:1007, 1998). However, it requires thoracoscopy and general anesthesia. Doxycycline or minocycline can be instilled in the pleural space at the bedside without thoracoscopy or general anesthesia. If, after 48 hours, the chest tube drainage remains high (>100 ml/day), a second dose of the sclerosing agent can be administered. Bleomycin appears to be less effective and more expensive than other drugs. Systemic analgesics and the administration of lidocaine in the sclerosing agent solution help to decrease the appreciable discomfort associated with the procedure (*Ann Intern Med* 120:56, 1994).

3. **Pleurectomy or pleural abrasion** requires thoracotomy and should be reserved for patients with a good prognosis when pleurodesis has been ineffective.

4. **Chemotherapy and mediastinal radiotherapy** may control effusions in responsive tumors such as lymphoma or small-cell bronchogenic carcinoma but are seldom useful in metastatic carcinoma.

5. **Observation** without invasive interventions may be appropriate for some patients.

Chronic Obstructive Pulmonary Disease

Chronic obstructive pulmonary disease (COPD) is a syndrome of chronic dyspnea with expiratory airflow limitation that, unlike asthma, does not fluctuate markedly. The term *COPD* includes chronic bronchitis and emphysema. However, other diseases, such as cystic fibrosis (CF), bronchiectasis, or bronchiolitis obliterans, are associated with airflow obstruction. COPD affects approximately 15 million people in the United States; it is the fourth leading cause of death, and its mortality continues to rise. The American Thoracic Society has published its standards for the diagnosis and care of patients with COPD (*Am J Respir Crit Care Med* 152:77S, 1995).

I. **Diagnosis and evaluation**

A. **History and physical examination.** Patients typically have a chronic productive cough for many years, followed by slowly progressive breathlessness brought on with decreasing amounts of exertion. COPD is unusual in the absence of a history of cigarette smoking. α_1-Antitrypsin deficiency should be considered in nonsmokers or young patients (younger than 50) with emphysema. Nocturnal symptoms are unusual in COPD unless associated with comorbidities, such as cardiac disease, obstructive sleep apnea (OSA), gastroesophageal reflux, or a marked reactive airway component. Weight loss frequently occurs in patients with severe emphysema. Tachypnea, pursed-lip breathing, and use of accessory muscles of respiration are common. The chest may be hyperresonant to percussion, breath sounds may be decreased, and adventitious sounds (wheezes, midinspiratory crackles, and large airway sounds) may be present. Signs of cor pulmonale may be present in severe or long-standing disease (see sec. **III.E**). Asterixis may be seen with severe hypercapnia.

B. **Chest radiographs** often show low, flattened diaphragms. In severe emphysema, the lung fields may be hyperlucent, with bullae and diminished vascular markings. Often, disease is most prominent in the upper lung zones except in α_1-antitrypsin deficiency, which may show a basilar predominance. Chest radiographs are valuable during an acute exacerbation to exclude such complications as pneumonia and pneumothorax.

C. **Pulmonary function testing.** The FEV_1 and all other measurements of expiratory airflow are reduced. The FEV_1 is the standard way of objectively assessing the clinical course and response to therapy as well as an important predictor of prognosis and mortality in patients with COPD. When the FEV_1 falls to less than 1 L, the 5-year survival is approximately 50%. Total lung capacity, functional residual capacity, and residual volume may be increased, indicating air trapping. The diffusion capacity of carbon monoxide, although reduced in the presence of emphysema, is not specific. In smokers, the rate of decline in the FEV_1 is approximately 60 ml/year and is proportional to the amount of smoking. Smoking cessation for more than a year leads to an improvement in lung function, with an FEV_1 decline equal to that of nonsmokers (approximately 20–30 ml/year) (*JAMA* 272:1497, 1994).

D. Arterial blood gases. Gas exchange abnormalities vary with the type and severity of ventilation-perfusion ($\dot{V}/\dot{Q}$) abnormalities. Perfusion of poorly ventilated areas of the lungs (i.e., areas with low $\dot{V}/\dot{Q}$) results in an increased alveolar-arterial oxygen tension [P(A-a)O_2] gradient and hypoxemia. A subpopulation of patients with severe airway obstruction have chronically increased arterial carbon dioxide tension (PaCO_2), but metabolic compensation (increased serum bicarbonate) maintains the arterial pH near normal. During an acute exacerbation of COPD, worsening airway obstruction, increased dead-space ventilation, and respiratory muscle fatigue may lead to rapid rises in PaCO_2, with subsequent acute respiratory acidosis.

II. Management of acute exacerbations. A variety of insults may provoke bronchospasm or an increase in mucous secretion with plugging. The resulting increase in airway obstruction may cause worsening dyspnea, fatigue, and sometimes respiratory failure. Infections are the most common identifiable cause of acute exacerbations; the most common organisms implicated are *Haemophilus influenzae, Streptococcus pneumoniae, Moraxella catarrhalis, Mycoplasma pneumoniae,* and such viruses as influenza and adenovirus. In addition, pulmonary emboli, pulmonary edema, oversedation, and pneumothorax may worsen gas exchange and increase breathlessness in patients with COPD.

A. Maintenance of adequate gas exchange

1. **Oxygen** should be administered to achieve and maintain an arterial oxygen tension (PaO_2) of 55–60 mm Hg (88–90% oxyhemoglobin saturation). The effectiveness of supplemental oxygen should be evaluated by serial ABG determinations. Adequate oxygenation must be maintained, even in the face of increasing hypercapnia (see Chap. 9). The requirement for high concentrations of supplemental oxygen suggests a complicating condition.

2. **Mechanical ventilation** should be considered in patients with acute ventilatory failure (see Chap. 9). Noninvasive ventilation with positive pressure delivered via a nasal or face mask is an alternative to intubation in selected patients with acute exacerbation of COPD (*N Engl J Med* 333:817, 1995). Patients managed with noninvasive ventilation must be alert and cooperative, hemodynamically stable, and capable of controlling their airway and clearing respiratory secretions (see Chap. 9).

B. Inhaled β_2-adrenergic agonists continue to be first-line therapy for rapid symptomatic improvement in patients with acute bronchoconstriction. Although oral and parenteral forms are available, reversal of airflow obstruction is achieved most effectively and safely by the repetitive administration of inhaled β_2-agonist bronchodilators. Inhaled β_2-adrenergic agonists, such as metaproterenol, terbutaline, or albuterol, have reduced duration of action in exacerbations of COPD and, therefore, can be given q30–60min as tolerated (*Am J Respir Care Med* 152:577, 1995); subsequent treatments can be decreased to 2–4 puffs q4h as the acute exacerbation of COPD starts resolving (Table 10-2). Use of a metered-dose inhaler (MDI) with a spacer device or reservoir is as effective as delivery of the drug by a nebulizer (*Chest* 98:822, 1987). The various β_2 agonists that are available for inhalation are of equivalent effectiveness. Patient instruction and supervised administration are essential to ensure that effective delivery is achieved (*BMJ* 303:1426, 1991).

C. Anticholinergic agents (see sec. **III.B.1**) such as ipratropium bromide have equivalent efficacy to β_2-adrenergic agonists in the treatment of acute exacerbations of COPD, but no consistent synergistic bronchodilation is obtained with combination therapy (*Chest* 98:835, 1990). However, other factors besides the bronchodilating effect suggest that combination therapy may have advantages. The combination of β_2-adrenergic agonist and an anticholinergic agent provides the rapid onset of the former plus the more

Table 10-2. Aerosolized bronchodilators

Drug	Formulation	Adult dosage	Duration (hrs)
β_2-Adrenergic agonists			
Metaproterenol (Alupent, others)	Nebulized 5% solution	0.2–0.3 ml	3–6
	MDI (650 μg/puff)	2–3 puffs q3–4h prn	
Albuterol (Proventil, Ventolin, others)	Nebulized 5% solution	2.5–5.0 mg	4–6
	MDI (90 μg/puff)	2–3 puffs q4–6h prn	
	Powder inhaler (200 μg Ventolin Rotacaps)	1–2 caps q4–6h prn	
Terbutaline (Brethaire)	MDI (200 μg/puff)	2–3 puffs q4–6h prn	4–6
Pirbuterol (Maxair)	MDI (200 μg/puff)	2–3 puffs q4–6h	4–6
Bitolterol mesylate (Tornalate)	MDI (370 μg/puff)	2–3 puffs q4–6h	4–6
Salmeterol (Serevent)	MDI (21 μg/puff)	2 puffs q12h	12
Formoterol*	MDI	2 puffs q12h	12
Anticholinergics			
Atropine sulfate	Nebulized 1% solution	0.5–2.5 mg	4–6
Ipratropium bromide (Atrovent)	MDI (18 μg/puff)	2 puffs q4–6h	4–6
	Nebulized 0.02% solution	2.5 ml	6–8
Combination			
Albuterol and ipratropium (Combivent)	MDI (120 μg and 21 μg/puff, respectively)	2 puffs q4–6h	4–6

MDI = metered-dose inhaler.
*Not available in the United States.

prolonged action of the latter. Side effects may be decreased compared to using large doses of β_2-adrenergic agonists. In addition, anticholinergic agents have no tendency to produce hypoxemia, as is sometimes seen with β_2-adrenergic agents (*Am Rev Respir Dis* 136:1091, 1987). During acute exacerbations, the usual dose of ipratropium, 2 puffs qid, can be increased to 4–6 puffs q4–6h to produce maximal bronchodilation. Ipratropium is also available in solution for nebulization (see Table 10-2). Tiotropium is a long-acting anticholinergic agent that may have a potential role as a once-daily maintenance treatment. Its role and effectiveness in COPD is gradually emerging (*Chest* 117:67S, 2000).

   D. Glucocorticoids, such as methylprednisolone, 125 mg IV q6h for 3 days, can be used in patients who are hospitalized with COPD exacerbation. Moderate improvement in clinical outcomes has been demonstrated compared with placebo, although the treatment group had an increased risk of hyperglycemia (*N Engl J Med* 340:1941, 1999). Oral prednisone, 40–60 mg PO qd, usually is

Table 10-3. Dosage of methylxanthines

IV administration

Loading dose of theophylline (aminophylline is equivalent to 80% anhydrous theophylline)

If no previous theophylline use: theophylline, 5 mg/kg (ideal body weight) over 20 mins

If previously taking theophylline (level not available): 3 mg/kg over 20 mins

If theophylline level known: theophylline, 1 mg/kg bolus for every 2 μg/ml desired increase in theophylline level

Maintenance IV infusion (mg/kg/hr)

Smoking adult: 0.6

Nonsmoking adult: 0.4

Elderly: 0.2

Cor pulmonale: 0.2

Pregnant: 0.3

Congestive heart failure: 0.2

Liver disease: 0.2

Oral administration

Daily oral theophylline dose (mg)(divided doses) = total dose (mg) of IV theophylline/24 hrs

Start therapy at relatively low dose (400–600 mg/day); increase by 100–200 mg/day following serum levels and therapeutic response

---

substituted after a few days and is tapered as tolerated. The role of glucocorticoids for acute exacerbations in outpatients with COPD is controversial.

E. Theophylline administration in patients with COPD is controversial. Considerable evidence suggests that theophylline provides therapeutic benefit to some patients, improving airway function and dyspnea. Theophylline also may improve mucociliary clearance and central respiratory drive. The decision to use oral or IV theophylline in the acute setting should be individualized and weighed against the risk of tachyarrhythmias (Table 10-3). Serum levels should be maintained in the low therapeutic range (8–12 mg/L) to avoid toxicity.

F. The role of **antimicrobial therapy** for COPD exacerbations is not well defined. For routine exacerbations of COPD in the absence of pneumonia, no current method reliably can differentiate bacteria-caused exacerbations from those produced by other agents. A benefit of antibiotic therapy is seen most often in patients who have more severe underlying lung disease and in those who experience more severe exacerbations (*JAMA* 273:957, 1995). Traditional first-line antibiotic regimens for acute bacterial exacerbations of chronic bronchitis (see Chap. 14) consist of a 7- to 10-day course of oral therapy [e.g., trimethoprimsulfamethoxazole, 160 mg/800 mg (one double-strength tablet) PO bid; amoxicillin, 250 mg PO tid; or doxycycline, 100 mg PO bid]. An increasing incidence of penicillin-resistant *S. pneumoniae* and beta-lactamase–producing bacteria, better profiles of tissue and respiratory secretion penetration, and concerns over patient compliance have rendered such alternative agents as azithromycin (500 mg PO on day 1 and 250 mg PO on days 2–5), clarithromycin (500 mg PO bid), or newer quinolones with pneumococcal coverage, such as levofloxacin (500 mg PO qd) or gatifloxacin (400 mg PO qd), reasonable choices despite higher costs (*Thorax* 50:249, 1995).

G. Chest physiotherapy may improve clearance of secretions in patients with copious respiratory secretions (>50 ml/day). However, increased hypoxemia during chest percussion or postural drainage may occur.

III. **Long-term management** is aimed not only at relievin managing acute exacerbations but, more important, at slowir of airflow obstruction and loss of vital capacity, preventin prolonging survival. Although the therapeutic armamentari only smoking cessation and the correction of hypoxemia impro

A. **Smoking cessation** interventions include (1) pharmacother: counseling on the preventable health risks of smoking and advice to stop smoking, (3) encouraging patients to make further attempts to stop smoking even after previous failures, (4) providing smoking cessation materials to patients, and (5) using smoking status as a "vital sign" (*JAMA* 275:1270, 1996). Pharmacotherapy doubles the quit rate and should be made available to all smokers. Currently available medications for smoking cessation include (1) nicotine-containing chewing gum, 2 or 4 mg chewed slowly over 20–30 minutes, repeated up to 60 mg/day; (2) transdermal nicotine patches, the usual regimen for which is 6 weeks of a high-dose patch, 21 mg/day, followed by 2–4 weeks of an intermediate-dose patch, 14 mg/day, and 2–4 weeks of a low-dose patch, 7 mg/day; (3) nicotine nasal spray, two sprays (equivalent to 1 mg) as needed not to exceed five doses/hour or 40 doses/day; and (4) nicotine inhaler, 6–16 cartridges/day for 12 weeks, followed by tapering over 6–12 weeks. Either form of pharmacotherapy is most effective when used in conjunction with formal smoking cessation programs or close medical follow-up (*JAMA* 281:72, 1999). Bupropion hydrochloride started 1 week before quitting smoking (150 mg PO qd for 3 days, then 150 mg PO bid for 7–12 weeks) increases the smoking cessation rate when used with a behavior modification program and can be combined with nicotine replacement (*N Engl J Med* 340:685, 1999).

B. The optimal **bronchodilator regimen** for long-term management of COPD has not been established. The main goal of therapy is symptomatic relief, as neither inhaled anticholinergic agents nor β-adrenergic antagonists have been shown to improve survival.

1. **Anticholinergic agents** are considered the first-line drug for most patients with stable COPD on the basis of studies showing that ipratropium is as effective as are β$_2$-adrenergic agonists and has a longer duration of action and less toxicity. The usual dosage of 2 puffs q4–6h can be doubled or tripled to achieve maximal bronchodilation (*N Engl J Med* 328:1017, 1993); minor side effects include cough and dry mouth. The combination of inhaled anticholinergic and adrenergic agents has been shown to provide more bronchodilation at 2 hours than do anticholinergics alone (*Chest* 107:401, 1995). Ipratropium bromide can improve nocturnal oxygen saturation and sleep quality in patients with moderate to severe COPD (*Chest* 115:1338, 1999).

2. **β-Adrenergic agonists** still are used commonly; however, safety of long-term administration of β-adrenergic agonists is controversial. In addition to the well-known adrenergic side effects, concerns regarding tolerance (tachyphylaxis), acute or long-term rebound bronchoconstriction, and deterioration of pulmonary function have been raised (*Arch Intern Med* 153:814, 1993). On-demand use of bronchodilators appears not to differ from continuous use with respect to decline in lung function, bronchial hyperresponsiveness, and number of exacerbations (*Am J Respir Crit Care Med* 151:131, 1995). Long-acting β-adrenergic agonists (salmeterol, 2 puffs bid) can improve respiratory symptoms, morning peak expiratory flows, and use of rescue bronchodilator therapy in patients with COPD (*Chest* 115:957, 1999).

3. **Oral theophylline** preparations provide therapeutic benefit to some COPD patients (*Chest* 105:1089, 1994). Administration of long-acting preparations in the evening may improve the overnight decline in lung function and morning respiratory symptoms (*Am Rev Respir Dis* 145:540, 1992; see Table 10-3).

C. **Glucocorticoids** produce a response in only a minority (10–25%) of outpatients with stable COPD. Many of those who respond have significant improvements (e.g., >50% improvement in FEV_1). In addition, inhaled corticosteroids may increase FEV_1 initially, although long term effects have not been demonstrated (*N Engl J Med* 340:1948, 1999). No method can predict glucocorticoid responsiveness with certainty, but patients who respond to β-adrenergic inhalation are more likely to benefit (*Chest* 108:1568, 1995). A trial of glucocorticoids (prednisone, 30–60 mg/day for 2 weeks) with spirometric evaluation before and after the trial may help to identify these patients. Therapy should be continued with the lowest effective dose only if pulmonary function test (PFT) values improve significantly (e.g., 15% improvement in FEV_1) on repeat testing in 2–3 weeks. Inhaled glucocorticoids should be substituted for systemic glucocorticoids when possible.

D. Oxygen therapy improves survival and quality of life in patients with COPD and chronic hypoxemia (*N Engl J Med* 333:710, 1995). The need for supplemental oxygen should be determined by ABGs. PaO_2 should be maintained at approximately 60 mm Hg or oxygen saturation at 90% or more. More oxygen may be required with exercise or sleep. Criteria for continuous or intermittent long-term oxygen therapy include a PaO_2 of consistently less than 55 mm Hg or oxyhemoglobin saturation of less than 88% by pulse oximetry at rest, with exercise, or during sleep, despite optimal medical therapy, or a PaO_2 of 55–59 mm Hg with evidence of cor pulmonale or secondary polycythemia (hematocrit >55%). The prescription for oxygen should include the source of supplemental oxygen, the type of delivery system, and the flow rate at rest and during exercise and sleep. Patient education with emphasis on the outcome benefits of long-term oxygen therapy, absence of "addiction" to oxygen, and safety issues is needed universally. A 1- to 3-month period of observation with reassessment of oxygenation to ensure clinical stability is recommended before committing patients to long-term oxygen therapy. After they attain stability, patients who are receiving long-term oxygen therapy need routine re-evaluation no more frequently than every 6 months (*Chest* 107:358, 1995).

E. Pulmonary hypertension and cor pulmonale in patients with COPD may present clinically as a progressive decrease in exercise tolerance in the absence of worsening airflow limitation. An ECG, echocardiography with Doppler measurement of the tricuspid jet, and radionuclide ventriculography can provide useful information regarding right ventricular function. The primary approach to treatment is to optimize the use of inhaled bronchodilators and to provide oxygen therapy. Digoxin should be considered only for patients in whom left ventricular failure also is present. Diuretics should be used cautiously, as they may be tolerated poorly in patients dependent on preload. In addition, diuretics may precipitate a metabolic alkalosis that can be deleterious in the hypercapnic patient. Phlebotomy should be considered when, despite supplemental oxygen, the hematocrit is greater than 50% in the presence of pulmonary vascular or CNS compromise. Therapy with vasodilators has not shown a survival benefit and is not recommended (*Am J Respir Crit Care Med* 155:781, 1997).

F. A comprehensive pulmonary rehabilitation program may help to improve the patient's exercise tolerance and sense of well-being beyond the benefit provided by education alone (*Am J Respir Crit Care Med* 159:1666, 1999).

G. Influenza vaccine and pneumococcal vaccine are recommended for patients with COPD (see Appendix F).

H. Psychoactive drugs should be used with caution in patients with COPD. Buspirone (5–10 mg PO tid) is an anxiolytic agent unrelated to benzodiazepines and usually is well tolerated; however, it requires several weeks to become effective. Selective serotonin reuptake inhibitors may be a reasonable choice given their low side effect profile. However, caution is advised in patients who are receiving theophylline, as some serotonin reuptake inhibitors prolong its elimination (*Can Med Assoc J* 151:1289, 1994).

I. α_1-**Protease inhibitor augmentation therapy** may be appropriate in patients who are older than 18 years and have documented alpha$_1$-protease inhibitor deficiency (<11 μmol/L) and airflow obstruction (FEV$_1$ between 30% and 50% of normal) and who have stopped smoking. Weekly IV administration of human alpha$_1$-protease inhibitor, 60 mg/kg, is safe and effective in achieving normal plasma levels of antitrypsin; however, its long-term benefit has not been established (*Am J Respir Crit Care Med* 158:48, 1998).

IV. **Surgical consideration.** Surgery in patients with COPD is associated with increased risk of morbidity and mortality. The evaluation of pulmonary patients in preparation for surgery must determine the risk factors that are amenable to improvement and must consider alternatives to surgery in the high-risk population. In addition to providing a complete history and physical examination, preoperative PFTs help clinicians make decisions regarding management of lung resection candidates (*Ann Intern Med* 112:763, 1990). The impact of functional testing for nonthoracic procedures is less clear. Preoperative ABG testing may help to assess risk and to determine appropriate postoperative ventilator settings. However, no values preclude a lifesaving operation.

A. **Nonthoracic surgery** is associated with variable changes in lung function; the farther the procedure from the diaphragm, the lower is the risk for complications (*Clin Chest Med* 14:253, 1993). Elective surgery should be carried out when the patient has no intercurrent illness or respiratory exacerbation. Smoking cessation should begin at least 8 weeks before surgery. Optimization of bronchodilator therapy, antimicrobials for suspected bacterial infection, verification of therapeutic theophylline blood levels, and education regarding incentive spirometry should begin at least 24–48 hours preoperatively (*Am J Respir Crit Care Med* 152:577, 1995). In patients with severe COPD, postoperative care requires close attention to fluid balance, gas exchange, bronchial hygiene, and deep venous thrombosis (DVT) prophylaxis.

B. **Lung resection** for diagnostic or therapeutic indications is relatively common in patients with COPD. In evaluating patients for lung resection, one has to estimate the lung function that will remain after surgery and whether that amount of function is associated with an acceptable incidence of morbidity, mortality, and respiratory disability. A predicted postoperative FEV$_1$ of 800 ml has been regarded traditionally as the minimum acceptable level, but decisions must be individualized (*Am J Respir Crit Care Med* 153:1201, 1996). In general, an FEV$_1$ of more than 2 L or more than 60% of the predicted value is acceptable for pneumonectomy. Values below this suggest that further analysis with split-function quantitative lung scan and exercise testing are needed. The predicted postoperative FEV$_1$ can be calculated by multiplying the preoperative FEV$_1$ by the percentage of perfusion of the remaining lung or the number of functional segments within the lobe to be resected divided by the total number of segments in both lungs. Preoperative measurement of oxygen uptake during exercise may predict postoperative complications (*Ann Thorac Surg* 61:1494, 1996).

C. **Lung volume reduction surgery** is a promising therapeutic option for a very select group of patients with emphysema (*Semin Thorac Cardiovasc Surg* 8:99, 1996). Health-related quality of life improves after pulmonary rehabilitation and lung volume reduction surgery (*Chest* 115:383, 1999). However, the indications and selection criteria are controversial, and studies are ongoing.

D. **Lung transplantation** has evolved as a therapeutic option for selected patients with end-stage COPD. Patients with an FEV$_1$ of less than 25% of predicted and/or a PaCO$_2$ of 55 mm Hg or greater and/or cor pulmonale can be considered for evaluation (*Am J Respir Crit Care Med* 158:335, 1998). For patients with COPD, the 1-, 2-, and 3-year actuarial survivals after transplant are 81%, 62%, and 43%, respectively (*UNOS: Annual Report*, 1999).

Cystic Fibrosis

CF is the most common lethal genetic disease in white populations. It is autosomal recessive, with a median survival of approximately 30 years. Nearly 35% of persons with CF are 18 years old or older (*N Engl J Med* 335:179, 1996).

 I. **Diagnosis** of CF is confirmed when a person has either typical pulmonary or GI manifestations or a history of CF in the immediate family and an elevated sweat chloride (>60 mEq/L in children and >80 mEq/L in adults) using the pilocarpine iontophoresis method. Measurement of nasal potential difference and CF gene mutation analysis (CF transmembrane conductance regulator gene) are useful adjuncts to diagnosis in atypical cases, and their use may become more widespread in the future (*N Engl J Med* 336:487, 1997).

 II. **Clinical manifestations** of CF reflect the abnormal composition of exocrine secretions, resulting in excessively thick and tenacious mucus, obstruction of the pancreatic ducts with inspissated secretions, and elevated sweat chloride and sodium concentrations.

   A. **Pulmonary** disease is characterized by chronic airway infection and the development of bronchiectasis and chronic obstructive lung disease and accounts for most of the morbidity and mortality associated with CF. The presenting symptoms of cough, purulent sputum, wheezing, and dyspnea are variable and depend on the extent of superimposed infection. Its course is chronic and progressive, with superimposed acute pulmonary exacerbations. Allergic bronchopulmonary aspergillosis may be present in up to 10% of patients with CF, with massive hemoptysis and pneumothorax being more common in the adult population.

   B. The most important **extrapulmonary** manifestation of CF is pancreatic insufficiency, which affects approximately 90% of persons with CF and results in fat malabsorption, steatorrhea, and malnutrition. Other extrapulmonary systems affected by CF are GI (constipation, intussusception, distal intestinal obstruction syndrome, rectal prolapse), endocrine (diabetes mellitus, affecting ≈ 10% of adults), hepatobiliary (cholelithiasis, cholecystitis, focal biliary cirrhosis, portal hypertension), skeletal (hypertrophic osteoarthropathy, retardation of growth and bone age, demineralization), upper respiratory tract (nasal polyps, chronic sinusitis), and genitourinary (sterility and infertility in men secondary to bilateral absence of the vas deferens). Although fertility may be decreased in women with CF secondary to thickened cervical mucus, many women with CF have tolerated pregnancy well (*Thorax* 50:170, 1995).

   C. **Laboratory studies**
     1. **Chest radiograph** usually reveals increased interstitial reticular markings, bronchiectasis, and hilar adenopathy. Generally, the upper lobes are more involved than are the lower lobes.
     2. **PFTs** typically are consistent with an obstructive abnormality. Patients also may exhibit bronchial hyperreactivity. Later in the disease, hypoxemia and progressive hypercapnia develop.
     3. **Cultures and sensitivities of the sputum** are mandatory during exacerbations. Early in life, the most characteristic organisms associated with CF are *Staphylococcus aureus* and *H. influenzae*. By adulthood, infection with mucoid strains of *Pseudomonas aeruginosa* predominate. Infection with *Burkholderia cepacia* has been associated with a rapid deterioration in some patients and may preclude transplantation at some centers.

 III. **Therapy.** The goals of therapy for the pulmonary disease in CF are to decrease the burden of infection, to provide bronchopulmonary hygiene, to aid in the clearance of secretions, and to maintain adequate nutrition. As the disease progresses, supplemental oxygen may be required, and referral for lung transplantation is appropriate for many patients.

A. **Antibiotics.** IV antibiotics are the treatment of choice for acute exacerbations of CF. Because *P. aeruginosa* is the pathogen encountered most frequently in adults, a combination of a semisynthetic penicillin or a cephalosporin with antipseudomonal activity (ceftazidime, 2 g IV q8h, or cefepime, 2 g IV q12h) and an aminoglycoside, such as tobramycin (3 mg/kg q8h), usually is selected, pending results from sputum cultures and sensitivities. The use of chronic prophylactic and suppressive oral antibiotics remains controversial. Inhaled tobramycin (300 mg bid) in patients with clinically stable disease has been shown to improve pulmonary function, decrease the density of *P. aeruginosa*, and reduce the need for IV antibiotics and hospitalizations. Voice alteration (13%) and tinnitus (3%) are potential adverse events associated with long-term inhaled tobramycin (*N Engl J Med* 340:23, 1999).

B. **Bronchial hygiene**
   1. **Chest physiotherapy** consisting of postural drainage with percussion, autogenic drainage, forced expiratory techniques (e.g., huffing), and participation in an exercise program has been shown to have short-term clinical utility in the clearance of mucous secretions and improvement of physical performance. Chest compression with an inflatable vest and such devices as positive expiratory pressure valves, intrapulmonary percussive ventilation devices, and airway oscillators (i.e., flutter valve) offer patients greater independence. One should be alert to the possibility of oxygen desaturation and exercise-induced bronchospasm when using these techniques.
   2. **Bronchodilators** are used for patients with bronchial hyperreactivity and may facilitate adequate respiratory toilet.
   3. **Dornase alfa,** the generic designation of recombinant human deoxyribonuclease I, acts by digesting extracellular DNA, released from dead neutrophils, which is present in increased amounts in CF sputum; this decreases the viscoelasticity of the sputum. Dornase alfa has been shown to improve pulmonary function and to decrease the risk of respiratory tract infections that require parenteral antibiotics (*N Engl J Med* 335:179, 1996). The recommended dosage is 2.5 mg q12–24h inhaled via a jet nebulizer. Generally, it is well tolerated; however, reported adverse effects have included pharyngitis, laryngitis, voice alteration, rash, chest pain, and conjunctivitis. In a small proportion of patients, serum antibodies develop, but their clinical significance is unknown. **Dornase alfa cannot be mixed with other nebulized medications.**

C. **Anti-inflammatory therapy.** Because some of the lung damage in CF is attributable to an excessive inflammatory response to chronic infection, it has been proposed that the natural history of the disease can be moderated if the inflammatory response can be controlled. Short-term courses of corticosteroid therapy may be useful in some patients; however, adverse effects preclude their long-term use. In one trial with high-dose ibuprofen, the rate of decline in FEV_1 was slowed, being most pronounced in children with mild lung disease (*N Engl J Med* 332:848, 1995).

D. **Oxygen therapy** is indicated in patients with hypoxemia at rest, at night, during exercise, or with evidence of pulmonary hypertension (see Chronic Obstructive Pulmonary Disease, sec. **III.D**).

E. **Nutritional support.** An important component of any CF management program is nutritional support, including pancreatic enzyme replacement (500–2000 units of lipase per kilogram per meal), nutritional supplements, and supplementation of fat-soluble vitamins.

F. **Lung transplantation.** The majority of patients with CF die from pulmonary disease. Referral for lung transplantation should be considered when the FEV_1 has decreased to approximately 30% of the predicted value.

Sequential bilateral lung transplantation is the procedure of choice because of the risk of spillover infection from the remaining native lung. The actuarial 1-, 2-, and 3-year survival for CF patients after lung transplantation is 81%, 58%, and 49%, respectively (*UNOS: Annual Report*, 1999).

Pulmonary Embolism

Pulmonary thromboembolism (PE) is an important cause of morbidity and mortality, especially among hospitalized patients. The majority of clinically significant PEs arise from DVTs in the iliofemoral system; many of the remainder arise in the pelvic venous plexus as postsurgical or gynecologic complications. Axillosubclavian vein thrombosis is recognized more commonly because of the increasingly frequent use of indwelling subclavian vein catheters (*Clin Chest Med* 16:341, 1995). Predisposing factors for thromboembolic disease include venous disease of the lower extremities, cancer, heart failure, recent major surgery, prolonged immobilization, paralysis, paresis or immobilization in plaster casts, a strong family history of thrombosis, and pregnancy. The clinical manifestations of acute PE and DVT lack sensitivity and specificity and provide little value in establishing the diagnosis. The most common symptoms are dyspnea, pleuritic chest pain, apprehension, and cough; frequent physical findings include tachypnea, tachycardia, accentuation of the pulmonic component of the second heart sound, and inspiratory crackles. Pleuritic chest pain and hemoptysis suggest pulmonary infarction. Localized tenderness in the distribution of the deep venous system and thigh and calf swelling on the symptomatic side may suggest DVT.

I. **Diagnosis of thromboembolism** is based on clinical suspicion, ancillary laboratory data, and the results of specific diagnostic studies. It is important to consider PE and the antecedent DVT as one clinical entity, wherein the diagnosis of either component establishes the indication for treatment.

   A. **A general diagnostic evaluation** should include a baseline CBC, coagulation studies, and ABG analysis, which may demonstrate an increased $P(A-a)O_2$. Arterial hypoxemia with a PaO_2 below 80 mm Hg occurs in the majority of patients and usually is accompanied by hypocapnia. However, a normal $P(A-a)O_2$ can occur in up to 14% of patients with acute PE (*Chest* 107:139, 1995). D-Dimer can be useful in excluding thromboembolic disease in patients with a low pretest probability of PE or a nondiagnostic lung scan (*Ann Intern Med* 129:1006, 1998). In several studies, a quantitative D-dimer (performed by enzyme-linked immunosorbent assay) of less than 500 ng/ml has been shown to effectively exclude PE. Echocardiography may be useful in patients with hemodynamic compromise (*Int J Cardiol* 47:273, 1995). Chest radiographs generally are not useful except to exclude alternate diagnoses. Classic signs of pulmonary infarction such as Hampton hump or decreased vascularity (Westermark sign) are suggestive but infrequent.

   B. **Specific diagnostic studies** are necessary in patients suspected of having PE. The patient's clinical status and previously obtained data determine which tests to order and the sequence in which they should be performed (*Am J Respir Crit Care Med* 160:1043, 1999).

      1. **Ventilation-perfusion ($\dot{V}/\dot{Q}$) lung scans** have traditionally been a pivotal test for suspected PE. However, the $\dot{V}/\dot{Q}$ scan is rarely interpreted as normal or high probability to be of diagnostic value. Furthermore, the information obtained depends not only on the quality and interpretation of the scan but on the clinician's estimation of the probability of PE in the patient being studied (pretest probability; Table 10-4).

Table 10-4. Presence of pulmonary embolism (%) by angiogram combining pretest probability and ventilation-perfusion ($\dot{V}/\dot{Q}$) lung scan results

$\dot{V}/\dot{Q}$ scan category	Clinical pretest probability (%)			
	80–100	20–79	0–19	All
High probability	96	88	56	87
Intermediate probability	66	28	16	30
Low probability	40	16	4	14
Near normal or normal	0	6	2	4
Total	68	30	9	28

Source: Data from PIOPED Investigators. Value of the ventilation/perfusion scan in acute pulmonary embolism: results of the Prospective Investigation of Pulmonary Embolism Diagnosis (PIOPED). *JAMA* 263:2753, 1990.

2. **Evaluation for DVT** may support a diagnosis of thromboembolic disease in patients in whom a $\dot{V}/\dot{Q}$ scan is nondiagnostic. Impedance plethysmography and compression ultrasonography are noninvasive techniques for the diagnosis of DVT in the thigh (*Ann Intern Med* 122:47, 1995). However, both these methods have a low sensitivity (24–38%) in asymptomatic patients (*Arch Intern Med* 151:2167, 1991; *Ann Intern Med* 117:735, 1992), patients after orthopedic surgery, and for the detection of calf-vein thrombosis (*N Engl J Med* 335:1816, 1996). Venous duplex scanning, which provides ultrasonic venous imaging with Doppler blood-flow imaging, may have greater accuracy than does either technique. However, a negative study using any of these methods does not rule out the presence of a pelvic vein thrombus. Venography may be needed to make a definitive diagnosis, in patients with a high clinical probability but negative ultrasonography. Other modalities that have been shown to detect pelvic and lower extremity deep vein thrombus include CT and MRI.

3. **Contrast agent–enhanced spiral (helical) CT** can be considered, although its role in the evaluation of patients with suspected PE is still evolving. Spiral CT has the greatest sensitivity for emboli in the main, lobar, or segmental pulmonary arteries. The importance of subsegmental emboli (~6% of patients) as well as the diagnostic accuracy of pulmonary angiography for emboli of this size is questionable. One particular advantage of CT is in the ability to assess simultaneously the secondary parenchymal changes associated with acute or chronic PE. Although there is high specificity (81–97%) for the diagnosis of acute PE, sensitivity (53–60%) is suboptimal (*Radiology* 209:235, 1998). Therefore, its exact role is uncertain, and studies are ongoing.

4. **Pulmonary angiography** should be performed whenever clinical data and noninvasive tests are equivocal or contradictory (*Circulation* 85:462, 1992). In addition, pulmonary angiography is appropriate in patients with a high probability of PE by $\dot{V}/\dot{Q}$ scan, if the risks of anticoagulation are high, or if vena cava interruption or thrombolytic therapy is being considered. Pulmonary angiography may be the appropriate initial diagnostic test in patients who are hemodynamically unstable.

II. **Treatment**

A. **Supportive care.** Supplemental oxygen should be given to correct hypoxemia. Patients with hypotension and reduced cardiac output who do not respond rapidly to IV saline infusion should be treated with norepinephrine or dopamine and should be considered for thrombolytic therapy or surgical intervention (see sec. **II.C**).

B. Prevention of recurrent emboli

1. **Anticoagulation** (see Chap. 19) with standard unfractionated IV heparin should be started immediately on the basis of clinical suspicion of PE and without waiting for definitive studies to be obtained, unless an absolute contraindication for anticoagulation exists. A bolus of heparin (80 units/kg) followed by a continuous infusion (18 units/kg/hour) titrated individually to an activated partial thromboplastin time between one and a half and two and a half times the control value (therapeutic range may vary depending on reagents used) is continued for 5–10 days (*Ann Intern Med* 119:874, 1993). Rapid achievement of therapeutic activated partial thromboplastin time values decreases the risk of recurrence. Low-molecular-weight heparins have equal (or greater) antithrombotic efficacy, with less likelihood of causing thrombocytopenia than unfractionated heparin (*Am J Respir Crit Care Med* 159:1, 1999; see Chap. 19). Oral warfarin can be given with the initiation of heparin. A starting dose of 5 mg/day for the first 2 days is followed by daily dosing adjusted to an international normalized ratio of 2.0–3.0 (*Ann Intern Med* 126:133, 1997). Warfarin then is continued for longer than 3 months or indefinitely if risk factors are still present or if thromboembolism is recurrent (*N Engl J Med* 340:901, 1999).

2. **Inferior vena cava** interruption should be considered in the following settings: (1) PE in patients for whom anticoagulants are absolutely contraindicated; (2) documented recurrent embolic events in patients who are anticoagulated adequately; (3) massive PE with hemodynamic compromise, especially with evidence of residual thrombus in a lower extremity; (4) patients with compromised cardiac or pulmonary function who may not survive a recurrent event; (5) patients undergoing pulmonary embolectomy; (6) patients with paradoxical emboli via a patent foramen ovale; or (7) septic pulmonary emboli from lower extremities or pelvic veins. Anticoagulation therapy should be continued (unless otherwise contraindicated), as it will prevent extension of an already existing clot and decrease the risk of postphlebitic venous insufficiency.

C. Specific therapy

1. **Systemic thrombolytic therapy** with streptokinase or recombinant tissue-plasminogen activator hastens the resolution of thrombi and reduces the morbidity from the postthrombotic syndrome but has not yet been shown to reduce mortality in patients with DVT or PE. Thrombolytic therapy should be considered in the treatment of patients who have a low risk of bleeding with extensive iliofemoral venous thrombosis or those with acute massive embolism and hemodynamic instability or right ventricular failure.

2. **Pulmonary embolectomy** (catheter or surgical) should be considered only in the rare patient who has angiographically proven pulmonary emboli and who remains in shock despite thrombolytic therapy and supportive care or in whom thrombolytic therapy would be appropriate but is contraindicated.

III. Chronic thromboembolic pulmonary hypertension occurs in a minority of patients who fail to resolve a thromboembolic pulmonary event, with resultant pulmonary vascular obstruction and consequent pulmonary hypertension. The syndrome should be considered in patients with unexplained dyspnea on exercise in association with physical findings of pulmonary hypertension. The lung perfusion scan may help to differentiate this condition from primary pulmonary hypertension (PPH). Subsequent invasive evaluation, including cardiac catheterization, angiography, or angioscopy, is best conducted by experienced medical teams who can perform pulmonary thromboendarterectomy. For selected patients, this surgical intervention offers substantial improvement in survival

(75% at >6 years), function, quality of life, and minimal disease-related health care utilization (*Am J Respir Crit Care Med* 160:523, 1999).

Pulmonary Aspiration Syndromes and Lung Abscess

I. **Pneumonia.** Diagnosis and treatment of pneumonia are discussed in Chap. 14.

II. **Pulmonary aspiration syndromes** occur most often in patients with a decreased level of consciousness, impaired pharyngeal or laryngeal function (e.g., myopathy, neuropathy, or immediately after extubation), increased intragastric pressure or volume (e.g., nausea, vomiting, ileus, tube feeding), or esophageal disorders that predispose them to reflux. **Aspiration** of gastric contents may have a variety of consequences.

A. **Aspiration of inert liquids or foreign bodies** may cause a syndrome of airway obstruction and manifest clinically as acute respiratory distress or hypoxemia. Radiographic evidence of pulmonary infiltrates, atelectasis, or lobar collapse may be present. The possible presence of aspirated food particles must always be considered in patients with known aspiration of gastric contents and focal infiltrates. Frequently, early bronchoscopy is indicated, especially if the patient has signs of parenchymal volume loss or has localized wheezing.

B. **Chemical pneumonitis** occurs if the pH of the aspirate is low (<2.5) or the volume of acidic aspirate is large. Symptoms of cough, dyspnea, and wheezing vary depending on the patient's level of consciousness. Tachypnea, tachycardia, hypotension, and fever may be seen in association with rales, increased $P(A-a)O_2$, and pulmonary infiltrates. If aspiration is massive, acute respiratory distress syndrome may develop. With the exception of use for treatment of aspiration associated with intestinal obstruction, severe gingivitis and periodontitis, or immunocompromised status, antibiotics should be withheld until evidence of bacterial superinfection is seen.

C. **Aspiration pneumonia** occurs in approximately 40% of patients who aspirate, most commonly 2–5 days after the initial event, and often is caused by mixed aerobic-anaerobic organisms. It may be difficult to discriminate between bacterial pneumonia and chemical pneumonitis. Although penicillin G, amoxicillin/clavulanate, or clindamycin is usually effective in outpatients, broader coverage with (1) a beta-lactam–beta-lactamase inhibitor alone or in combination with a fluoroquinolone, (2) a cephalosporin with clindamycin, or (3) imipenem or meropenem should be considered in hospitalized patients, because they are more likely to be infected with mixed flora including anaerobes gram-negative bacilli, and *S. aureus*. (*Clin Infect Dis* 31:347, 2000; see Chap. 14).

III. **Lung abscess** most often follows aspiration of oropharyngeal contents that contain large numbers of anaerobes. Extensive gingival and dental disease predisposes to such infections. The onset of illness may be insidious, with constitutional symptoms, fever, and weight loss. Foul-smelling sputum suggests infection with anaerobic bacteria.

A. **Evaluation.** Other causes of cavitary lung disease should be considered, including tuberculosis, fungal disease, actinomycosis, acute necrotizing pneumonia (e.g., gram-negative bacilli and *S. aureus*), carcinoma, lymphoma, vasculitis, septic embolism, and PE with infarction. Sputum should be cultured for mycobacteria and fungi, and skin testing with an intermediate-strength purified protein derivative should be performed. Bronchoscopy is indicated if an obstructing tumor or foreign body is suspected.

B. **Therapy.** Postural drainage of the involved segment is performed to facilitate removal of secretions. Antibiotic treatment with aqueous penicillin G,

1.5–2.0 million units IV q4h, is satisfactory, although treatment with clinda-mycin may hasten the resolution of anaerobic lung abscesses. Therapy can be switched to oral penicillin VK, 500 mg PO q6h, or clindamycin, 300–450 mg PO tid, once a definite clinical response is observed and should be continued until the cavity closes. Healing may take 6–12 months. Surgical resection or percutaneous drainage of a lung abscess is required only rarely for a nonresolving abscess with persistent fevers and leukocytosis despite appropriate medical therapy, the development of a bronchopleural fistula, empyema, persistent hemoptysis, evidence of an enlarging cavity, or mechanical ventilation dependence (*Ann Thorac Surg* 44:356, 1987; *Radiology* 178:347, 1991).

IV. **Empyema** is discussed in Pleural Effusion, sec. **II.B.**

Interstitial Lung Disease

The interstitial lung diseases are a heterogeneous group of disorders, pathologically characterized by acute, subacute, or chronic infiltration of the alveolar walls by cells, fluid, and connective tissue. If left untreated, the initial intra-alveolar and interstitial inflammation may progress to irreversible fibrosis, altered alveolar architecture, and impaired gas exchange. The differential diagnosis of interstitial lung disease is extensive (Table 10-5).

I. **Clinical manifestations**
   A. **General.** Patients typically present with breathlessness and a nonproductive cough. The physical examination, chest radiograph, PFTs, and ABG abnormalities vary depending on the underlying etiology.
   B. **Clinical manifestations of idiopathic pulmonary fibrosis (IPF)** (*Am J Respir Crit Care Med* 161:646, 2000). Physical examination reveals bibasilar end-inspiratory crackles; clubbing of the digits is present in 40–80%. Evidence of pulmonary hypertension develops in 30–40% of cases. Chest radiographs usually demonstrate diffuse bilateral reticular infiltrates; however, 14% of patients may have normal chest radiographs. Early gas exchange abnormalities include a decrease in the diffusion capacity of carbon monoxide and oxygen desaturation during exercise. ABGs may show variable degrees of hypoxemia at rest and a chronic respiratory alkalosis; with more severe disease, $PaCO_2$ may rise, and acidosis may occur. PFTs demonstrate a restrictive abnormality, with decreased lung volumes (especially total lung capacity) but usually no evidence of airflow obstruction (ratio of FEV_1 to forced vital capacity >0.75). However, in smokers, bronchiolar or emphysematous changes may complicate the pathologic and functional changes caused by IPF (*Am J Respir Crit Care Med* 151:1180, 1995).

II. **Initial evaluation** includes a careful history, focusing on possible reversible causes of lung injury. Particular attention should be given to exposure to dusts, fumes, and drugs with known pulmonary toxicity. In addition, the duration of illness should be estimated by noting the rate of progression of symptoms and especially by reviewing previous chest radiographs. High-resolution, thin-section CT scans may be useful for the radiographic detection of interstitial lung disease, determining the optimal biopsy site, and assessing suspected etiologies (e.g., infection, malignancy) (*Radiology* 191:669, 1994). Although the etiology may be suspected from the initial evaluation, diagnosis often requires microscopic examination of lung tissue. A pathologic diagnosis should be obtained before initiation of glucocorticoid or immunosuppressive therapy. The method of lung biopsy used depends on the suspected diagnosis.
   A. **Fiberoptic bronchoscopy with transbronchial lung biopsy** provides small samples but should be the initial procedure if the leading diagnostic possibilities are infection, cancer, sarcoidosis, or other conditions with specific,

Table 10-5. Causes of interstitial lung disease

Known etiologies

Occupational or environmental inhalants: dusts (organic, inorganic), gases (oxygen toxicity), fumes

Drugs (e.g., cytotoxic agents, amiodarone, nitrofurantoin, gold)

Radiation

Infections (viral, bacterial, fungal, parasites)

Giant-cell interstitial pneumonia (hard-metal pneumoconiosis)

Lymphocytic interstitial pneumonitis (LIP)

Hypersensitivity pneumonitis

Pulmonary edema (cardiogenic or noncardiogenic)

Neoplasms (e.g., lymphangitic spread of carcinoma, lymphoma, alveolar cell carcinoma)

Metabolic causes

Unknown etiologies

Sarcoidosis

Idiopathic pulmonary fibrosis (cryptogenic fibrosing alveolitis)

    Usual interstitial pneumonia (UIP)

    Desquamative interstitial pneumonia (DIP)/respiratory bronchiolitis interstitial lung disease (RBILD)

    Acute interstitial pneumonia (AIP) (Hamman-Rich disease)

    Nonspecific interstitial pneumonia (NSIP)

Interstitial disease associated with collagen vascular disorders

Pulmonary vasculitis

Pulmonary hemorrhage syndromes (e.g., Goodpasture's, idiopathic hemosiderosis)

Eosinophilic granuloma

Alveolar proteinosis

Amyloidosis

Veno-occlusive disease

Microlithiasis

Neurofibromatosis, tuberous sclerosis, lymphangioleiomyomatosis

Bronchiolitis obliterans organizing pneumonia (BOOP)

---

        well-defined, widespread histologic abnormalities (*Am J Respir Crit Care Med* 151:909, 1995).

    B. Open-lung biopsy requires thoracoscopy or thoracotomy but provides an opportunity to study a relatively large amount of tissue for diagnosis. Open-lung biopsy is the procedure of choice when transbronchial lung biopsy is nondiagnostic or contraindicated or when IPF or another syndrome with a variable and patchy histologic appearance is likely. The pathologic classification of IPF (see Table 10-5) aids in assessing prognosis and choosing therapy (*Am J Respir Crit Care Med* 157:1301, 1998).

III. Monitoring of disease activity. Serial evaluation of the severity of breathlessness, radiographic changes (including high-resolution thin-section CT scan), and physiologic derangements (as judged by PFTs, ABGs, and physiologic response to exercise) are used to assess the rate of progression of disease and to facilitate decisions concerning therapy. Serial measurements of exercise gas exchange are the most sensitive physiologic indicator of the clinical course of IPF.

IV. Therapy

A. General therapy. Potentially injurious occupational, environmental, and drug exposures should be discontinued. Appropriate therapy should be directed toward management of heart failure, infection, or other treatable comorbidities of interstitial lung disease.

B. Supplemental oxygen with appropriate increases during sleep and exercise should be prescribed when needed (see Chronic Obstructive Pulmonary Disease, sec. **III.D**).

C. Treatment of specific interstitial lung diseases

    1. Sarcoidosis is a granulomatous disease of unknown etiology, with protean clinical manifestations and an unpredictable natural course. Up to two-thirds of patients who present with sarcoidosis experience resolution or improvement in symptoms or radiographic abnormalities over the following several years, with chronic disease developing in only a minority of patients. Because of the waxing and waning nature of the illness and the lack of controlled studies, it has been difficult to prove that glucocorticoids actually improve outcome (*Am J Respir Crit Care* 149:893, 1994). **However, glucocorticoids are indicated for significant extrapulmonary organ involvement** (e.g., heart, brain, kidney, and eye or progressive liver involvement or hypercalciuria).

      a. Initial evaluation after diagnosis should include an ECG, formal ophthalmologic examination, liver function tests, serum calcium tests, and 24-hour urine calcium determination (*Semin Respir Med* 13:402, 1992). Cardiac involvement is clinically evident in only 5% of the patients, most of whom have extensive extracardiac disease. However, it is the most common cause of death attributed to sarcoidosis and frequently is unrecognized antemortem (*Chest* 103:253, 1993).

      b. The **asymptomatic patient** with no evidence of clinical or radiologic progression should be followed closely without treatment. In an asymptomatic patient with parenchymal infiltrates and a mild to moderate restrictive defect, decisions regarding initiation of therapy should be individualized. Bilateral hilar lymphadenopathy (stage I) seldom requires glucocorticoid therapy. When pulmonary infiltrates with or without lymphadenopathy (stages II and III) occur in patients with sarcoidosis, the appropriate therapy is controversial.

      c. Symptomatic patients and those with progressive objective deterioration warrant a trial of glucocorticoids (prednisone, 30–40 mg PO qd for 4–8 weeks). When therapy is effective, a clinical and radiologic response is obtained in 2–4 weeks. If no response is obtained in 4–8 weeks, it is reasonable to discontinue treatment gradually (*Am Rev Respir Dis* 147:1598, 1993). If a clinical response is obtained, prednisone should be tapered to the lowest dose that maintains the clinical response (usually >15 mg qod) and maintained for approximately 1 year before therapy is discontinued completely. Serial evaluation should be performed every 2 months initially, gradually lengthening the intervals to 4–5 months; patients should be followed carefully for at least 2 years after glucocorticoids have been discontinued. Relapse occurs in up to 20–50% of cases after discontinuation of the treatment. Chloroquine, hydroxychloroquine, azathioprine, and methotrexate have been used successfully in the management of severe mucocutaneous sarcoidosis and in patients who either do not respond to prednisone or have severe side effects (*Am J Respir Crit Care Med* 160:736, 1999). Other immunosuppressive agents that have been tried (e.g., chlorambucil, cyclosporine, cyclophosphamide, ketoconazole) have been shown to have limited benefit in sarcoid lung disease.

2. **IPF** has a highly variable but progressive course, with a median survival of less than 5 years from presentation. Relatively good prognostic factors include young age, female gender, recent onset of symptoms, less severe breathlessness, infiltrates at presentation, predominantly cellular histology (as opposed to fibrosis), and initial responsiveness to glucocorticoids (*Am J Respir Crit Care Med* 149:450, 1994; *Am J Respir Crit Care Med* 161:646, 2000).

   a. **Glucocorticoids** (prednisone, 1.0–1.5 mg/kg PO qd) should be initiated early in the course of the illness and, if a response occurs, the dosage should be decreased to 0.5–1.0 mg/kg PO qd after 3–6 months and then to 0.25 mg/kg PO qd for 6 additional months. After 1 year, prednisone is tapered slowly to the minimal dosage that maintains clinical stability (*J Respir Dis* 14:1244, 1993). Fifty percent of treated patients have a subjective improvement, whereas 25% demonstrate objective improvement (*Thorax* 38:349, 1983).

   b. **Cyclophosphamide**, 1–2 mg/kg PO qd, not to exceed 200 mg/day PO (adjusted to maintain a WBC count >4000/µl), or azathioprine, 3 mg/kg PO qd, not to exceed 200 mg/day, in combination with low-dose glucocorticoids, may result in improvement in some cases that are unresponsive to glucocorticoids alone (*Am Rev Respir Dis* 144:291, 1991; *Chest* 102:1090, 1992). Cyclosporine (5–10 mg/kg PO qd) has been suggested for patients with IPF who are awaiting lung transplantation (*J Heart Lung Transplant* 12:909, 1993).

   c. **Novel potential therapeutic interventions** include antifibrotic agents (pirfenidone), immunomodulating agents (interferon-gamma, interferon-beta, suramin), antioxidants, and thalidomide (*Am J Respir Crit Care Med* 160:1771, 1999). Other immunosuppressive agents (colchicine, methotrexate, penicillamine) are less useful (*Am J Respir Crit Care Med* 155:395, 1997). Interferon gamma-1b may improve lung function and oxygenation in those patients with IPF who had no response to glucocorticoids alone (*N Engl J Med* 341:1264, 1999).

   d. **Single-lung transplantation** remains a therapeutic option for selected patients with IPF. Referral for lung transplantation should be considered when the pulmonary function is abnormal even though the patient may be only minimally symptomatic (*Am J Respir Crit Care Med* 158:335, 1998). The actuarial 1-, 2-, and 3-year survival after transplantation is 67%, 52%, and 35%, respectively (*UNOS: Annual Report*, 1999).

3. **Radiation pneumonitis** is a subacute inflammatory pneumonitis that occurs in response to radiation exposure to the lung. Usually, symptoms are cough, dyspnea, and low-grade fevers. Radiographically, the presence of an infiltrate corresponding to the region of radiation exposure is characteristic. The incidence, severity, and time of onset of symptoms depend on several factors, the most important of which are the total radiation dose, fractionation schedule, volume of lung irradiated, and concomitant administration of bleomycin or other cytotoxic therapy. In general, the onset of symptoms occurs 6–12 weeks after completion of radiotherapy; however, the onset can range from 1–6 months. Management of radiation pneumonitis involves excluding other causes of pulmonary infiltrates, especially infections, recurrent tumors, and lymphangitic carcinomatosis. Mild symptoms can be managed with cough suppressants, antipyretics, and rest. Patients with more severe symptoms and a deterioration in gas exchange should be treated with glucocorticoids. Prednisone is started at 60–100 mg/day, continued until symptoms and gas exchange improve (usually 3–5 days), and then tapered to 20–40 mg PO qd. After 4 weeks of treatment, attempts should be made gradually to taper the prednisone dosage completely.

Only half of patients with radiation pneumonitis will respond to gluco-corticoid therapy.

Pulmonary Hypertension

Pulmonary hypertension may result from a variety of underlying diseases, including pulmonary venous hypertension (e.g., left ventricular dysfunction, mitral stenosis), chronic hypoxemia (e.g., COPD; see Chronic Obstructive Pulmonary Disease, sec. **III.E**), left-to-right shunts (e.g., atrial septal defects), or vascular diseases of the lungs (e.g., thromboembolic disease). It can occur also in patients with portal hypertension, HIV infection, collagen vascular diseases, history of appetite-suppressant drugs (fenfluramine, dexfenfluramine), or cocaine or amphetamine use (*N Engl J Med* 336:111, 1997). **PPH** is an uncommon disease of unknown etiology characterized by sustained elevation of pulmonary artery pressure (mean, >25 mm Hg at rest or >30 mm Hg with exercise) that is not attributed to any other cause.

I. **The diagnosis of PPH** is one of exclusion. It occurs most often in young women with complaints of dyspnea, fatigue, and occasionally syncope. Evaluation of the patient should include chest radiography, PFTs, exercise testing, echocardiography, $\dot{V}/\dot{Q}$ scanning, and pulmonary artery catheterization. Pulmonary angiography may be appropriate in some patients.

II. **Therapy for PPH** is limited. Typically, the natural history is characterized by hemodynamic worsening over time, with no available cure. The median survival after diagnosis is approximately 2.5 years but may improve with treatment (*N Engl J Med* 327:76, 1992).

   A. **Supportive measures** include supplemental oxygen for hypoxemic patients and judicious use of diuretics in the presence of fluid overload.

   B. **Vasodilator therapy** is effective in some patients with PPH, but individual responses are difficult to predict. An initial vasodilator trial under hemodynamic monitoring is recommended before one embarks on a long-term course of therapy (*N Engl J Med* 336:111, 1997). The potential direct benefits of vasodilator therapy for PPH include improved pulmonary hemodynamics, right ventricular function, and oxygen delivery, which may lead to clinical improvement (*Chest* 105:17S, 1994). IV epoprostenol (prostacyclin), IV adenosine, oral calcium channel blockers, or inhaled nitric oxide have been used for vasoreactivity challenge testing. In responsive patients, long-term therapy with the oral vasodilators, nifedipine (30–240 mg/day) or diltiazem (120–900 mg/day), prolongs survival (*Ann Intern Med* 121:409, 1994). Epoprostenol by continuous IV infusion improves hemodynamics, exercise tolerance, quality of life, and survival in patients in the New York Heart Association functional classes III and IV. Drug-induced side effects include jaw pain, cutaneous erythema, diarrhea, and arthralgias. Intermittent therapy with nebulized or oral iloprost, a stable analog of prostacyclin, offers new therapeutic options for selected patients (*Ann Intern Med* 132:435, 2000). Atrial septostomy can improve the hemodynamic status in selected patients with severe PPH (*J Am Coll Cardiol* 32:297, 1998; *Am J Cardiol* 84:682, 1999). In cases of secondary pulmonary hypertension such as scleroderma, systemic lupus erythematosus, Eisenmenger's syndrome, or portopulmonary hypertension, continuous epoprostenol therapy has been shown to improve exercise capacity and cardiopulmonary hemodynamics. (*Ann Intern Med* 132:425, 2000).

   C. **Anticoagulation with warfarin** in doses adjusted to keep an international normalized ratio of approximately 2.0 is recommended in most patients with PPH, owing to the increased risk of microvascular thrombosis, venous stasis, and limitation in physical activity. Warfarin has been shown to improve survival (*Chest* 105:175, 1994).

D. **Lung transplantation or heart-lung transplantation** is the ultimate therapeutic alternative for selected patients. Even markedly depressed right ventricular function improves considerably after single- or double-lung
   transplantation (*Circulation* 84:2275, 1991). Referral should be considered
   for patients with a New York Heart Association functional class III or IV,
   mean right atrial pressure of greater than 15 mm Hg, mean pulmonary
   arterial pressure of greater than 55 mm Hg, and a cardiac index of less than
   2 L/minute/m^2 (*Am J Respir Crit Care Med* 158:335, 1998). The actuarial
   1-, 2-, and 3-year survival for PPH after lung transplantation is 65%, 55%,
   and 44%, respectively (*UNOS: Annual Report*, 1999).

Sleep Apnea Syndrome

Sleep apnea syndrome, clinically defined by frequent episodes of apnea,
hypopnea, and symptoms of functional impairment, is associated with significant adverse health effects and increased mortality (*Chest* 97:27, 1990).
Approximately 2% of women and 4% of men between ages 30 and 60 years meet
diagnostic criteria for sleep apnea syndrome (*N Engl J Med* 328:1230, 1993).
Obstructive Sleep Apnea (OSA) is caused by repetitive inspiratory occlusion of
the upper airway during sleep. This occlusion results in respiratory efforts
without airflow, hypoxemia, disrupted sleep pattern, and an array of potentially
serious physiologic consequences (*Am Rev Respir Dis* 134:791, 1986).

I. **Diagnosis.** Disorders commonly associated with OSA include obesity, nasal
   obstruction, adenoidal or tonsillar hypertrophy, micrognathia, retrognathia,
   macroglossia, acromegaly, hypothyroidism, vocal cord paralysis, and bulbar
   involvement from neuromuscular disease (*Otolaryngol Clin North Am* 23:727,
   1990). Overlap is also significant between OSA and hypertension, CHF, and
   cardiac arrhythmias (*Clin Chest Med* 19:99, 1998).

   A. **Clinical presentation.** Snoring and excessive daytime sleepiness are the car-
      dinal features of OSA. Patients may complain also of personality changes,
      intellectual deterioration, morning headaches, automatic behavior, and loss
      of libido. Systemic hypertension, pulmonary hypertension, and cardiac
      arrhythmias are the consequences of repetitive oxygen desaturation.
      Hypoxemia, hypercapnia, polycythemia, and cor pulmonale may complicate
      the late stage of the disease, especially when obesity and chronic lung dis-
      ease are present (*Mayo Clin Proc* 65:1087, 1990).

   B. **Polysomnography.** Performed at night in a qualified sleep laboratory by a
      trained technician, polysomnography is the diagnostic gold standard (*Am
      Rev Respir Dis* 139:559, 1989). The indications for a sleep study include
      (1) excessive daytime sleepiness, (2) unexplained pulmonary hypertension
      or polycythemia, (3) disturbances of respiratory control in patients with
      daytime hypercapnia, (4) titration of optimal nasal continuous positive
      airway pressure (CPAP) therapy, and (5) assessment of objective response
      to therapeutic interventions.

II. **Management.** The therapeutic approach to OSA depends on the severity of the
    disease, underlying medical condition, cardiopulmonary sequelae, and expected
    degree of patient compliance. The treatment must be highly individualized, with
    special attention to correcting potentially reversible exacerbating factors. These
    include weight reduction when appropriate, avoidance of alcohol and sedatives,
    nasal decongestants if needed, assessment of nighttime oxygenation, and specific
    therapy for other conditions (e.g., COPD, hypertension, hypothyroidism). All
    patients should have a thorough nose and throat examination to detect sources of
    upper airway obstruction that are surgically correctable (e.g., septal deviation,
    enlarged tonsils, enlarged uvula). Nasal CPAP, with its level optimized
    individually in the sleep laboratory, is the treatment of choice for most patients
    with OSA. Side effects, including nasal and eye complaints, discomfort, and

intolerance to machine noise, affect compliance. Newer mask designs, variable inspiratory and expiratory airway pressure devices, and quieter and smaller CPAP units have improved long-term tolerance to nasal CPAP (*Chest* 98:317, 1990). Mandibular advancement using oral devices benefits some patients. Tracheostomy is the most effective treatment for OSA. However, it is invasive and interferes with speech, exercise, social interactions, and mucociliary clearance. Suitable patients for tracheostomy are those who have life-threatening hypoxemia or cardiac arrhythmias, disabling hypersomnolence, and intolerance or noncompliance with other therapies.

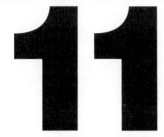

Allergy and Immunology

Anne Pittman and
Mario Castro

Drug Reactions

Adverse reactions to drugs are a very common problem. Only a subset of reactions are mediated immunologically. Other drug reactions include toxic or idiosyncratic reactions. Many different mechanisms can account for immunologically mediated drug reactions (Table 11-1). These reactions can occur with relatively low doses of the drug, usually after an initial exposure with a latent period. Re-exposure to the drug results in the allergic or immunologic reaction.

I. **Beta-lactam sensitivity.** Penicillins and other beta-lactam antibiotics are commonly associated with immunologically mediated drug reactions.

   A. **Penicillins** have a high incidence of immunologic reactivity as a result of their chemical structure. The core structure consists of a reactive bicyclic beta-lactam ring that serves as a hapten by covalently binding to tissue carrier proteins. Ninety-five percent of tissue-bound penicillin is found to be haptenated as the benzylpenicilloyl form and is called the **major determinant.** Five percent of tissue-bound penicillin consists of three non–cross-reactive metabolites, termed the **minor determinants.** Immediate allergic reactions are most often related to the **major determinant.** In addition, some modified penicillins can also produce allergic reactions in which the antigenic determinant is the side chain. Skin testing is available if there is a question of penicillin sensitivity. Accurate penicillin skin testing requires having available the appropriate reagents, which consist of the penicillin molecule, the minor and major determinants, and the appropriate modified penicillins. In 97% of patients with a negative skin test to penicillin, an immediate hypersensitivity reaction to penicillin will not develop. A non–immunoglobulin E (IgE)–mediated reaction (e.g., a morbilliform rash) may develop in these patients. **No case of penicillin-induced anaphylaxis has been reported in a patient who is skin test negative.** Seventy-five percent of patients who report a history of penicillin sensitivity are negative on skin testing and are not at risk for anaphylaxis. Moreover, 4% of patients with unknown or negative histories of penicillin reactions have positive skin tests and are at risk for having an IgE-mediated event. Skin testing should be performed by an allergist who is familiar with the protocol.

   B. **Cephalosporins** share cross reactivity with penicillins because of their related structure. Studies report a four- to eightfold increased risk of hypersensitivity reactions to cephalosporins in penicillin-allergic patients. The degree of cross reactivity is related to the generation of the cephalosporin (first more than second more than third generation). The overall reaction rate to cephalosporins of penicillin skin test–positive patients is approximately 3%. Although many of the reactions to second- and third-generation cephalosporin are directed at the side chains, skin testing to penicillin in these patients can be quite helpful, as most severe anaphylactic reactions

Table 11-1. Immunologically mediated drug reactions

Type of reaction	Representative examples	Mechanism
Anaphylactic	Anaphylaxis Urticaria Angioedema	IgE-mediated degranulation of mast cell with resultant mediator release
Cytotoxic	Autoimmune hemolytic anemia Interstitial nephritis	IgG or IgM antibodies against cell antigens and complement activation
Immune complex	Serum sickness Vasculitis Hemolytic anemia	Immune complex deposition and subsequent complement activation
Cell mediated	Contact dermatitis Photosensitivity dermatitis	Activated T cells against cell-surface–bound antigens

IgE = immunoglobulin E; IgG = immunoglobulin G; IgM = immunoglobulin M.

are directed at the reactive bicyclic core. Patients with a history of a severe reaction to penicillin should be considered sensitive to cephalosporin unless they are skin test negative. Although it may be appropriate to give a second- or third-generation cephalosporin to patients with a history of a nonanaphylactic reaction to penicillin, it is advisable to precede the dose with an oral provocation dose challenge.

- **C. Other related antibiotics**
    - **1. Monobactams. Aztreonam** is the prototype antibiotic with a monocyclic structure. No significant cross reactivity is found between this group and the beta-lactams.
    - **2. Carbapenems. Imipenem** is the prototype member of this antibiotic group. A very high degree of cross reactivity (50%) is found between imipenem determinants and penicillin determinants.
    - **3. Carbacephems** (e.g., loracarbef) are structurally related to cephalosporins. Few data exist in regard to cross reactivity, but they should be assumed to be related antigenically and should be avoided in severely penicillin-sensitive patients.
- **II. Radiocontrast sensitivity reactions** mimic anaphylaxis but are not IgE mediated. The contrast medium probably causes a direct degranulation of mast cells in susceptible patients. Reactions can occur in 5–10% of patients, with a fatal reaction occurring in 1 in 40,000 procedures. The following risk factors have been identified: age over 50 years, pre-existing cardiovascular or renal disease, a personal history of allergy, and a history of a radiocontrast reaction. No evidence has been found that sensitivity to seafood or iodine predisposes to reactions to radiocontrast media. Although no predictive tests are available, if patients have a history of a reaction, the use of a low-ionic-strength contrast medium and premedication is strongly suggested. Subsequent reactions can be decreased substantially by pretreatment with antihistamines and corticosteroids in the following manner: Prednisone at 50 mg PO is given 13 hours, 7 hours, and 1 hour before the procedure. Diphenhydramine at 50 mg PO also is given 1 hour before the procedure. H_2 blockers can also be given 1 hour before the procedure. It is important to remember that this is not 100% effective and that appropriate precautions should be taken.
- **III. Stevens-Johnson syndrome** (also known as erythema multiforme major) is a rare, self-limited inflammatory disorder of the skin and mucous membranes

that is caused by a variety of agents, usually drugs or infections, and is characterized by a variety of morphologic cutaneous lesions. The incidence rate ranges from 2.6–7.1 cases per one million population per year. Mucosal lesions (oropharynx, lips, and conjunctivae) that involve multiple mucosal surfaces are common. Severe cases can involve the eyes, nares, tracheobronchial tree, and esophagus and have been reported to evolve into a clinical syndrome that resembles toxic epidermal necrolysis. Treatment focuses on the discontinuation of suspected drugs (unless this maneuver is life threatening) and treating any underlying infection. Other therapeutic maneuvers are directed to symptoms and may include hydration to maintain fluid balance, antihistamines to decrease pruritus, analgesics to relieve pain, and wet dressings to débride crusted erosions. Systemic corticosteroids are used, but their efficacy is unproved.

IV. **Management of the patient with a history of drug reactions.** Prevention is the most effective way to minimize the morbidity and mortality from drug reactions. Drug use should always be avoided unless a definite medical indication exists. A careful history of drug reactions including the type and magnitude is helpful in defining the potential risk of a reaction. The risk of a drug reaction can be delineated by evaluating the type of reaction that occurred. **Toxic reactions** such as nausea secondary to macrolide antibiotics or codeine are not immunologic reactions and do not necessarily predict problems with other members in their respective class. Other toxic effects, such as **"red man syndrome"** seen with rapid vancomycin infusions can be avoided by slowing the rate of infusion and do not preclude further use of the drug. **True immunologic reactions** require special consideration because re-exposure to even small amounts of the drug can result in a severe reaction. A history of anaphylaxis or other IgE-mediated reactions tends to increase the likelihood of further IgE-mediated reactions. The history of a **maculopapular reaction** to a drug may not be associated with an increased risk of an IgE-mediated event. A past immunologic reaction tends to predict the type of future reactions. **If no alternative drug is available** and the patient gives a history of an IgE-mediated reaction, penicillin skin testing should first be performed. If the drug in question is a penicillin or a cephalosporin, penicillin skin testing should first be performed. **If the patient has a positive skin test,** penicillin desensitization by an allergist should be performed. If the drug in question is not a beta-lactam, **incremental challenge testing** can be undertaken. This test involves the administration of a very low dose of the drug (e.g., <1 mg) and then a slow increase in the dose (usually a doubling of the previous dose) q15min until a therapeutic dose is reached. Once a therapeutic dose is reached, the drug should be administered at least q12h to avoid precipitation of allergic reaction with subsequent doses.

V. **Treatment of drug reactions.** Discontinuation of the suspected drug or drugs is the most important initial approach in managing an allergic reaction. If the patient is taking the drug for a life-threatening illness (e.g., meningitis) and the reaction is a mild skin reaction, it may be reasonable to continue the medication and treat the reaction symptomatically. If the rash is progressive, the drug must be discontinued to avoid a desquamative process such as Stevens-Johnson syndrome.

Anaphylaxis

Anaphylaxis is an IgE-mediated, rapidly developing, systemic allergic reaction. Anaphylactoid reactions result from the direct release of mast cell mediators.

I. **The clinical manifestations of anaphylaxis and anaphylactoid reactions** are the same. Most serious reactions occur within minutes after exposure to the antigen. However, the reaction may be delayed for hours. Some patients experience a biphasic reaction characterized by a recurrence of symptoms after 4–8 hours. A few patients have a protracted course that requires several hours of continuous treatment.

A. Manifestations include pruritus, urticaria, angioedema, respiratory distress (due to laryngeal edema, laryngospasm, or bronchospasm), hypotension, abdominal cramping, and diarrhea. **The most common cause of death is airway obstruction,** followed by hypotension. The spectrum of reactions ranges from very severe and life threatening to mild. However, left untreated, all reactions have the potential to become severe very rapidly. **A previous mild reaction does not predict a mild reaction with re-exposure to the offending agent.**

B. Immediate treatment of anaphylaxis and anaphylactoid reactions

1. **Epinephrine is the mainstay of therapy** and should be administered immediately. A dose of 0.3–0.5 mg (0.3–0.5 ml of a 1:1000 solution) SC should be administered and repeated at 20-minute intervals if necessary. Patients with major airway compromise or hypotension can be given epinephrine sublingually (0.5 ml of a 1:1000 solution), via a femoral or internal jugular vein (3–5 ml of a 1:10,000 solution), or via an endotracheal tube (3–5 ml of a 1:10,000 solution diluted to 10 ml with normal saline). For protracted anaphylaxis that requires multiple doses of epinephrine, an IV epinephrine drip may be useful. The infusion is titrated to blood pressure (see Appendix D).

2. **Airway management** should be a priority. Supplemental 100% oxygen therapy should be administered. Endotracheal intubation may be necessary. If laryngeal edema is not rapidly responsive to epinephrine, cricothyroidotomy or tracheotomy may be required.

3. **Volume expansion** with IV fluids may be necessary. An initial bolus of 500–1000 ml normal saline should be followed by an infusion that is titrated to BP and urine output.

4. **β-Adrenergic antagonist therapy increases the risk of anaphylactoid reaction and anaphylaxis** and renders the reaction more difficult to treat (*Ann Intern Med* 115:270, 1991). Glucagon, given as a 1-mg (1 ampule) bolus and followed by a drip of up to 1 mg/hour, provides inotropic support for patients who are taking β-adrenergic antagonists. **α-Adrenergic agonist vasopressors must be avoided in this setting because of unopposed alpha-mediated vasoconstriction.**

C. Additional treatment of anaphylaxis and anaphylactoid reactions

1. **Inhaled β-adrenergic agonists** [albuterol, 0.5 ml (2.5 mg), or metaproterenol, 0.3 ml (15 mg) in 2.5 ml normal saline] should be used to treat resistant bronchospasm. Aminophylline can be used as a second-line drug (see Chap. 10).

2. **Glucocorticoids** have no significant immediate effect. However, they may prevent relapse of severe reactions. Methylprednisolone, 125 mg IV, or hydrocortisone, 500 mg IV, can be administered.

3. **Antihistamines** relieve skin symptoms but have no immediate effect on the reaction. They may shorten the duration of the reaction. The addition of an H_2 antagonist may be useful.

II. Observation for a minimum of 6 hours is indicated for patients with mild reactions limited to urticaria, angioedema, or mild bronchospasm. Patients with moderate to severe reactions should be admitted to the hospital for close observation of a possible biphasic reaction.

III. Recurrent anaphylaxis. Prevention of recurrent episodes requires identification and avoidance of the offending antigen. Medications, *Hymenoptera* stings, and foods are the most common causes of anaphylaxis. Radiocontrast medium is the most common cause of anaphylactoid reactions. An exhaustive diagnostic evaluation is not indicated after a single episode of anaphylaxis if a cause is not suggested by the history. In patients with recurrent episodes and no obvious

Table 11-2. Conditions that can present as refractory asthma

Upper airway obstruction
  Tumor
  Epiglottitis
  Vocal cord dysfunction
  Obstructive sleep apnea
Tracheomalacia
Endobronchial lesion
Foreign body
Congestive heart failure
Gastroesophageal reflux
Sinusitis
Herpetic tracheobronchitis
Adverse drug reaction
  Aspirin
  β-Adrenergic antagonist
  Angiotensin-converting enzyme inhibitors
  Inhaled pentamidine
Allergic bronchopulmonary aspergillosis
Hyperventilation with panic attacks

etiologic finding, other possible diagnoses should be considered. An elevated serum tryptase during an episode confirms a diagnosis of anaphylaxis.

A. Self-administered epinephrine should be prescribed for all patients with a history of anaphylaxis to a food or *Hymenoptera* sting. The patient should be instructed in its use. Patients with a history of anaphylaxis to *Hymenoptera* also should be referred to an allergist for desensitization.

B. Mastocytosis should be considered in those patients with recurrent anaphylaxis and no finding of other obvious etiology. The diagnosis is confirmed by demonstration of persistently elevated levels of mast cell mediators, such as serum tryptase, during times that the patient is asymptomatic.

Asthma

Asthma is a disease of the airways characterized by airway inflammation and increased responsiveness (hyperreactivity) to a wide variety of stimuli (triggers). This hyperreactivity leads to obstruction of the airways, the severity of which may be widely variable in the same individual. As a consequence, patients have paroxysms of cough, dyspnea, chest tightness, and wheezing. Asthma is an episodic disease, with acute exacerbations that are interspersed with symptom-free periods. Other conditions may present with wheezing and must be considered, especially in patients who are not responsive to therapy (Table 11-2).

I. Clinical manifestations and evaluation of asthma
  A. Attacks are episodes of shortness of breath or wheezing that last minutes to hours. Patients may be completely symptom free between attacks. Typically,

attacks are triggered by acute exposure to irritants, such as perfume, cleaning solution, smoke, or allergens.

B. Exacerbations occur when airway reactivity is increased and lung function becomes unstable. During an exacerbation, attacks occur more easily and are more severe and persistent. Exacerbations are associated with factors that increase airway hyperreactivity, such as viral infections, allergens, and occupational exposures.

C. Nasal polyps. Patients with asthma and polyps should avoid aspirin and all nonsteroidal anti-inflammatory drugs because of the possibility of a severe systemic reaction.

D. Pulmonary function tests (PFTs) are essential to diagnose asthma. In patients with asthma, PFTs demonstrate an obstructive pattern, the hallmark of which is a decrease in expiratory flow rates. Patients experience a reduction in the forced expiratory volume over 1 second (FEV_1) and a proportionally smaller reduction in the forced vital capacity (FVC). This produces a decreased FEV_1/FVC ratio (<0.75). With mild obstructive disease that involves only the small airways, the FEV_1/FVC ratio may be normal, and the only abnormality may be a decrease in airflow at midlung volumes (forced expiratory flow 25–75%). Patients with lung hyperinflation have an increased residual volume and residual volume–total lung capacity ratio. The flow volume loop demonstrates a decreased flow rate for any lung volume and is useful to rule out other causes of dyspnea, such as upper airway obstruction or restrictive lung disease. The clinical diagnosis of asthma is supported by an obstructive pattern that improves after bronchodilator therapy. Improvement is defined as an increase in FEV_1 of more than 12% and 200 cc after 2–3 puffs of short-acting bronchodilator. In patients with chronic, severe asthma, the airflow obstruction may no longer be completely reversible. In these patients, the most effective way of establishing the maximal degree of airway reversibility is to repeat PFTs after a course of oral corticosteroids (usually 40 mg/day for 10 days). The lack of demonstrable airway obstruction or reactivity does not rule out a diagnosis of asthma. In cases in which spirometry is normal, the diagnosis can be made by showing heightened airway responsiveness to methacholine or histamine.

E. A chest radiograph should be obtained to eliminate other causes of dyspnea, cough, or wheezing.

II. Evaluation and treatment of an acute asthma attack

A. Assessment of severity

1. **History.** Recent emergency room visits and current oral corticosteroid use may indicate an exacerbation that has become refractory to outpatient management. Previous attacks that have required the use of oral corticosteroids, a previous episode of respiratory failure, use of more than two canisters per month of inhaled short-acting bronchodilator, and seizures with asthma attacks have been associated with severe and potentially fatal asthma. Most patients have a progressive worsening of symptoms over a period of days or weeks. A precipitous onset of symptoms should raise the possibility of gastroesophageal reflux or a reaction to acute ingestion of aspirin or a nonsteroidal anti-inflammatory agent.

2. **Physical examination.** A rapid assessment should be performed to identify those patients who require immediate intervention. **The presence or intensity of wheezing is an unreliable indicator of the severity of an attack.** A **severe attack** is suggested by respiratory distress at rest, difficulty in speaking in sentences, diaphoresis, or agitation. A respiratory rate greater than 28 breaths/minute, a pulse greater than 110 beats/minute, or a pulsus paradoxus greater than 25 mm Hg indicates a severe episode. Patients with depressed mental status require intubation. Subcutaneous emphysema should alert the examiner to

the presence of a pneumothorax or pneumomediastinum. Impending respiratory muscle fatigue may cause a depressed respiratory effort, paradoxical diaphragmatic movement, and alternating abdominal and ribcage breathing.

3. **Laboratory evaluation**

   a. **An objective measurement of airflow obstruction** is essential to the evaluation of an asthma attack. The severity of the exacerbation should be classified as **mild-moderate** [peak expiratory flow (PEF) or FEV_1 >50% of predicted], **severe** (PEF or FEV_1 <50%), or impending or actual respiratory arrest. Hospitalization is recommended if the response to treatment is poor or incomplete. A low threshold for admission is appropriate for patients with recent hospitalization, a failure of aggressive outpatient management (with oral corticosteroids), or a previous life-threatening attack. When spirometry is not available, peak flow rates can be obtained easily with a peak flowmeter. Generally, hospitalization is recommended if the PEF or FEV_1 is less than 50% of predicted, arterial carbon dioxide tension ($PaCO_2$) is greater than 42 mm Hg, the symptoms are severe, or the patient is drowsy or confused; however, the decision to hospitalize needs to be individualized. The response to initial treatment (60–90 minutes after three doses of a short-acting bronchodilator) is a better predictor of the need for hospitalization than is the severity of an exacerbation.

   b. **Arterial blood gas measurement** should be considered in patients in severe distress or with an FEV_1 of less than 30% of predicted values after initial treatment. An arterial oxygen tension of less than 60 mm Hg is a sign of severe bronchoconstriction or of a complicating condition. Initially, the $PaCO_2$ is low, owing to an increase in respiratory rate. With a prolonged attack, the $PaCO_2$ may rise as a result of severe airway obstruction, increased dead-space ventilation, and respiratory muscle fatigue. **A normal or increased $PaCO_2$ is a sign of impending respiratory failure and necessitates hospitalization.** The patient requires aggressive bronchodilator therapy and should be monitored closely (often in an ICU) to assess the need for mechanical ventilation.

B. **Therapy**

   1. **Supplemental oxygen** should be administered to the patient who is awaiting an assessment of arterial oxygen tension and should be continued to maintain an oxygen saturation of greater than 90% (95% in patients with coexisting cardiac disease or pregnancy).

   2. **Bronchodilators** are first-line therapy in an asthma attack. Reversal of airflow obstruction is achieved most effectively by frequent administration of inhaled β_2-adrenergic agonists.

      a. Albuterol is administered either via metered-dose inhaler (MDI) or nebulizer. For a **mild-moderate exacerbation,** initial treatment starts with 6–12 puffs of albuterol via MDI or 2.5 mg via nebulizer and repeated q20min until improvement is obtained or toxicity is noted. For **severe exacerbation**, albuterol, 2.5–5.0 mg, with ipratropium bromide, 0.5 mg via nebulizer, should be administered q20min. Alternatively, albuterol, 10.0–15.0 mg, administered continuously over an hour may be more effective in severely obstructed adults. The subsequent dosing schedule is adjusted according to the patient's symptoms and clinical presentation. Often, patients require β_2-adrenergic agonists q2–4h during an acute attack. The use of an MDI with a spacer device under the supervision of trained personnel is as effective as aerosolized solution by nebulizer. Patient cooperation may not be possible in the patient with severe airflow obstruction.

b. **Parenteral administration of bronchodilators** is unnecessary if inhaled medications can be administered quickly. In rare settings, aqueous epinephrine (0.3 ml of a 1:1000 solution SC q20min) for up to three doses can be used. If epinephrine is administered, ECG monitoring is necessary.

3. **Systemic corticosteroids** speed the resolution of a severe exacerbation of asthma and should be administered to all patients admitted for treatment of such exacerbation.

   a. **Methylprednisolone** is the drug of choice for IV therapy. IV methylprednisolone, 125 mg, given in the emergency room (on initial presentation) decreases the rate of return to the emergency room of those patients who are discharged.

   b. **The ideal dose of corticosteroid** needed to speed recovery and limit symptoms is still not defined well. Currently, methylprednisolone, 40–60 mg IV q6h, is recommended. Oral corticosteroid administration may be as effective if given in equivalent doses (prednisone, 60 mg PO q6–8h).

   c. **For maximal therapeutic response, tapering of high-dose corticosteroids should not take place** until objective evidence of clinical improvement is observed (usually 36–48 hours). Initially, patients are given a daily dose of oral prednisone, which then is reduced slowly. Dosing oral steroids twice a day may minimize symptoms. A 7- to 14-day tapering dosage of prednisone usually is successful in combination with an inhaled corticosteroid that has been instituted at the beginning of the tapering schedule. In patients with severe disease or with a history of respiratory failure, a slower reduction in dosage is appropriate.

   d. **Patients discharged from the emergency room should receive oral corticosteroids.** A dose of prednisone, 40 mg/day for 5 days, can be substituted for a tapering schedule in selected patients. Either regimen should be accompanied by the initiation of an inhaled corticosteroid (or an increase in the previous dose of inhaled corticosteroid).

4. **Methylxanthines** are not generally recommended.

5. **Close follow-up** is required for patients discharged from the hospital or emergency room, because baseline airway hyperreactivity persists for 4–6 weeks after an asthma exacerbation. A return visit to the physician should be scheduled within 5–7 days.

III. Daily asthma management

A. **The goals of daily management** are to control symptoms while maintaining normal activity and pulmonary function, to prevent exacerbations, and to minimize medication toxicity. Successful management requires patient education, objective measurement of airflow obstruction, and a medication plan for daily use and for exacerbations.

   1. **Patient education** should focus on the chronic and inflammatory nature of asthma, with identification of factors that contribute to increased inflammation. The consequences of ongoing exposure to chronic irritants or allergens and the rationale for therapy should be explained. Patients are instructed to avoid factors that aggravate their disease. Verbal and written instruction should be provided.

   a. **A number of factors increase airway hyperresponsiveness** and cause an acute and chronic increase in the severity of the disease. Dust mites, cockroaches, and pet dander cause an increase in airway inflammation and symptoms in allergic patients. Many occupational allergens and irritants cause asthma, even in small doses. Viral upper respiratory tract infections and sinusitis are important causes of asthma exacerbations. Gastroesophageal reflux can cause cough and wheezing in some patients. Some factors, such as tobacco and wood smoke, trigger acute bronchospasm and should be avoided by all patients.

    b. Cold air and exercise can increase symptoms. Prophylactic use of cromolyn, nedocromil, or an inhaled β_2-adrenergic agonist (3 puffs 20 minutes before exposure) can minimize exercise-induced symptoms.

    c. Aspirin and nonsteroidal anti-inflammatory medications can cause the sudden onset of severe airway obstruction. Patients with aspirin sensitivity and nasal polyps typically have the onset of asthma in the third or fourth decade of life.

  2. PEF monitoring provides an objective measurement of airflow obstruction and should be considered in patients who require daily medication. Ideally, the PEF should be measured in the early morning and again after 12 hours, with additional measurements taken before and 20 minutes after bronchodilator therapy. For many patients, monitoring PEF intermittently is sufficient. The personal best PEF (the highest PEF obtained when the disease is under control) is identified, and the PEF is checked when symptoms escalate or in the setting of an asthma trigger. Patients should learn to anticipate situations that cause increased symptoms. In addition, it is useful for patients to monitor their PEF during times in which medications are changed.

  3. It is important for patients to recognize signs of poorly controlled disease. These signs include an increased need for β_2-adrenergic agonists, limitation of activity, waking at night because of asthma symptoms, and variability in the PEF. Specific instructions about handling these symptoms (asthma action plan), including criteria for seeking emergency care, should be provided. Poorly controlled asthma is characterized by a greater response to bronchodilator therapy (increased difference between PEF before and after bronchodilator) and by an increase in the circadian variation in PEF.

B. Medical management involves chronic management and a plan for acute exacerbations. Most often it includes the daily use of an anti-inflammatory, disease-modifying medication **(long-term-control medications)** and as-needed use of a short-acting bronchodilator **(quick-relief medications)**.

  1. The **severity** of asthma varies over time in individual patients. Consequently, medication requirements vary over time. The National Heart, Lung, and Blood Institute consensus report classified asthma into four different stages (mild intermittent, mild, moderate, and severe persistent) (*NHBLI*, July 1997, NIH publication 97-4051). It is preferred to start therapy at a level higher than the patient's severity to gain control and then to decrease the therapy in follow-up once control has been achieved.

    a. Mild intermittent asthma. This disorder is characterized by infrequent asthma symptoms ($\leq$two times a week) and awakening at night fewer than two times a month. In this setting, a short-acting β_2-adrenergic agonist used on an as-needed basis (e.g., albuterol, 2–3 puffs) is appropriate.

    b. Mild persistent asthma. These patients have asthma symptoms more than two times a week but less than one time a day and nocturnal awakenings due to asthma more than two times a month. PEF or FEV_1 is usually 80% or greater than predicted. In addition to the short acting β_2-adrenergic agonist, a long-acting control medication is required for these patients. A low dose of inhaled corticosteroid (Table 11-3) or leukotriene antagonist is an appropriate long-term controller medication for this severity.

    c. Moderate persistent asthma. These patients have asthma symptoms daily and nocturnal awakenings due to asthma more than one time a week. PEF or FEV_1 may be >60 to <80% predicted. A medium dose of inhaled corticosteroid (see Table 11-3) or the addition of a long-acting bronchodilator (salmeterol, 2 puffs bid) to low-medium dose inhaled corticosteroid is appropriate.

Table 11-3. Comparative daily dosages for inhaled corticosteroids

Drug	Low dose	Medium dose	High dose
Triamcinolone (100 µg/ puff)	4–10 puffs	10–20 puffs	>20 puffs
Beclomethasone dipropionate (42, 84 µg/puff)	4–12 puffs: 42 µg	12–20 puffs: 42 µg	>20 puffs: 42 µg
	2–6 puffs: 84 µg	6–8 puffs: 84 µg	>10 puffs: 84 µg
Budesonide Turbuhaler (DPI: 200 µg/dose)	1–2 inhalations	2–3 inhalations	>3 inhalations
Flunisolide (250 µg/puff)	2–4 puffs	4–8 puffs	>8 puffs
Fluticasone (MDI: 44, 110, 220 µg/puff)	2–6 puffs: 44 µg	2–6 puffs: 100 µg	>6 puffs: 100 µg
	2 puffs: 110 µg		>3 puffs: 220 µg
DPI: 50, 100, 250 µg/ dose	2–6 inhalations: 50 µg	3–6 inhalations: 100 µg	>6 inhalations: 100 µg
			>2 inhalations: 250 µg

DPI = dry powder inhaler; MDI = metered-dose inhaler.

> **d. Severe persistent asthma.** These patients have asthma symptoms continuously, are limited in their physical activity, and have frequent nocturnal awakenings because of their asthma. PEF or FEV_1 may be less than 60% predicted. A high dose of inhaled corticosteroid (see Table 11-3) and a long-acting bronchodilator are appropriate. Alternatively, sustained-release theophylline can be added. These patients often require long-term oral corticosteroids, although repeat attempts should be made to reduce the dose while they are receiving high-dose inhaled corticosteroids.
> 2. **Inhaled corticosteroids** are safe and effective for the treatment of chronic asthma (see Table 11-3). They should be administered with a spacing device, and patients should be instructed to rinse their mouth with water after each administration to minimize oral deposition of the steroid and to reduce the possibility of oral candidiasis and hoarseness. The dose is increased as necessary according to symptoms and PEF. In patients with frequent β_2-adrenergic agonist use or other signs of poorly controlled disease, the dose is increased by 50–100% until symptoms are controlled. If symptoms are severe, accompanied by nighttime awakening, or have a PEF of less than 65% of predicted values, a short course of oral corticosteroid (40–60 mg/day for 5 days) might be necessary to get control of the disease quickly. Attempts should be made to decrease the dose of inhaled corticosteroid by 25% every 2–3 months to the lowest possible dose to maintain control.
> 3. **Cromolyn sodium** and **nedocromil sodium** are anti-inflammatory inhaled medications that are useful in children with mild persistent asthma, especially allergic asthma. The usual dosage is 8–12 puffs/day in three to four divided doses. Maximum improvement may be delayed for 4–6 weeks after initiation of therapy. Little additional benefit accrues from using these medications with an inhaled steroid.
> 4. **Leukotriene antagonists.** Montelukast (10 mg PO qd) and zafirlukast (20 mg PO bid) are oral leukotriene receptor antagonists. These agents provide effective control of mild-moderate persistent asthma in the majority of patients. In comparison with inhaled beclomethasone in

patients with mild to moderate persistent asthma, montelukast was found to have a more rapid initial response, whereas beclomethasone had a larger overall effect (*Ann Intern Med* 130:487, 1999). Leukotriene antagonists should be strongly considered for patients with aspirin-induced asthma or for individuals who cannot master MDI technique.

5. **Methylxanthines.** Theophylline provides mild bronchodilation in asthmatics. Sustained-release theophylline may be useful as adjuvant therapy to an anti-inflammatory agent in persistent asthma, especially for controlling nighttime symptoms. It is essential that serum concentrations of theophylline be monitored on a regular basis, aiming for a level of 5–15 μg/ml. Theophylline has a narrow therapeutic range with significant toxicities. One should always consider potential interactions when adding medications (especially antibiotics) for asthma patients on theophylline.

6. The addition of a **long-acting bronchodilator**, such as salmeterol (2 puffs bid), leukotriene antagonist, or theophylline, has been shown to reduce the required dose of inhaled corticosteroid inhaler in patients with moderate persistent asthma. Inhaled, short-acting, β_2-adrenergic agonists should be used on an as-needed basis. The regular use of a short-acting bronchodilator is an indication of poorly controlled asthma and requires the institution of, or increase in, an anti-inflammatory medication.

7. **Nocturnal symptoms.** These symptoms may necessitate the addition at night of either a long-acting inhaled β-adrenergic agonist (e.g., salmeterol, 2 puffs qhs) or sustained-release theophylline. Increased circadian variability in airflow obstruction (nighttime awakening) is a sign of heightened airway hyperreactivity; thus, an increase in the dose of anti-inflammatory medication also should be considered in these patients.

8. Patients who have **severe persistent asthma** and in whom control is inadequate despite the use of oral or high-dose inhaled corticosteroids (see Table 11-3) typically have daily symptoms, chronic limitation of activity, and frequent nocturnal symptoms and require frequent bronchodilator use. The goal of therapy is to minimize symptoms and to minimize the need for oral corticosteroids.

   a. In patients who require high-dose inhaled corticosteroids or regular use of oral corticosteroid, **fluticasone**, 220 μg per puff, or **budesonide**, 200 μg/puff, is very effective in reducing symptoms and in minimizing the effects of oral corticosteroid use. Higher doses (**4** puffs bid) have been used successfully in selected patients with corticosteroid-dependent asthma.

   b. **Systemic corticosteroid absorption** can occur in patients who use inhaled corticosteroids. Consequently, prolonged therapy with high-dose inhaled corticosteroids should be reserved for those patients with severe disease or for those who otherwise require oral corticosteroids. Repeated efforts should be made at tapering the dose.

   c. **Medications to reduce the need for oral corticosteroids,** such as methotrexate, cyclosporin, or troleandomycin, have been studied and may be useful in some patients.

Urticaria and Angioedema

Urticaria (hives) are raised, flat-topped, well-demarcated skin lesions with surrounding erythema. An individual lesion usually lasts minutes to hours. If an individual lesion lasts for longer than 24 hours, a different diagnosis must be entertained. Central clearing can cause an annular lesion and often is seen after antihistamines have been taken. Angioedema is a deeper lesion causing areas of skin-colored, localized swelling. It can involve any area but most often involves the tongue, lips, or eyelids. Often, patients have angioedema and urticaria at the same time. When angioedema occurs without urticaria, often it is related to the ingestion of angiotensin-converting enzyme inhibitors (or angiotensin-receptor antagonists) or is a symptom of hereditary angioedema.

I. Acute urticaria and angioedema

A. Acute urticaria or angioedema is defined as an episode lasting less than 6 weeks. Usually, it is caused by an allergic reaction to a medication or food or is a prodrome to an infection. Aspirin and nonsteroidal anti-inflammatory agents are among the most common causes of urticaria, as are penicillins, cephalosporins, sulfonamides, and other antibiotics. A patient can develop a sensitivity to a food, medication, or self-care product that previously had been used without difficulty.

B. Treatment

1. **Severe urticaria and angioedema**

    a. **In the presence of systemic symptoms** suggesting hypotension, laryngeal edema, or bronchospasm, epinephrine (0.3–0.5 ml of a 1:1000 solution SC) should be administered (see Anaphylaxis).

    b. **SC epinephrine** occasionally can also be useful for acute, severe urticaria (hives) in the absence of systemic symptoms. In these situations, diphenhydramine, 25–50 mg IM or PO, often is administered as well.

2. **The ideal treatment of acute urticaria and angioedema** is to identify and eliminate their cause. Most cases resolve within 1 week. **All potential causes should be eliminated** until the lesions resolve. In some instances, it is possible to reintroduce an agent cautiously that is believed not to be the cause. This trial should be done in the presence of the physician, with epinephrine available.

    a. **Medications,** especially aspirin, are common offenders. **Patients who react to aspirin will react to other nonsteroidal anti-inflammatory medications.** In addition, these agents and angiotensin-converting enzyme inhibitors and beta-blockers may potentiate urticaria caused by other agents.

    b. **Self-care products,** such as shampoos, soaps, lotions, laundry detergents, and dryer softener sheets, often cause urticaria.

    c. **Foods** that commonly cause a reaction include peanuts and other nuts, shellfish and fish, milk, eggs, wheat, soybeans, and fruits. However, any food can cause an allergic reaction.

    d. **In hospitalized patients,** medications, IV contrast media, and latex should be considered as possible causes. Latex exposure may cause urticaria and anaphylaxis. It should be considered in the differential diagnosis of intraoperative anaphylaxis or urticaria in the health care worker.

3. **Oral antihistamines** should be administered to patients around the clock for 72 hours, or longer if their hives have not cleared. Hydroxyzine usually is effective at 25 mg qid and can be increased to 50 mg qid. After 72 hours, antihistamines can be taken as needed. Combinations of traditional and nonsedating antihistamines work well to control urticaria in patients intolerant of the sedating side effects of hydroxyzine alone. Cetirizine (10 mg PO qd), loratadine (10 mg PO qd), or fexofenadine (60 mg PO bid) can be used during the day with hydroxyzine, 25–50 mg, as an evening dose.

4. **Oral corticosteroids** should be prescribed for patients with systemic symptoms of anaphylaxis, those who have had previous episodes of anaphylaxis with urticaria, and those with facial involvement or severe symptoms that have not responded to antihistamines.

II. Evaluation of chronic urticaria

A. Chronic urticaria is defined as episodes of hives that persist for longer than 6 weeks. The etiology remains unidentified in more than 80% of cases. Innumerable causes can trigger chronic urticaria and angioedema; medications, foods, and self-care products are the most common causes.

B. The initial evaluation of chronic urticaria should include a careful history and physical examination to rule out systemic causes. If the history or examination suggests a cause, further testing may be appropriate. Often, urticaria is part of a viral prodrome. The early stages of mononucleosis and viral hepatitis may be associated with urticaria. Hives also can accompany parasitic infections. Testing may include a CBC with absolute eosinophil count, stool culture for ova and parasites, liver chemistries, and a hepatitis profile. A skin biopsy is indicated when individual lesions last for more than 24 hours or are resistant to therapy.

   1. **Urticarial vasculitis** should be considered in patients who have individual lesions that are refractory to antihistamine therapy. Often, hypocomplementemia and an elevated erythrocyte sedimentation rate are observed. The individual lesions typically last for more than 24 hours. Diagnosis requires a biopsy.

   2. **Hereditary angioedema** should be considered in patients with isolated angioedema. A complement profile should reveal a low C4 even between attacks. A low C1 esterase inhibitor level confirms the diagnosis.

   3. **Malignancy or connective tissue disease** may cause urticaria. Furthermore, an acquired C1 esterase deficiency causing angioedema has been associated with malignancy and connective tissue diseases. In the absence of other signs or symptoms of these conditions, an extensive workup to search for occult malignancy or rheumatologic disease is not recommended.

C. Treatment of chronic urticaria

   1. **An elimination diet,** restricting foods to lamb and rice, or elemental supplements can be useful in ruling out food allergy as a cause of chronic urticaria. If the lesions do not resolve within 7 days on a restrictive diet, food allergy is unlikely.

   2. **Elimination of all self-care products,** with the exception of those that contain no methylparaben, fragrance, or preservative, is useful when sensitivity to these products is possible. If the lesions do not resolve within 7 days, allergy to these products is unlikely.

   3. **All over-the-counter medications should be eliminated.** Careful consideration should be given to the elimination or substitution of each prescription medication. If a patient reacts to one medication in a class, the reaction likely will be triggered by all medications in that class.

   4. **Antihistamines usually are sufficient to control chronic urticaria.** Once a combination is identified as preventing the hives, that regimen should be continued for a period of 2 months. If the patient continues to do well, dosages can be reduced to that amount necessary for symptom control.

      a. **Nonsedating antihistamines,** such as loratadine, fexofenadine, and cetirizine, are well tolerated and should be used as first-line agents.

      b. **Classic antihistamines,** such as hydroxyzine, 25 mg PO q4–6h around the clock or prn, can be added for better control of lesions or for breakthrough lesions. This dose can increase by 25 mg/dose to a total of 400 mg/day. The dose usually is limited by sedation.

      c. **Doxepin,** an antidepressant with H_1- and H_2-blocking effects, is a useful addition and often is less sedating than is hydroxyzine. The usual starting dose is 10 mg PO bid. It can be increased by 10 mg/dose until hives are suppressed. The maximum dose is 150 mg bid.

      d. **H_2-blocking agents** may be helpful in addition to H1 antihistamines to control breakthrough hives.

      e. **Oral corticosteroids** should be reserved for those patients in whom adequate control cannot be achieved with a combination of the aforementioned agents. Steroids should be used only for short periods.

Immunodeficiency

Immunodeficiency diseases are characterized by an increased susceptibility to infection. The type of infection and age of onset provide the first clues as to the type of immune defect. The most common disease of immune deficiency is AIDS (see Chap. 15). Children and young adults present with abnormalities in T and B cells and are at risk for severe viral and bacterial infections. Adults usually present with defects in humoral immunity and are at increased risk of sinus or pulmonary infection from encapsulated bacteria.

I. Humoral immune deficiency

A. **Immunoglobulin A (IgA) deficiency** is the most common immune deficiency, with 1 in 500 people having the disorder. Patients may be asymptomatic or present with recurrent sinus and pulmonary infections. Therapy is directed at early treatment with antibiotics because IgA replacement is not available. In 15% of cases an associated immunoglobulin G (IgG) subclass deficiency is present. IgA-deficient patients are at risk for developing a severe transfusion reaction because of the presence in some individuals of anti-IgA IgE antibodies and therefore should be transfused with washed RBCs.

B. **Common variable immunodeficiency (CVID).** This diagnosis includes a heterogeneous group of disorders in which patients present in the second to fourth decade of life with recurrent sinus and pulmonary infections and are discovered to have low or absent IgG, IgA, and immunoglobulin M (IgM) antibodies. They also have a decreased ability to produce immunoglobulin after immunization. Patients with CVID may have associated autoimmune abnormalities, most commonly autoimmune hemolytic anemia, immune thrombocytopenic purpura, pernicious anemia, and rheumatoid arthritis. B-cell numbers are usually normal. In addition, the incidence of malignancy, especially lymphoid malignancy, is increased. Therapy consists of supportive care as well as prompt treatment of infections with antibiotics and IV immunoglobulin (IVIG) replacement therapy (see sec. **III**).

C. **Subclass deficiency.** Deficiencies of each of the IgG subclasses (IgG_1, IgG_2, IgG_3, and IgG_4) have been described. These patients present with similar complaints as the CVID patients. Total IgG levels may be normal. A strong association with IgA deficiency exists (see sec. **I.A**).

D. **Hyper-IgE syndrome** (Job's syndrome) is characterized by recurrent pyogenic infections of the skin and lower respiratory tract. This infection can result in severe abscess and empyema formation. The most common organism is *Staphylococcus aureus*, but other bacteria and fungi have been reported. Patients present with recurrent infection and have an associated pruritic dermatitis, coarse facies, growth retardation, and hyperkeratotic nails. Laboratory data reveal the presence of normal levels of IgG, IgA, and IgM but markedly elevated levels of IgE. A marked increase in tissue and blood eosinophils is also observed. The pathogenesis of the disorder is unknown, but it appears to be transmitted in an autosomal mode of inheritance with variable penetrance. No specific therapy exists except for early treatment of infection with antibiotics.

E. **Immunodeficiency may be caused by hypercatabolism of immunoglobulin molecules.** The majority of immune defects of humoral immunity represent disorders in synthesis. However, there are states associated with infection that represent increased degradation or catabolism of immunoglobulin. Increased utilization of immunoglobulin may be seen in patients with severe underlying infection. Therefore, any formal diagnosis and evaluation of humoral immunodeficiency should be postponed until infections are adequately treated. Protein-losing gastroenteropathy and renal glomerular defects as seen in nephrotic syndrome can result in the loss of large amounts of serum proteins, giving rise to hypoalbuminemia as well as hypogammaglobulinemia.

II. **Evaluation of suspected immunodeficiency.** Increased frequency of sino-pulmonary infections is the most common problem confronted in clinical practice that requires an evaluation for possible humoral immune deficiency. Workup consists of a **CBC, immunoglobulin** levels, **complement levels,** and an **HIV test.** If levels of immunoglobulin are normal and other possible precipitating factors such as allergy and anatomic abnormalities are ruled out, further evaluation should be pursued. This includes checking IgG subclass levels as well as an evaluation of B-cell function. An evaluation of B-cell function should also be performed in patients with recurrent infection and low immunoglobulin levels to distinguish CVID from hypercatabolism. B-cell response to immunization with a protein antigen, such as tetanus, and a polysaccharide antigen, such as pneumococcus, is tested because of the differences in the way in which proteins and polysaccharides are processed and presented by T cells. Titers of specific antibody are measured before and 4 weeks after immunization, with a good response being a fourfold increase in antibody titer. Multiple serotypes of pneumococcus should be evaluated. A good response would be expected in greater then three of the serotypes. A patient with normal or low immunoglobulin and a poor response to immunization is classified as having CVID.

III. **Treatment of humoral immunodeficiency.** Specific replacement therapy does not exist for the treatment of IgA deficiency. These patients should be treated promptly at the first sign of infection with an antibiotic that covers *Streptococcus pneumoniae* or *Haemophilus influenzae*. Patients with subclass deficiency and CVID can be treated with IVIG. Numerous preparations of IVIG are available, all of which are treated with viral inactivation steps. Replacement should be initiated with 400 mg/kg and infused slowly according to the manufacturer's suggestions. Some data suggest that rapid infusions can be performed in most individuals. Patients, especially those with no detectable IgA, need to have vital signs monitored q15min initially, as **anaphylaxis from anti-IgA IgE antibodies** can develop in these individuals. In those patients with low or absent IgA, it is best to use an IVIG preparation that is documented to contain very little IgA, such as Gammagard. Infusions generally are done at monthly intervals, but it is best to document that adequate IgG levels are maintained between infusions. In some individuals infusions may be required q3wk.

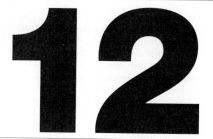

Renal Diseases

Shubhada N. Ahya
and Daniel W. Coyne

Evaluation of the Patient
with Renal Disease

The first indication of renal disease frequently is abnormal routine laboratory data, such as an elevated serum creatinine (Cr) level or a urinalysis with proteinuria, hematuria, or pyuria. Renal function should be assessed in patients with symptoms of malaise, edema, or urinary complaints. A careful history and physical examination are essential and often lead to the correct diagnosis. Initial evaluation should determine the need for emergent dialysis and then should be directed at identifying reversible causes of renal dysfunction.

I. **Initial studies** should include a urine dipstick for proteinuria, hematuria, pyuria, and pH, and microscopic examination of a freshly voided specimen. Hematuria may reflect a variety of conditions, including infection or inflammation of the prostate or bladder, malignancy (e.g., bladder or renal cell carcinoma), renal stones (see Nephrolithiasis), polycystic kidney disease, trauma with or without the presence of a bleeding diathesis, papillary necrosis, or glomerular disease (see Glomerulonephropathies). Dirty brown sediment with epithelial cells and granular casts is seen with ischemic damage of the tubules. Pyuria is seen with urinary tract infection or interstitial nephritis. WBC casts may be seen in pyelonephritis and interstitial nephritis, and RBC casts are indicative of glomerulonephritis (GN). The presence of crystals may indicate stone disease or certain alcohol poisonings (see Chap. 26). Serum chemistries should include electrolytes, Cr, BUN, calcium, magnesium, phosphate, uric acid, and protein. If the serum Cr is stable, the glomerular filtration rate (GFR) can be estimated by using the following empiric formula for CR clearance (Cl_{Cr}):

$$Cl_{Cr}(ml/minute) = [(140 - age) \times weight(kg)]/[72 \times serum \ Cr(mg/dl)]$$
$$\times 0.85(for \ women)$$

This equation provides only a rough estimate of GFR and should not be used in place of a 24-hour urine collection for Cl_{Cr}. Weight should reflect ideal body weight.

II. **Supplementary studies** can be useful to assess renal function further and may aid in identifying specific disorders.

A. **Twenty-four-hour urine studies** include measurement of urine volume, Cr, and protein. The GFR can be estimated by calculation of the Cl_{Cr}:

$$Cl_{Cr}(ml/minute) = [urine \ Cr(mg/dl) \times volume(ml)]/[serum \ Cr(mg/dl)$$
$$\times time(minutes)]$$

This value is useful in adjusting drug dosage in renal insufficiency, in predicting remaining renal function, and in timing the placement of dialysis access. In adults under the age of 50 years, if the 24-hour Cr for women is less than 15–20 mg/kg lean body weight and for men is less than 20–25 mg/kg lean body weight, the collection may be incomplete, leading to an underestimation of the GFR. In severe renal failure, the measured Cl_{Cr} may overestimate the true GFR. In this setting, the mean of the Cl_{Cr} and urea clearance is a more accurate reflection of GFR. Twenty-four–hour protein studies are necessary for confirmation of the nephrotic syndrome and are useful for following the response to treatment of certain glomerular diseases. Alternatively, the total protein (mg/dl) to Cr (mg/dl) ratio on a random urine specimen grossly estimates proteinuria (g/1.73 m^2 body surface area/day) in most patients; a ratio of greater than 3:1 suggests nephrotic range proteinuria. Measurements of 24-hour urinary volume, Cr, sodium, citrate, calcium, phosphate, oxalate, and uric acid are indicated in the evaluation of some patients with nephrolithiasis. However, this evaluation is best performed in the outpatient setting when the patient is on a usual diet.

B. **Other laboratory evaluation.** Blood tests—including the erythrocyte sedimentation rate; antinuclear, anti–glomerular basement membrane (anti-GBM), and antineutrophil cytoplasmic antibodies; complement levels; cryoglobulin studies; hepatitis B and C serologies; and antistreptococcal antibody titers—may be useful in evaluating glomerular disease. Serum and urine protein electrophoresis should be performed in selected patients with proteinuria to exclude multiple myeloma and amyloid disease. Of note, a routine dipstick urinalysis is less sensitive to proteins other than albumin. Urine eosinophils are seen in allergic interstitial nephritis, rapidly progressive GN (RPGN), acute prostatitis, and renal atheroemboli. Urine osmolality may be useful in the evaluation of hyponatremia.

C. **Renal ultrasonography** can assess kidney size, determine the presence of hydronephrosis, and identify renal cysts. Small kidneys generally reflect chronic renal disease, although kidney size may not be diminished in some common chronic processes such as diabetes, HIV, amyloidosis, and multiple myeloma. The presence of hydronephrosis suggests obstructive nephropathy that may be chronic or acute in nature. Multiple bilateral cortical cysts are highly suggestive of autosomal dominant polycystic kidney disease.

D. **IV urography** is useful in the evaluation of nonglomerular hematuria, stone disease, and voiding disorders.

E. **Radionuclide scanning** uses predominantly technetium isotopes to define renal filtration and tubular secretion. The renal scan allows an assessment of the relative contribution of each kidney to overall renal function and provides important information if unilateral nephrectomy is being considered. Renal scanning is useful when disruption of renal blood flow is suspected; the absence of perfusion of either kidney should prompt further investigation of the renal vasculature. In addition, radionuclide studies can be used to follow renal function, leaks, and rejection in transplanted kidneys.

F. **MRI and magnetic resonance angiography** can be helpful in evaluating renal masses, detecting main renal artery stenosis, and diagnosing renal vein thrombosis. Unlike **standard arteriography,** magnetic resonance angiography does not require nephrotoxic contrast agents and possesses high sensitivity and specificity for atherosclerotic disease that involves the proximal renal arteries.

G. **Renal biopsy** can determine diagnosis, guide therapy, and provide prognostic information.

    1. **Biopsy may be indicated** in adults with glomerular diseases that present with proteinuria greater than 2 g/day (or overt nephrotic syndrome), hematuria, or RBC casts. It can be helpful in diseases such as systemic lupus erythematosus (SLE), pulmonary-renal syndromes, and paraproteinemias with renal involvement. Biopsy should also be considered in patients with renal failure and kidneys of normal size when other studies are nondiagnostic.

    2. **Preparative measures for biopsy** include establishing the presence of two kidneys and sterility of the urine, controlling hypertension, and correcting abnormalities of hemostasis. Packed RBCs should be available for transfusion. The patient should not take medications that interfere with platelet function (e.g., aspirin) before or immediately

Table 12-1. Causes of acute renal failure

Prerenal (ischemic) failure

Volume contraction

Hypotension

Heart failure (severe)

Liver failure (?; see Chap. 18)

Intrinsic renal failure

Acute tubular necrosis (prolonged ischemia; nephrotoxic agents such as heavy metals, aminoglycosides, radiographic contrast media)

Arteriolar injury

    Accelerated hypertension

    Vasculitis

    Microangiopathic disorder (thrombotic thrombocytopenic purpura, hemolytic-uremic syndrome)

Glomerulonephritis

Acute interstitial nephritis (drug induced)

Intrarenal deposition or sludging (uric acid, myeloma)

Cholesterol embolization (especially after an arterial procedure)

Postobstructive failure

Ureteral obstruction (clot, calculus, tumor, sloughed papillae, external compression)

Bladder outlet obstruction (neurogenic bladder, prostatic hypertrophy, carcinoma, calculus, clot, urethral stricture)

---

after the biopsy. Patients on dialysis who require a biopsy should have their dialysis sessions scheduled so as to avoid heparin anticoagulation immediately after the biopsy.

Acute Renal Failure

Acute renal failure (ARF) presents clinically as a rapidly rising Cr level or a decline in urine output. ARF is incited by many causes (Table 12-1), but all result in a sudden decline in the ability of the kidney to maintain fluid and electrolyte homeostasis. Renal failure may be oliguric (urine output <500 ml/day) or nonoliguric. **The approach to patients with ARF is simplified by classifying it as prerenal, intrinsic, or postobstructive.** Table 12-2 includes laboratory tests that are helpful in differentiating oliguric prerenal azotemia from oliguric, intrinsic acute tubular necrosis. Serum and urine should be obtained simultaneously before a fluid challenge or diuretic use is initiated. **Examination of a fresh urine sample is essential,** as it reflects current renal function.

  I. **Prerenal azotemia** is the clinical result of renal hypoperfusion due to a decrease in effective arterial blood volume. Decreased arterial blood volume may result from volume depletion, peripheral vasodilation, or low cardiac output. Volume expansion, BP support, or treatment of heart failure may result in reversal of renal insufficiency. In prerenal states, the kidney avidly retains sodium, usually resulting in low urine sodium and a fractional excretion of sodium (FE_{Na}) of less than 1%. Other conditions in which a FE_{Na} of less than 1% may be observed are radiocontrast-induced renal failure, acute GN, liver failure (see Chap. 18),

Table 12-2. Laboratory examination in oliguric acute renal failure

Diagnosis	U/P_{Cr}	U_{Na}	FE_{Na} (%)	U osmolality
Prerenal azotemia	>40	<20	<1	>500
Oliguric ATN	<20	>40	>1	<350

ATN = acute tubular necrosis; FE_{Na} = fractional excretion of sodium; P = plasma; U = urine.

heme-induced nephrotoxicity, early obstructive nephropathy, vasculitis, and normal renal function. FE_{Na} is particularly helpful in oliguric ARF. FE_{Na} is calculated as follows:

$$FE_{Na} = [(U_{Na} \times P_{Cr})/(P_{Na} \times U_{Cr})] \times 100$$

where U = urine and P = plasma. However, prolonged hypoperfusion may lead to **acute tubular necrosis.** This intrinsic tubular damage results in sodium loss and an FE_{Na} of greater than 1%. This calculation may not be diagnostic in patients who are elderly, who have received diuretics, or who have pre-existing renal disease.

- **A. Hemodynamic monitoring** may be of value to assure adequate volume expansion while avoiding overexpansion and to assess and manage poor cardiac function. Invasive monitoring with a central venous pressure or pulmonary artery catheter is indicated if an accurate assessment of intravascular volume cannot be obtained by physical examination and an initial volume challenge.
- **B. Fluid challenge** may be appropriate in oliguric patients who are not volume overloaded. The quantity of fluid to be given must be determined on an individual basis, but typically 500–1000 ml normal saline is infused over 30–60 minutes. Frequent cardiopulmonary examination is necessary. Some cases of intrinsic renal failure also may respond with increased urine output. If no response is obtained, volume infusion can be followed by furosemide, 100–400 mg IV, to promote urine flow. Occasionally, the addition of metolazone, 5–10 mg PO, facilitates initiation of diuresis induced by volume repletion and furosemide. If successful, the lowest effective dose of furosemide can be continued in the volume-replete patient, with careful monitoring to avoid volume depletion. Diuretic administration may convert oliguric ARF to non-oliguric ARF, which simplifies management and may improve prognosis. However, large doses of IV furosemide for prolonged periods should be used with caution, as hearing loss may occur.
- **C. Dopamine** (<3 µg/kg/minute, a dosage that preferentially dilates the renal vasculature) occasionally initiates natriuresis and diuresis. However, clear evidence for a renal protective effect of dopamine is lacking and hence is not routinely recommended in ARF (*Kidney Int* 50:4, 1996).

II. **Obstructive nephropathy** in the upper or lower urinary tract may incite ARF.
- **A. Early diagnosis and relief of obstruction** are essential to prevent permanent renal damage. **Lower tract obstruction** can be assessed (and relieved) by temporary bladder catheterization, whereas renal ultrasonography usually identifies lower and **upper tract obstruction.** Urine flow often increases dramatically after relief of bilateral obstruction. This postobstructive diuresis frequently is physiologic and reflects excretion of fluid, urea, and sodium accumulated during the period of obstruction; however, inappropriate loss of volume and electrolytes may occur after relief of severe, acute bilateral obstruction. If the postobstructive diuresis appears excessive, fluid and electrolytes should be replaced. The appropriate initial replacement fluid in such cases is usually 0.45% saline.
- **B. Micro-obstructive uropathy** with associated pyuria and eosinophiluria **may be caused by indinavir, a protease inhibitor used in the treatment of HIV disease.** Discontinuation of the drug can restore renal function.

III. Intrinsic renal failure results from a variety of injuries to the renal blood vessels, glomeruli, tubules, or interstitium (see Table 12-1). These insults may be toxic, immunologic, or idiopathic. They may be iatrogenic or develop as part of a systemic disorder or as a primary renal disease.

A. Radiocontrast nephropathy occurs with increased frequency in patients with long-standing diabetes mellitus or pre-existing renal insufficiency. Volume depletion, multiple myeloma, heart failure, and age greater than 65 years may also be risk factors. The ARF of contrast nephropathy tends to be oliguric, and the serum Cr peaks in the first 72 hours. Patients often recover renal function over 7–14 days. To reduce the incidence of ARF, patients at risk should be hydrated beginning 12–24 hours before the contrast study and ending 12 hours after the study. Infusion rates need to be individualized but should be approximately 75–150 ml/hour of 0.45% saline, the goal being a slightly volume-expanded patient with a high urine output. Furosemide should be reserved for patients in whom volume overload develops during hydration. Acetylcysteine (600 mg PO bid; four doses total, starting 1 day before procedure) may reduce the incidence and severity of contrast nephropathy (*N Engl J Med* 343:180, 2000).

B. Aminoglycoside nephrotoxicity may cause ARF that is often nonoliguric and results from direct toxicity to the proximal tubules. Predisposing factors include prolonged exposure to these drugs, advanced age, volume depletion, liver disease, and pre-existing renal disease. Patients in whom ARF develops from aminoglycoside therapy usually have received the medication for at least 5 days. The risk of aminoglycoside nephrotoxicity appears to be lower when the extended-interval dosing method is used (see Chap. 13).

C. Pigment-induced renal injury occurs during hemolysis or rhabdomyolysis. In **rhabdomyolysis,** it may be beneficial to expand volume aggressively to replace the fluid that is lost into necrotic muscle and to establish high urine flow. If sufficient urine flow can be established, attempts to raise the urine pH to greater than 6.5 to increase the solubility of heme pigments can be accomplished with an IV infusion of 2–3 ampules of $NaHCO_3$ in 1 L 5% dextrose in water.

D. Acute uric acid nephropathy (tumor lysis syndrome) may occur from cell lysis, with consequent hyperuricemia during cytotoxic therapy for hematologic malignancies. Uric acid production can be decreased by administration of allopurinol, 600 mg PO, before cytotoxic therapy, followed by 100–300 mg/day. The dosage should be adjusted for renal function (see Appendix E). Forced alkaline diuresis to maintain a urine pH of 6.5–7.0 also helps to prevent uric acid precipitation; this can be accomplished with acetazolamide, 250 mg PO qid, or with IV infusion of 2–3 ampules of $NaHCO_3$ in 1 L 5% dextrose in water. If tumor lysis results in hyperphosphatemia, urine alkalinization greater than pH 7.0 increases the risk of calcium phosphate precipitation and thus should be avoided.

E. Acute interstitial nephritis secondary to drugs may present with the classic signs of fever, rash, and renal dysfunction. When present, eosinophilia and eosinophiluria suggest the diagnosis. A high index of suspicion for interstitial nephritis must be maintained in patients who are taking drugs such as the penicillins, sulfonamides, quinolones, and nonsteroidal anti-inflammatory drugs. In most cases, renal insufficiency resolves with discontinuation of the offending agent. A 1-week course of prednisone, 60 mg PO qd, may hasten recovery. Streptococcal infections, leptospirosis, viral infections, and sarcoidosis have also been implicated as causes of interstitial nephritis.

F. Hemolytic-uremic syndrome/thrombotic thrombocytopenic purpura may be induced by bacterial toxin, medications such as mitomycin C, cyclosporine, tacrolimus (see Chap. 16), OKT3, or radiation therapy, or may be associated with pregnancy or certain malignancies of the GI tract. Diagnosis and therapy are discussed in Chap. 19.

G. Bone marrow transplant (BMT)–associated nephropathy refers to renal failure that develops at least 3 months after autologous or allogeneic bone marrow transplantation. **Acute BMT nephropathy** presents with marked hypertension, peripheral edema, microangiopathic hemolytic anemia, thrombocytopenia, and elevated lactic acid dehydrogenase. Renal function typically declines rapidly and is often associated with severe proteinuria. **Chronic BMT nephropathy** is characterized by less severe manifestations of the acute form, with initial steady reduction in renal function within the first 12–24 months followed by stabilization. Radiation is frequently implicated in the pathogenesis of the disease. Treatment is generally supportive and includes good BP control.

H. **Cholesterol emboli** are seen in patients with diffuse atherosclerotic disease who undergo aortic or other large arterial manipulation or who are receiving warfarin or thrombolytic therapy. Physical findings may include retinal arteriolar plaques, lower extremity livedo reticularis, or necrotic areas of the distal digits. Laboratory findings that may aid in the diagnosis include eosinophilia, eosinophiluria, and hypocomplementemia. No specific therapy is available; anticoagulation can worsen embolic disease.

I. **Scleroderma kidney** is characterized by acute onset of renal failure with moderate to severe hypertension that, if left untreated, progresses to end-stage renal disease within 1–2 months. Clinical features are discussed in Chap. 24. The mainstay of therapy is aggressive antihypertensive therapy with angiotensin-converting enzyme (ACE) inhibitors.

J. **Acute GN** can result in ARF. **RPGN** presents with an acute deterioration in renal function, proteinuria (sometimes in the nephrotic range), and an active urinary sediment with hematuria and RBC casts. Oliguria may be present. Many patients with idiopathic RPGN note a preceding viral-like illness. RPGN can be further characterized by the presence of immune deposits [e.g., SLE, poststreptococcal GN, immunoglobulin A (IgA) nephropathy, endocarditis], the paucity of immune deposits (e.g., Wegener's granulomatosis, microscopic polyangiitis, Churg-Strauss syndrome, idiopathic), or the presence of anti-GBM disease (see Glomerulonephropathies). Pathology is notable for crescent formation in more than 50% of glomeruli. As many as 75% of patients with idiopathic RPGN may respond to high-dose, pulse glucocorticoid therapy—methylprednisolone, 7–15 mg/kg/day in divided doses for 3 days, followed by prednisone, 1 mg/kg/day for 1 month, gradually tapered over the next 6–12 months. In patients with extrarenal disease that is suggestive of vasculitis or a renal biopsy that demonstrates necrotizing GN, the addition of cyclophosphamide, 2 mg/kg/day PO, may be beneficial.

IV. **Management of ARF** requires the repeated assessment of clinical and laboratory data and appropriate interventions to maintain fluid and electrolyte homeostasis.

A. **Conservative medical management** of ARF requires complete fluid intake and output records, daily weights, and frequent (at least three times a week) measurements of serum electrolytes, BUN, Cr, calcium, and phosphate. Intravascular volume should be clinically assessed at least daily.

1. **Fluid management** is essential to avoid volume depletion, which may contribute to ARF by decreasing renal perfusion. When clinical assessment is unclear, invasive hemodynamic monitoring may be required (see sec. **I.A**). Once any volume deficit has been corrected, fluid and sodium balance must be carefully regulated to avoid volume overload. Fluid replacement (usually 0.45% saline if IV) should be equal to insensible loss (approximately 500 ml/day in afebrile patients) plus urinary and other drainage losses. Increased urine output and diuretic responsiveness in nonoliguric ARF allow more liberal administration of fluids (and nutrients). Because patients with nonoliguric ARF may lose significant amounts of fluid and electrolytes in the urine, careful attention to volume status and serum electrolyte levels is necessary to avoid electrolyte and water depletion. Hyponatremia in patients with ARF usually is secondary to volume expansion with hypotonic fluid, whereas hyper-

natremia is caused most often by overly aggressive diuresis in combination with inadequate intake of free water.

2. **Dietary modification. Total caloric intake** should be 35–50 kcal/kg/day to avoid catabolism. Patients who are highly catabolic (e.g., postsurgical and burn patients) or malnourished require higher protein intake and should be considered for early institution of dialysis (see sec. **IV.B**). **Salt intake** should be restricted to 2–4 g/day to facilitate volume management. **Potassium intake** should be restricted to 40 mEq/day, and **phosphorus intake** should be restricted to 800 mg/day. Ingestion of magnesium-containing compounds should be avoided.

3. **Hyperkalemia** is common and, if mild (<6 mEq/L), can be treated with dietary restriction (see sec. **IV.A.2**) and potassium-binding resins (e.g., sodium polystyrene sulfonate). Marked hyperkalemia or hyperkalemia accompanied by ECG abnormalities requires immediate medical therapy (e.g., calcium chloride, insulin, glucose, and bicarbonate; see Chap. 3). **Hyperkalemia that is refractory to medical therapy is an indication for dialysis.**

4. **Phosphorus and calcium levels** are frequently abnormal due to reduced renal excretion and excess release of cellular phosphate, despite dietary restriction. Serum calcium often is low but rarely requires specific treatment. The calcium-phosphate product should be kept at less than 60 to avoid metastatic calcification (see Chronic Renal Failure for therapy).

5. **Metabolic acidosis** that is mild (serum bicarbonate level ≥16 mEq/L) does not require therapy. More marked acidosis should be corrected with sodium bicarbonate, 650–1300 mg PO tid. Severe uncompensated acidosis (serum pH <7.2) requires prompt medical therapy with parenteral sodium bicarbonate (see Chap. 3) and a search for the underlying etiology. Sodium bicarbonate therapy should be used with care, as it may exacerbate volume overload and cause tetany by decreasing the ionized calcium concentration. **Acidosis that is unresponsive to medical therapy is an indication for dialysis** (see sec. **IV.B**).

6. **Hypotension** should be promptly evaluated and corrected with volume expansion or vasopressors, depending on the patient's intravascular volume status. **Hypertension** should be managed aggressively. Volume overload frequently contributes to hypertension and should be avoided. Antihypertensive medications that do not decrease renal blood flow (e.g., clonidine, prazosin, or calcium channel antagonists) are preferred. Hypertensive crisis can be managed with IV labetalol or IV sodium nitroprusside with monitoring of thiocyanate levels in patients with renal insufficiency (see Chap. 4).

7. **Drug dosages** of agents excreted by the kidney must be adjusted for the level of renal function (see Appendix E).

8. **Anemia** is common in ARF and usually is caused by decreased RBC production and increased blood loss. GI bleeding is common in ARF, probably due to uremic platelet dysfunction and GI mucosal changes. Major bleeding sources should be excluded. Desmopressin acetate (DDAVP) is appropriate for patients with active bleeding, whereas transfusion is appropriate for patients with active bleeding or symptoms referable to anemia (see Chap. 20). Erythropoietin is expensive and not effective as short-term therapy for anemia.

9. **Infection** is the most common cause of death in patients with ARF. Antimicrobial therapy is dictated by the infectious process, and potentially nephrotoxic agents should not be withheld if their use is otherwise indicated. Most antimicrobial dosages need to be adjusted for the degree of renal failure (see Appendix E).

B. **Indications for dialysis.** A patient with ARF should be evaluated daily to assess the need for dialysis. Technical aspects of dialysis are considered under Renal Replacement Therapies.

1. **Severe hyperkalemia, acidosis, or volume overload that is refractory to conservative therapy** mandates the initiation of dialysis.
2. **Additional indications** for initiation of dialysis include uremic pericarditis, encephalopathy, neuropathy, and nutritional requirements (e.g., hyperalimentation) that would precipitate volume overload or uremia, and certain alcohol and drug intoxications (see Chap. 26).
3. **Uremic signs and symptoms** become prominent as BUN rises. Neurologic manifestations, such as lethargy, seizures, myoclonus, asterixis, and peripheral polyneuropathies, may develop with uremia and are an indication for dialysis. **Uremic pericarditis** often is manifested only as a pericardial friction rub and should be treated with dialysis; heparin use during dialysis should be minimized in these patients. If pericarditis fails to resolve with dialysis, or if signs of pericardial tamponade develop, pericardial drainage is indicated.

V. **Management of the recovery phase of ARF** usually requires careful monitoring of serum electrolytes, volume status, and urinary fluid and electrolyte losses. As with obstructive nephropathy, a diuretic phase may occur during recovery. Management is similar to that for postobstructive diuresis (see sec. **II**). Renal function may continue to improve over weeks to months.

Glomerulonephropathies

Glomerular disease may be primary or secondary to a systemic process. The clinical presentation is broad and includes **isolated hematuria or proteinuria, nephritic syndrome, or nephrotic syndrome. The nephritic syndrome** is characterized by hematuria, RBC casts, proteinuria, hypertension, edema, and deteriorating renal function. **The nephrotic syndrome** is characterized by proteinuria (>3.5 g/day), hypoalbuminemia, hyperlipidemia, and edema. These syndromes may appear as a manifestation of primary glomerular disease or may be associated with systemic diseases such as diabetes mellitus, amyloidosis, multiple myeloma, SLE, or many other disorders. Renal biopsy often provides useful diagnostic, therapeutic, and prognostic information. Treatment of glomerulopathies is disease dependent but frequently involves glucocorticoids and, in many cases, cytotoxic drugs. Treatment of glomerulonephropathies with such agents should be done only in consultation with a nephrologist or other experienced physician. Initial dosages of cytotoxic drugs are suggested but may require adjustment to keep the WBC count above 3000–3500 µl. WBC counts should be checked at least weekly initially while cytotoxic agents are administered.

I. **Primary glomerulonephropathies**
   A. **Minimal-change disease (MCD)** presents with nephrotic syndrome. Certain neoplastic disorders such as Hodgkin's disease and non-Hodgkin's lymphoma have been associated with the development of MCD and should be considered in the appropriate setting. Progression to chronic renal failure (CRF) is rare.
      1. **The pathologic diagnosis** is made by normal light microscopy, negative immunofluorescence, and foot process fusion on electron microscopy.
      2. **Therapy.** Approximately 80% of adults with MCD respond to prednisone, 1 mg/kg/day PO, with a decrease in proteinuria to less than 3 g/day or a remission of the nephrotic syndrome. In patients who respond, steroids should be tapered over 3 months and then discontinued. Failure to respond may reflect an error in diagnosis; MCD most commonly is confused with early, focal, segmental glomerulosclerosis. Urinary protein should be carefully monitored during steroid taper. If relapse is documented, reinstitution of prednisone often is effective. Treatment with cytotoxic agents may be indicated in patients who are deemed steroid

dependent, steroid resistant, or frequent relapsers. Cyclophosphamide, 2 mg/kg/day PO for 8 weeks; chlorambucil, 0.2 mg/kg/day PO for 8–12 weeks; or cyclosporine, 5 mg/kg/day for 6–12 months is a typical regimen (*Kidney Int* S70:1, 1999).

B. Focal segmental glomerulosclerosis is an idiopathic glomerular disorder that is usually characterized by hypertension, hematuria, renal insufficiency, and nephrotic syndrome. The disease slowly progresses to CRF within 5–10 years of diagnosis.

  1. Pathology reveals focal and segmental sclerosis of glomeruli.

  2. Therapy has generally not proved to be effective in the treatment of this disorder, but a trial of prednisone, 60 mg PO qd for at least 2–3 months, may be appropriate in an effort to reduce proteinuria and slow progression to CRF. Some authors recommend a combination of glucocorticoids and agents such as cyclosporine, 5 mg/kg/day, or cyclophosphamide to induce remission (*Kidney Int* S70:26, 1999).

C. Membranous nephropathy usually presents with the nephrotic syndrome, although some patients have isolated proteinuria. Membranous nephropathy may be a primary renal disease or associated with a systemic disease (e.g., malignancy, SLE, or infections such as hepatitis B, syphilis, hepatitis C, or schistosomiasis) or drug ingestions (e.g., penicillamine, gold). The GFR generally is normal or near normal, and the urinary sediment often is unremarkable. Approximately one-third of patients with membranous nephropathy progress to end-stage renal disease; the remainder enter remission or have stable or very slowly declining renal function. Because of the generally good outcome, treatment usually is reserved for patients with poor prognostic factors (age, male gender, hypertension, reduced GFR, proteinuria >10 g/day, or marked interstitial fibrosis on renal biopsy).

  1. Pathologic examination demonstrates thickening of the glomerular capillary wall secondary to subepithelial deposits of immunoglobulin G and C3.

  2. Treatment options include high-dose alternate-day glucocorticoids in conjunction with a cytotoxic agent (e.g., chlorambucil, 0.2 mg/kg/day, or cyclophosphamide, 1.5–2.5 mg/kg/day) for 6–12 months and, in nonresponders, cyclosporine, 3.5 mg/kg/day for 12 months.

D. IgA nephropathy is most often an idiopathic disorder that is typically characterized by asymptomatic microscopic hematuria with mild proteinuria or recurrent episodes of gross hematuria that may shortly follow (within 1–3 days) an upper respiratory infection. Renal biopsy may be indicated if evidence of renal insufficiency (e.g., proteinuria >1 g/day) is found. IgA nephropathy may be associated with hepatic cirrhosis, gluten enteropathy, dermatitis herpetiformis, or Henoch-Schönlein purpura. Patients with **Henoch-Schönlein purpura** may present with the tetrad of palpable purpura (usually in the lower trunk or extremities), abdominal pain, joint inflammation, and renal failure due to IgA nephropathy.

  1. Pathology is notable for increased mesangial cellularity and matrix; immunofluorescence and electron microscopy reveal mesangial deposition of IgA and C3.

  2. Therapy with glucocorticoids may be helpful in patients who do not have stable disease. The use of omega-3 fatty acids found in fish oil may be beneficial in preventing the deterioration of renal function.

II. Secondary glomerulonephropathies

  A. Diabetic nephropathy is the most common cause of end-stage renal disease in the United States (see Chap. 22).

  B. SLE may involve the kidney and can present as slowly progressive azotemia with urinary abnormalities, as nephrotic syndrome, or as rapidly progressive renal insufficiency. Renal biopsy is useful in SLE for evaluating disease activity and assessing irreversible changes such as glomerular sclerosis, tubular atrophy, and interstitial fibrosis.

1. A wide variety of **pathologic changes** may be seen on renal biopsy, including mesangial, membranous, focal or diffuse proliferative, and crescentic GN. A predominance of irreversible changes with little acute inflammation portends a poor response to therapy and should modify the aggressiveness of immunosuppressive treatment.

2. **Treatment** for patients with severe renal disease is methylprednisolone, 500 mg IV q12h for 3 days, followed by oral prednisone, 0.5–1.0 mg/kg PO qd. Prednisone should then be tapered over 6–8 weeks to the lowest dosage that controls disease activity, preferably using an alternate-day regimen. The addition of cyclophosphamide, 0.5–1.0 g/m^2 IV monthly for 6 months, then quarterly, improves the likelihood of remission and appears to reduce the likelihood of progressive renal failure.

C. **MPGN** exhibits a variety of clinical presentations, including acute GN, nephrotic syndrome, and asymptomatic hematuria and proteinuria. The diagnosis should be suspected if these clinical findings are associated with low complement levels. Hepatitis C accounts for most cases of MPGN (see sec. **II.E**) and is often associated with **cryoglobulinemia** (see Chap. 24). MPGN progresses slowly to renal failure.

1. **Pathology** includes mesangial proliferation and alterations of the GBM with subendothelial (type I) or intramembranous (type II) deposits.

2. **Therapy** for idiopathic MPGN has not been shown to improve disease-free survival.

D. **Dysproteinemias** include amyloidosis, light chain and heavy chain deposition diseases, and fibrillary/immunotactoid glomerulopathies, and may be associated with multiple myeloma, Waldenström's macroglobulinemia, and certain B-cell malignancies. The diagnosis is often suggested by an abnormal serum protein electrophoresis (SPEP) or urine protein electrophoresis (UPEP). **Amyloidosis** is characterized by the extracellular deposition of fibrils comprised of the variable region of monoclonal immunoglobulin light chains (typically lambda) in a beta-pleated configuration. **Light chain deposition disease** is characterized by the extracellular deposition of the constant region of monoclonal immunoglobulin (kappa >80% of the time) light chains, whereas heavy and light chains are seen in **heavy chain deposition disease.** Patients with amyloidosis and light chain and heavy chain diseases often have cardiac, hepatic, and neuropathic in addition to renal involvement.

1. **Pathologic diagnosis of amyloidosis** can be made by Congo red–positive staining of the beta-pleated fibrils. In **light chain deposition disease,** a granular pattern of deposition that is negative for Congo red staining is seen. Immunofluorescence staining for lambda and kappa light chains and heavy chains aids in making the appropriate diagnosis. Electron microscopy is also helpful in diagnosis; fibrils are typically 10 nm in diameter in amyloidosis, 20–30 nm in fibrillary glomerulopathy, and 30–50 nm in immunotactoid glomerulopathy.

2. **Therapy** with melphalan and prednisone has proved to be beneficial for amyloidosis and light chain deposition disease. For dysproteinemias associated with multiple myeloma, high-dose chemotherapy with or without BMT may be effective aggressive therapy in some patients. Colchicine has also been used in the treatment of AA amyloidosis associated with familial Mediterranean fever. No effective therapy is known for fibrillary/immunotactoid glomerulopathies.

E. **Infection-related GN** may occur in association with a variety of infectious processes, including **bacterial endocarditis, visceral abscesses, and infected shunts.** Treatment of the infection usually leads to the resolution of the active GN. **Poststreptococcal GN** may follow group A beta-hemolytic streptococcal infection of the upper respiratory tract or skin and is usually self-limited. **Hepatitis C** may cause MPGN, usually in association with **cryoglobulinemia.**

Treatment with interferon-alpha can be attempted (see Chap. 18), but its effectiveness in resolving the renal manifestations of hepatitis C is unclear.

F. Pulmonary-renal syndromes

1. The most common cause of pulmonary-renal syndrome is **pneumonia with acute tubular necrosis.**

2. **Anti-GBM antibody disease** may present with pulmonary and renal involvement **(Goodpasture's syndrome)** or with renal disease alone. Anti-GBM disease often is rapidly progressive.

   a. **Diagnosis** is based either on the presence of anti-GBM antibodies in the serum or on linear deposition of antibody along the basement membrane on renal biopsy. Of these patients, 10–30% may have a positive antineutrophil autoplasmic antibody (ANCA).

   b. **Standard therapy** is to clear anti-GBM antibodies from the serum while also suppressing formation of new antibodies. Daily total volume plasmapheresis for approximately 2 weeks, in combination with cyclophosphamide, 2 mg/kg PO qd for 8 weeks, and methylprednisolone, 7–15 mg/kg/day for 3 days followed by prednisone, 60 mg PO qd tapered over 8 weeks, is usually effective. Frequent clinical evaluation and measurement of anti-GBM antibody titers monitor progress. Immunosuppression should be continued until the anti-GBM antibody is undetectable. Relapse is common and tends to occur within the first several months. Therapy may not be effective if the patient is already oliguric, is receiving dialysis, or has a Cr level of greater than 6.5 mg/dl.

3. **Wegener's granulomatosis** (see Chap. 24)

   a. **Diagnosis** is made by tissue biopsy showing granulomatous inflammation. Immunofluorescence on kidney biopsy shows a paucity of immune deposits. Patients have a positive cytoplasmic ANCA in 90% of cases.

   b. **Therapy** includes a combination of cyclophosphamide, 2 mg/kg/day PO continued for at least 1 year beyond the induction of remission and subsequently tapered, plus prednisone, 1 mg/kg PO qd for 4 weeks followed by slow taper and conversion to alternate-day therapy over the next 6–9 months. Trimethoprim-sulfamethoxazole, 160 mg/800 mg (double strength) bid, has been shown to reduce relapses in patients with Wegener's granulomatosis (*N Engl J Med* 335:16, 1996).

4. **Microscopic polyarteritis nodosa** (microscopic polyangiitis)

   a. **Diagnosis** can be confirmed on biopsy of an affected kidney by the presence of focal necrotizing GN with crescent formation similar to what is observed in Wegener's granulomatosis. Perinuclear ANCA serology is often positive. **Churg-Strauss syndrome** can be distinguished from microscopic polyangiitis and Wegener's granulomatosis by the presence of asthma and eosinophilia.

   b. **Therapy** involves the combination of prednisone and cyclophosphamide similar to that used in the treatment of Wegener's granulomatosis.

G. Sickle cell nephropathy may present with microscopic or gross hematuria (which in some cases may be due to papillary necrosis), proteinuria, tubular dysfunction, and sclerosing glomerulopathy. Treatment may include maintenance of high urine output, alkalinization of urine, and correction of fluid and electrolyte derangements as needed. ACE inhibitor therapy is beneficial in reducing proteinuria and possibly progression of sclerotic glomerular lesions.

H. HIV-associated nephropathy is characterized by proteinuria, edema, and hematuria with or without azotemia. The histologic appearance on biopsy is similar to that of focal segmental glomerulosclerosis. Antiretroviral therapy may stabilize renal function and reduce proteinuria. Prednisone, 60 mg/day for 3 months, may also improve renal function, whereas ACE inhibitors may be beneficial in reducing proteinuria. HIV infection has also been associated with other renal diseases, including membranous, membranoproliferative,

proliferative, and crescentic GN; thrombotic thrombocytopenic purpura/ hemolytic-uremic syndrome; and tubulointerstitial nephritis.

Chronic Renal Failure

CRF may result from many different etiologies and is often asymptomatic until severe renal insufficiency develops. The decline in GFR may be followed by plotting the reciprocal of serum Cr versus time. The resulting plot usually is linear, unless there is a superimposed renal insult, and is useful in end-stage planning and in predicting the time when dialysis is needed (typically when GFR is <10 ml/minute in individuals without diabetes and <15 ml/minute in patients with diabetes). Avoidance of factors that are known to cause an acute decline in renal function and early referral to a nephrologist for implementation of conservative medical treatment of CRF may preserve renal function and postpone the need for dialysis.

I. **Acute deterioration in CRF** (i.e., a sudden decline in GFR that is more rapid than expected) should prompt a search for a superimposed, reversible process.

   A. **Decreased renal perfusion** may be due to volume depletion or compromise of cardiac output, or both. Ideally, CRF patients should be volume expanded, as suggested by the presence of a small amount of pedal edema, and cardiac output should be optimized. Afterload reduction may be particularly useful in these patients, but caution should be taken to avoid decreased renal perfusion pressure. Hypotension induced by antihypertensive agents can exacerbate CRF, as can poorly controlled hypertension. Thus, all significant fluctuations in BP control should be investigated, especially if they are associated with a reduction in renal function.

   B. **Drugs** may cause direct toxicity to renal structures (e.g., aminoglycosides), decreased renal perfusion (e.g., nonsteroidal anti-inflammatory drugs), or allergic interstitial nephritis (e.g., allopurinol). Careful attention to drug dosing in patients with decreased GFR and avoidance of unnecessary use of nephrotoxic agents are appropriate.

   C. **Urinary tract obstruction and infections** should be considered in any patient with an unexplained sudden decline in renal function.

   D. **Progression of renal artery stenosis** may worsen pre-existing renal failure.

   E. **Cholesterol embolization** may worsen CRF and is seen most often in patients after procedures requiring arterial catheterization.

   F. **Renal vein thrombosis** may occur in nephrotic patients and exacerbate CRF and proteinuria.

II. **Conservative management** of CRF includes measures to correct and prevent metabolic derangements of renal failure and preserve remaining renal function.

   A. **Dietary modification**

      1. **Protein restriction** reduces accumulation of nitrogenous waste products. In addition, a low-protein diet may slow the progression of renal failure. Intake should be reduced to 0.6–0.8 g/kg/day of high-biological-value protein when the GFR falls below 30 ml/minute. Adequate caloric intake (35–50 kcal/kg/day) must be provided to avoid endogenous protein catabolism; thus, patients should be followed carefully for evidence of malnutrition. In nephrotic patients, an amount of protein equal to that lost in the urine should be added to their daily allowance calculated previously. Addition of an ACE inhibitor can reduce proteinuria and hence protein losses. Angiotensin II receptor blockers may have similar efficacy in patients who are unable to tolerate ACE inhibitor therapy.

      2. **Potassium** should be restricted to 40 mEq/day when GFR falls below 20 ml/minute.

      3. **Phosphorus and calcium** levels are altered in CRF due to (1) phosphorus retention, resulting in a rise in serum phosphorus levels and a reciprocal fall in calcium levels, with resultant stimulation of parathyroid

hormone (PTH) secretion; (2) decreased generation of 1,25-dihydroxyvitamin D_3, further contributing to low serum calcium levels and decreasing suppression of PTH release; and (3) skeletal resistance to the action of PTH. Consequently, PTH secretion is increased (i.e., **secondary hyperparathyroidism**) and contributes to **renal osteodystrophy** (see sec. **III**). Hyperphosphatemia may also play a role in the progression of renal failure. The goal is to maintain predialysis serum phosphorus levels between 4.0 and 5.0 mg/dl. Dietary phosphorus should be restricted to 800–1000 mg/day when GFR is less than 50 ml/minute. As GFR falls further, phosphate restriction becomes less effective, and the addition of phosphate binders that prevent GI phosphate absorption is indicated. Calcium carbonate, 500 mg–2 g PO with meals, is effective in most patients. Serum calcium should be checked regularly. If the serum phosphate level cannot be reduced to 4–5 mg/dl with $CaCO_3$, or the initial phosphate level is greater than 7 mg/dl, aluminum hydroxide antacids (e.g., Amphojel or Basaljel), 15–30 ml or one to three capsules PO with meals, should be used. Chronic use of aluminum-containing antacids can lead to aluminum accumulation in CRF patients and can cause osteomalacia (see sec. **III**). Sevelamer, a phosphate binder that lacks aluminum and calcium, can be used alternatively. Lack of dietary phosphate restriction is the most common reason that phosphate binders fail to control hyperphosphatemia. $CaCO_3$ should be stopped if the calcium phosphate product is consistently greater than 60, to avoid the possibility of metastatic calcification. If hypocalcemia (corrected for serum albumin) persists after phosphate has been controlled, nighttime $CaCO_3$ and 1,25-dihydroxyvitamin D_3 may be indicated (see Chap. 3).

4. **Sodium and fluid restriction** must be determined on an individual basis, taking the patient's cardiovascular status into consideration. For most patients, a no-added-salt diet (NaCl, 8 g/day) is palatable and adequate. If necessary, 24-hour urinary sodium loss can be determined to aid in sodium intake planning. Once a patient has reached an acceptable volume status, fluid intake should equal daily urine output plus an additional 500 ml for insensible losses. Fluid restriction is appropriate only in patients with dilutional hyponatremia. The presence of heart failure or refractory hypertension requires greater restriction of salt and water. In **nephrotic patients with edema,** salt restriction (2–3 g/day) and judicious use of diuretics should be implemented. Despite massive edema, these patients are subject to intravascular volume depletion, and excessive diuretic therapy may lead to severe volume contraction with decreased renal perfusion. Nevertheless, furosemide alone or in combination with a thiazide or metolazone should be used to control edema causing respiratory compromise, skin breakdown, or difficulty in ambulation. Hypokalemia is common and should be treated. Occasionally, parenteral furosemide is necessary, sometimes preceded by an infusion of albumin to mobilize fluid into the vascular space.

5. **Magnesium** is excreted by the kidney and accumulates in CRF. Extradietary intake of magnesium (e.g., some antacids and cathartics) should be avoided.

B. **Hypertension** accelerates the rate of decline of renal function in patients with CRF and should be treated aggressively (see Chap. 4). Target BP in most forms of CRF should be 125/75 or less. ACE inhibitors should be used whenever possible, as they appear to have renoprotective properties beyond their antihypertensive effect. Angiotensin II receptor blockers may have similar efficacy with fewer side effects. Diuretic use must be carefully monitored to avoid volume depletion. Loop diuretics (e.g., furosemide) remain effective when the GFR is less than 25 ml/minute.

C. **Acidosis** is treated with oral sodium bicarbonate, 325–650 mg PO tid, when serum bicarbonate falls below 18–20 mEq/L. The additional sodium load from such therapy may require further dietary sodium restriction or administration of a diuretic. Although citrate is converted by the liver to bicarbonate, it should not be used in CRF because it dramatically enhances GI absorption of aluminum and can lead to acute aluminum neurotoxicity.

D. Anemia is responsible for many symptoms of CRF and can be corrected with use of recombinant human erythropoietin in dialysis and in predialysis patients after ensuring iron stores are adequate. Treatment should be initiated in most patients with a hematocrit of less than 30%. The initial dose is 50–100 units/kg SC two to three times a week, with a target hematocrit of 31–36% (see Chap. 20). In patients who are receiving erythropoietin, hematocrit should be checked at least monthly.

E. Additional management of nephrotic syndrome. The nephrotic syndrome increases the risk of cardiac (e.g., atherosclerosis) and noncardiac (e.g., infection) comorbidities.

    1. Hyperlipidemia in patients with long-standing nephrotic syndrome may increase the risk for atherosclerotic disease, and, therefore, dietary restriction of cholesterol and saturated fat is prudent. 3-Hydroxy-3-methylglutaryl (HMG) coenzyme A reductase inhibitors (see Chap. 5) are effective in improving the lipoprotein profile in these patients.

    2. Thromboembolic complications. The nephrotic syndrome produces a hypercoagulable state, and the clinician should maintain a high index of suspicion for thromboemboli. Thrombi in adults usually are venous and may involve the renal veins in addition to lower and upper extremities. If embolization occurs, anticoagulation with heparin, followed by long-term warfarin therapy, is indicated (see Chap. 19).

F. Permanent vascular access should be considered by identifying the non-dominant forearm. The patient should be instructed to avoid any needle-sticks and blood draws to that arm for future AV fistula or graft placement.

III. Renal osteodystrophy refers to skeletal disorders seen in CRF and end-stage renal disease. It includes **high bone turnover diseases** such as osteitis fibrosa and mixed bone turnover disease and **low bone turnover diseases** such as osteomalacia and adynamic bone disease. Therapy should be initiated early in the course of progressive renal failure. Goals include (1) maintenance of normal serum calcium and phosphorus levels, (2) prevention of the development of PTH hyperplasia and consequent suppression of secondary hyperparathyroidism, (3) prevention of extraskeletal calcification, and (4) maintenance of normal bone histology.

A. Osteitis fibrosa is caused by **secondary hyperparathyroidism** (see sec. **II.A.3**). Clinical manifestations include bone pain, fractures, skeletal deformity, proximal muscle weakness, pruritus, and extraskeletal calcification. Serum PTH, measured by immunoassay for intact hormone, is markedly elevated. Radiographic studies typically show subperiosteal resorption and patchy osteosclerosis. A bone biopsy may be indicated to confirm the presence of osteitis fibrosa and exclude aluminum-related bone disease. Specific therapy includes the following.

    1. Correction of hyperphosphatemia (see sec. **II.A.3**)

    2. Normalization of serum calcium levels and suppression of PTH to 1–2 times the upper limit of normal in CRF patients and 1.5–4.0 times the upper limit of normal in dialysis-dependent patients.

        a. These can be achieved with the use of vitamin D preparations such as **calcitriol** (0.25–1.0 μg PO qd) or **1-hydroxy vitamin D$_{12}$.** Hypercalcemia is a major side effect of both preparations and should be avoided. Serum calcium levels should be measured at least monthly, and the dose should be adjusted accordingly at 1- to 2-month intervals. In HD patients, IV administration of **19-nor-1,25-dihydroxy vitamin D$_2$** (paricalcitol), a synthetic vitamin D analog that reduces the incidence of hypercalcemia and hyperphosphatemia, three times a week may suppress hyperparathyroidism more effectively than calcitriol.

    b. Parathyroidectomy may be required to control severe hyperparathyroidism. Indications include (1) **calciphylaxis** (ischemic necrosis of skin or soft tissue associated with vascular calcification), (2) persistent severe hypercalcemia (after other causes of hypercalcemia are excluded), (3) progressive extraskeletal calcification, and (4) severe hyperparathyroidism (PTH >1000) in spite of medical therapy.

B. Mixed bone turnover disease also occurs in the setting of hyperparathyroidism. It may be seen in patients with previously established osteitis fibrosa and with osteomalacia related to aluminum exposure.

C. Low bone turnover disease includes **osteomalacia** and **adynamic bone lesions** and occurs in the setting of relatively low PTH levels. Aluminum intoxication as a cause of low bone turnover disease is now rare; the risk of this disease has fallen because of the decreased use of aluminum-containing dialysate and phosphate binders. Serum aluminum levels do not reflect tissue aluminum content, and, hence, definitive diagnosis requires bone biopsy. Pseudofractures and spontaneous fractures are seen. In symptomatic patients with biopsy-proven aluminum-related bone disease, all sources of aluminum exposure should be eliminated. When necessary, **deferoxamine mesylate** should be given at the lowest possible dose (e.g., 0.5 g/week IM or IV), followed 8–12 hours later with HD using a high-flux dialyzer. Side effects of deferoxamine include nausea, vomiting, hypotension, cataracts and other visual abnormalities, and predisposition to bacteremia and mucormycosis.

Renal Replacement Therapies

Renal replacement therapy in CRF is indicated when metabolic abnormalities can no longer be controlled with conservative management or when signs and symptoms of uremia develop. A variety of therapeutic options are available to the patient with end-stage renal disease.

I. Hemodialysis (HD) works by diffusion of small-molecular-weight solutes across a semipermeable membrane. Fluid removal occurs via ultrafiltration. Dialysis usually is performed three times a week. Because urea distributes through total body water, larger patients require longer treatment times; hence, the duration of each treatment is adjusted to achieve at least a 65% reduction in urea, with most treatments lasting 3–4 hours. When HD is instituted, dietary protein should be increased to 1.0–1.2 g/kg/day, and fluid intake should be adjusted to permit a weight gain of approximately 2 kg between dialysis sessions. Antihypertensive medication may have to be reduced, and often short-acting antihypertensives should be withheld on dialysis days. Some complications of HD are described in the following sections.

    A. Vascular access for blood outflow and return is necessary. Permanent vascular access requires creation of a primary arteriovenous (AV) anastomosis or a synthetic AV graft. **Primary AV fistulas** are considered the optimal form of permanent access; they have the lowest incidence of infection and thrombosis. Fistulas should be placed 3–6 months before anticipated dialysis because they take time to mature fully. In contrast, because **synthetic grafts** must merely heal and become incorporated, they usually are placed 1–3 months before anticipated dialysis. **Tunneled silastic catheters** placed in the internal jugular vein are increasingly used for long-term access; they have lower rates of infection and venous complications (stenosis, compromise of future arm grafts) than do those placed in the subclavian veins. Temporary access is usually via an internal jugular or femoral venous catheter.

        1. Infections via vascular access sites are common and may produce local or systemic signs. Careful examination and ultrasonography of the access site may reveal a local abscess, which should be cultured and drained. Fevers, especially during an HD treatment, should be promptly evaluated. Blood cultures should be obtained, and empiric antibiotic coverage should be considered even in patients who lack an obvious source of infection. Initial therapy must include coverage for staphylococci and should be continued for at least 4 weeks. Removal of an infected access often is necessary.

   2. **Thrombosis** of a vascular access site can be recanalized by balloon catheter embolectomy, thrombolysis, or thrombectomy. The access site usually can be used immediately after declotting.

B. **Hypotension during dialysis** is most commonly due to intravascular volume depletion and, less commonly, to use of antihypertensives or nitrates before dialysis, allergic reactions to the dialyzer, left ventricular dysfunction, or autonomic insufficiency. Acute treatment includes infusion of normal saline and reduction of the ultrafiltration rate. Other causes of hypotension, such as myocardial infarction, cardiac tamponade, sepsis, and bleeding, should be considered.

C. **Active bleeding and coagulopathies** may be exacerbated by the systemic anticoagulation used in HD. The heparin dosage used for HD can usually be minimized or even withheld in patients with such disorders, or a change to peritoneal dialysis (PD) should be considered. The platelet dysfunction seen in many uremic patients causes prolongation of the bleeding time and can be improved by the use of IV desmopressin (diamino-8-D-arginine-vasopressin, 0.3 µg/kg in 50 ml saline q4–8h), IV conjugated estrogen (0.6 mg/kg/day for 5 days), or intranasal diamino-8-D-arginine-vasopressin (see Chap. 19).

D. **Pericarditis** may occur in patients who are undergoing dialysis and appears to be different from uremic pericarditis. Treatment involves intensification of dialysis to six to seven times a week. If this therapy fails or if evidence of tamponade is found, pericardiectomy is indicated. Anticoagulation during HD should be minimized or discontinued until pericarditis resolves.

E. **Dialysis disequilibrium** is a syndrome that may occur during the first few treatments of profoundly uremic patients and is attributed to CNS edema from rapid osmolar shifts. Symptoms include nausea, emesis, and headache, with occasional progression to confusion and seizures. This complication can be prevented or ameliorated by using lower blood flows and shorter treatment duration during initial dialysis sessions. **Dialysis dementia** is a progressive syndrome that occurs secondary to CNS accumulation of aluminum. Hesitant, nonfluent speech is frequently the presenting sign. It is infrequently seen, owing to the decreased use of aluminum-containing phosphate binders.

II. **Peritoneal dialysis**

A. **Modalities.** PD can be used in ARF and end-stage renal disease. It uses the peritoneum as a dialysis membrane, with solutes removed by diffusion into the dialysate. Fluid removal is controlled by adjusting the dextrose concentration in the dialysate (1.5%, 2.5%, or 4.25% glucose) to create an osmotic gradient. Higher dextrose concentrations and more frequent exchanges increase the rate of fluid removal. A typical dialysis exchange is performed by infusion of 2 L fluid into the peritoneal cavity, followed by an equilibration period and dialysate drainage. In ARF, PD exchanges can be performed as often as every hour. **Continuous ambulatory PD** involves 2- to 3-L exchanges performed four to five times a day by the patient. **Continuous cycling PD** uses an automatic cycler to perform exchanges during sleep. It can be supplemented by daytime exchanges. PD should be avoided in patients with recent abdominal surgery or a history of multiple surgeries with adhesions. Strict sterile technique is mandatory when exchanges are being performed. Compared with HD, PD is less efficient and less useful in highly catabolic patients. PD usually is better tolerated by patients with dilated cardiomyopathies because it causes fewer abrupt changes in BP and

Table 12-3. Intraperitoneal antibiotics in peritoneal dialysis

Antibiotic	Continuous dose (add to every exchange)	Intermittent dose (add to one exchange each day)
Cefazolin and cephalothin	Loading dose: 500 mg/L Maintenance dose: 125 mg/L	500 mg/L (or 15 mg/kg) If UO >500 ml/day, increase by 0.6 mg/kg body weight
Ceftazidime	Loading dose: 250 mg/L Maintenance dose: 125 mg/L	1000 mg/day in one exchange
Gentamicin, netilmicin, tobramycin	Loading dose: 8 mg/L Maintenance dose: 4 mg/L	If UO >500 ml/day, give 1.5 mg/kg loading dose, then 0.6 mg/kg/day* If UO ≤500 ml/day, give 0.6 mg/kg/day without load
Imipenem	Loading dose: 500 mg/L Maintenance dose: 200 mg/L	1000 mg intraperitoneally bid

UO = urine output.
*Adjust dose based on blood levels.

electrolytes, and fluid removal is continuous. PD also offers greater independence to chronic dialysis patients than does HD.

B. Complications of PD

1. **Infections** are the most significant problem in PD and include peritonitis, infection of the catheter tunnel, and infection of the catheter exit site. **Peritonitis** typically causes increasing abdominal pain and cloudy peritoneal fluid. It is usually secondary to a break in sterile technique. Patients generally are trained to save cloudy fluid for cell count and culture and then to initiate antibiotic therapy on an outpatient basis. Because of the emergence of vancomycin resistance, initial empiric therapy should consist of cefazolin plus ceftazidime (Table 12-3) added to the PD fluid, which then should dwell for 5–6 hours (*Peritoneal Dialysis Int* 20:396, 2000). Further antibiotic therapy should be guided by Gram stain and cultures. Fluid balance must be closely monitored and dialysate concentration adjusted to avoid dehydration or volume overload. Hospitalization is indicated in patients with frank sepsis, resistant or recurrent infections, or suspicion of organ perforation or abscess formation. **Tunnel or exit site infections** involve skin organisms, frequently are difficult to treat, and may require catheter removal and temporary HD until the infection resolves.

2. **Hyperglycemia** may occur as a result of absorption of glucose in PD fluid. If necessary, regular insulin can be added directly to the dialysate (e.g., 2 units added to 2 L 1.5% dextrose, 6 units added to 2 L 4.25% dextrose). In diabetic patients, intraperitoneal insulin is effective in controlling blood glucose. Conversion from SC insulin to intraperitoneal insulin is best accomplished in the hospital, where proper glucose monitoring can be ensured. Initially, the patient's usual total daily SC insulin dose is divided by the number of exchanges that he or she will receive and is given as regular insulin in each continuous ambulatory PD exchange. Additional insulin to cover glucose in the PD fluid should be included. The insulin dose required is one and a half to four times the previously required SC dose.

    3. Protein loss in PD can be excessive, and therefore dietary protein intake should be increased to 1.2–1.4 g/kg/day.

III. Ultrafiltration and hemofiltration remove large volumes of fluid with minimal removal of metabolic wastes. These filtration techniques are useful for removing fluid in patients with renal insufficiency and volume overload who do not need concomitant dialysis.

    A. Ultrafiltration is performed in a manner similar to standard HD, except that no dialysate is used. Negative pressure applied across the dialyzer membrane causes an ultrafiltrate of plasma to form and be removed. Large volumes of fluid are removed in a short period. The patient may experience hypotension.

    B. Slow, continuous renal replacement therapies include **continuous veno-venous hemofiltration** (CVVH) alone or with HD (CVVHDF) and continuous AV hemofiltration (CAVH) alone or with HD (CAVHDF). These modalities were developed to treat critically ill patients in an ICU setting. Continuous treatment permits slow but large volume and solute removal with minimal hemodynamic compromise. In CAVH and CAVHDF, blood flows from an arterial catheter into the dialyzer and is returned to the patient via a venous catheter. The patient's BP provides the driving force for filtration; no blood pump is needed. CVVH and CVVHDF use a specialized dialysis machine that circulates blood though a double-lumen dialysis catheter, avoiding the need for an arterial line. Both modalities usually require systemic anticoagulation, and patients are bed bound. Fluid balance, electrolytes, and glucose must be closely monitored. Drug clearance may be higher than with HD or PD, and therefore drug levels should be monitored whenever possible.

IV. Renal transplantation offers patients a lifestyle closest to normal and may lead to improved survival over HD and PD. One-year graft survival rates are 80% for cadaver allografts and 90% for living, related donor grafts.

    A. Pretransplantation evaluation of the recipient includes assessment of cardiovascular status and structural abnormalities of the urinary tract, correction of potential sources of infection (e.g., dental hygiene problems), human lymphocyte antigen typing, and evaluation for preformed antibodies against potential donor antigens. The latter, along with blood group compatibility testing, should prevent hyperacute rejection in most cases. Contraindications to transplantation include most malignancies, active infections, and significant cardiac or pulmonary disease.

    B. Immunosuppression, infectious, and long-term complications are discussed in Chap 16.

Nephrolithiasis

I. Clinical manifestations of nephrolithiasis include hematuria, predisposition to urinary tract infection, and pain (usually flank) with passage of the stone. Renal stones may also be an incidental finding on radiographic studies. Oliguria and ARF may occur when both collecting systems are blocked by stones.

II. Diagnostic evaluation of an acute episode of flank pain and hematuria should include a plain abdominal radiogram, as most renal stones are radiopaque. Exceptions include cystine stones, which may be of intermediate opacity, and uric acid stones, which are radiolucent. IVP should be performed acutely if renal colic is severe and obstruction is suspected. IVP or renal ultrasound is useful in evaluating the anatomy of the kidneys and collecting systems. Urine should be cultured and examined for pH and crystals. Other initial studies include serum electrolytes, Cr, calcium, uric acid, and phosphorus levels. Urine should be strained and all passed stones should be saved for analysis. After resolution of the acute episode, further diagnostic evaluation can be guided by stone composition. The extent of the metabolic evaluation that should be undertaken for the patient with a single calcium stone has not been established, but recurrent calcium nephrolithiasis warrants complete investigation. Patients with noncalcium stones should undergo complete evaluation after the first episode. Additional studies may include PTH levels (if hypercalcemia is present) and 24-hour urine studies for measurement of calcium, phosphate, urate, oxalate, citrate, Cr, sodium, urea nitrogen, and cystine. Yearly follow-up examination of the patient with nephrolithiasis includes abdominal radiographs to check for new stone formation or growth of existing stones and repeat metabolic studies to assess the effects of specific therapies.

III. **Treatment** of nephrolithiasis includes immediate analgesia and hydration. If the stone is obstructing outflow or is accompanied by infection, removal is indicated. After passage of a stone, treatment is directed at prevention of recurrent stone formation. In most patients, the foundation of general therapy is maintenance of high urine output (>2.5 L/day) through oral hydration and avoidance of dietary excesses. Evaluation and management depend on the type of stone and are best performed in the outpatient setting.

13

Antimicrobials

Raymond M. Johnson and
David J. Ritchie

For most antibiotics there are two or three choices of dosages/intervals. In general this decision should be based on size of the patient (<50 kg vs. >50 kg) and severity of illness. One should always err on the side of higher dosing. Many antibiotics can be given intramuscularly in addition to intravenously (see specific agents). This can be used in difficult cases when IV access cannot immediately be (re)established. Many antibiotics have major drug interactions (see Appendix C) or require alternate dosing in renal insufficiency, or both (see Appendix E). As a general note, **uncomplicated urinary tract infections (UTIs) rarely require IV therapy;** therefore, the lowest IV doses referred to by manufacturers have been left out, as these are suitable only for treating UTIs. Nearly all antibiotics have been associated with **pseudomembranous colitis,** and this diagnosis should be pursued for all patients in whom profuse diarrhea or diarrhea plus one or more of the following develop: blood in the stool, abdominal pain, or relapse of fever. For HIV antiretroviral and antiparasitic agents, see Chap. 15.

Antibacterial Agents

I. **Penicillins (PCN)** are among the oldest antimicrobial agents in use. They irreversibly bind PCN-binding proteins, components of the bacterial cell wall, causing osmotic rupture and death. Once the mainstay of antimicrobial therapy, these agents have a reduced role today because of acquired resistance in many bacterial species through alterations in the PCN-binding proteins or expression of hydrolytic enzymes. PCNs remain among the drugs of choice for syphilis, group A *Streptococcus, Listeria monocytogenes, Pasteurella multocida, Actinomyces,* susceptible enterococcus species, and some anaerobic infections.

   A. **Aqueous penicillin G** [2–4 million units (μ) IV q4h or 18–24 μ qd by continuous infusion] is the IV preparation of PCN. It is the therapy of choice for **neurosyphilis.** Although the potassium salt is more common, the sodium salt is available and should be given in the setting of hyperkalemia or azotemia.

   B. **Procaine penicillin G** is an IM repository form of penicillin G that is rarely used today.

   C. **Benzathine penicillin** is a long-acting repository form of penicillin G that is commonly used for treating early syphilis [<1-year duration (one dose 2.4 μ IM)] and late latent syphilis [unknown duration or >1 year (2.4 μ IM qwk for 3 doses)]. It is occasionally given for group A streptococcal pharyngitis and prophylaxis after acute rheumatic fever or poststreptococcal glomerular nephritis.

   D. **Penicillin V** (250–500 mg PO qid) is an oral version of PCN that is typically used to treat group A streptococcal pharyngitis.

   E. **Ampicillin** (2–3 g IV q4–6h) is the **drug of choice** for susceptible enterococcus species and *L. monocytogenes.* Oral ampicillin (250–500 mg PO qid) is commonly used for uncomplicated sinusitis, pharyngitis, otitis media, and UTIs. **Ampicillin/sulbactam** (1.5–3.0 g IV q6h) combines ampicillin with the beta-lactamase inhibitor sulbactam, thereby extending its spectrum to include

oxacillin-sensitive *Staphylococcus aureus* **(OSSA)**, anaerobes, and gram-negative upper airway pathogens. It is effective for upper and lower respiratory tract, genitourinary tract, and polymicrobial soft-tissue infections. It is the IV antibiotic of choice for serious cellulitis due to human or animal bites.

F. **Amoxicillin** (250–500 mg PO tid) is an oral antibiotic similar to ampicillin that is commonly used for uncomplicated sinusitis, pharyngitis, otitis media, and UTIs. **Amoxicillin/clavulanic acid** (875 mg PO bid or 500 mg PO tid) combines amoxicillin with the beta-lactamase inhibitor clavulanate and is an oral antibiotic similar to ampicillin/sulbactam. It is useful for treating complicated sinusitis, otitis media, and skin infections and is the antibiotic of choice for prophylaxis in human or animal bites after appropriate local treatment. It is often used as a step-down therapy from IV ampicillin/sulbactam. The 875-mg PO bid dosing regimen causes less diarrhea.

G. **Nafcillin and oxacillin** (2 g IV q4–6h) are penicillinase-resistant synthetic PCNs that are the drugs of choice for treating OSSA infections. These drugs have little activity against enterococci or gram-negative bacteria. Dose reduction by one-half should be considered in decompensated liver disease. **Dicloxacillin and cloxacillin** (250–500 mg PO qid) are oral antibiotics with a spectrum of activity similar to that of nafcillin and oxacillin. They are typically used to treat localized skin infections without systemic signs or symptoms.

H. **Mezlocillin, ticarcillin, and piperacillin** (3 g IV q4h or 4 g IV q6h) are penicillin derivatives with improved gram-negative activity. Ticarcillin and piperacillin have reasonable antipseudomonal activity but require coadministration of an aminoglycoside for serious infections. Mezlocillin and piperacillin have good enterococcal activity and accumulate to high levels in bile, making them useful drugs for ascending cholangitis and prophylaxis before manipulations of the biliary tree.

   1. **Ticarcillin/clavulanic acid** (3.1 g IV q4–6h) combines ticarcillin with the beta-lactamase inhibitor clavulanate. This combination extends the spectrum to include most Enterobacteriaceae and anaerobes, making it a useful antibiotic for intra-abdominal infections. It is second-line therapy for complicated soft-tissue infections. Ticarcillin/clavulanic acid may have a unique role in treating *Stenotrophomonas* (*Chemotherapy* 44:293, 1998). Alternative therapy with imipenem, cefepime, or a quinolone should be used when bacteria with *AmpC*-inducible beta-lactamases (i.e., *Enterobacter, Citrobacter, Serratia, Providencia, Acinetobacter,* and *Morganella* species) are identified as principal pathogens. Ticarcillin/clavulanic acid has a high sodium load for salt-sensitive patients.

   2. **Piperacillin/tazobactam** (3.375 g IV q4–6h) combines piperacillin with the beta-lactamase inhibitor tazobactam. It has a similar spectrum and indications as ticarcillin/clavulanate plus activity against ampicillin-sensitive enterococci. **Ticarcillin/clavulanate and piperacillin/tazobactam are not reasonable monotherapy for serious infections caused by** *Pseudomonas aeruginosa* **or nosocomial pneumonias; an aminoglycoside should be coadministered.**

I. **Adverse effects.** All penicillin derivatives have been associated with anaphylaxis, interstitial nephritis, anemia, and leukopenia. Oxacillin and nafcillin can cause hepatitis. Ticarcillin can aggravate bleeding by interfering with platelet adenosine diphosphate receptors. Prolonged high-dose therapy (>2 weeks) is typically monitored with weekly serum creatinine and blood counts [liver function tests (LFTs) are included with oxacillin/nafcillin]. All patients should be asked about PCN or cephalosporin allergy. These agents should not be used in a patient with a reported allergy without prior skin testing or desensitization, or both.

II. **Cephalosporins** kill bacteria by interfering with cell wall synthesis by the same mechanism as PCNs. These agents are popular because of their low toxicity and broad spectrum of activity.

A. **First-generation cephalosporins** have activity against staphylococci, streptococci, and community-acquired *Escherichia coli, Klebsiella,* and *Proteus* species. They have limited efficacy against the other enteric gram-negative rods and anaerobes. These agents are commonly used for treating OSSA osteomyelitis, pharyngitis, UTIs, and skin/soft-tissue infections. **Cefazolin** (1–2 g IV/IM q8h), and **cephalothin, cephapirin, and cephradine** (1–2 g IV/IM q4–6h), have similar spectrums of activity and indications. **Cefadroxil** (500 mg–1 g PO bid), **cephalexin, and cephadrine** (500 mg–1 g PO qid) are oral preparations of the parenteral first-generation cephalosporins.

B. **Second-generation cephalosporins** have expanded coverage against enteric gram-negative rods. They are divided into above-the-diaphragm and below-the-diaphragm agents.

1. **Cefuroxime** (1.5 g IV/IM q8h), **cefonicid** (1–2 g IV/IM qd), and **cefamandole** (1–2 g IV/IM q4–6h) are useful antibiotics above the diaphragm. They have reasonable staphylococcal and streptococcal activity in addition to an extended spectrum against gram-negative aerobes and are typically used for skin/soft-tissue infections, complicated UTIs, and community-acquired pneumonia (cefuroxime). They do not cover *Bacteroides fragilis*.

2. **Cefoxitin** (1–2 g IV q4–8h), **cefotetan** (1–3 g IV/IM q12h), and **cefmetazole** (2 g IV q6–12h) are below-the-diaphragm antibiotics. They do not have dependable staphylococcal or streptococcal activity. They have an extended spectrum against gram-negative aerobes and anaerobes including *B. fragilis*. These antibiotics are typically used for intra-abdominal or gynecologic surgical prophylaxis and infections, including diverticulitis and pelvic inflammatory disease. Cefoxitin has a unique role in the treatment of atypical mycobacterial infections.

3. **Cefuroxime axetil** (250–500 mg PO bid), **cefprozil** (250–500 mg PO bid), **cefdinir** (300 mg PO bid), and **cefaclor** (250–500 mg PO bid) are oral second-generation cephalosporins that are typically used for bronchitis, sinusitis, otitis media, UTIs, local soft-tissue infections, and step-down therapy for pneumonia or cellulitis that is responsive to parenteral second-generation cephalosporins. Cefdinir is approved for treating uncomplicated community-acquired pneumonia (when an atypical agent is not suspected). **Loracarbef** (200–400 mg PO q12–24h), technically a carbacephem rather than a cephalosporin, is used for the same indications as the oral second-generation cephalosporins, with the additional indication for uncomplicated pyelonephritis.

C. **Third-generation cephalosporins** have the broadest coverage for enteric, aerobic gram-negative rods and retain good activity against streptococci other than enterococci. They have moderate anaerobic activity but do not cover *B. fragilis*. Ceftazidime is the only third-generation cephalosporin that is useful for treating serious *P. aeruginosa* infections. Several of these agents have good CNS penetration and are useful in treating meningitis (see Chap. 14). **Third-generation cephalosporins are not reliable for treatment of organisms with the *AmpC*-inducible beta-lactamases regardless of the results of susceptibility testing.** These microbes should be treated with cefepime, carbapenems, or quinolones.

1. **Ceftriaxone** (1–2 g IV/IM q12–24h), **cefotaxime** (1–2 g IV/IM q4–12h), **ceftizoxime** (1–4 g IV/IM q8–12h), and **cefoperazone** (2–4 g IV q12h) are very similar to one another in spectrum and efficacy. They are used as empiric therapy for pyelonephritis, urosepsis, pneumonia, intra-abdominal infections (combined with metronidazole), gonorrhea, and meningitis (ceftriaxone and cefotaxime). They are also used for osteomyelitis, septic arthritis, endocarditis, and soft-tissue infections once an organism has been identified. OSSA should be treated with oxacillin or a first-generation cephalosporin rather than these agents. **Ceftizoxime is the most convenient agent in dialysis patients, as it is eliminated exclusively by the kidneys.** Dialysis patients with infections other than meningitis should receive a 2-g initial dose followed by 1–2 g at the end of each dialysis session. This

feature can be exploited to avoid placement of additional venous access.

2. **Cefixime** (400 mg PO qd), **cefpodoxime proxetil** (100–400 mg PO bid), and **ceftibuten** (400 mg PO qd) are oral third-generation cephalosporins. They are useful drugs for bronchitis and complicated sinusitis, otitis media, and UTIs. These agents are reasonable step-down therapy for pneumonia that is responsive to the parenteral third-generation cephalosporins. Cefpodoxime proxetil is approved for uncomplicated community-acquired pneumonia. Cefixime and cefpodoxime have roles in the management of gonorrhea.

3. **Ceftazidime** (1–2 g IV/IM q8h) is a drug of choice for infections caused by susceptible *P. aeruginosa*. *Pseudomonas* UTIs can be treated with lower doses (500 mg IV/IM q12h).

D. **Cefepime** (500 mg–2 g IV/IM q8–12h) is a **fourth-generation cephalosporin** that has excellent aerobic gram-negative rod coverage, including *P. aeruginosa* and bacteria with *AmpC*-inducible beta-lactamases. Its gram-positive spectrum and anaerobe coverage are similar to those of the third-generation cephalosporins. Cefepime is routinely used for empiric therapy in febrile neutropenic patients. It has a role in treating antibiotic-resistant gram-negative bacteria and polymicrobial infections in any site except the CNS, where clinical experience is lacking. Metronidazole should be given with cefepime for intra-abdominal infections.

E. **Adverse effects.** All cephalosporins have been associated with anaphylaxis, interstitial nephritis, anemia, and leukopenia. All patients should be asked about PCN or cephalosporin allergies. Patients who are allergic to PCNs have a 10% incidence of a cross-hypersensitivity reaction to cephalosporins. These agents should not be used in a patient with a reported allergy without prior skin testing or desensitization, or both. Prolonged therapy (>2 weeks) is typically monitored with a weekly serum creatinine and CBC. Ceftriaxone (and possibly cefoperazone) can cause biliary sludging and symptomatic gallbladder disease, requiring discontinuation of the medication. Cefamandole, cefmetazole, cefoperazone, and cefotetan have an *N*-methylthiotetrazole side chain that interferes with vitamin K–dependent clotting factor metabolism and is associated with disulfiram-like reactions with ethanol intake. *N*-methylthiotetrazole–containing cephalosporins should be avoided when a prolonged course of therapy is likely, as a significant coagulopathy may develop.

III. **Aztreonam** (1–2 g IV/IM q6–12h) is a monobactam that is active only against aerobic gram-negative rods including *P. aeruginosa*. It has no gram-positive or anaerobic activity. Aztreonam is useful in patients with known PCN or cephalosporin allergies, as no apparent cross reactivity is present.

IV. **Carbapenems** kill bacteria by interfering with cell wall synthesis, similar to PCNs and cephalosporins. They are among the antibiotics of choice for infections caused by organisms with the *AmpC*-inducible beta-lactamases and have good activity against *P. aeruginosa*. They are important agents for treatment of antibiotic-resistant bacterial infections at any site except the CNS, where drug penetration is borderline and seizures likely. They are commonly used for severe polymicrobial infections including Fournier's gangrene, intra-abdominal catastrophes, and sepsis in compromised hosts. Carbapenems are active against most gram-positive and gram-negative bacteria including anaerobes. Notably resistant bacteria include ampicillin-resistant enterococci, oxacillin-resistant *S. aureus* (ORSA), *Stenotrophomonas*, and *Burkholderia* species.

A. **Imipenem** (500 mg–1 g IV/IM q6–8h) and **meropenem** (1 g IV q8h) are the two currently available parenteral carbapenems and have a similar spectrum of activity, toxicity, and indications.

B. **Adverse effects.** Carbapenems can precipitate seizure activity or confusion, or both, in older patients, patients on dialysis, and patients with pre-existing seizure disorders or CNS pathology. Carbapenems should be avoided in these patients unless no reasonable alternative therapy is available. Like cephalosporins, carbapenems have been associated with anaphylaxis, interstitial nephritis, anemia, and leukopenia. All patients should be asked about PCN or cephalosporin allergy. Patients who are allergic to PCNs/cephalosporins infrequently have a cross-hypersensitivity reaction to carbapenems; however, these agents should not be used in a patient with a reported severe allergy without prior skin testing, desensitization, or both. Prolonged therapy (>2 weeks) is typically monitored with a weekly serum creatinine, LFTs, and CBC.

V. **Aminoglycosides** kill bacteria by binding to the bacterial ribosome, causing misreading during translation of bacterial messenger RNA into proteins. These drugs are commonly used in severe infections caused by gram-positive and gram-negative aerobes as a second agent until the patient's condition stabilizes. Prolonged therapy is indicated for patients with endovascular infections caused by enterococcus species or PCN/cephalosporin-resistant streptococci. Aminoglycosides tend to be synergistic with cell wall–active antibiotics such as penicillins, cephalosporins, and vancomycin. They are ineffective in the low pH/low oxygen environment of abscesses and do not have activity against anaerobes. Use of these antibiotics is limited by significant nephro- and ototoxicities. Resistance to one aminoglycoside is not routinely associated with resistance to all members of this class, and in cases of serious infections, susceptibility testing with each aminoglycoside is appropriate.

A. **Traditional dosing** of aminoglycosides is q8h, with the upper end of the dose range reserved for life-threatening infections. Peak and trough levels should be obtained with the third or fourth dose and then every 3–4 days, along with a serum creatinine. **Increasing serum creatinine or peak/troughs out of the acceptable range requires** *immediate* **attention.** Traditional dosing should be used for pregnant patients and for those with endocarditis, burns that cover more than 20% of the body, cystic fibrosis (CF), anasarca, and creatinine clearance (Cl_{Cr}) of less than 20 ml/minute. For all other indications extended-interval dosing is more convenient for the patient and the physician.

B. **Extended-interval dosing** of aminoglycosides is an alternative method of administration. Extended-interval doses are given in the following sections with each drug. A drug level is obtained 6–14 hours after the first dose, and the nomogram (Fig. 13-1) is consulted to determine the dosing interval. Monitoring includes obtaining a drug level at 6–14 hours after the dosage every week and a serum creatinine three times a week. In patients who are not responding to therapy, a 12-hour level should be checked, and if that level is undetectable, extended-interval dosing should be abandoned in favor of traditional dosing. For obese patients [actual weight >20% above ideal body weight (IBW)] (see Chap. 2 for calculation of IBW) an **obese dosing weight** must be used for determining doses in either traditional or extended-interval dosing.

Obese dosing weight = IBW + 0.4 (actual weight – IBW)

C. **Specific agents**
   1. **Gentamicin** is the least expensive antibiotic in this class. Traditional dosing is an initial loading dose of 2 mg/kg IV (3 mg/kg in the critically ill) followed by 1.0–1.7 mg/kg IV q8h (peak, 4–10 µg/ml; trough, <2 µg/ml). Extended-interval dosing is 5 mg/kg, with interval determined by nomogram.
   2. **Tobramycin** tends to be favored by physicians who treat CF patients. Traditional dosing is an initial loading dose of 2 mg/kg IV (3 mg/kg in the critically ill) followed by 1.0–1.7 mg/kg IV q8h (peak, 4–10 µg/ml; trough, <2 µg/ml). Extended-interval dosing is 5 mg/kg, with interval determined by nomogram. Tobramycin is also available as an inhalational agent for adjunctive therapy for patients with CF or bronchiectasis complicated by *P. aeruginosa* infection (300-mg inhalation bid).
   3. **Amikacin** has an additional unique role in mycobacterial and *Nocardia* infections. Traditional dosing is an initial loading dose of 5.0–7.5 mg/kg

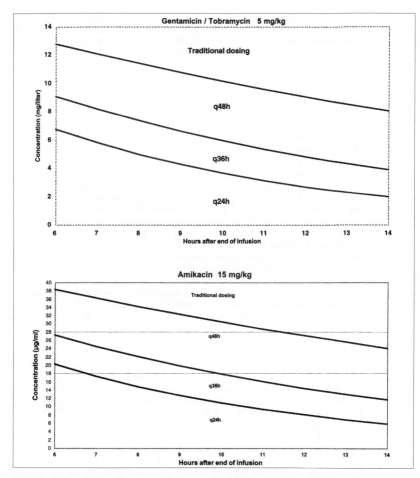

Fig. 13-1. Nomograms for extended-interval aminoglycoside dosing. (Adapted from RM Reichley, JR Little, TC Bailey, Barnes-Jewish Hospital and Washington University School of Medicine.)

IV (9 mg/kg in the critically ill) followed by 5 mg/kg IV q8h or 7.5 mg/kg IV q12h (peak, 20–35 µg/ml; trough, <10 µg/ml). Extended-interval dosing is 15 mg/kg, with the interval determined by nomogram.

4. **Streptomycin** is most commonly used for treating drug-resistant tuberculosis (TB; 15 mg/kg/day IM; maximum dose per day is 1 g for daily dosing and 1.5 g for twice- or thrice-weekly dosing) and enterococcal endocarditis (7.5 mg/kg IM/IV q12h; maximum, 500 mg q12h). It generally has less gram-negative activity than the other aminoglycosides and no activity against *P. aeruginosa*. Other indications for streptomycin (tularemia, brucellosis, plague) have largely been supplanted by gentamicin or nonaminoglycoside antibiotic therapy.

D. **Adverse effects.** Nephrotoxicity is the major adverse effect of aminoglycosides. If possible, prolonged therapy with aminoglycosides should be monitored by physicians who routinely administer home IV therapy with systematic monitoring of patients' laboratory studies. Nephrotoxicity is reversible when detected early but can be permanent, especially in patients with tenuous renal function due to other medical conditions. Aminoglycosides should be avoided in patients with decompensated liver disease except for life-threatening infections (*Gastroenterology* 82:97, 1982). Ototoxicity (vestibular or cochlear) is less of a problem but requires weekly hearing tests with extended therapy (>7–14 days). Streptomycin is unique in that it causes more ototoxicity with a lower risk of nephrotoxicity. One should avoid giving aminoglycosides with other known nephrotoxic agents (i.e., amphotericin, foscarnet, nonsteroidal anti-inflammatory drugs, pentamidine, polymyxins, cidofovir, and cisplatin).

VI. **Vancomycin** (15 mg/kg IV q12h; 30 mg/kg IV q12h for meningitis) is a glycopolypeptide antibiotic that kills gram-positive bacteria by interfering with cell wall synthesis. The goal trough should be 5 μg/ml or greater. Peak levels should only be measured in critically ill patients, with a goal of 20–40 μg/ml. Dialysis patients should receive a single dose and then be redosed when the level drops below 10–15 μg/ml. It binds a D-alanyl-D-alanine precursor that is critical for peptidoglycan cross linking in most gram-positive (not gram-negative) bacterial cell walls. Vancomycin is bacteriostatic for enterococci. Vancomycin was the only antibiotic with efficacy against many enterococci and ORSA until the approval of quinupristin/dalfopristin and linezolid. Several factors, including the emergence of resistant nosocomial pathogens, the low toxicity of vancomycin, and its ease of administration, led to an overuse of vancomycin and the evolution of vancomycin-resistant bacteria.

A. **Indications for usage.** Today, most hospitals have serious problems with vancomycin-resistant *Enterococcus faecium* (VRE), and reports of vancomycin intermediate-sensitivity *S. aureus* (VISA) are increasing. With the continued use of vancomycin, it is possible that *S. aureus* will acquire vancomycin resistance, generating a difficult-to-treat, virulent nosocomial pathogen. Therefore, vancomycin should be restricted to use in the following circumstances: (1) treatment of serious infections caused by ORSA, (2) treatment of serious infections caused by ampicillin-resistant enterococci, (3) treatment of serious infections caused by gram-positive bacteria in patients who are allergic to all other appropriate therapies, (4) oral treatment of *Clostridium difficile* colitis that has not responded to two courses (10 days each) of metronidazole or failing metronidazole with a potentially life-threatening colitis, (5) surgical prophylaxis for placement of prosthetic devices at institutions with known high rates of ORSA or in patients who are known to be colonized with ORSA, (6) empiric use in meningitis until an organism has been identified and sensitivities done if the pathogen is pneumococcus, and (7) life-threatening sepsis syndrome in a patient with known ORSA colonization or extended hospitalization until pathogen(s) are identified. Vancomycin should not be used routinely in the following circumstances: (1) routine surgical prophylaxis, (2) empiric therapy for nonseptic neutropenic fever, (3) treatment of single blood culture isolates of coagulase-negative staphylococcus or treatment of coagulase-negative staphylococcus blood cultures in cases in which the site of infection is inconsistent with the organism (e.g., community-acquired pneumonia and intra-abdominal infection), (4) routine treatment of *C. difficile* colitis, (5) to complete a course of therapy in the absence of ORSA or ampicillin-resistant enterococci, (6) to prophylax against catheter infection, and (7) use in topical application or irrigation. **In dialysis patients,** vancomycin use should be avoided in clinical situations in which ORSA is unlikely. Vancomycin should also be avoided in small localized infections (e.g., cellulitis, carbuncles) well away from graft sites or catheters. Ceftizoxime (2 g IV/IM, then 1–2 g after hemodialysis) is convenient therapy for community-acquired pneumonia, intra-abdominal infections (with metronidazole), and many soft-tissue infections. For more serious infections ceftizoxime can be given with a single dose of aminoglycoside (gentamicin or tobramycin, 1.5–2.0 mg/kg). For uncomplicated soft-tissue infections, cefprozil (500 mg PO q12h for 2 doses, then 500 mg PO qd), cefdinir (300 mg PO q12h for 2 doses, then 300 mg PO qd), dicloxacillin (500 mg PO qid), or clindamycin (450 mg PO tid) are reasonable therapies for dialysis patients with good insight and follow-up.

B. Adverse effects. Vancomycin is typically given by slow infusion over at least 1 hour. Infusion rates of greater than 10 mg/minute can cause the red man syndrome (flushing of the upper body).

VII. Fluoroquinolones kill bacteria by inhibiting bacterial DNA gyrase and topoisomerase, which are critical for DNA replication. In general these antibiotics are well absorbed orally, with serum levels that approach those of parenteral therapy. With the addition of new fluoroquinolones, the spectrum of activity in this class of antibiotics rivals that of the cephalosporins. These agents typically have poor activity against enterococci, although they may have some efficacy for UTIs when other agents are inactive or contraindicated. Newer fluoroquinolones have activity against OSSA but should be considered only when oxacillin, nafcillin, and first-generation cephalosporins are contraindicated or inactive. Enoxacin (400 mg), ciprofloxacin (500 mg), or ofloxacin (400 mg) can be used as single-dose therapy to treat gonorrhea. **Aluminum- and magnesium-containing antacids, sucralfate, bismuth, oral iron, oral calcium, and oral zinc preparations can markedly impair absorption of oral quinolones.**

A. Norfloxacin (400 mg PO q12h), **enoxacin** (200–400 mg PO q12h), and **lomefloxacin** (400 mg PO qd) are useful for the treatment of UTIs caused by gram-negative rods. These agents are not used to treat systemic infections.

B. Ciprofloxacin (250–750 mg PO q12h or 200–400 mg IV q12h) and **ofloxacin** (200–400 mg IV or PO q12h) are active against gram-negative aerobes including *AmpC* pathogens. Ciprofloxacin is the most active quinolone against *P. aeruginosa* and is the quinolone of choice for serious infections with that pathogen. It has relatively poor activity against gram-positive cocci and anaerobes and should not be used for empiric therapy for community-acquired pneumonia or for treating OSSA. These agents are commonly used for UTIs, pyelonephritis, infectious diarrhea, prostatitis, and intra-abdominal infections (with metronidazole). They are second-line agents for TB therapy. Oral and IV therapy give similar maximum serum levels.

C. Levofloxacin (250–500 mg PO or IV q24h), **sparfloxacin** (400 mg PO once, then 200 mg PO qd), **gatifloxacin** (400 mg PO/IV qd), and **moxifloxacin** (400 mg PO qd) are newer fluoroquinolones with improved coverage of aerobic gram-positive bacteria (streptococci, staphylococci, and enterococci), with less gram-negative activity (especially against *P. aeruginosa*) than ciprofloxacin. Sparfloxacin, gatifloxacin, and moxifloxacin also have reasonable anaerobic activity, possibly expanding their role in mixed aerobic/anaerobic infections. Overall, these agents can be thought of as above-the-diaphragm quinolones that are useful for sinusitis, bronchitis, or chronic obstructive pulmonary disease exacerbations; community-acquired pneumonia; UTIs; and pyelonephritis. They are reasonable therapy for soft-tissue infections if penicillins or cephalosporins are inactive or contraindicated. The newer quinolones should not be used routinely to treat diabetic foot infections/osteomyelitis until clinical trials support their use for this indication. Some of these agents have reasonable activity against mycobacteria and have a potential role in treating drug-resistant TB and atypical mycobacterial infections.

D. Trovafloxacin/alatrofloxacin (200–400 mg PO/IV; PO and IV dosing are equivalent) has the broadest spectrum of the quinolones including gram-positive aerobes/anaerobes and gram-negative aerobes/anaerobes including *B. fragilis*. Its spectrum of activity is comparable to that of the carbapenems and can be used for polymicrobial infections at any site except the CNS and osteomyelitis, where clinical experience is lacking. This antibiotic should be reserved for severe pulmonary, intra-abdominal, and soft-tissue infections. This agent is one of the drugs of choice for severely ill patients with PCN or cephalosporin allergies. Unfortunately, since its original approval trovaflox-acin has been associated with rare cases of hepatotoxicity, resulting in liver transplant or death. For this reason its use has been restricted to "treat-ment of serious infections in hospitalized patients where alternative thera-pies are not available." LFTs should be performed every 3–4 days and therapy limited to 14 days.

E. **Adverse effects.** The principal adverse reactions with fluoroquinolones include nausea, CNS disturbances (drowsiness, headache, restlessness, and dizziness, especially in the elderly), rashes, and phototoxicity. The use of sparfloxacin and lomefloxacin requires an explicit warning to patients about photosensitivity reactions. Sparfloxacin and moxifloxacin can cause prolon-gation of the QT interval and should not be used in patients with known conduction abnormalities on ECG or in those who are taking medications that prolong the QT interval or induce bradycardia. Sparfloxacin and moxi-floxacin should be used cautiously in the elderly, in whom asymptomatic conduction disturbances are more common. Trovafloxacin/alatrofloxacin requires careful monitoring of the liver function profile because of rare, fatal drug-associated hepatitis. **Fluoroquinolones should not be used in patients younger than 18 years or in pregnant or lactating women.** They cause an age-related arthropathy and should be discontinued in patients in whom joint pain or tendonitis (Achilles tendon) develops. **This class of anti-biotics has major drug interactions** (see Appendix C).

VIII. **Macrolide antibiotics** are bacteriostatic agents that block protein synthesis in bacteria by binding the 50S subunit of the bacterial ribosome. These antibiotics are commonly used to treat pharyngitis, otitis media, sinusitis, and bronchitis, especially in PCN-allergic patients. They are also among the drugs of choice for treating *Legionella*, *Chlamydia*, and *Mycoplasma* infections. The newer macrolides are reasonable therapy for community-acquired pneumonia and have a unique role in the treatment of *Mycobacterium avium* complex (MAC) infections in HIV patients. This class of antibiotics has good activity against gram-positive cocci and upper respiratory gram-negative bacteria, with no meaningful activity against enteric gram-negative rods.

A. **Erythromycin** (250–500 mg PO qid or 0.5–1.0 g IV q6h; poorly tolerated through peripheral veins) is commonly used to treat bronchitis, pharyngitis, sinusitis, otitis media, and soft-tissue infections in PCN-allergic patients. It has good activity against gram-positive cocci except enterococci. Erythromy-cin is effective for treatment of atypical respiratory tract infections due to *Legionella pneumophila* (1 g IV q6h), *Chlamydia pneumoniae*, and *Myco-plasma pneumoniae*. It is also used in treatment of *Chlamydia trachomatis* (500 mg PO qid × 7 days) and as an alternate therapy for syphilis in PCN-allergic patients. Usefulness of this antibiotic for upper and lower respiratory tract infections is hampered by significant resistance among *Haemophilus influenzae* and *Moraxella catarrhalis* isolates.

B. **Dirithromycin** (500 mg PO qd) has a similar spectrum of activity and clini-cal application as erythromycin with the convenience of once-a-day dosing. It is not used in treatment of sexually transmitted diseases. It does not have the numerous drug interactions seen with erythromycin and clarithromycin and can be used instead of erythromycin to avoid drug interactions.

C. **Clarithromycin** (250–500 mg PO bid) has a spectrum of activity similar to that of erythromycin but with enhanced activity against upper respiratory pathogens (*Moraxella* and *Haemophilus*). It is commonly used to treat bron-chitis, sinusitis, otitis media, pharyngitis, soft-tissue infections, and commu-nity-acquired pneumonia. It has a prominent role in treating MAC infections in HIV patients and is an important component of regimens used to eradicate *Helicobacter pylori* (see Chap. 17).

D. **Azithromycin** [500 mg PO × 1 day, then 250 mg PO qd × 4 days (Zpack); 250–500 mg PO qd; 500 mg IV qd] is very similar to clarithromycin in spectrum and indications. It has a prominent role in MAC prophylaxis (1200 mg PO qwk) and treatment (250–500 mg PO qd) in HIV patients. It is commonly used to treat *C. trachomatis* infections (1 g PO × 1 day). It does not have the numerous drug interactions seen with erythromycin and clarithromycin.

E. Clindamycin (150–450 mg PO tid–qid or 600–900 mg IV q8h) is a lincosamide with a predominantly gram-positive spectrum similar to that of erythromycin plus activity against most anaerobes including *B. fragilis*. It has excellent oral bioavailability, 90%, and penetrates into bone and abscess cavities. Clindamycin is commonly used in children to treat osteomyelitis. In adults it is used as monotherapy for lung abscesses. A significant number of ORSA isolates remain susceptible to clindamycin. It is typically used as the second agent in combination therapy when anaerobic infections (peritonsillar/retropharyngeal abscesses, necrotizing fasciitis, recurrent group A streptococcal pharyngitis) are suspected. Metronidazole is more commonly used for intra-abdominal infections. Clindamycin has additional uses, including treatment of babesiosis (in combination with quinine), treatment of toxoplasmosis (in combination with pyrimethamine), and treatment of *Pneumocystis carinii* pneumonia (PCP; in combination with primaquine).

F. Adverse effects. Macrolides are associated with nausea, abdominal cramping (less common with clarithromycin, azithromycin, and clindamycin), and LFT abnormalities. Liver function profiles should be checked intermittently during extended therapy. Hypersensitivity reactions with prominent skin rash are more commonly seen with clindamycin, as is pseudomembranous colitis. **Erythromycin and clarithromycin have multiple drug interactions, including potentially fatal arrhythmias, when used with certain medications (i.e., cisapride, digoxin). This class of antibiotics has major drug interactions** (see Appendix C).

IX. Sulfamethoxazole, sulfadiazine, sulfisoxazole, trimetrexate, and trimethoprim slowly kill bacteria by inhibiting folic acid metabolism. This class of antibiotics is most commonly used for uncomplicated UTIs, sinusitis, and otitis media. They have unique roles in treatment of PCP, *Nocardia*, *Toxoplasma*, and *Stenotrophomonas* infections.

A. Sulfamethoxazole (2 g PO, then 1 g PO q12h), **sulfisoxazole** (1 g PO q6h), and **trimethoprim** (100 mg PO bid) are occasionally used to treat UTIs as monotherapy. These drugs are more logically used in combination preparations outlined in the following sections. Trimethoprim in combination with dapsone is an alternate therapy for mild PCP pneumonia (see Chap. 15).

B. Trimethoprim-sulfamethoxazole is a combination antibiotic (IV or PO) with a 1:5 ratio of trimethoprim to sulfamethoxazole. The IV preparation is dosed at 5 mg/kg IV q8h (based on the trimethoprim content) for serious infections. The oral preparations [160 mg trimethoprim/800 mg sulfamethoxazole per double-strength (DS) tablet] are almost completely bioavailable, and similar drug levels can be obtained by taking 5 mg/kg q8h PO. Both components have excellent tissue penetration, including bone, prostate, and CNS. The combination has a broad spectrum of activity but typically does not inhibit *P. aeruginosa* or anaerobes. It is the therapy of choice for PCP pneumonia (see Chap. 15), *Stenotrophomonas maltophilia*, *Trophermyma whippleii*, and *Nocardia* infections. It is commonly used for treating sinusitis, otitis media, bronchitis, prostatitis, and UTIs (1 DS PO bid). Some strains of ORSA remain susceptible to trimethoprim-sulfamethoxazole. It is used as PCP prophylaxis (1 DS PO twice a week, 3 times a week, or daily) in transplant patients, bone marrow transplant patients, patients receiving fludarabine, and HIV patients. IV therapy is routinely converted to the PO equivalent for patients who require prolonged therapy (PCP, *Actinomyces*, *Nocardia*). For serious infections such as *Nocardia* brain abscesses, it is useful to monitor sulfamethoxazole peaks (100–150 µg/ml) and troughs (50–100 µg/ml) occasionally during the course of therapy and to adjust dosing accordingly. In patients with renal insufficiency, doses can be adjusted by following trimethoprim peaks (5–10 µg/ml).

Prolonged therapy can cause bone marrow suppression, requiring treatment with leucovorin, 5–10 mg PO qd until cell counts normalize.

C. **Sulfadiazine** (1.0–1.5 g PO q6h) in combination with pyrimethamine (200 mg PO followed by 50–75 mg PO qd) and leucovorin (10–20 mg PO qd) is the therapy of choice for toxoplasmosis. Sulfadiazine is occasionally used in *Nocardia* infections.

D. **Trimetrexate** (45 mg/m^2 IV qd) combined with leucovorin (20 mg/m^2 PO or IV q6h continued for 3 days after the last dose of trimetrexate) is an alternate therapy for PCP pneumonia. Bone marrow suppression, renal insufficiency, and hepatotoxicity may occur.

E. **Adverse effects.** These drugs are associated with cholestatic jaundice, bone marrow suppression, interstitial nephritis, and severe hypersensitivity reactions (Stevens-Johnson/erythema multiforme). Nausea is common with higher doses. All patients should be asked whether they are allergic to "sulfa drugs," and specific commercial names should be mentioned (i.e., Bactrim or Septra).

X. **Chloramphenicol** (12.5–25.0 mg/kg IV q6h; maximum, 1 g IV q6h) is a bacteriostatic antibiotic that binds to the 50S ribosomal subunit, blocking protein synthesis in susceptible bacteria. It has broad activity against aerobic and anaerobic gram-positive and gram-negative bacteria, including *S. aureus*, enterococci, and enteric gram-negative rods. It also is active against *Spirochetes*, *Rickettsia*, *Mycoplasma*, and *Chlamydia*. Today it is used almost exclusively for serious VRE infections. **Adverse effects** include idiosyncratic aplastic anemia (~1/30,000) and dose-related bone marrow suppression as the principal toxicities. Peak drug levels (1 hour postinfusion) should be checked every 3–4 days (goal peak <25) and doses adjusted accordingly. Dosage adjustment is necessary in the presence of significant liver disease. **This class of antibiotics has major drug interactions** (see Appendix C).

XI. **Metronidazole** (250–750 mg PO/IV q8h) kills anaerobic bacteria and some protozoa by accumulation of toxic metabolites that interfere with multiple biological processes. It has excellent tissue penetration, including abscess cavities, bone, and CNS. Metronidazole has greater activity against gram-negative than gram-positive anaerobes but is active against *Clostridium perfringens* and *difficile*. It is used as monotherapy to treat *C. difficile* colitis and bacterial vaginosis and in combination with other antibiotics to treat intra-abdominal infections and brain abscesses (see Chap. 14). Protozoan infections that are routinely treated with metronidazole include *Giardia*, *Entamoeba histolytica*, and *Trichomonas vaginalis*. A dose reduction may be warranted for patients with decompensated liver disease. **Adverse effects** include nausea, dysgeusia, disulfiram-like reactions to alcohol, and mild CNS disturbances (headache, restlessness). Rarely, this medication is associated with seizures and peripheral neuropathy.

XII. **Tetracyclines** are bacteriostatic antibiotics that bind the 30S ribosomal subunit blocking protein synthesis. These agents have unique roles in the treatment of *Rickettsia*, *Chlamydia*, *Nocardia*, and *Mycoplasma* infections. They are used as therapy for Lyme-related arthritis and as alternate therapy for syphilis and *P. multocida* in PCN-allergic patients. Their general use is limited because of widespread resistance among more common bacterial pathogens.

A. **Tetracycline** (250–500 mg PO q6h) is commonly used for severe acne and some *Helicobacter pylori* eradication regimens (see Chap. 17). Aluminum- and magnesium-containing antacids and preparations containing oral calcium, oral iron, or other cations can significantly impair oral absorption. Milk and antacids should be avoided within 2 hours of the dose. It can be used for treatment of acute Lyme borreliosis, Rocky Mountain spotted fever, psittacosis, *Mycoplasma* pneumonia, *Chlamydia* pneumonia (TWAR), and chlamydial infections of the eye or genitourinary tract, but these infections are generally treated with doxycycline or other antibiotics.

B. **Doxycycline** (100 PO/IV q12h) is the most commonly used tetracycline. It is standard therapy for *C. trachomatis*, Rocky Mountain spotted fever, ehrlichiosis, and psittacosis.

C. Minocycline (200 mg IV/PO, then 100 mg IV/PO q12h) is similar to doxycy-cline in its spectrum of activity and clinical indications. It is second-line therapy for pulmonary nocardiosis and cervicofacial actinomycosis.

D. Adverse effects. Nausea and photosensitivity are common side effects. Patients should be warned about sun exposure. Rarely, these medications are associated with pseudotumor cerebri. They cannot be given to children because they can cause tooth enamel discoloration.

XIII. Streptogramins are a new class of marginally bactericidal antimicrobial agents that complex with bacterial ribosomes to inhibit protein synthesis.

A. Quinupristin/dalfopristin (7.5 mg/kg IV q8h) is the only U.S. Food and Drug Administration (FDA)-approved drug in this class. This antibiotic combination gained FDA approval largely because of its activity against antibiotic-resistant gram-positive organisms, especially VRE, ORSA, VISA, and antibiotic-resistant strains of *Streptococcus pneumoniae*. It has some activity against gram-negative upper respiratory pathogens (*Haemophilus* and *Moraxella*) and anaer-obes, but more appropriate antibiotics are available to treat these infections. Quinupristin/dalfopristin should be reserved for serious infections with ORSA and *S. pneumoniae* when vancomycin cannot be tolerated. Quinupristin/dalfo-pristin is bacteriostatic for enterococci. It may be first-line therapy for serious infections with VISA and VRE (it has little activity against *Enterococcus faeca-lis*), although chloramphenicol remains reasonable therapy for VRE in settings in which it remains susceptible. For VRE peritonitis in continuous ambulatory peritoneal dialysis patients, IV therapy is combined with 25 mg/L quinupristin/ dalfopristin in alternate dialysis bags (*Lancet* 344:1025, 1994). In polymicrobial infections (in which a resistant organism has been identified or strongly sus-pected), consideration should be given to an additional agent such as a qui-nolone or cephalosporin to improve the gram-negative coverage. This antibiotic (or linezolid) may be the drug of choice if the much-feared debut of vancomycin-resistant *S. aureus* comes to pass.

B. Adverse effects include arthralgias and myalgias, which occur frequently and can force discontinuation of therapy. IV site pain and thrombophlebitis are common when the drug is administered through a peripheral vein. Quinupristin/dalfopristin has been associated with increased bilirubin lev-els. It is primarily cleared by hepatic metabolism and likely requires dose adjustment with significant hepatic impairment, but data are currently lacking. This drug should be avoided if possible in the setting of decompen-sated liver disease. **Quinupristin/dalfopristin is similar to erythromycin in regard to drug interactions** (see Appendix C).

XIV. Oxazolidinones are a new class of marginally bactericidal antibiotics that block assembly of bacterial ribosomes to inhibit protein synthesis. **Linezolid** (600 mg IV/PO bid; IV/PO drug levels are equivalent) is the only FDA-approved drug in this class. It has good activity against aerobic and anaerobic gram-positive bacteria, including drug-resistant enterococci, staphylococci, and streptococci. It has no meaningful activity against the Enterobacteriaceae and borderline activity against *Moraxella* and *H. influenzae*. A second agent such as a cephalosporin or quinolone should be considered for mixed infections. Clinical experience with this antibiotic has not been extensive. In early use it has shown excellent activity in VRE infections. Its activity against ORSA is comparable to that of vancomycin. Its use should be restricted to serious infections with VRE, patients with an indication for vancomycin therapy who are intolerant of that medication, and possibly for ORSA cellulitis (400 mg PO bid) when IV access is an issue. Use of this medication for other applications such as osteomyelitis and endocarditis cannot be recommended without supporting data. Resistance does develop to this antibiotic, and it is imperative that abscesses be adequately drained to minimize this risk. Linezolid is well tolerated. Its principal **adverse effects** are diarrhea, nausea, headaches, and thrombocytopenia that rarely limit therapy. A CBC, serum creatinine, and LFTs should probably be checked every 1–2 weeks during prolonged therapy with this new agent. Linezolid is a mild monoamine oxidase inhibitor. Patients should be advised to avoid over-the-counter cold remedies that contain pseudoephedrine or phenylpropanolamine, as coadministration with linezolid can elevate blood pressure. Linezolid does not require dose adjustments for renal or hepatic dysfunction.

XV. **Fosfomycin** (3-g sachet dissolved in cold water PO once) is a bactericidal oral antibiotic approved for treatment of uncomplicated UTIs. It kills bacteria by inhibiting an early step in cell wall synthesis and has an impressive spectrum of activity that includes all the major urinary pathogens and difficult-to-treat organisms, including *P. aeruginosa*, *Enterobacter* species, and enterococci (including VRE). It has formal FDA approval for treating uncomplicated UTIs in women with susceptible strains of *E. coli* and *E. faecalis*. It should not be used to treat pyelonephritis or systemic infections. It should only be administered once, as therapeutic drug levels are maintained in the urine for approximately 48 hours and repeat dosing does not improve clinical outcomes. No guidelines have been formulated for its use in significant renal impairment. Diarrhea is the most common adverse effect. Fosfomycin should not be taken with metoclopramide or cisapride, as they interfere with fosfomycin absorption.

XVI. **Nitrofurantoin macrocrystals** (50–100 mg PO qid for 5–7 days) are a bactericidal oral antibiotic useful for uncomplicated UTIs except those caused by *Proteus* species. The drug is metabolized by bacteria into toxic intermediates that inhibit multiple bacterial processes. This drug has had a modest resurgence, as it is frequently effective against uncomplicated VRE UTIs. It has no activity against *P. aeruginosa* or *Serratia* species. Although the drug was commonly used in the past for "UTI suppression" therapy, this should be avoided, as prolonged therapy is associated with chronic pulmonary syndromes that can be fatal. This drug should not be used for pyelonephritis or any other systemic infections. **Adverse effects** include nausea as the most common side effect. The drug should be taken with food to minimize this problem. Patients should be warned that their urine may become brown secondary to the medication. It should not be used with elevated serum creatinine, as the risk for development of treatment-associated neuropathy may be increased. Pulmonary toxicities are associated with prolonged therapy. Nitrofurantoin should not be given with probenecid, as this combination decreases the concentration of nitrofurantoin in the urine.

XVII. **Methenamine [methenamine hippurate or methenamine mandelate;** 1 or 2 tablets (depending on the specific preparation) PO qid] is a urine/bladder antiseptic that is converted into formaldehyde in the urine when the pH is less than 6.0. The pharmacy or package insert for the specific preparation should be consulted for dosing. Because the active drug is formaldehyde, nearly all bacteria and fungi are potentially susceptible to therapy. The formaldehyde is generated while the urine is retained in the bladder; therefore, methenamine is effective only in the lower urinary tract, and its efficacy is impaired in the setting of a draining Foley catheter. These drugs are rarely used because of the large number of alternative antibiotics that are available today. They do have a limited role in treating uncomplicated UTI caused by multiple drug–resistant bacteria or yeast. Urine pH should be obtained once early in therapy. **Adverse effects** include bladder irritation, dysuria, and hematuria with prolonged use. Therapy should be limited to a maximum of 3 weeks at a time. This drug is contraindicated in the setting of glaucoma, significant renal insufficiency, and acidosis. It should not be given concomitantly with sulfonamides, as these drugs form an insoluble precipitate in the urine.

XVIII. **Colistimethate** (**polymyxin E;** IV therapy is 2.5–5.0 mg/kg/day divided into 2–4 doses; maximum dose, 5 mg/kg/day) and **polymyxin B** [12,000–15,000 units/kg/day by continuous infusion (500,000 units in 500 ml 5% dextrose in water, adjust rate to achieve desired daily dosing)] are bactericidal polypeptide antibiotics that kill by disrupting the cell membrane of gram-negative bacteria. These drugs have roles in the treatment of multiple drug–resistant gram-negative rods, predominantly *P. aeruginosa*, in patients with CF or bronchiectasis. **These medications should only be given under the guidance of an experienced clinician, as parenteral therapy has significant CNS side effects and potential nephrotoxicity. Inhaled colistimethate** (75 mg given by standard nebulizer tid) is better tolerated, with only mild upper airway irritation, and has some efficacy as adjunctive therapy for *P. aeruginosa* (*J Antimicrob Chemother* 19:831, 1987). **Adverse effects** with parenteral therapy include paresthesias, slurred speech, peripheral numbness, tingling, and significant dose-dependent nephrotoxicity. The package insert or appropriate text should be consulted for dosing for patients with renal insufficiency, as overdosage in this setting can result in neuromuscular blockade and apnea. If CNS side effects are significant with bid dosing of colistimethate, qid dosing or continuous infusion (total daily dose in 500 ml 5% dextrose in water infused over 24 hours) should be arranged. Serum creatinine should be monitored daily early in therapy and then at a regular interval for the duration of therapy. These antibiotics should not be coadministered with aminoglycosides, other known nephrotoxins, or neuromuscular blockers.

Antituberculous Agents

Effective therapy of *Mycobacterium* TB (MTB) infections requires combination chemotherapy designed to prevent the emergence of resistant organisms. Increased resistance to the conventional antituberculous agents has led to the use of more complex regimens and has made susceptibility testing an integral part of TB management (see Chap. 14).

I. **Isoniazid** (INH, 300 mg PO qd) kills susceptible mycobacteria by interfering with the synthesis of the lipid components of the cell wall. It is well absorbed orally and has good penetration throughout the body including the CNS. It is a component of nearly all treatment regimens and can be given twice a week in directly observed therapy (15 mg/kg/dose; 900 mg maximum). INH remains the drug of choice for recent purified protein derivative conversions (300 mg PO qd for 9 months). **Adverse effects** include mild elevations in liver transaminases (20%). Elevations of greater than threefold necessitate holding therapy. The INH-induced hepatitis is potentiated by rifampin. It can be idiosyncratic but is usually seen in the setting of underlying liver disease or concomitant consumption of alcohol. Hepatic transaminases should be obtained at baseline and monthly in patients over 35 and in alcoholics. Patients with known liver dysfunction should have weekly LFTs during the initial stage of therapy. INH antagonizes vitamin B_6, potentially causing a peripheral neuropathy. This can be avoided or minimized by coadministration of pyridoxine, 25–50 mg PO qd, especially in the elderly, in pregnant women, and in patients with diabetes, renal failure, alcoholism, and seizure disorders.

II. **Rifamycins** kill susceptible mycobacteria by inhibiting the DNA-dependent RNA polymerase, thereby shutting down transcription.

   A. **Rifampin** (600 mg PO qd or twice a week) is active against many gram-positive and gram-negative bacteria in addition to MTB. It is also used as adjunctive therapy in prosthetic valve endocarditis due to coagulase-negative staphylococci (300 mg PO q8h). The drug is well absorbed orally and is widely distributed throughout the body including the cerebrospinal fluid (CSF).

   B. **Rifabutin** (300 mg PO qd) is principally used to treat TB and MAC infections in HIV-positive patients who are receiving highly active antiretroviral therapy. It has less deleterious effects on protease inhibitor metabolism than does rifampin (see Chap. 15).

   C. **Rifapentine** (600 mg PO twice a week for 2 months, then qwk to complete therapy) is a rifamycin that appears to be associated with more relapses than rifampin; therefore, it is typically not used as a first-line drug.

D. **Adverse effects.** Patients should be warned about reddish-orange discoloration of body fluids (and contact lenses). Rash, GI disturbances, hepatitis, and interstitial nephritis can occur. Uveitis has been associated with rifabutin and hyperuricemia with rifapentine. **This class of antibiotics has major drug interactions** (see Appendix C).

III. **Pyrazinamide** (15–30 mg/kg PO qd; maximum, 2 g or 50–75 mg/kg PO twice a week; maximum, 4 g/dose) kills mycobacteria replicating in macrophages by an unknown mechanism. It is well absorbed orally and widely distributed throughout the body including the CSF. Pyrazinamide is typically used for the first 2 months of therapy. **Adverse effects** include hyperuricemia and hepatitis.

IV. **Ethambutol** (15–25 mg/kg PO qd or 50–75 mg/kg PO twice a week; maximum, 2.5 g/dose) is bacteriostatic with an unknown mechanism of action. It is included in initial TB regimens in areas where the incidence of INH-resistant TB is greater than or equal to 4%. The lower dose should be used with initial therapy. **Adverse effects** includes optic neuritis, which manifests as decreased red-green color perception, decreased visual acuity, or visual field deficits. Baseline and monthly visual examinations should be performed during therapy.

V. **Streptomycin** is an aminoglycoside that is used as a substitute for ethambutol and for drug-resistant MTB. It does not penetrate the CNS and cannot be used for TB meningitis (see Antibacterial Agents, sec. **V.C.4**).

Antiviral Agents

Current antiviral agents only suppress viral replication. Viral containment or elimination requires an intact host immune response.

I. **Anti-influenza drugs** include two new drugs, zanamivir and oseltamivir, that block the influenza A and B neuraminidases. This enzymatic activity is necessary for successful viral egress and release from infected cells. These drugs have modest activity in clinical trials (1- to 2-day improvement in symptoms), and no studies have addressed the use of these agents in high-risk patients. They are well tolerated. Their role in treating influenza infections remains to be determined. Annual vaccination remains the intervention of choice for all high-risk patients.

A. **Amantadine** and **rimantadine** (100 mg PO bid for both; dose reduction to 100 mg PO qd is warranted in elderly patients and patients on dialysis or with decompensated liver disease) prevent influenza A entry into cells by blocking endosomal acidification, which is necessary for fusion of the viral envelope with the host cell membrane. These agents have no effect against influenza B. They are effective when therapy is initiated within 48 hours of initial symptoms and continued for 7–10 days. In the absence of complicating medical conditions or a new pandemic, influenza A infection usually resolves within 3–7 days if untreated. Patients at high risk of complications (e.g., immunocompromised patients, the elderly, diabetics, dialysis patients, and patients with pulmonary or cardiac disease) should probably be treated even after 48 hours of symptoms in the absence of studies that specifically address the treatment of high-risk patients. These drugs can be used for influenza A prophylaxis in nonimmune individuals who have been exposed to the virus and in patients and staff members of nursing homes or hospitals during an epidemic. All patients and staff who would meet the criteria for prophylaxis during outbreaks should be vaccinated annually unless they have known egg allergies. **Adverse effects** include GI disturbances and CNS dysfunction, including dizziness, nervousness, confusion, slurring of speech, blurred vision, and sleep disturbances. Rimantadine has fewer drug interactions than amantadine.

B. **Zanamivir** [10 mg (2 inhalations) q12h for 5 days, started within 48 hours of the onset of symptoms] is an inhaled neuraminidase inhibitor that is active against influenza A and B. Zanamivir is FDA approved for treatment of uncomplicated acute influenza infection in adults and adolescents over age 12 who have been symptomatic for less than 48 hours. When used within 30 hours of the onset of influenza symptoms, zanamivir reduces the duration of symptoms by an average of 1–2 days. The agent has also been used successfully for influenza prophylaxis, although it is not yet FDA approved for use in this setting. **Adverse effects** of zanamivir include headache, GI disturbances, dizziness, and upper respiratory symptoms. Bronchospasm or declines in lung function, or both, may occur in patients with underlying respiratory disorders and may require a rapid-acting bronchodilator for control.

   C. **Oseltamivir** (75 mg PO bid for 5 days) is an orally administered neuraminidase inhibitor that is active against influenza A and B. Oseltamivir is FDA approved for treatment of uncomplicated acute influenza in adults who have been symptomatic for less than 2 days. When used within 40 hours of the onset of influenza symptoms, oseltamivir was associated with a 1.3-day reduction in median time to clinical improvement. The most common **adverse effects** are nausea, vomiting, and diarrhea. Dizziness and headache may also occur.

II. **Antiherpetic agents** are nucleotide analogs that inhibit viral DNA synthesis.

   A. **Acyclovir** [400 mg PO tid for herpes simplex virus (HSV), 800 mg PO 5 times a day for localized varicella zoster virus (VZV) infections, 5 mg/kg IV q8h for severe HSV infections, and 10 mg/kg IV q8h for severe VZV infections and HSV encephalitis] is active against HSV and VZV. The drug has no effect on herpes viruses that are latent. Acyclovir is indicated for treatment of primary and recurrent genital herpes, severe herpetic stomatitis, and herpes simplex encephalitis. It is also used for herpes zoster ophthalmicus, disseminated primary VZV in adults (significant morbidity compared to the childhood illness), and severe disseminated primary VZV in children. It can be used as prophylaxis in patients who have frequent HSV recurrences (400 mg PO bid). **Adverse effects** including reversible crystalline nephropathy may occur; pre-existing renal failure, dehydration, and IV bolus dosing increase the risk of this effect. Rare cases of CNS disturbances, including delirium, tremors, and seizures, may also occur, particularly with high doses, in patients with renal failure and in the elderly.

   B. **Valacyclovir** (1000 mg PO q8h for herpes zoster, 1000 mg PO q12h for initial episode of genital HSV infection, and 500 mg PO q12h for recurrent episodes of HSV) is an orally administered prodrug of acyclovir that is used for treatment of acute herpes zoster infections and treatment or suppression of genital HSV infection. The most common **adverse effect** is nausea. Valacyclovir rarely causes CNS disturbances. High doses (8 g/day) have been associated with development of hemolytic-uremic syndrome/thrombotic thrombocytopenic purpura in immunocompromised patients, including those with HIV and bone marrow and solid organ transplants.

   C. **Famciclovir** (500 mg PO q8h for herpes zoster and 125 mg PO q12h for recurrent episodes of genital HSV infection) is an orally administered antiviral agent used for the treatment of acute herpes zoster reactivation and for treatment or suppression of genital HSV infections. **Adverse effects** include headache, nausea, and diarrhea.

   D. **Ganciclovir** [5 mg/kg IV q12h for 14–21 days for induction therapy of cytomegalovirus (CMV) retinitis, followed by 6 mg/kg IV for 5 days every week or 5 mg/kg IV qd; the oral dose is 1000 mg PO tid with food] is used to treat CMV. It has activity against HSV and VZV, but safer drugs are available to treat those infections. The drug is widely distributed in the body, including the CSF. Ganciclovir is indicated for treatment of CMV retinitis in immunocompromised patients and may be useful for other CMV diseases. Indefinite maintenance therapy generally is required to suppress CMV disease in patients with AIDS. Oral ganciclovir CMV prophylaxis is rarely used since the advent of highly active antiretroviral therapy in HIV care. The major **adverse effect** that limits therapy is neutropenia, and this may require the addition of granulocyte colony-stimulating factor for management (300 µg SC qwk–qd). Thrombocytopenia, rash, confusion, headache, nephrotoxicity, and GI disturbances may also occur. Blood counts and electrolytes should be monitored weekly while the patient is receiving therapy. **Other agents with nephrotoxic or bone marrow suppressive effects may enhance the adverse effects of ganciclovir.**

E. **Foscarnet** (60 mg/kg IV q8h or 90 mg/kg IV q12h for 14–21 days as induction therapy, followed by 90–120 mg/kg IV qd as maintenance therapy for CMV; the dose for acyclovir-resistant HSV and VZV is 40 mg/kg IV q8h) is used to treat CMV retinitis in patients with AIDS. It is typically considered for use in patients who are not tolerating or responding to ganciclovir. It is occasionally used for CMV disease in bone marrow transplant patients to avoid bone marrow suppression. Foscarnet has a role in treatment of acyclovir-resistant HSV/VZV infections or ganciclovir-resistant CMV infections. The major **adverse effect** is nephrotoxicity. A Cl_{Cr} should be obtained at baseline and repeated monthly during prolonged therapy. Electrolytes (PO_4, Ca^{2+}, Mg^{2+}, serum creatinine) should be checked twice a week. Normal saline (500–1000 ml) should be given before and during infusions to minimize nephrotoxicity. This drug should be avoided in patients with a serum creatinine of greater than 2.8 or baseline Cl_{Cr} of less than 50 ml/minute. Foscarnet chelates divalent cations and can cause tetany even with normal serum calcium levels. Other side effects include seizures, phlebitis, rash, and genital ulcers. Prolonged therapy with foscarnet should be monitored by experienced physicians who perform home IV therapy and systematically monitor patients' laboratory results. **One should avoid concomitant use of other nephrotoxins (amphotericin, aminoglycosides, pentamidine, nonsteroidal anti-inflammatory drugs, cisplatin, or cidofovir). Use of foscarnet with pentamidine can cause severe hypocalcemia.**

F. **Cidofovir** (5 mg/kg IV qwk for 2 weeks as induction therapy, followed by 5 mg/kg IV q14d chronically as maintenance therapy) is used to treat CMV retinitis in patients with AIDS. Efficacy of the drug is not established for CMV in other organ systems or in patients without AIDS. It can be administered through a peripheral IV line. Nephrotoxicity is the most important **adverse effect,** and the drug should be avoided in patients with a Cl_{Cr} of less than 55 ml/minute, a serum creatinine greater than 1.5 mg/dl, significant proteinuria, or a recent history of receipt of other nephrotoxic medications. Each cidofovir dose should be administered with probenecid (2 g PO 3 hours before the infusion and then 1 g at 2 and 8 hours after the infusion) along with 1 L normal saline IV 1–2 hours before the infusion to minimize nephrotoxicity. Patients should have serum creatinine and urine protein checked before each dose of cidofovir is given. These patients should be followed by experienced physicians who routinely administer therapy that requires systematic monitoring of patients' laboratory studies.

Antifungal Agents

I. **Amphotericin B** kills fungi by interacting with ergosterol to disrupt the fungal plasma membrane. Reformulation of this agent in various lipid complexes has decreased some of its adverse side effects.

A. **Amphotericin B deoxycholate** (standard; 0.3–1.25 mg/kg/day as a single infusion over 2–4 hours) is the mainstay of antifungal therapy for severely ill patients with fungal disease. The total dose for noncandidal species is 1.0–1.5 g. It is not effective for *Pseudallescheria boydii* and some other uncommon fungal pathogens. Amphotericin B is available as an oral suspension for treating thrush in HIV-positive patients (100 mg swish and swallow qid).

B. Lipid complexed preparations of amphotericin B including **amphotericin B lipid complex** (5 mg/kg IV qd), **liposomal amphotericin B** (3–5 mg/kg IV qd), and **amphotericin B colloidal dispersion** (3–4 mg/kg IV qd) have decreased nephrotoxicity and less frequent fever, chills, nausea, and CNS side effects. Despite these advantages, lipid complexed preparations have not yet been directly compared to standard amphotericin B therapy for most fungal infections. Studies have shown lipid preparations to be at least equivalent and possibly slightly superior to standard amphotericin B for empiric therapy in neutropenic fevers. However, no survival difference has been found. On the other hand, a lipid complexed preparation of amphotericin B showed disappointing effectiveness in HIV-positive patients with cryptococcal meningitis (*Clin Infect Dis* 22:315, 1996) and paracoccidioidomycosis (*Am J Trop Med Hyg* 60:837, 1999). Lipid complexed preparations of amphotericin B are very expensive. Based on currently available clinical data, no clear evidence exists for increased efficacy with the use of lipid complexed preparations. No good studies are available for comparing the lipid complexed preparations to each other. Lipid complexed amphotericin B is indicated primarily in patients who do not tolerate or respond to therapy with standard amphotericin B. As a general rule, all patients with normal serum creatinine should receive standard amphotericin B. Patients who have diabetes or known significant vascular disease, or require other nephrotoxic drugs require additional considerations. Minimum indications for using or switching to lipid complex preparations would be a serum creatinine of greater than 2.0, a doubling of the serum creatinine, or both.

C. The major **adverse effect** of amphotericin B is nephrotoxicity. Patients should receive 500–1000 ml normal saline before infusion to minimize nephrotoxicity that appears to be related to vasospasm in animal models. Other common side effects are fever/chills, nausea, headache, and myalgias. Premedication with 500–1000 mg acetaminophen controls many of these symptoms. More severe reactions can be premedicated with hydrocortisone, 25–100 mg IV. Intolerable infusion-related chills can be managed with meperidine, 25–50 mg IV. Amphotericin B therapy is associated with potassium and magnesium wasting that requires supplementation. Serum creatinine and electrolytes (including Mg^{2+} and K^+) should be monitored at least twice a week. Irreversible renal failure appears to be related to cumulative dosing. **One should avoid coadministration of other known nephrotoxins.**

II. Flucytosine (5-FC, 25.0–37.5 mg/kg PO q6h) kills susceptible *Candida* species and cryptococci by interfering with DNA synthesis. Its main clinical uses are for treatment of cryptococcal meningitis and *Candida* endocarditis in combination with amphotericin B. Less toxic azole therapy is used for candidal UTIs. **Adverse effects** include dose-related bone marrow suppression and bloody diarrhea due to intestinal flora conversion of 5-FC to 5-fluorouracil. Peak drug levels should be monitored to keep peak levels between 50 and 100 µg/ml. Dose adjustment and close monitoring by levels are critical in the setting of renal insufficiency. LFTs should be done at least once a week.

III. Azoles are fungistatic agents that inhibit ergosterol synthesis. **These agents should not be given with cisapride, as this combination can cause fatal arrhythmias. Coadministration with digoxin requires careful monitoring of levels.**

A. Itraconazole (200–400 mg PO qd or 200 mg IV q12h for 4 doses, then 200 mg IV qd) is a triazole with broad-spectrum antifungal activity. It is commonly used to treat histoplasmosis, blastomycosis, and *Sporothrix* infections. It may be the therapy of choice for fungi that are resistant to amphotericin B such as *P. boydii*. It is second-line therapy for *Aspergillus*, but it is being used more often as primary therapy or to "consolidate" a course of conventional amphotericin B. It can be used to treat infections caused by dermatophytes including onychomycosis of the toenails (200 mg PO qd for 12 weeks) and fingernails (200 mg PO bid for 1 week, with a 3-

week interruption, and then a second course of 200 mg PO bid for 1 week). The capsules require food/gastric acidity for absorption, whereas the elixir is better absorbed on an empty stomach.

B. Fluconazole (100–400 mg PO/IV qd) is typically the drug of choice for local-ized candidal infections such as UTIs, thrush, esophagitis, peritonitis, and hepatosplenic infection. It remains a second-line agent in severe dissemi-nated candidal infections behind amphotericin B. It is also a second-line agent for treatment of cryptococcal meningitis (400 mg PO qd for 10–12 weeks, then 200 mg PO qd). It is commonly used to suppress cryptococcal meningitis in immunocompromised patients (200 mg PO qd) after initial therapy with amphotericin B and flucytosine. Single-dose therapy is effec-tive for vaginal yeast infections (150 mg PO once). Fluconazole is not active against *Aspergillus* species. Its absorption is not dependent on gastric acid.

C. Ketoconazole (200–600 mg PO qd) is useful for treating histoplasmosis, blas-tomycosis, and chromomycosis infections outside of the CNS. It is not effec-tive for *Aspergillus* species. Its absorption is dependent on gastric acidity.

D. The most common **adverse effects** are nausea, diarrhea, and rashes. Hepa-titis is a rare but serious complication. Therapy must be monitored closely in the setting of compromised liver function (weekly LFTs). Itraconazole levels should be checked after 1 week of therapy to confirm absorption. IV itraconazole should be avoided in patients with a Cl_{Cr} of less than 30 ml/minute to avoid excessive accumulation of the hydroxyl-beta-cyclodextrin vehicle. Ketoconazole antagonizes testosterone metabolism, and antiandro-gen side effects can occur with prolonged therapy. **This class of antibiotics has major drug interactions** (see Appendix C).

IV. Terbinafine (250 mg PO qd for 6–12 weeks) is an allylamine antifungal agent that kills fungi by inhibiting ergosterol synthesis. It is approved for the treatment of onychomycosis of the fingernail (6 weeks of treatment) or toenail (12 weeks of treatment). It is not used for systemic infections. The main **adverse effects** are headache, GI disturbances, rash, LFT abnormalities, and taste disturbances. Terbinafine should not be used in patients with hepatic cirrhosis or a Cl_{Cr} of less than 50 ml/minute because of inadequate data. Terbinafine has only moderate affinity for cytochrome P-450 hepatic enzymes and does not significantly inhibit the metabolism of cyclosporine (15% decrease) or warfarin.

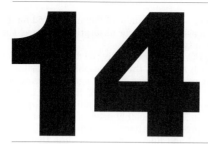

Treatment of Infectious Diseases

Linda M. Mundy

Principles of Therapy

The decision to institute antimicrobial chemotherapy should be made carefully. Aside from the expense and potential for adverse effects associated with any drug, indiscriminate use of antimicrobials has hastened the development of drug resistance. When antimicrobial therapy is indicated, a number of factors must be considered. When antimicrobial agents are not readily available due to industry-related shortages, consultation with an infectious disease expert for alternative therapeutic options is prudent. For dosing of antimicrobial agents in patients with renal insufficiency, see Appendix E.

I. **Choice of initial antimicrobial therapy.** The infecting organism often is unknown when therapy is initiated. In these cases, empiric therapy should be directed against the most likely pathogens, using a regimen that possesses the narrowest spectrum that adequately covers the predicted organisms. Therapy should then be altered in accordance with the patient's course and laboratory results.

   A. **During the initial evaluation,** a Gram stain of potentially infected material often permits a rapid presumptive diagnosis and may be essential for interpretation of subsequent culture results.

   B. **Local susceptibility patterns** must be considered in selecting empiric therapy because patterns vary widely among communities and individual hospitals.

   C. **Cultures** are usually necessary for precise diagnosis and are required for susceptibility testing. Whenever organisms with special growth requirements are suspected, the microbiology laboratory should be consulted to ensure appropriate transport and processing of cultures.

   D. **Antimicrobial susceptibility testing** facilitates a rational selection of antimicrobial agents and should be performed on nearly all significant positive cultures.

II. **Status of the host.** The clinical status of the patient determines the speed with which therapy must be instituted, the route of administration, and the type of therapy (*Clin Infect Dis* 29:264, 1999). Patients should be evaluated promptly for hemodynamic stability, rapidly progressive or life-threatening infections, and immune defects.

   A. **Timing of the initiation of antimicrobial therapy.** In acute clinical scenarios, empiric therapy usually is begun immediately after appropriate cultures have been obtained. However, if the patient's condition is stable, delaying the empiric use of antimicrobials might permit specific therapy based on the results of culture and susceptibility testing and might avoid adverse effects from the use of unnecessary drugs. Urgent therapy is indicated in febrile patients who are neutropenic or asplenic. In other immunosuppressed patients, fever alone seldom warrants urgent therapy; rather, the overall clinical assessment determines the need for empiric antimicrobials (see Chap. 21). Sepsis, meningitis, and rapidly progressive anaerobic or necrotizing infections should also be treated promptly with antimicrobials.

B. **Route of administration.** Patients with serious infections should be given antimicrobial agents intravenously. In less urgent circumstances, IM or oral therapy often is sufficient. Oral therapy is acceptable when it can be tolerated by the patient and when it is likely to produce adequate drug concentrations at the site of infection.

C. **Type of therapy.** Bactericidal therapy is indicated for patients with immunologic compromise or life-threatening infection. It is preferred also for infections characterized by impaired regional host defenses, such as endocarditis, meningitis, and osteomyelitis.

D. **Pregnancy and the puerperium.** Although no antimicrobial is known to be completely safe in pregnancy, the penicillins and cephalosporins are used most often. **Tetracyclines and quinolones are among the agents specifically contraindicated,** and the sulfonamides and aminoglycosides should not be used if alternative agents are available (see Appendix B). Most antibiotics administered in therapeutic dosages appear in breast milk and therefore should be used with caution in patients who are breast-feeding.

III. **Antimicrobial combinations.** The indiscriminate use of antimicrobial combinations should be avoided because of the potential for increased toxicity, pharmacologic antagonism, and the selection of resistant organisms. The empiric use of multiple antimicrobials to provide broader coverage is justified in seriously ill patients when (1) the identity of an infecting organism is not apparent, (2) the suspected pathogen has a variable antimicrobial susceptibility, or (3) failure to initiate effective antimicrobial therapy will likely increase morbidity or mortality. In addition, antimicrobial combinations are specifically indicated to produce synergism (e.g., enterococcal endocarditis), to treat polymicrobial infections (e.g., peritonitis after rupture of a viscus), and to prevent the emergence of antimicrobial resistance [e.g., tuberculosis (TB)].

IV. **Assessment of antimicrobial therapy.** When therapy is initiated or is to be continued, one should consider the following questions: Is the isolated organism the etiologic agent? Is adequate antimicrobial therapy being provided? Is the antimicrobial agent penetrating to the site of infection? Have resistant pathogens emerged? Is a persistent fever due to underlying disease, an iatrogenic complication, a drug reaction, or another process?

V. **Duration of therapy.** The duration of therapy depends on the nature of the infection and the severity of the clinical presentation. Treatment of acute uncomplicated infections should be continued until the patient has been afebrile and clinically well for a minimum of 72 hours. Infections at certain sites (e.g., endocarditis, septic arthritis, osteomyelitis) require more prolonged therapy.

Fever and Rash

Petechial, purpuric, and macular skin eruptions are associated with several important systemic infections. Because many of these infections are due to meningitis-causing organisms or present with a headache as well as a rash, a lumbar puncture frequently is a necessary part of the routine evaluation of these illnesses.

I. **Initial therapy** of the severely ill patient with fever and a disseminated rash must include coverage for the more common and life-threatening diseases that can present in this way, including meningococcemia, pneumococcemia, and Rocky Mountain spotted fever. Unless the initial history and physical examination strongly suggest a particular diagnosis, a reasonable empiric regimen is ceftriaxone, 2 g IV q12h, plus doxycycline, 100 mg IV or PO q12h. Antimicrobial coverage can be altered once the results of additional studies (e.g., cultures and susceptibility tests) are available.

II. **Specific considerations**

A. *Neisseria meningitidis* **septicemia (meningococcemia)** should be considered in any febrile patient with a petechial, purpuric, or macular rash because of its high mortality and potentially rapid course. The diagnosis can frequently be made from a Gram stain of petechial scrapings, a peripheral blood buffy-coat specimen, or cerebrospinal fluid (CSF) if concomitant meningitis is present. The treatment of choice for confirmed meningococcemia is penicillin G, 300,000 units/kg/day (maximum, 24 million units/day), divided into q2h doses. Antimicrobial susceptibility testing should be performed; PCN-resistant strains require cephalosporin administration. Chloramphenicol can be used in the severely beta-lactam–allergic patient.

B. Encapsulated bacteria such as *Streptococcus pneumoniae* and *Haemophilus influenzae* may produce a clinical presentation similar to that of meningococcemia, primarily in asplenic patients (see Meningitis).

C. Rocky Mountain spotted fever due to *Rickettsia rickettsii* typically begins with fever, chills, headache, and myalgias. A characteristic macular rash develops 1–5 days later. With time, the rash may become petechial. Treatment with doxycycline, 100 mg IV or PO q12h for 14 days, or chloramphenicol, 1 g IV q6h for 14 days, is recommended (see Zoonoses and Arthropod-Borne Diseases, sec. **I.A**).

D. Ehrlichiosis, due to *Ehrlichia chaffeensis* and other *Ehrlichia* species, may present with a rash and be clinically indistinguishable from Rocky Mountain spotted fever. Treatment consists of doxycycline, 100 mg IV or PO q12h. Chloramphenicol is not effective (see Zoonoses and Arthropod-Borne Diseases, sec. **I.B**).

E. Other infections associated with macular, maculopapular, or petechial rashes include typhoid fever (rose spots), endocarditis, disseminated gonorrhea, and disseminated candidiasis in the neutropenic host. Noninfectious causes include drug reactions [e.g., trimethoprim-sulfamethoxazole (TMP/SMX)] and collagen vascular disease (e.g., systemic lupus erythematosus). Self-induced disease must be considered in patients with persistent, refractory skin lesions.

Sepsis

I. Septic shock is caused by bacteremia more often than fungemia or viremia. Two phases can occur clinically: an early hyperdynamic phase and a later hypodynamic phase (see Chap. 9).

II. Early antimicrobial treatment is essential. If a probable source of infection is evident, antimicrobials can be selected to treat the most likely pathogens originating from that site. If no obvious source is discovered, empiric antimicrobial selection should be based on the clinical situation. Before therapy is initiated, specimens of potentially infected body fluids should be collected for Gram stain and culture. Two sets of blood cultures should be obtained from separate venipuncture sites. Empiric coverage usually includes a beta-lactam antimicrobial agent plus an aminoglycoside.

A. For community-acquired sepsis with no obvious underlying disease, a first-generation cephalosporin plus an aminoglycoside covers most potential pathogens.

B. Asplenic patients are at particular risk for fulminant sepsis with encapsulated organisms such as *S. pneumoniae*, *H. influenzae*, and *N. meningitidis*. Penicillin G, 2 million units IV q2–4h, or vancomycin, 1 g IV q12h, plus a third-generation cephalosporin (e.g., ceftriaxone, 2 g IV q12h) should be administered promptly. A Gram stain of a buffy-coat specimen can subsequently be performed, which sometimes reveals the pathogen.

C. Catheter-associated nosocomial septicemia usually is due to *Staphylococcus aureus*, coagulase-negative staphylococci, aerobic gram-negative bacilli, or enterococci. Vancomycin plus an aminoglycoside is appropriate initial therapy (see Catheter-Related Infections).

D. Neutropenic hosts, in whom *Pseudomonas aeruginosa* sepsis may be likely, usually are treated with an antipseudomonal beta-lactam antimicrobial agent plus an aminoglycoside. The addition of an antistaphylococcal agent such as vancomycin may be warranted in patients with indwelling central venous catheters (CVCs) (see Chap. 21).

Catheter-Related Infections

CVCs are increasingly used in acute and chronic health care delivery today. While providing convenient and beneficial venous access, CVCs contribute to more than 200,000 catheter-related bloodstream infections (CR-BSIs) annually, with associated increases in mortality, hospital stay, and medical costs.

I. **Diagnostic measures.** Clinical findings that increase the clinical suspicion of CR-BSIs are local inflammation or phlebitis at the CVC insertion site, sepsis, endophthalmitis, lack of other source of bacteremia, and resolution of fever after catheter removal. Blood cultures should initially be drawn through the catheter and from peripheral venipuncture.

II. **Therapy.** Typical (*S. aureus*, *Staphylococcus epidermidis*) and unusual (*Pseudomonas cepacia*, *Enterobacter agglomerans*, *Enterobacter cloacae*, *Candida albicans*) pathogens have been associated with CR-BSIs.

   A. **Initial empiric antimicrobial therapy.** Host factors such as comorbidities, infusates, severity of illness, multidrug-resistant colonization, prior infections, and current antimicrobial agents are important considerations when selecting the initial antimicrobial regimen.

   B. **Pathogen-specific therapy.** Once the pathogen has been identified, antimicrobial therapy should be narrowed to the most effective regimen. Duration of treatment should be longer if the CVC remains in situ.

   C. **Isolated catheter-related candidemia** in immunocompetent hosts can be treated with a short course of amphotericin B (0.5 mg/kg/day IV for a total of 250–500 mg) if the candidemia resolves promptly with catheter removal. Fluconazole (200–400 mg PO qd for 14 days) is an alternative.

   D. **CVC removal** may involve complex decision making with consideration of host status, ongoing vascular access, and the identified pathogen. CVCs should always be removed if local inflammation or phlebitis is present at the insertion site. Immunosuppressed patients with CVCs who have fever, neutropenia, and hemodynamic instability should have CVCs removed immediately. The majority of septic patients with short-term CVCs should have CVCs removed at the first signs of sepsis. Decisions for removal of long-term catheters are tailored to the clinical scenario. All catheter-associated yeast infections and essentially all CR-BSIs due to gram-negative pathogens and *S. aureus* require catheter removal.

III. **Prevention**

   A. **Placement.** Aseptic insertion techniques are imperative with CVC placement. Tincture of iodine skin preparation can reduce the risk of pseudobacteremia from coagulase-negative staphylococci (*Am J Med* 107:119, 1999). In addition, the location of the CVCs can have an impact on the risk for CR-BSIs. Internal jugular CVCs are associated with higher CR-BSIs than are subclavian venous catheters, presumably due to proximity to oropharyngeal secretions, higher skin temperature, and difficulties in immobilizing the CVC and maintaining occlusive dressings. Emergent line placement is also a risk factor for CR-BSI. SC tunneling of the CVCs can reduce the incidence of internal jugular CR-BSIs in critically ill patients (*JAMA* 276:1416, 1996). Femoral CVCs have the highest rates of CR-BSIs and should be removed within 72 hours of placement. The incidence of femoral CR-BSIs in critically ill patients can be reduced by using SC tunneling (*Ann Intern Med* 130:729, 1999).

B. **Antiseptic impregnated CVCs** appear to be associated with lower incidences of catheter colonization and CR-BSIs (*Ann Intern Med* 127:257, 1997; *JAMA* 281:261, 1999).

C. **Catheter care.** Strategies to decrease the incidence of CR-BSIs include the use of transparent dressings, strict adherence to aseptic technique and handwashing, antiseptic impregnated catheter cuffs, topical antiseptic solutions, and routine catheter changes by experienced health care workers. Topical antimicrobial ointment, in-line membrane filters, and frequent dressing changes are interventions that have not been associated with reduced CR-BSIs. Exchange of CVCs over guidewires is controversial and not routinely recommended.

Meningitis

Acute bacterial meningitis is a medical emergency. Meningitis should be considered in any patient with fever and neurologic symptoms, especially if he or she has a history of other infection or head trauma. Prognosis depends on the interval between the onset of disease and the initiation of antimicrobial therapy. Antimicrobial therapy should be instituted without delay, and appropriate diagnostic procedures should follow.

I. **Diagnostic measures.** In the absence of focal neurologic signs, a lumbar puncture for CSF opening pressure and a CSF specimen should be obtained. A CT scan of the head, preferably with contrast medium, is indicated in the patient with focal neurologic signs or a diminished level of consciousness.

A. **Cultures.** CSF specimens should be taken to the laboratory immediately. Blood, nasal swabs, and aspirates of skin lesions should be handled similarly. If viral meningitis is a possibility, CSF specimens should be cultured promptly. If prompt culturing is not possible, CSF and serum should be frozen at –70°C. Viral cultures of the throat and stool may provide additional evidence for the cause of the meningitis. Culture of the CSF remains the gold standard for pathogen identification. *S. pneumoniae* and *N. meningitidis* are responsible for most cases of adult bacterial meningitis.

B. **CSF examination** should include cell counts (including a WBC differential count) and a Gram stain of the centrifuged sediment. CSF pleocytosis with negative cultures might be associated with viral meningoencephalitis, parameningeal infection, neoplastic disease, subarachnoid hemorrhage, trauma, and partially treated bacterial meningitis. Chronic meningitis due to fungi or mycobacteria also should be considered if initial cultures for bacteria are negative. Neutrophilic pleocytosis usually is seen in bacterial meningitis but might also be present early in viral meningitis. In very early bacterial meningitis, pleocytosis may be absent. A cryptococcal antigen test and an acid-fast stain should be examined if Gram staining does not yield a diagnosis. A wet-mount examination of the sediment may reveal motile amebas in amebic meningoencephalitis. The CSF protein commonly is elevated and the glucose level is decreased in bacterial meningitis and in tuberculous and fungal meningitis. Detection of capsular polysaccharide antigens is possible for *S. pneumoniae, H. influenzae* type B, *N. meningitidis* (groups A and C), and group B streptococci; however, these are rarely performed because of false-positive and false-negative results. In contrast, the detection of capsular polysaccharide of *Cryptococcus neoformans* in CSF by latex agglutination is sensitive and specific when positive at a dilution of 1:4 or greater (see Systemic Mycoses, sec. **V**).

II. **Supportive measures.** Among supportive measures are maintenance of electrolyte balance, airway patency, and fluid restriction for seizure prophylaxis. Use of glucocorticoids as adjuvant treatment to antimicrobial therapy of meningitis in adults is controversial.

III. **Initial antimicrobial therapy.** When bacterial meningitis is suspected, high-dose parenteral antimicrobial therapy should be administered. If the cause of the meningitis is unclear, antimicrobials should be chosen on the basis of the clinical setting and the CSF Gram stain (*N Engl J Med* 336:708, 1997). If no organisms are seen on the Gram stain, use of a third-generation cephalosporin (e.g., ceftriaxone, 2 g IV q12h, or cefotaxime, 2 g IV q4h) is prudent while culture results are pending. In areas where pneumococcal penicillin resistance is higher than 5%, vancomycin should be combined with the ceftriaxone or cefotaxime until culture and susceptibility data are available. *Listeria* species should be considered in immunocompromised adults and those patients older than 50 years, and therapy should include ampicillin. In the postneurosurgical setting, or after head or spinal trauma, broad-spectrum coverage with vancomycin and ceftazidime is indicated. Empiric antibiotic regimens should be altered once culture and sensitivity data are known.

IV. **Therapy for specific infections**
  A. **For *S. pneumoniae*,** penicillin G, 300,000 units/kg/day (maximum, 24 million units/day) divided into q2h or q4h doses for 10–14 days, is appropriate when the isolate is fully susceptible to penicillin. Penicillin-allergic patients can be given a skin test and desensitized, treated with ceftriaxone or cefotaxime (if the allergic reaction was mild), or treated with chloramphenicol, 1.0–1.5 g IV q6h, unless the isolate is penicillin resistant. Alternatively, vancomycin, 1 g IV q12h, can be used. Therapy for penicillin-resistant pneumococci depends on the results of cephalosporin sensitivity testing; combination therapy of ceftriaxone, 2 g IV q12h, and vancomycin, 1 g IV q12h, is recommended (*N Engl J Med* 336:708, 1997; *Antimicrob Agents Chemother* 39:2171, 1995).
  B. **For *N. meningitidis*,** penicillin G, 300,000 units/kg/day (maximum, 24 million units/day) divided into q2h doses, should be continued for at least 5 days after the patient has become afebrile. Penicillin-allergic patients can be given a skin test and desensitized; treated with ceftriaxone, 2 g IV q12h, or cefotaxime, 2 g IV q4h (if the allergic reaction was mild); or treated with chloramphenicol. Patients with meningococcal meningitis should be placed in a private room on respiratory isolation for at least the first 24 hours of treatment. Close contacts (e.g., persons living in the same household) should receive prophylaxis with rifampin (RIF), 600 mg PO bid for 2 days, or single-dose therapy with either ciprofloxacin, 500 mg PO, or ceftriaxone, 250 mg IM. Terminal component complement deficiency (C6–C9) should be ruled out in patients with recurrent meningococcal infections.
  C. ***H. influenzae*** is a rare cause of meningitis in adults. Cefotaxime or ceftriaxone is effective as initial therapy. Chloramphenicol is the preferred alternative for patients allergic to penicillin and cephalosporins. Ampicillin, 2 g IV q4h, is the drug of choice for beta-lactamase–negative strains. Treatment should continue for at least 10 days.
  D. ***S. aureus*** is a rare cause of meningitis and produces high mortality despite treatment. It can be caused by high-grade staphylococcal bacteremia, direct extension from a parameningeal focus, a neurosurgical procedure, or skull trauma. Initially, oxacillin, 2 g IV q4h, should be given. First-generation cephalosporins should not be used because they do not enter the CSF. Vancomycin, 1 g IV q12h, is the drug of choice for penicillin-allergic patients and when oxacillin resistance is likely or is confirmed by susceptibility testing. Documentation of adequate CSF levels may be prudent, particularly in patients who respond poorly to therapy. RIF may be beneficial in cases of oxacillin-resistant *S. aureus* meningitis that does not respond to vancomycin alone.
  E. ***S. epidermidis*** (and other coagulase-negative staphylococci) meningitis usually is secondary to an infected ventricular shunt. Vancomycin, 1 g IV q12h, is the drug of choice. Intraventricular vancomycin, 10 mg qd–qod, may be a useful adjunct. A combination of RIF and vancomycin has not shown superiority over vancomycin alone. Removal of an infected shunt is often necessary for cure.
  F. **Gram-negative bacillary meningitis** occurs as a result of head trauma and neurosurgical procedures and in neonates, the elderly, and debilitated

patients. Third-generation cephalosporins such as cefotaxime or ceftriaxone are indicated for susceptible pathogens. TMP/SMX, chloramphenicol, and ampicillin are alternatives. Ceftazidime, 2 g IV q8h, has been used effectively for *P. aeruginosa* meningitis but should probably be combined with IV aminoglycoside therapy.

G. *Listeria monocytogenes* is a cause of meningitis in immunosuppressed adults and the elderly. Treatment is with ampicillin, 2 g IV q4h (or penicillin G, 2 million units IV q2h), in combination with a systemically administered aminoglycoside for at least 3–4 weeks. TMP/SMX (TMP, 5 mg/kg IV q6h) is an alternative for the penicillin-allergic patient.

H. **Acute aseptic meningitis** is defined as any infectious or noninfectious meningitis for which the etiology is not apparent after the initial clinical evaluation and CSF analysis with routine stains and cultures. The differential diagnosis includes enteroviruses, arboviruses, mumps virus, lymphocytic choriomeningitis virus, herpesvirus, HIV, and drug-induced inflammatory processes. Following colonization or exposure, hematogenous dissemination is often followed by CNS invasion. CSF pleocytosis is common and CSF PCR can detect enteroviruses and herpesviruses. For enteroviruses, the treatment is supportive care. For suspected herpesvirus meningitis, high-dose acyclovir is empirically started until CSF PCR studies are negative.

Infective Endocarditis

Infective endocarditis (IE) usually is caused by gram-positive cocci. Parenteral drug users and patients with catheter-associated sepsis are at an increased risk for contracting staphylococcal disease. Gram-negative and fungal endocarditides are infrequent and usually occur in IV drug abusers or in patients with prosthetic valves. Clinical features are influenced by the causative organism. Patients may present acutely (within 3–10 days) with critical illness **(acute bacterial endocarditis)** or subacutely **(subacute bacterial endocarditis)** with symptoms of fatigue, weight loss, low-grade fever, immune complex disease (nephritis, arthralgias), and emboli (renal, splenic, and cerebral infarcts; petechiae; Osler's nodes; Janeway lesions). A deformed or previously damaged valve is the usual focus of infection in subacute bacterial endocarditis. Left-sided endocarditis occurs most commonly with pre-existing valvular disease. Dental procedures and bacteremia from distant foci of infection are frequent seeding events; instrumentation of the genitourinary or GI tract is a less common cause. Right-sided endocarditis, involving the tricuspid or pulmonic valves, is seen most frequently in parenteral drug abusers and in hospitalized patients with vascular catheters.

I. **Diagnosis.** The most reliable diagnostic criterion is continuous bacteremia in a compatible clinical setting.

A. **Blood cultures** are positive in at least 90% of patients. The yield can be reduced if the patient has received antimicrobial therapy within 1–2 weeks. Three culture samples should be taken from separate sites over at least a 1-hour period before empiric therapy is begun.

B. **Echocardiography** is not a routine diagnostic test for IE. Patients with IE and vegetations seen by conventional echocardiography are at higher risk of embolism, heart failure, and valvular disruption. A normal echocardiogram does not exclude the diagnosis of IE. Likewise, false-positive findings occur with myxomatous valvular degeneration, ruptured chordae tendineae, and atrial myxomas. Echocardiography is used, however, in the Duke criteria for endocarditis (*Am J Cardiol* 77:403, 1996). **Transesophageal echocardiography** is more sensitive than M-mode or two-dimensional techniques. Visualization of vegetations alone does not mandate surgical intervention.

Vegetations visualized by echocardiography may persist unchanged for at least 3 years after clinical cure.

II. **Treatment** of bacterial endocarditis of native valves requires high doses of antimicrobials for extended periods. Quantitative susceptibility testing of the responsible organism(s) to multiple antibiotics is more reliable than disk diffusion testing and is essential to ensure that optimal treatment is administered. Measurement of the serum bactericidal titer (SBT) is recommended for endocarditis with inherently resistant or tolerant organisms (e.g., enterococci) or when response to therapy is suboptimal. Interpretation of the SBT is controversial, but peak and trough SBTs of at least 1:64 and 1:32, respectively, correlate with bacteriologic cure, and attainment of an SBT titer of 1:8–1:16 is recommended. **Baseline audiometry** is recommended for patients who will receive 7 or more days of aminoglycoside therapy, with follow-up audiometry contingent on the duration of treatment or symptom development.

A. **Acute bacterial endocarditis** requires empiric antimicrobial treatment before culture results become available. *S. aureus* and gram-negative bacilli are the most likely pathogens. Treatment for *S. aureus* should include oxacillin, 2 g IV q4h, plus gentamicin or tobramycin, 1.0–1.5 mg/kg IV q8h. Therapy can then be modified on the basis of culture and susceptibility data.

B. **Subacute bacterial endocarditis (SBE)** is caused most often by streptococci. Penicillin therapy typically results in cure rates of more than 90%. *Streptococcus bovis* bacteremia and endocarditis are associated with lower GI disease, including neoplasms. Group B and G streptococcal endocarditis may also be associated with lower intestinal pathology.

1. **For viridans streptococci,** penicillin G, 2 million units IV q4h for 4 weeks, is effective for penicillin-susceptible strains [minimal inhibitory concentration (MIC) <0.1 μg/ml]. Therapy with parenteral penicillin and an aminoglycoside for 2 weeks is an alternative, but extended aminoglycoside treatment should be avoided in the elderly and in patients who cannot tolerate the potential nephrotoxicity or ototoxicity (*Clin Infect Dis* 27:1470, 1998). If the penicillin MIC equals or exceeds 0.1 μg/ml but is not more than 0.5 μg/ml, the addition of streptomycin or gentamicin may be appropriate for the first 2 weeks of therapy, followed by penicillin G alone for 2 weeks. Patients with endocarditis caused by streptococci with penicillin MICs in excess of 0.5 μg/ml may require combination therapy similar to that given for enterococcal IE (*JAMA* 274:1706, 1995). In patients who are allergic to penicillin, skin testing and desensitization should be considered. Vancomycin is an acceptable alternative.

2. **Group A beta-hemolytic streptococci and *S. pneumoniae*** should be treated with penicillin G, 2–4 million units IV q4h for 4–6 weeks. Penicillin-resistant pneumococci should be treated with ceftriaxone daily for 4–6 weeks.

3. ***Enterococcus* species** cause 10–20% of cases of subacute bacterial endocarditis. Recommended treatment regimens are ampicillin, 2 g IV q4h, or penicillin G, 3–5 million units IV q4h, in combination with gentamicin, 1.0–1.5 mg/kg IV q8h for 4–6 weeks. In susceptible strains, vancomycin in combination with an aminoglycoside is effective and should be used for penicillin-allergic patients or patients with beta-lactamase–producing strains. Aminoglycoside and vancomycin levels should be monitored. Baseline and weekly audiometry also is recommended. SBTs should be determined to optimize therapy. In enterococcal endocarditis, high-level resistance to either or both gentamicin and streptomycin occurs. Isolates that are resistant to gentamicin and to streptomycin are resistant to all aminoglycosides. The optimal management in the face of high-level resistance to all aminoglycosides is unclear. Isolates from patients with enterococcal endocarditis should be screened for beta-lactamase production and vancomycin resistance.

4. **S. aureus** should be treated with oxacillin, 2 g IV q4h for 6 weeks. An aminoglycoside can be added during the first 3–5 days of therapy or in patients who do not respond to beta-lactam therapy alone. The prognosis is better in young parenteral drug abusers with right-sided endocarditis, in whom treatment with oxacillin for 4 weeks might be sufficient. Older patients with aortic valve infection have a high mortality and often require surgical intervention. For IE caused by oxacillin-resistant *S. aureus*, vancomycin is the drug of choice. Cephalosporins should not be used in such cases, even if the isolate is sensitive in vitro.

5. **S. epidermidis** infection leading to endocarditis primarily occurs in patients with valvular prostheses. These organisms often are resistant to penicillin, semisynthetic penicillins, and the cephalosporins. Pending susceptibility studies, the treatment of choice is vancomycin, 1 g IV q12h, in combination with RIF, 300 mg PO q8h for at least 6–8 weeks, along with gentamicin, 1 mg/kg IV q8h for the first 2 weeks of therapy. Vancomycin and aminoglycoside levels should be monitored. Because detection of beta-lactam resistance in coagulase-negative staphylococci is potentially difficult, beta-lactam therapy for serious coagulase-negative staphylococci infections is controversial.

6. **HACEK** is an acronym for a group of fastidious, slow-growing gram-negative bacteria (*Haemophilus*, *Actinobacillus*, *Cardiobacterium*, *Eikenella*, and *Kingella* species) that have a predilection for infecting heart valves. The treatment of choice is ceftriaxone (or another third-generation cephalosporin). Four weeks of therapy is standard for native valve infection. Penicillin or ampicillin plus an aminoglycoside can be substituted.

7. **When IE is suspected but routine cultures are negative,** efforts should be made to isolate more fastidious organisms such as fungi and nutritionally deficient streptococci. Therapy can be initiated despite negative cultures with penicillin G, 2–3 million units IV q4h, or ampicillin, 2 g IV q4h, plus an aminoglycoside for 4–6 weeks. Vancomycin can be substituted in penicillin-allergic patients.

C. **Prosthetic valve endocarditis (PVE)** occurs in 1–4% of patients. Early infections (within 2 months of surgery) commonly are caused by *S. aureus*, *S. epidermidis* (see sec. **II.B.5**), gram-negative bacilli, *Candida* species, and other opportunistic organisms. The diagnosis is difficult, because fever and transient bacteremia often occur in the postoperative period. PVE must be considered in any patient with sustained bacteremia after valve surgery. Treatment for oxacillin-sensitive *S. aureus* consists of combination therapy with oxacillin, 2 g IV q4h, plus RIF, 300 mg PO q8h for at least 6 weeks. For oxacillin-resistant *S. aureus*, vancomycin, 1 g IV q12h, with RIF is used. Gentamicin, 1 mg/kg IV q8h, should be given for the initial 2 weeks of therapy in either case. Therapy should also be guided by the results of MIC and SBT studies. Late PVE (i.e., >2 months after surgery) usually is caused by organisms similar to those seen on native valves.

III. **Role of surgery.** Indications for urgent cardiac surgery include (1) uncontrolled infection as manifested by sustained bacteremia, (2) refractory heart failure, (3) an unstable prosthetic valve, or (4) prosthetic valve obstruction. Surgical intervention might also be necessary when native valve endocarditis is complicated by recurrent systemic emboli, mycotic aneurysm, persistent conduction defects, chordae tendineae or papillary muscle rupture, or early closure of the mitral valve on echocardiography, or when PVE is complicated by a periprosthetic leak. In addition, fungal endocarditis is refractory to medical therapy and requires surgery. Endocarditis due to gram-negative bacilli may be refractory to antimicrobials alone. Although a 10-day course of preoperative antimicrobials is desirable, surgery must not be delayed in patients whose condition is deteriorating.

IV. **Response to antimicrobial therapy.** Frequently, clinical improvement is seen within 3–10 days. Daily blood cultures should be obtained until sterility is

Table 14-1. Endocarditis prophylaxis

Situation	Drug and dosage
Regimens for dental, oral, respiratory tract, or esophageal procedures	
Standard prophylaxis	Amoxicillin, 2 g PO 1 hr before procedure
Unable to take PO	Ampicillin, 2 g IM or IV within 30 mins before procedure
Penicillin-allergic patients	Clindamycin, 600 mg PO 1 hr before procedure, or cephalexin or cefadroxil,* 2 g PO 1 hr before procedure, or clarithromycin or azithromycin, 500 mg PO 1 hr before procedure
Penicillin-allergic and unable to take PO	Clindamycin, 600 mg IV within 30 mins before procedure, or cefazolin,* 1 g IV within 30 mins before procedure
Regimens for GI and genitourinary procedures	
High-risk patients	Ampicillin, 2 g IM or IV, plus gentamicin, 1.5 mg/kg (max 120 mg) within 30 mins before procedure; 6 hrs later, ampicillin, 1 g IM or IV, or amoxicillin, 1 g PO
High-risk, penicillin-allergic patients	Vancomycin, 1 g IV, plus gentamicin, 1.5 mg/kg (max 120 mg), timed to be completed within 30 mins before procedure
Moderate-risk patients	Amoxicillin, 2 g PO 1 hr before procedure, or ampicillin, 2 g IM or IV within 30 mins before procedure
Moderate-risk, penicillin-allergic patients	Vancomycin, 1 g IV timed to finish within 30 mins before procedure

*Cephalosporins should not be used in patients with anaphylactic or urticarial reactions to penicillin.
Source: Adapted from AS Dajani, KA Taubert, W Wilson, et al. Prevention of bacterial endocarditis. Recommendations by the American Heart Association. *JAMA* 277:1794, 1997.

documented. Persistent or recurrent fever usually represents extensive cardiac infection but also might be due to septic emboli or drug hypersensitivity. Such fever seldom represents the development of antimicrobial resistance, and drug therapy should be altered only if clear evidence exists of another infection or drug hypersensitivity.

V. Prophylaxis (*Ann Intern Med* 129:829, 1998). The American Heart Association recommends that prophylaxis for IE be provided to patients at high risk (e.g., those with prosthetic cardiac valves or other intravascular prostheses, a history of IE, or complex cyanotic heart disease) or moderate risk (e.g., those with other congenital cardiac malformations, rheumatic valvular disease or other acquired valvular dysfunction, hypertrophic cardiomyopathy, or mitral valve prolapse with valvular regurgitation or thickened leaflets) (Table 14-1). Even in these patients, the need for prophylaxis depends on the procedure being done. Dental procedures that warrant prophylaxis include dental extractions, periodontal or endodontal procedures, and professional teeth cleaning. Some dental procedures such as filling cavities do not warrant prophylaxis. GI tract procedures that warrant prophylaxis include esophageal sclerotherapy, esophageal stricture dilatation, and endoscopic retrograde cholangiography with biliary obstruction. For transesophageal echocardiography or routine endoscopy with or without biopsy, prophylaxis is optional for high-risk patients. Prophylaxis is not recommended for routine endotracheal intubation. For bronchoscopy with a flexible bronchoscope with or without biopsy, prophylaxis is optional for high-risk patients. Prophylaxis is not indicated for a cesarean section; for a vaginal delivery it is optional for high-risk patients. Cardiac catheterization, pacemaker placement, or the incision or biopsy of surgically scrubbed skin does not warrant prophylaxis (*JAMA* 277:1794, 1997). One should note that the most recent recommendations do not include postprocedure antibiotics except for high-risk patients who are undergoing GI or genitourinary procedures.

Respiratory Tract Infections

I. Upper respiratory tract infections

A. Most cases of **pharyngitis** are viral, although distinction from bacterial pharyngitis might be impossible on clinical grounds. Noninfectious causes include pemphigus and systemic lupus erythematosus.

1. Diagnosis

a. Throat cultures in adults can be reserved for patients with a history of rheumatic fever, symptomatic patients exposed to a patient with streptococcal pharyngitis, patients with significant infection (i.e., fever, pharyngeal exudate, and cervical adenopathy), and patients whose pharyngeal infection fails to clear despite symptomatic therapy. Group A beta-hemolytic streptococci (GABHS), which require therapy to prevent acute pyogenic complications or rheumatic fever, can be identified by either culture or antigen detection tests. Antigen detection tests, although specific, vary in sensitivity. A positive test permits early diagnosis and treatment, but a negative test does not safely exclude GABHS, making a culture necessary.

b. Serology for infectious mononucleosis (e.g., a test for heterophil agglutinin or a monospot) and a differential WBC count to detect atypical lymphocytes should be performed when infectious mononucleosis is suspected. With pharyngitis, atypical lymphocytosis, and a negative heterophil test, the differential diagnosis includes primary cytomegalovirus infection and acute HIV infection.

2. Treatment. Most cases of pharyngitis are self-limited and do not require antimicrobial therapy (for gonococcal pharyngitis, see Sexually Transmitted Diseases). Treatment for GABHS should be initiated in the setting of a positive culture or antigen detection test, if the patient is at high risk for development of rheumatic fever, or if the diagnosis is strongly suspected, pending the results of culture. Treatment schedules include penicillin V, 250 mg PO qid or 500 mg PO bid, for 10 days; erythromycin, 250 mg PO qid for 10 days; or benzathine penicillin G, 1.2 million units IM as a one-time dose. Hospitalization and parenteral therapy are indicated if a patient is unable to take oral fluids or if airway obstruction is present. Surgical intervention might be necessary in the latter case.

3. Secondary prophylaxis against GABHS infection is indicated for the prevention of recurrent infection in patients at high risk (e.g., children, parents of young children, schoolteachers, medical and military personnel, patients in crowded living conditions) and for those who have had rheumatic fever within the last 5 years. Prophylaxis regimens include benzathine penicillin G, 1.2 million units IM every 4 weeks (regimen of choice); penicillin V, 125–250 mg PO bid; sulfadiazine, 1 g PO qd (for adults with normal renal function); or erythromycin, 250 mg PO bid indefinitely for those at high risk.

B. Epiglottitis should be considered in the febrile patient who complains of severe sore throat and dysphagia but in whom minimal findings are noted on inspection of the pharynx.

1. Diagnosis. If epiglottitis is suspected, a lateral soft-tissue radiograph of the neck to assess airway occlusion and throat and blood cultures should be obtained.

2. **Treatment. Hospitalization and prompt otolaryngologic consultation for airway management are suggested in all suspected cases.** Antimicrobial therapy should include an agent that is active against *H. influenzae*. In areas where ampicillin resistance is common, ceftriaxone (1–2 g IV q24h), cefotaxime (1–2 g q6–8h), or cefuroxime (0.75–1.5 g IV q8h) is an appropriate agent.

C. **Sinusitis** is caused by blockage of the ostiomeatal complex. The goals of intensive medical therapy for acute and chronic sinusitis are to control infection, reduce tissue edema, facilitate drainage, maintain patency of the sinus ostia, and break the pathologic cycle that leads to chronic sinusitis.

1. **Acute sinusitis** in adults is most often caused by *S. pneumoniae*, *H. influenzae*, rhinoviruses, and anaerobes.

   a. **Diagnosis.** Cough and purulent postnasal discharge occur in the majority of patients, but fever occurs in fewer than 50%. Pain over the affected sinus that worsens with percussion or movement may be present.

   b. **Treatment.** First-line empiric therapy includes a 10-day regimen of amoxicillin/clavulanate, TMP/SMX [160 mg/800 mg—i.e., one double-strength (DS) tablet, PO bid], loracarbef, or cefuroxime axetil. Useful adjunctive measures include systemic decongestants, topical decongestants (phenylephrine or oxymetazoline) for no more than 3–5 days, and nasal irrigation with saline spray.

2. **Chronic sinusitis**

   a. **Diagnosis.** The primary complaint in patients with chronic sinusitis is nasal congestion or obstruction. Secondary complaints include pain, pressure, postnasal discharge, and fatigue. Posttreatment coronal sinus CT with bone windows is the radiographic modality of choice; plain films are not recommended. Nasal endoscopy may complement CT scan by visualization of the surface mucosa of the ethmoid air cells. The etiologic agents include those for acute sinusitis, as well as *S. aureus*, *Corynebacterium diphtheriae*, *Bacteroides* species, and *Veillonella* species.

   b. **Treatment.** Antimicrobial therapy should include anaerobic antimicrobial coverage and, possibly, a nasal steroid spray. Some chronic cases require endoscopic surgery.

II. **Lower respiratory tract infections**

A. **Acute bronchitis**

1. **Diagnosis.** Acute bronchitis involves inflammation of the bronchi that causes acute onset of cough and sputum production and symptoms of upper respiratory tract infection with or without fever. The usual causes are viral agents such as coronavirus, rhinovirus, influenza, or parainfluenza. Rare causes include *Mycoplasma pneumoniae*, *Chlamydia pneumoniae*, and *Bordetella pertussis*.

2. **Treatment.** Treatment is symptomatic and directed most often at controlling cough (dextromethorphan, 15 mg PO q6h). Routine antimicrobial use is controversial. For pertussis, erythromycin, 500 mg PO qid, is recommended; alternatively, TMP/SMX, ampicillin, or chloramphenicol can be used. For atypical organisms, no clearly defined benefit to therapy exists. For patients who have a persistent cough, erythromycin, 250–500 mg PO qid, or doxycycline, 100 mg PO bid for 14 days, may be effective. During epidemics, patients presenting with presumptive influenza A infection may benefit from amantadine or rimantadine.

B. **Exacerbations of chronic bronchitis**

1. **Diagnosis.** Exacerbations of chronic bronchitis (cough and sputum production for at least 3 months per year for 2 consecutive years) are marked by an increase in volume or purulence of sputum with increased cough or dyspnea (see Chap. 10). *S. pneumoniae* and *H. influenzae* are

the major pathogens recovered in sputum culture from patients with acute exacerbations of chronic bronchitis (AECB). Many episodes of AECB are incited by tobacco exposure, air pollution, occupational exposure, subclinical asthma, viral infection, or allergies.

  2. Treatment. Agents with some established merit include TMP/SMX, one DS tablet PO bid; doxycycline, 100 mg PO bid; amoxicillin/clavulanate, 875 mg PO bid; or some select third-generation fluoroquinolones.

C. Pneumonia occurs from inflammation of the pulmonary parenchyma caused by a microbial agent. The three routes of infection are inhalation, microaspiration, and large-volume aspiration.

  1. Community-acquired pneumonia (*N Engl J Med* 333:1618, 1995; *Clin Infect Dis* 31:347, 2000)

   a. Diagnosis. The diagnosis of community-acquired pneumonia is made in patients whose chest radiograph reveals a new pulmonary infiltrate, usually combined with fever and respiratory symptoms (cough, sputum production, pleurisy, dyspnea). Physical examination reveals fever, tachypnea, crackles, or consolidation on auscultation. Most (80%) patients are treated as outpatients, although all should be evaluated for severity of illness, comorbid factors, and oxygenation. Assessment of etiologic agents in hospitalized patients should include pretreatment expectorated sputum for Gram stain and culture and blood cultures. Fiberoptic bronchoscopy is used for detection of associated anatomic lesions, biopsy for histopathologic workup, or quantitative cultures of conventional bacteria. For the atypical agents *Legionella pneumophila*, *C. pneumoniae*, and *M. pneumoniae*, rapid diagnostic tests such as throat-swab polymerase chain reaction (PCR) are in transition from investigational to clinical use. Documented seroconversion, with acute and convalescent sera, might be diagnostic but is not useful when therapeutic decisions are required. Thoracentesis of pleural effusions should be performed with analyses of pH, cell count, Gram stain and culture, protein, and lactate dehydrogenase (see Chap. 10).

   b. Treatment. The selection of antimicrobial agents should be pathogen directed. Empiric therapy for immunocompetent outpatients who are younger than 40 years and who lack comorbidity should be doxycycline. Older immunocompetent hosts and those with comorbidities should receive either a macrolide, doxycycline, or a fluoroquinolone with enhanced activity against *S. pneumoniae*. Outpatients older than 60 years or those who have comorbidities should be treated with a second-generation cephalosporin, amoxicillin, or amoxicillin/clavulanate with or without a macrolide. For hospitalized patients, a second- or third-generation cephalosporin or beta-lactam/beta-lactamase inhibitor with or without a macrolide or fluoroquinolone is recommended. For critically ill patients, a macrolide or fluoroquinolone should be included for treatment of possible *L. pneumophila*.

  2. Nosocomial pneumonia

   a. Diagnosis. Nosocomial pneumonia occurs in 0.3–0.7% of hospitalized patients. It is defined as a new pulmonary infiltrate in patients with fever, with or without cough, that occurs more than 48 hours after admission. Optimal specimens are uncontaminated sterile body fluids (pleural or blood), bronchoscopy aspirates (cultured quantitatively), or aspirates from endotracheal tubes. The most frequent pathogens are gram-negative bacilli and *S. aureus*. Fiberoptic bronchoscopy may be diagnostic (quantitative cultures) and therapeutic (re-expansion of lung segment) in these patients.

    b. Treatment. Initial empiric treatment should include gram-negative antimicrobial coverage. Targeted therapy should be based on in vitro sensitivity test results. Empyemas require drainage.

D. Lung abscess (see Chap. 10)

Gastrointestinal and Abdominal Infections

I. Enteric infections that cause diarrheal disease usually are self-limited. The diagnosis and treatment of these infections are discussed in Chap. 17.

II. *Helicobacter pylori*–associated disease is discussed in Chap. 17.

III. Peritonitis

    A. Primary or spontaneous peritonitis usually occurs in patients with cirrhosis and ascites. *Escherichia coli*, *S. pneumoniae*, other streptococci, and Enterobacteriaceae account for the majority of infections, although anaerobic bacteria and *Mycobacterium tuberculosis* might occasionally be responsible. Initial therapy with a third-generation cephalosporin that has good activity against streptococci is appropriate.

    B. Secondary peritonitis may be due to perforation of the GI tract or contiguous spread from a visceral infection or abscess. Enterobacteriaceae, obligate anaerobes, and enterococci are common pathogens, but staphylococci, *M. tuberculosis*, and *Neisseria gonorrhoeae* also are seen. Empiric antimicrobial therapy should include broad-spectrum coverage while culture results are awaited. For peritonitis from a presumed GI source, a variety of regimens appear to be effective. These include (1) ampicillin plus an aminoglycoside plus either clindamycin or metronidazole; (2) an aminoglycoside plus cefoxitin, cefotetan, clindamycin, or chloramphenicol; (3) cefoxitin or cefotetan alone; or (4) a carbapenem when more resistant organisms are likely to be present. Abscess formation is common and requires surgical or percutaneous drainage in most cases. Peritonitis complicating peritoneal dialysis is discussed in Chap. 12.

IV. Hepatobiliary infections

    A. Cholecystitis

        1. Diagnosis. Biliary colic usually is the predecessor of acute cholecystitis and lasts from 30 minutes to 3 hours. Patients present with fever, right upper quadrant or epigastric pain, nausea, vomiting, and signs of localized peritonitis. Older patients might present with sepsis and altered mental status. Acalculous cholecystitis occurs in 5–10% of patients. Ultrasonography and technetium-99m–hydroxy iminodiacetic acid (HIDA) scanning are the diagnostic imaging modalities of choice.

        2. Treatment. Treatment includes parenteral fluids, broad-spectrum antimicrobial therapy, and analgesia. In approximately 30% of patients, complications develop or surgery is required. The timing of surgery is controversial in uncomplicated cholecystitis, but usually an operation is performed within 6 days of a patient's initial presentation or is delayed for 6 weeks in patients whose condition stabilizes with nonoperative management.

    B. Hepatitis (see Chap. 18)

    C. Cholangitis

        1. Diagnosis. This inflammatory process comprises several different disease entities, including acute cholangitis, recurrent cholangitis, and primary (idiopathic) cholangitis. The mechanism of cholangitis includes infected bile in the setting of partial or complete obstruction of the common bile duct. Acute cholangitis may present as Charcot's triad of fever, right upper quadrant abdominal pain, and jaundice. The organisms found in the biliary tract often are the same as the normal intestinal flora. The competing differential diagnosis is cholecystitis.

2. **Treatment.** Most patients can be managed medically with a regimen that includes parenteral fluids, correction of any coagulopathy, antimicrobial agents, and, possibly, nasogastric decompression. Patients whose condition does not improve with medical therapy might require endoscopic retrograde cholangiopancreatography (ERCP) or surgical biliary drainage (see Chap. 17). Initial antibiotic regimens should include ampicillin, an aminoglycoside, and metronidazole, or an extended-spectrum ureidopenicillin such as piperacillin.

V. Appendicitis requires surgical intervention, usually with adjuvant antimicrobial therapy.

VI. Diverticulitis is primarily a medical disease. The causative organisms include gram-negative bacilli and anaerobes. The standard regimen is TMP/SMX, 160 mg/800 mg (DS) PO bid, and metronidazole, 500 mg PO bid, for 10 days. Surgical intervention is warranted for a perforated viscus (see Chap. 17).

VII. Intra-abdominal abscesses develop as complications of primary or secondary peritonitis. The infections are predominantly polymicrobial and consistent with normal intestinal flora. Ultrasonography or abdominal CT scans may be useful diagnostic techniques. Effective management includes adequate drainage combined with antimicrobial therapy. Comparable antimicrobial regimens include cefoxitin with or without an aminoglycoside, piperacillin, ampicillin/sulbactam, clindamycin plus an aminoglycoside, and imipenem.

Skin, Soft-Tissue, and Bone Infections

I. Skin infections

A. Erysipelas is a superficial, erythematous, edematous, sharply demarcated lesion almost always caused by GABHS. The treatments of choice are penicillin, 0.5–1g PO qid; procaine penicillin G, 600,000 units IM bid; or penicillin G, 2–6 million units/day IV, depending on the severity of illness. In patients who are allergic to penicillin, erythromycin, 500 mg PO qid, or vancomycin, 1 g IV q12h, is an alternative.

B. Cellulitis typically is more deep seated and has less distinct margins than does erysipelas and, in normal hosts, usually is caused by GABHS or *S. aureus*; these pathogens are clinically indistinguishable. Initial therapy is oxacillin, 1–2 g IV q6h, or cefazolin, 1–2 g IV q8h. If *Streptococcus* is documented as the cause of infection, treatment is as recommended for erysipelas (see sec. **I.A**). Lower extremity cellulitis associated with cutaneous ulcers in diabetic patients may be polymicrobial in origin. Agents with activity against anaerobes (e.g., metronidazole or clindamycin) can be added when cellulitis is being treated in this setting. Alternatively, cefoxitin, 1–2 g IV q8h, can be used as single-agent therapy for these patients.

C. Scabies is an ectoparasitic infestation with *Sarcoptes scabiei*. Transmission occurs through direct contact. Patients present with a pruritic papular rash involving the finger webs, wrists, elbows, axillary folds, trunk, buttocks, and genitalia.

1. **Clinical diagnosis** is made on the basis of a typical rash and a history of recent exposure to scabies. Microscopic diagnosis requires scraping of a skin lesion and visualization of the scabies mite, eggs, or feces under low-power light microscopy.

2. **Treatment** requires application of lindane 1% [lotion (1 oz) or cream (30 g)] or permethrin cream 5% to the body from the neck down for 8–14 hours. A second application might be required. Clothes, sheets, and other linens must be laundered in hot water.

II. Soft-tissue infections

A. Myositis

1. **Pyomyositis** is due to *S. aureus* (90%), *Streptococcus pyogenes*, *E. coli*, or *S. pneumoniae*. Large-bore needle aspiration might allow for diagnosis, but surgical drainage is required in most cases. Pathogen-specific therapy should continue for at least 2–3 weeks.

2. **Anaerobic myonecrosis (gas gangrene)** usually is due to *Clostridium perfringens*, *Clostridium septicum*, *S. aureus*, GABHS, or other anaerobes. Distinguishing this condition from necrotizing fasciitis often requires gross inspection of the involved muscle at the time of surgery. Treatment requires prompt surgical débridement and combination antimicrobial therapy with penicillin and clindamycin.

B. Necrotizing fasciitis is a serious, invasive, soft-tissue infection in which thrombosis of the microcirculation leads to gangrene. It is uncommon but often life threatening. The outcome is better with upper limb involvement than with involvement of the abdomen, groin, or perineum (Fournier's gangrene).

1. **Diagnosis.** Pathogens in the infected site are usually the normal flora of the site. Anaerobic bacteria outnumber aerobic bacteria at all body sites. Certain clinical findings correlate with some bacteria: edema with the *Bacteroides fragilis* group, *Clostridium* species, *S. aureus*, *Prevotella* species, and GABHS; gas and crepitation in tissues with Enterobacteriaceae and *Clostridium* species; and foul odor with *Bacteroides* species.

2. **Treatment.** Rapid parenteral fluids, broad-spectrum antimicrobial coverage, and aggressive surgical débridement are imperative.

III. Osteomyelitis should be considered in patients with localized bone pain who are febrile or septic. Diagnosis is made by culturing the pathogen from bone. If a causative organism is not identified, antimicrobial therapy should be selected on the basis of the most likely pathogens. Cure typically requires at least 6 weeks of high-dose antimicrobial therapy. Parenteral therapy should be given initially, but oral regimens can be considered after 2–3 weeks, provided the causative agent is susceptible and adequate bactericidal levels can be achieved.

A. Acute hematogenous osteomyelitis is caused most frequently by *S. aureus*. Blood cultures often are positive. In the absence of vascular insufficiency or a foreign body, acute osteomyelitis can usually be treated with antimicrobial therapy alone, on the basis of culture and susceptibility results. Vertebral osteomyelitis commonly involves two adjacent vertebral bodies and may be due to *S. aureus*, gram-negative bacilli, or *M. tuberculosis*, presumably arising by dissemination via communicating veins or Batson's plexus. Complications include paraspinal abscesses.

B. Osteomyelitis associated with contiguous foci (e.g., postoperative infections) may be due to *S. aureus* or gram-negative bacilli.

C. Osteomyelitis associated with vascular insufficiency (e.g., in diabetic patients) seldom is cured by drug therapy alone; revascularization, débridement, or amputation often is required.

D. Osteomyelitis in the presence of internal fixation devices usually cannot be eradicated by antimicrobials alone. Cure typically requires the removal of the foreign material.

E. Osteomyelitis associated with hemoglobinopathies is caused most often by *S. aureus* or *Salmonella* species. *Salmonella* osteomyelitis may require surgical treatment and parenteral administration of high-dose ampicillin or chloramphenicol, 1 g IV q6h.

F. **Chronic osteomyelitis** usually is associated with a sequestrum of dead necrotic bone. Eradication requires a combination of medical and surgical treatment to remove the persistent nidus of infection. Long-term, continuous, suppressive antimicrobial therapy can be used if surgery is not feasible.

Genitourinary Infections

Genitourinary infections, by definition, vary by gender. The diagnostic and therapeutic approach to adults with urinary tract infections (UTIs) can be simplified by dividing patients into the groups described in the following sections (*N Engl J Med* 335:468, 1996).

I. **Lower UTI** is characterized by pyuria, often with dysuria, urgency, or frequency. A rapid presumptive diagnosis can be made by microscopic examination of a fresh, unspun, clean-voided urine specimen. A urine Gram stain can be helpful in guiding initial antimicrobial choices. Bacteriuria (more than one organism per oil-immersion field) or pyuria (more than eight leukocytes per high-power field) correlates well with the presence of infection. Quantitative culture often yields more than 10^5 bacteria/ml, but colony counts as low as 10^2–10^4 bacteria/ml may indicate infection in women with acute dysuria.

A. **Acute uncomplicated cystitis in women** is caused by *E. coli* in 80% of cases and by *Staphylococcus saprophyticus* in 5–15% of cases.

   1. **Diagnosis.** The diagnosis is based on presenting symptoms and microscopic examination of urine. In the face of a narrow spectrum of organisms and relatively predictable antimicrobial susceptibilities, empiric therapy is advocated.

   2. **Treatment.** If pyuria is present microscopically or by leukocyte esterase testing, empiric treatment with TMP/SMX, 160 mg/800 mg PO bid for 3 days, is recommended. In patients who are intolerant of sulfa, TMP, 100 mg PO bid, can be used. Fluoroquinolones are more costly than is TMP/SMX but are an alternative. Because single-dose regimens are associated with higher relapse rates, 3-day regimens are more cost effective. A pretreatment urine culture is recommended for diabetics, patients who are symptomatic for more than 7 days, patients with recurrent UTI, women who use a contraceptive diaphragm, and individuals older than 65 years. Therapy should be extended to 7 days in this subset of patients.

B. **Recurrent cystitis in women** is due to varying host-dependent risk factors, which vary for young women, healthy postmenopausal women, and older women who are institutionalized (*Clin Infect Dis* 30:152, 2000).

   1. **Diagnosis.** The diagnosis is made on the basis of the presenting symptoms and microscopic examination of the urine.

   2. **Treatment.** Relapses with the original infecting organism that occur within 2 weeks of cessation of therapy should be treated for 2 weeks or more and may indicate a urologic abnormality. An alternative method of contraception might decrease the frequency of reinfection in women who use a diaphragm and spermicide.

   3. **Prophylaxis.** Prophylactic therapy might be helpful for patients who experience frequent reinfection. Sterilization of the urine with a standard treatment regimen is necessary before prophylaxis is initiated. For women with relapses that correlate with sexual intercourse, TMP/SMX, 80 mg/400 mg (one single-strength tablet), or cephalexin, 250 mg, after coitus may provide adequate prophylaxis. TMP/SMX, 40 mg/200 mg qd or qod, usually is sufficient to decrease recurrences unrelated to coitus.

C. **UTIs in men** are rare and do not necessarily indicate a urologic abnormality. In men, risk factors for UTI include anal intercourse, lack of circumcision, and intercourse with a partner whose vagina is colonized by uropathogens.

1. **Diagnosis.** The diagnosis may be made on the basis of symptoms, if present, combined with microscopic examination of the urine. A pretreatment urine culture should be obtained.
2. **Treatment.** If no complicating factors are present, a 7-day course of TMP/SMX, TMP alone, or a fluoroquinolone can be prescribed. If the response to therapy is prompt, a urologic evaluation is unlikely to be useful. Urologic studies are appropriate when treatment fails, in the event of recurrent infections, or when pyelonephritis occurs.

D. **Asymptomatic bacteriuria in adults**
1. **Diagnosis** of asymptomatic bacteriuria is defined as two successive cultures with greater than or equal to 10^5 colony-forming units/ml in patients without symptoms.
2. **Treatment** for asymptomatic bacteriuria is justified only before urologic surgery and in pregnant women. No evidence supports the routine screening of urine or treatment in other settings.

E. **Catheter-associated bacteriuria** is a common source of gram-negative bacteremia in hospitalized patients.
1. **Prevention measures** include aseptic technique for urinary catheter insertion, use of a closed drainage system, and removal of the catheter as soon as possible. Condom catheters may be associated with UTIs in the setting of poor personal hygiene and condom catheter changes that occur less than once a day.
2. **Treatment.** In patients with chronic indwelling catheters, the development of bacteriuria is inevitable, and long-term antimicrobial suppression simply selects for multidrug-resistant bacteria. Such patients should be treated with systemic antimicrobials only when symptomatic infection is evident.

F. **Acute urethral syndrome**
1. **Diagnosis.** Acute urethral syndrome occurs in women who have lower UTI symptoms and pyuria with fewer than 10^5 bacteria/ml urine. These patients may have bacterial cystitis or urethritis caused by *Chlamydia trachomatis*, *Ureaplasma urealyticum*, or, less frequently, *N. gonorrhoeae*. Specific cultures of the endocervix for sexually transmitted diseases (STDs) should be performed (see Sexually Transmitted Diseases).
2. **Treatment.** If no specific etiology is found, doxycycline, 100 mg PO bid for 7 days, is recommended. Azithromycin, 1 g PO in a single dose, is an alternative. Erythromycin, 500 mg PO qid for 7 days, should be used in pregnant women with nongonococcal urethritis. Adjunctive measures include hydration and analgesia with phenazopyridine, 200 mg PO tid. Analgesia should not be given for longer than 7 days because it may obscure persistent infection.

G. **Prostatitis**
1. **Diagnosis.** Acute prostatitis is characterized by fever, chills, dysuria, and a tense or boggy, extremely tender prostate on examination. Patients with chronic prostatitis are usually asymptomatic, but some experience low back pain, perineal or testicular discomfort, mild dysuria, and recurrent bacteriuria. Quantitative urine cultures before and after prostatic massage may be necessary to diagnose these infections. Prostatitis often is associated with fewer than 10^3 bacteria/ml fluid. Infections usually are caused by enteric gram-negative bacilli.
2. **Treatment.** TMP/SMX, 160 mg/800 mg (DS) PO bid for 14 days, is an effective, economical treatment for acute infections. Quinolones are useful alternatives. Patients with chronic bacterial prostatitis should receive prolonged therapy (for at least 1 month with the quinolones or 3 months with TMP/SMX).

H. **Epididymitis** usually is caused by *N. gonorrhoeae* or *C. trachomatis* in sexually active young men and by gram-negative enteric organisms in older men. Diagnosis and therapy should be directed accordingly, with ceftriaxone and doxycycline in young men and TMP/SMX or ciprofloxacin in men older than 40 years.

I. **When candiduria is present,** it is crucial to distinguish colonization from infection. Pyuria and candiduria in an immunocompromised host may be best treated with optimization of host status (glucose control in diabetics, removal or change of Foley catheter). In symptomatic patients, fluconazole, 100 mg PO qd for 3 days, can be tried. Amphotericin continuous bladder irrigations have not been proven to be efficacious for candiduria and are not recommended.

II. **Pyelonephritis**

A. **Acute uncomplicated pyelonephritis**

1. **Diagnosis.** Patients present with fever, flank pain, and lower UTI symptoms. Urine specimens characteristically demonstrate significant bacteriuria, pyuria, and occasional leukocyte casts. Urine cultures should be obtained in all suspect patients. Blood cultures should be obtained in those who are hospitalized, as bacteremia will be detected in 15–20%. The causative agent usually is *E. coli*.

2. **Treatment.** Patients with mild to moderate illness who are able to take oral medication can be safely treated as outpatients with TMP/SMX or fluoroquinolones for 10–14 days. Patients with more severe illness, those who are nauseated and vomiting, and pregnant patients should be treated initially with parenteral therapy. Appropriate empiric parenteral regimens include TMP/SMX, third-generation cephalosporins, fluoroquinolones, or aminoglycosides (with or without a beta-lactam antimicrobial). If enterococcal infection is suspected on the basis of a urine Gram stain, ampicillin, 1 g IV q6h, with or without gentamicin, 1 mg/kg IV q8h, is appropriate.

B. **In patients who do not respond to initial empiric treatment** within 48 hours, antimicrobial therapy should be changed to treat the pathogen detected by the initial urine culture, and the presence of an anatomic abnormality should be considered.

1. **Evaluation for anatomic abnormalities.** Noninvasive studies, such as ultrasonography, CT scan, or IVP, should be considered to rule out intrarenal abscess, emphysematous pyelonephritis, or a foreign body (renal calculi).

2. **Treatment.** Intrarenal abscesses may require drainage or prolonged antimicrobial therapy. Emphysematous pyelonephritis requires immediate nephrectomy. The approach to renal calculi depends on stone size and location. Analgesic therapy and consideration of stone retrieval are important.

Toxin-Mediated Infections

I. **Clostridial infections**

A. **Botulism**

1. **Diagnosis.** Botulism presents as the acute onset of weakness in muscles innervated by cranial nerves, resulting in dysphasia, dysphagia, and diplopia or blurred vision. The diagnosis can be confirmed by either detection of toxin in serum, stool, or a sample of a food consumed before the onset of illness or by recovery of *Clostridium botulinum* from a gastric, wound, or stool specimen.

2. **Treatment.** Specific treatment includes infusion of botulism antitoxin. The Centers for Disease Control and Prevention, Atlanta, recommend administration of two vials of trivalent botulism antitoxin as soon as this diagnosis is suspected (before it is confirmed).

B. **Tetanus**

1. **Diagnosis.** The clinical presentation of tetanus is progressive generalized rigidity and convulsive spasm of skeletal muscles. This presentation is followed by trismus, dysphagia, or autonomic dysfunction. A

prior injury or wound has usually occurred. Meningitis should be excluded by lumbar puncture.

  2. **Treatment.** Treatment often includes prolonged ICU management, often with tracheostomy and ventilator support. Administration of anti-tetanus toxoid and human tetanus immune globulin is routine, and intrathecal tetanus immune globulin (250 IU) has been shown to decrease morbidity and mortality (*J R Soc Med* 87:135, 1994). The role of antimicrobial therapy remains controversial.

II. **Toxic shock syndrome** is caused by an exotoxin produced by *S. aureus*, but a similar syndrome may be seen with invasive streptococcal infections. Although first recognized in menstruating women who used tampons, nonmenstrual toxic shock syndrome can complicate staphylococcal colonization of surgical wounds.

  A. **Diagnosis.** The clinical presentation includes fever, a diffuse macular erythroderma involving the palms and soles that often desquamates 1–2 weeks after the illness, hypotension, conjunctivitis, vomiting, and diarrhea. Blood cultures should be routinely obtained but often are negative.

  B. **Treatment.** Supportive care is the mainstay of acute therapy. Antistaphylococcal therapy does not appear to affect the acute illness but might prevent progression of local infection and decrease the rate of relapse. Discontinuation of tampon use also might reduce recurrences.

Sexually Transmitted Diseases

Because infection with multiple organisms is common in STDs, studies for gonorrhea, chlamydial infection, and syphilis should be included in all evaluations. In addition, HIV testing and counseling are recommended by the United States Public Health Service. An STD that apparently is refractory to treatment may represent reinfection, a concomitant previously undiagnosed STD, or antimicrobial resistance. Patients with STDs should be reported to the local health department. Sex partners of patients with certain STDs should be referred to the health department for evaluation and possible treatment.

I. **Ulcerative diseases**

  A. **Genital herpes** is caused by human herpes simplex virus, usually type 2, and is characterized by painful grouped vesicles in the anogenital region that rapidly ulcerate and form shallow tender lesions. The initial episode may be associated with inguinal adenopathy, fever, headache, myalgias, and aseptic meningitis; recurrences usually are less severe than the initial episode.

  1. **Diagnosis.** The diagnosis of herpes simplex virus infection requires culture confirmation. Culture of first-episode lesions is recommended, but culture of recurrent lesions is optional if the presentation is characteristic. Because of the frequency of herpetic infection, all undiagnosed genital ulcer lesions should be subjected to viral culture.

  2. **Treatment.** Acyclovir, 400 mg PO tid (or 200 mg PO 5 times a day) for 7–10 days, is recommended for all primary genital herpes infections if begun within 1 week of symptoms. Treatment may be indicated for severe recurrences and may include acyclovir, 400 mg PO tid (or 200 mg PO 5 times a day) for 5 days; valacyclovir, 500 mg PO bid for 5 days; or famciclovir, 125 mg PO bid for 5 days. Suppressive therapy (acyclovir, 400 mg PO bid) of culture-confirmed genital herpes infections may be indicated for severe or frequent recurrences. Topical acyclovir has no proven benefit in the treatment or prophylaxis of herpes simplex infection.

  B. **Syphilis** is caused by *Treponema pallidum*. Primary syphilis may develop within several weeks of exposure and involves one or more painless, indurated, superficial ulcerations (chancre). Secondary syphilis might develop after the chancre resolves and might include a rash, mucocutaneous lesions, adenopathy, and constitutional symptoms. Tertiary syphilis includes cardiovascular, gummatous, and neurologic disease (general paresis, tabes dorsalis, or meningovascular syphilis).

1. **Diagnosis.** In **primary syphilis,** dark-field microscopy of the lesion exudate, a nontreponemal serologic test (e.g., rapid plasma reagin (RPR) test, VDRL test), and a treponemal serologic test [e.g., fluorescent treponemal antibody absorption test (FTA), microhemagglutinin antigen–*Treponeum pallidum* (MHA-TP)] are used for confirmation. Diagnosis of **secondary syphilis** is made on the basis of positive serologic studies and the presence of compatible clinical illness. **Latent syphilis** is diagnosed serologically in the absence of disease as early latent disease if serology has been positive for less than 1 year and as late latent disease if serology has been positive for more than 1 year. Diagnosis of **tertiary disease** requires clinical correlation with cardiovascular, neurologic, and systemic symptoms. Lumbar puncture should be performed in the presence of neurologic or ophthalmic signs or symptoms, evidence of tertiary disease, treatment failure, or serum rapid plasma reagin or VDRL of 1:32 or greater (unless the duration of infection is less than 1 year). Patients with HIV and syphilis of more than 1 year's duration also should undergo a lumbar puncture.

2. **Treatment.** To treat primary, secondary, and early latent disease, benzathine penicillin G, 2.4 million units IM in a single dose, is used. Alternatives include doxycycline, 100 mg PO bid for 14 days, or erythromycin, 500 mg PO qid for 14 days. Treatment of disease of more than 1 year's duration (except neurosyphilis) should include benzathine penicillin G, 2.4 million units IM, one dose per week for 3 weeks; an alternative is doxycycline, 100 mg PO bid for 4 weeks. Neurosyphilis treatment should include aqueous penicillin G, 12–24 million units IV qd in divided doses for 10–14 days; an alternative is procaine penicillin, 2.4 million units IM qd, plus probenecid, 500 mg PO qid for 10–14 days. Some practitioners follow this standard neurosyphilis regimen with an additional IM injection of benzathine penicillin G.

C. **Chancroid** is caused by *Haemophilus ducreyi*. Disease is rare in the United States outside of endemic regions (e.g., New York City, the Southeast). Clinical symptoms include the development of a painful, nonindurated genital ulcer with undermined edges in conjunction with tender, bilateral inguinal adenopathy that may suppurate.

1. **Diagnosis** of chancroid requires culture of *H. ducreyi* from a genital lesion or lymph node aspirate. A presumptive diagnosis is provided by a lymph node aspirate with typical small, pleomorphic gram-negative bacilli.

2. **Treatment** might include ceftriaxone, 250 mg IM in a single dose; erythromycin, 500 mg PO qid for 7 days; azithromycin, 1.0 g PO in a single dose; or ciprofloxacin, 500 mg PO bid for 3 days.

II. **Vaginitis and vaginosis**

A. **Trichomoniasis** is a parasitic infection caused by *Trichomonas vaginalis*. Clinical symptoms include profuse, malodorous purulent vaginal discharge; dysuria; and genital inflammation.

1. **Diagnosis.** Physical examination reveals profuse frothy discharge and cervical petechiae. The pH of vaginal fluid usually is 4.5 or higher. Diagnosis requires visualization of motile trichomonads on a saline wet mount of discharge.

2. **Treatment.** Metronidazole, 2.0 g PO in a single dose, is effective; intravaginal metronidazole gel is not effective. In the event of single-dose treatment failure, patients should receive metronidazole, 500 mg PO bid for 7 days. No therapy for trichomoniasis is safe and effective during pregnancy, but intravaginal clotrimazole, 100 mg (suppositories) or cream qhs for 7 days, may relieve symptoms.

B. **Vulvovaginal candidiasis** is caused by *Candida* species and commonly develops in relation to oral contraceptive use and antibiotic therapy. Vulvovaginal candidiasis, particularly if recurrent, may be a presenting manifestation of unrecognized HIV infection. It presents with thick, cottage cheese–like vaginal discharge in conjunction with intense vulvar inflammation, pruritus, and external dysuria.

   1. **Diagnosis.** Physical examination reveals thick vaginal discharge and external genital inflammation. Definitive diagnosis requires visualization of fungal elements on a potassium hydroxide (KOH) preparation, but therapy often is initiated on the basis of the clinical presentation.

   2. **Treatment.** Oral fluconazole, 100 mg/day for 3 days, or any of the intravaginal imidazole regimens (e.g., clotrimazole vaginal cream or suppository, 100 mg qhs for 7 days or 200 mg qhs for 3 days) is effective. For recurrent infection, fluconazole, 100 mg PO, is effective. Duration of treatment is tailored to the individual case.

C. **Bacterial vaginosis** is characterized by an imbalance in the vaginal flora and presents with a malodorous vaginal discharge. An overgrowth of *Gardnerella* species, anaerobes, and *Mycoplasma* species occurs with the loss of hydrogen peroxide–producing lactobacilli in the vagina. Although, because of the symptoms, bacterial vaginosis is often grouped with STDs in discussions of genital infections, it is **not an STD.**

   1. **Diagnosis.** Clinical presentation includes a homogeneous, thin, milk-white vaginal discharge that smoothly coats the vaginal walls. Minimal external genital inflammation is present. Diagnosis requires that three of the following findings be made on examination of the vaginal discharge: fishy odor on addition of 10% KOH to a slide that contains vaginal discharge, pH of 4.5 or higher, homogeneous character of discharge, and presence of clue cells (epithelial cells studded with bacteria) on light microscopy.

   2. **Treatment.** Either metronidazole (500 mg PO bid for 7 days or as a 0.75% gel intravaginally bid for 5 days) or clindamycin (as a 2% cream intravaginally qhs for 7 days or 300 mg PO bid for 7 days) is effective. For poorly compliant patients, single-dose metronidazole, 2.0 g PO, can be used but is less effective.

III. **Cervicitis and urethritis** are frequent presentations of gonococcal or chlamydial infections. Most cases are due to infection with *N. gonorrhoeae* or *C. trachomatis*, but other agents implicated include *Mycoplasma hominis*, *U. urealyticum*, and *T. vaginalis*. Gonococcal and chlamydial infection frequently coexist, and their clinical presentations may be identical.

A. **Diagnosis.** Women with urethritis or cervicitis, or both, complain of mucopurulent vaginal discharge, dyspareunia, and dysuria. Men with urethritis complain of dysuria and a purulent penile discharge. A positive endocervical or urethral culture, a positive endocervical or urethral DNA probe test, or a positive PCR of an endocervical, urethral, or urinary specimen is required for diagnosis. For gonorrhea, a Gram stain of endocervical or urethral discharge that shows polymorphonuclear leukocytes with gram-negative diplococci might also establish the diagnosis.

B. **Treatment.** Because chlamydial infections frequently occur with gonorrhea, simultaneous therapy for both infections is recommended when gonorrhea is diagnosed. Single-dose antigonococcal therapies include ofloxacin, 400 mg PO; ciprofloxacin, 500 mg PO; ceftriaxone, 125 mg IM; cefixime, 400 mg PO; or spectinomycin, 2 g IM. Effective antichlamydial therapy includes azithromycin, 1 g PO in a single dose; doxycycline, 100 mg PO bid for 7 days; or erythromycin stearate, 500 mg PO qid (or enteric-coated erythromycin base, 666 mg PO tid) for 7 days.

IV. **Pelvic inflammatory disease (PID)** is an upper genital tract infection in women. It is characterized by pelvic pain, cervical discharge, and fever. Microbiological etiologies include *C. trachomatis*, *N. gonorrhoeae*, *Mycoplasma* species, and anaerobes. The clinical spectrum ranges from mild illness to pelvic peritonitis, perihepatitis, and tubo-ovarian abscess. Long-term consequences of untreated PID include chronic pain, infertility, and ectopic pregnancy.

A. Diagnosis. Symptoms include pelvic pain, dyspareunia, vaginal discharge, abnormal menstruation, and fever. Diagnosis requires the presence of lower abdominal tenderness, adnexal tenderness, and cervical motion tenderness. Endocervical cultures or probes for chlamydia and gonorrhea should be obtained. The presence of at least 10 WBCs per low-power field on Gram staining of an endocervical smear is consistent with PID; few or no WBCs suggest an alternative diagnosis. Criteria for hospitalization include an uncertain diagnosis, suspected pelvic abscess, PID in pregnancy or adolescence, PID with HIV infection, severe nausea or vomiting, intolerance of oral medication, lack of follow-up, and failure to respond to outpatient therapy.

B. Treatment. Inpatient therapy should include either cefoxitin, 2 g IV q6h, or cefotetan, 2 g IV q12h, plus doxycycline, 100 mg IV or PO q12h; or clindamycin, 900 mg IV q8h, plus gentamicin, 2 mg/kg loading dose followed by 1.5 mg/kg maintenance dose q8h (extended-interval dosing of gentamicin can also be used). Both IV regimens should be continued for at least 48 hours after the patient shows signs of improvement; subsequent treatment should include doxycycline, 100 mg PO bid for 14 days. For outpatient therapy, several regimens are effective: (1) cefoxitin, 2 g IM, with probenecid, 1 g PO, plus doxycycline, 100 mg PO bid for 14 days; (2) ceftriaxone, 250 mg IM, plus doxycycline, 100 mg PO bid for 14 days, plus metronidazole, 500 mg PO bid for 7 days; or (3) ofloxacin, 400 mg PO bid for 14 days, plus metronidazole, 500 mg PO bid for 14 days. Intrauterine devices should be removed. Patients should abstain from sexual intercourse during therapy. All patients must receive follow-up within 72 hours to ensure adequate response to therapy.

V. Pediculosis pubis ("crabs") is an ectoparasitic infestation caused by *Phthirus pubis*. Transmission usually requires intimate sexual contact. Patients present with pruritus of the pubic region, associated with pubic inflammation.

A. Diagnosis. Crab lice may be visible on pubic skin, and eggs may be visible on hair shafts. Light microscopy of lice and eggs might aid in making the diagnosis.

B. Treatment. Effective therapy requires application of lindane 1% shampoo for 4 minutes, permethrin 1% creme rinse for 10 minutes, or pyrethrins with piperonyl butoxide for 10 minutes to all skin between the chest and thighs, including the axillae. Patients must also launder all clothes, sheets, and other linens in hot water.

Tuberculosis

TB is a systemic disease caused by *M. tuberculosis*. Pulmonary disease is the most frequent clinical presentation. Lymphatic involvement, genitourinary disease, osteomyelitis, and miliary dissemination might occur, as well as meningitis, peritonitis, and pericarditis. In large U.S. cities, 30–40% of active TB cases are the result of reactivation of primary disease and 2% are confirmed as recently acquired. Patients with an increased likelihood of reactivation include those with HIV infection, silicosis, diabetes mellitus, chronic renal insufficiency, malignancy, malnutrition, and other forms of immunosuppression. The prevalence of TB is increased among immigrants from Southeast Asia, China, the Indian subcontinent, and Central America. Mycobacteria that are resistant to primary agents also are more common in these immigrants.

I. Diagnosis is established by culturing the organism. Positive fluorochrome or acid-fast smears are presumptive evidence of active TB, although nontuberculous mycobacteria and some *Nocardia* species may give positive results with these techniques. Use of radiometric culture systems and species-specific DNA probes can provide valuable information much faster than can traditional methods. Drug susceptibility testing should be performed on all initial isolates as well as on follow-up isolates from patients who do not respond to standard therapy.

II. **Treatment** does not have to take place in a hospital setting, but hospitalization to initiate therapy provides an opportunity for intensive patient education. If a patient is hospitalized, proper isolation in a negative-pressure room is essential. The local health department should be notified of all cases of TB so that contacts can be identified, compliance with therapy can be ensured by directly observed therapy (DOT), and follow-up can be provided.

A. **Chemotherapy.** At least two drugs to which the organism is susceptible must be used because of the high frequency with which primary drug resistance to a single drug develops. Extended therapy is necessary because of the prolonged generation time of mycobacteria. Because compliance with multidrug regimens for prolonged periods is difficult, DOT should be used for all patients.

1. **Initial therapy** of uncomplicated pulmonary TB (including cavitary disease) should include four drugs unless the likelihood of drug resistance is very low [i.e., the rate of isoniazid (INH) resistance in the community is less than 4%; the patient has not received prior therapy for TB, has not been exposed to any contacts with drug-resistant TB, and is not from an area where drug-resistant TB is prevalent]. INH (5 mg/kg; maximum, 300 mg PO qd), RIF (10 mg/kg; maximum, 600 mg PO qd), pyrazinamide (PZA, 15–30 mg/kg PO qd), and either ethambutol (EMB, 15 mg/kg PO qd) or streptomycin (15 mg/kg; maximum, 1.5 g IM qd) should be administered initially. If the isolate proves to be fully susceptible to INH and RIF, EMB (or streptomycin) can be dropped and INH, RIF, and PZA continued to finish 8 weeks, followed by 16 weeks of INH and RIF. After at least 2 weeks of daily therapy, the medications can be administered twice a week at adjusted doses. A variety of options for two or three times per week DOT are available (*Am J Respir Crit Care Med* 149:1359, 1994). All intermittent dosing regimens should be directly administered (DOT). Pyridoxine (vitamin B₆), 25–50 mg PO qd, should be given to those who are prone to neuropathy (diabetics, alcoholics, patients with dietary deficiencies) and considered in all patients.

2. **Organisms that are resistant** only to INH can be effectively treated with a 6-month regimen if a standard four-drug regimen consisting of INH, RIF, PZA, and EMB or streptomycin was started initially. When INH resistance is documented, the INH should be discontinued, and the remaining three drugs should be continued for the duration of therapy. Therapy for multidrug-resistant TB has been less well studied, and consultation with an expert in the treatment of TB should be considered. Therapy should include at least three drugs to which the organism is susceptible. Careful documentation of bacteriologic sputum culture conversion is important, and therapy should be continued for at least 12 months and possibly as long as 24 months after cultures convert to negative. Surgery should be considered for patients in whom the bulk of the disease is resectable.

3. **Extrapulmonary disease** in adults can be treated in the same manner as pulmonary disease, with 6- to 9-month short-course regimens.

4. **Pregnant patients** with drug-sensitive TB should be treated with INH and RIF for 9 months. EMB should also be used initially until sensitivities are known. Pyridoxine, 50 mg PO qd, should also be given. PZA and streptomycin should be avoided.

B. **Monitoring response to therapy.** Patients with pulmonary TB whose sputum smears are positive before treatment should submit sputum for acid-fast bacilli smear and culture every 1–2 weeks until smears become negative. Sputum should then be obtained monthly until negative cultures are documented. Conversion of cultures from positive to negative is the most reliable indicator of a response to treatment. Continued symptoms or persistently positive smears or cultures after 3 months of treatment should raise the suspicion of drug resistance or noncompliance and should prompt referral of the patient to an expert in the treatment of TB.

C. **Monitoring for adverse reactions.** Patients should have a baseline laboratory evaluation at the start of therapy that includes hepatic enzymes, bilirubin, CBC, and serum creatinine (Cr) level. Routine laboratory monitoring for patients with normal baseline values is probably unnecessary, but some experts check transaminases monthly in patients over 35 years of age. Monthly clinical evaluations with specific inquiries about symptoms of drug toxicity are essential. Patients who are taking EMB should be tested monthly for visual acuity and red-green color perception. Patients should be instructed to anticipate side effects and to call with questions as they arise.

D. **Glucocorticoid administration.** In TB, the administration of glucocorticoids is controversial. Prednisone, 1 mg/kg PO qd initially, has been used in combination with antituberculous drugs for life-threatening complications such as meningitis and pericarditis.

III. **Chemoprophylaxis.** Untreated, approximately 5% of persons with latent TB infection (LTBI) develop active TB disease within 2 years of infection. An additional 5% will develop TB disease during their lifetime. Adequate treatment (prophylaxis) can substantially reduce this risk. A positive tuberculin skin test (TST; 5TU administered by the Mantoux method) is the only means of diagnosing LTBI.

A. **Criteria for a positive TST** are (1) 5-mm induration in patients with HIV infection or another defect in cell-mediated immunity, close contacts of a known case of TB, patients with chest radiographs typical for TB, and patients with organ transplantation or other immunosuppression (>15 mg/day prednisone for >1 month); (2) 10-mm induration in immigrants from high-prevalence areas (Asia, Africa, Latin America, Eastern Europe), prisoners, the homeless, parenteral drug abusers, nursing home residents, the medically underserved, low-income populations, patients with chronic medical illnesses, and those people having frequent contact with these groups (e.g., health care workers, prison guards); and (3) 15-mm induration in individuals who are not in a high-prevalence group (*Am J Respir Crit Care Med* 161:S221, 2000; *Am J Respir Crit Care Med* 161:1376, 2000).

B. **Prophylactic therapy (treatment for LTBI)** should be administered only after active disease has been ruled out by a proper evaluation (chest radiography, sputum collection, or both). INH, 300 mg PO qd for 9 months, should be administered, regardless of age, to persons with LTBI who have risk factors for progression to active TB disease. Groups considered highest priority for treatment are (1) persons in whom a TST conversion develops within 2 years of a previously negative TST regardless of age; (2) persons with a history of untreated TB or chest radiographic evidence of previous infection; (3) persons with HIV infection, diabetes mellitus, end-stage renal disease, hematologic or lymphoreticular malignancy, conditions associated with rapid weight loss or chronic malnutrition, silicosis, or patients who are receiving immunosuppressive therapy; and (4) household members and other close contacts of patients with active disease who have a reactive TST. Persons with HIV who have had known contact with a patient with active TB should be treated for LTBI regardless of tuberculin status. Similarly, children (younger than 4 years) who are close contacts should be started on treatment for LTBI (INH, 10–20 mg/kg/day; maximum dose, 300 mg) even if tuberculin negative ("window prophylaxis"). In immunocompetent children, treatment can be stopped if a repeat TST at 3 months is negative. Contacts with a nonreactive TST should undergo a repeat TST 3 months after the last exposure to the infectious person. A 9-month course of INH is adequate for all patients with LTBI even among those who are HIV coinfected. Alternatives to the 9-month regimen of INH include RIF, 600 mg PO qd, with PZA, 20–25 mg/kg (maximum of 2 g) administered daily for 2 months, or RIF, 600 mg/day for 4 months. Immunosuppressed persons should receive 12 months of prophylactic treatment.

Referral to the health department for chemoprophylaxis is recommended to ensure compliance and to monitor for medication-related complications.

Systemic Mycoses

Fungal infections can often be identified by taking into account the clinical findings, site of infection, inflammatory response, and fungal appearance. Yeast-like fungi are typically round or oval and reproduce by budding, whereas molds are composed of tubular structures called hyphae that grow by branching and longitudinal extension. The clinical presentations are protean and not pathogen specific.

I. **Blastomycosis,** a major endemic mycosis in North America, is caused by *Blastomyces dermatitidis*.
   A. **Diagnosis.** The diagnosis of blastomycosis requires demonstration of large yeasts with broad-based buds or a positive culture from tissues or body fluids. Serologic studies are unreliable for diagnosis.
   B. **Treatment.** Itraconazole (200–400 mg PO qd) for a minimum of 6 months can be used for non–life-threatening, nonmeningeal blastomycosis. Amphotericin B (0.3–0.6 mg/kg/day for a total dose of 1.5–2.5 g) should be used for life-threatening or meningeal blastomycosis; a course of itraconazole can be used after amphotericin B therapy has been completed.

II. **Coccidioidomycosis,** a major endemic mycosis of the southwestern United States and Central America, is caused by *Coccidioides immitis*. Infection begins with inhalation of spores into the lung. Sixty percent of infected persons experience no symptoms or have nonspecific respiratory symptoms.
   A. **Diagnosis.** The diagnosis of coccidioidomycosis requires visualization of an endosporulating spherule in tissue or body fluids, positive culture, or positive complement fixation serology. Skin testing has a limited diagnostic role because anergy may occur and a positive test indicates only prior infection. Lumbar puncture should be performed in persons with severe disease, rapidly progressive disease, or disseminated disease, to rule out CNS involvement.
   B. **Treatment.** Fluconazole (400–600 mg PO qd) or itraconazole (200 mg PO bid) have been used successfully to treat mild or moderate nonmeningeal coccidioidomycosis; treatment should be continued for more than 6 months after the disease becomes inactive. Patients with severe disease, progressive disease, or disseminated disease should be treated with amphotericin B (1.0–1.5 mg/kg/day for a total of 1–3 g, depending on the clinical response). Some patients may require long-term therapy with itraconazole.

III. **Histoplasmosis,** a major endemic mycosis associated with bird and bat excrement in the Ohio and Mississippi River Valleys, is caused by *Histoplasma capsulatum*.
   A. **Diagnosis.** The diagnosis of histoplasmosis requires visualization of small yeasts in tissue or body fluids or a positive culture, associated with positive complement fixation and immunodiffusion serology. Detection of *Histoplasma* antigen in urine, serum, or CSF is reliable in the diagnosis of disseminated infection of cetain conditions (e.g., AIDS).
   B. **Treatment.** Itraconazole (200 mg PO tid loading dose for 3 days, followed by 200–400 mg PO qd for 6–12 months) is effective therapy in mild disease in immunocompetent hosts. Documentation of therapeutic levels of itraconazole is essential. Amphotericin B (total dose of 1.5–2.5 g) is the treatment of choice for moderate to severe disease or disease in immunocompromised hosts.

IV. **Sporotrichosis** follows traumatic inoculation, generally of extremities, after contact with soil or plant material, and lymphocutaneous disease is the usual manifestation. Untreated disease can persist and slowly progress over time; hematogenous dissemination occurs rarely in immunocompromised hosts, and pneumonia, arthritis, or meningitis can develop.
   A. **Diagnosis.** The diagnosis of sporotrichosis requires demonstration of yeast in tissue or body fluids, a positive culture, or positive serologic studies.

B. Treatment. A saturated solution of potassium iodide (5 drops PO tid, increased to 40 drops tid or until intolerance develops, for 1–2 months after clearing of lesions) is effective for lymphocutaneous disease, but treatment is poorly tolerated. Itraconazole (200 mg PO qd for 3–6 months) also is effective for lymphocutaneous disease and is better tolerated. Nonmeningeal extralymphocutaneous disease can be treated with itraconazole, 200 mg PO bid for 1–2 years. Documentation of therapeutic levels of itraconazole is essential. Severe and meningeal disease should be treated with amphotericin B, 1.5–2.5 g total.

V. Cryptococcosis is a mycosis that occurs worldwide and is caused by *C. neoformans*, a ubiquitous yeast associated with soil and pigeon excrement.

    A. Diagnosis. The diagnosis requires detection of encapsulated yeast in tissue or body fluids with culture confirmation. The latex agglutination test for cryptococcal antigen in serum or CSF provides a supportive diagnosis. Lumbar puncture generally is recommended in persons with systemic disease to exclude coexistent CNS disease (see Chap. 15).

    B. Treatment. Amphotericin B, 0.7 mg/kg/day IV, combined with flucytosine, 37.5 mg/kg PO q6h for 2 weeks, followed by a 6-month course of fluconazole, 400 mg PO qd, appears to be effective for the treatment of meningitis in immunocompetent and non-HIV immunocompromised hosts. An alternative is 6 weeks of amphotericin B plus flucytosine. Treatment of isolated pulmonary cryptococcosis in immunocompromised hosts has not been standardized (*Semin Respir Crit Care Med* 18:249, 1997).

VI. Aspergillosis includes a variety of clinical conditions caused by *Aspergillus* species, which are ubiquitous environmental fungi. Disease generally follows inhalation of spores into the lung, but cutaneous disease can follow direct inoculation. Clinical presentations can be divided into three categories: allergic aspergillosis, aspergilloma, and invasive aspergillosis.

    A. Allergic bronchopulmonary aspergillosis presents acutely with asthma, eosinophilia, and pulmonary infiltrates. The natural history includes remissions and exacerbations with eventual pulmonary bronchiectasis and fibrosis.

        1. Diagnosis generally requires the presence of asthma, documentation of eosinophilia, type I hypersensitivity to *Aspergillus* antigens, serum precipitins against *Aspergillus*, elevated serum immunoglobulin E and immunoglobulin G against *Aspergillus*, pulmonary infiltrates, or central bronchiectasis.

        2. Treatment requires allergen avoidance and might require the intermittent use of corticosteroids.

    B. Pulmonary aspergilloma has a variable natural history, including spontaneous resolution and locally invasive disease.

        1. Diagnosis is made in the setting of a characteristic radiographic presentation and serum *Aspergillus* precipitins.

        2. Treatment includes observation; surgical resection is reserved for those patients with massive hemoptysis.

    C. Invasive aspergillosis is a serious condition associated with vascular invasion, thrombosis, and ischemic infarction of involved tissues and progressive disease after hematogenous dissemination.

        1. Diagnosis requires characteristic histologic evidence of involved tissue and a positive culture.

        2. Treatment of serious invasive aspergillosis requires amphotericin B (1 mg/kg/day for 2.0–2.5 g total). Itraconazole (600 mg PO qd for 4 days, then 200–400 mg PO qd for 1 year) may be effective in mildly to moderately invasive aspergillosis, but its definitive role in therapy is not yet established.

VII. Candidiasis commonly involves an endogenous source (e.g., vagina, GI tract, mouth, skin) and presents as an opportunistic infection in immunocompromised hosts (see Chap. 15) and is also associated with concurrent antibiotic use, contraceptive use, immunosuppressant and cytotoxic therapy, and indwelling foreign bodies. Candidiasis may present as mucocutaneous or invasive disease (e.g., candidemia with or without tissue dissemination and with skin lesions, ocular disease, or osteomyelitis). Mucocutaneous disease may resolve after elimination of the causative condition (e.g., antibiotic therapy) or may persist and progress in the setting of immunosuppressive conditions. Although isolated candidemia can resolve spontaneously, particularly after catheter removal if disease is related to an infected catheter, serious complications can occur. Systemic antifungal therapy is recommended for all forms of invasive candidiasis.

A. Diagnosis. Mucocutaneous candidiasis is usually a clinical diagnosis, although a KOH preparation of exudate might provide confirmation. Invasive candidiasis usually is diagnosed by positive cultures of blood or tissue.

B. Treatment

1. **Oral candidiasis** responds to nystatin (500,000 units "swish and swallow" 3–5 times a day), clotrimazole troches (10 mg dissolved in the mouth 5 times a day), oral azole therapy (ketoconazole, 200–400 mg PO qd, or fluconazole, 100–200 mg PO qd), and low-dose amphotericin B (10–20 mg IV qd for 7–14 days). For mucocutaneous disease, the duration of therapy depends on clinical response and the reversibility of the underlying condition.

2. **Isolated catheter-related candidemia** can be treated with amphotericin B and catheter removal (see Catheter-Related Infections).

3. **Disseminated candidiasis** should be treated with more prolonged courses of amphotericin B (0.5 mg/kg/day IV for a total of 0.5–2.0 g). Fluconazole (200–400 mg IV or PO qd) is an alternative for nonneutropenic patients with invasive disease who are unable to tolerate amphotericin B, but non–*Candida albicans* species are less susceptible to azoles. **Liposomal amphotericin** may be indicated for patients who have documented or suspected severe systemic mycoses that are unsuitable for treatment with azoles, who have documented renal intolerance to conventional amphotericin B, or who have baseline renal insufficiency or risk factors for development of renal insufficiency, including a (1) Cr greater than 2.5 mg/dl or Cr clearance (Cl_{Cr}) of less than 40 ml/minute, (2) Cr greater than 2 mg/dl or Cl_{Cr} less than 60 ml/minute and receiving one nephrotoxic medication, or (3) Cr greater than 1.5 mg/dl or Cl_{Cr} less than 75 ml/minute and receiving at least two nephrotoxic medications. The nephrotoxic medications of most concern are cisplatin, cyclosporin A, aminoglycosides, foscarnet, pentamidine, cidofovir, and scheduled nonsteroidal anti-inflammatory drugs.

Zoonoses and Arthropod-Borne Diseases

I. Rickettsial disease

A. Rocky Mountain spotted fever is a serious, potentially fatal vasculitis due to infection with *R. rickettsii*. Most reported cases occur between April and September and are associated with a tick bite. Endemic regions in the United States include the South Atlantic states, the Midwest, and the West.

1. **Diagnosis.** *R. rickettsii* invade and multiply within endothelial cells of arteries and veins. The average incubation period for Rocky Mountain spotted fever is 7 days, and clinical manifestations include sudden onset of severe retrobulbar headache, fever, chills, myalgias, malaise, nausea, vomiting, and photophobia. A maculopapular rash is seen in 90% of patients, usually after 3–4 days of fever; the rash begins on the wrists and ankles and later spreads to the trunk, face, and remainder of the extremities, with development of petechiae. Thrombocytopenia and elevations of liver function tests are common. Diagnosis depends on heightened clinical suspicion in the appropriate epidemiologic setting.

Confirmation requires immunofluorescence staining of skin biopsy specimens or analysis of acute and convalescent serology.

2. **Treatment.** Doxycycline (100 mg PO or IV q12h), tetracycline (25–50 mg/kg PO divided qid), or chloramphenicol (50–75 mg/kg/day PO or IV divided qid; maximum, 4 g/day) can be administered, as all are effective. Chloramphenicol IV is preferred therapy if CNS manifestations are prominent. Fever and associated symptoms usually resolve within 72 hours, and therapy can be discontinued after 7 days.

B. **Ehrlichiosis,** a systemic illness caused by *Ehrlichia* species, exhibits features similar to those of Rocky Mountain spotted fever. Most cases occur between May and July and are associated with a tick bite. Endemic U.S. regions include the South, the South Atlantic, and the South Central states. Two similar syndromes are recognized: human monocytic ehrlichiosis (caused by *E. chaffeensis*; tropism for monocytes) and human granulocytic ehrlichiosis (caused by *Ehrlichia equi* and *Ehrlichia phagocytophilia*; tropism for granulocytes). The average incubation period of disease is 7 days. Onset of illness occurs with fever, chills, headache, myalgia, and malaise, followed by nausea and anorexia; a rash is seen in fewer than 50% of patients. Leukopenia, thrombocytopenia, and elevated liver function tests are common.

1. **Diagnosis** depends on a heightened clinical suspicion in a febrile patient with tick exposure during the summer months, particularly in the setting of leukopenia and thrombocytopenia. Visualization of morulae in monocytes or granulocytes is uncommon but, if obtained, might provide the diagnosis. Confirmation rests on analysis of acute and convalescent serology. PCR-based blood and CSF studies are currently investigational.

2. **Therapy** consists of tetracycline, 25 mg/kg/day PO, divided qid, or doxycycline, 100 mg PO or IV bid, for 7–14 days.

II. Spirochetal disease

A. **Lyme disease** is the leading tick-borne disease in the United States. It is a systemic illness of variable severity caused by *Borrelia burgdorferi* and has dermatologic, rheumatologic, neurologic, and cardiac manifestations. Most cases are reported between May and August and are associated with a tick bite, and more than 90% of cases have occurred in the Northeastern coastal states, the upper Midwest, and northern California. After an average incubation period of 7–10 days, early local disease is characterized by a macular dermatitis called erythema migrans and by mild constitutional symptoms. Manifestations of early disseminated disease occur within several weeks to months and include multiple skin lesions (erythema migrans), neurologic symptoms (e.g., seventh cranial nerve palsy, meningoencephalitis, peripheral neuropathy), cardiac symptoms [e.g., atrioventricular (AV) block, myopericarditis], and asymmetric oligoarticular arthritis. Late disease occurs after months to years and includes chronic dermatitis, chronic neurologic disease, and chronic asymmetric monoarticular or oligoarticular arthritis.

1. **Diagnosis** rests on clinical suspicion in the appropriate epidemiologic setting. Enzyme-linked immunosorbent assay is available but is poorly standardized, often resulting in false-positive findings; a positive result should be confirmed with a Western blot. Early treatment may inhibit the antibody response. Culture of *B. burgdorferi* from skin lesions provides a definitive diagnosis but is impractical.

2. **Treatment** for early Lyme disease, isolated seventh nerve palsy, and first-degree AV block includes tetracycline (250 mg PO qid for 10–21 days), doxycycline (100 mg PO bid for 10–21 days), or amoxicillin (500 mg PO tid for 10–21 days) with or without probenecid (500 mg PO tid). Ten-day therapy usually is reserved for isolated erythema migrans. Optimal therapy for early disseminated and chronic Lyme disease is not established. Regimens used include doxycycline (100 mg PO bid for 30 days), penicillin G (3–4 million units IV q4h for 14–21 days), and ceftriaxone (2 g IV qd for 14–21 days). Parenteral therapy is recommended for high-grade AV block.

B. **Leptospirosis** is a ubiquitous enzootic infection caused by *Leptospira interrogans*. Infection follows contact with contaminated animal tissues, fluids, excreta, or contaminated water sources. Reservoirs of infection include rodents, skunks, foxes, domestic livestock, dogs, and frogs. More than 50% of recent cases are a result of nonoccupational exposure. Disease prevalence peaks during the summer months. After an incubation period of 7–14 days, clinical manifestations of **anicteric leptospirosis** include fever, headache, myalgias, conjunctival suffusion, GI symptoms, pharyngitis, adenopathy, hepatomegaly, and rash. These manifestations usually last 1 week or less. Elevated liver function studies, elevated Cr level, and abnormal urinalysis are common. **Icteric leptospirosis** is a much more severe and prolonged illness than anicteric leptospirosis and involves hepatic and renal failure, hemorrhage, vascular collapse, and alterations in consciousness.

1. **Diagnosis.** The diagnosis is confirmed via blood culture, urine culture, or acute and convalescent serologic studies.

2. **Treatment.** Tetracycline (500 mg PO q6h for 7 days), doxycycline (100 mg PO or IV bid for 7 days), penicillin G (1.5 million units IV q4–6h for 7 days), amoxicillin (500 mg PO q6h for 7 days), and ampicillin (500–750 mg PO q6h for 7 days; 500–1000 mg IV q6h if severe) are effective in reducing clinical illness, particularly when given in the first few days of illness. IV therapy should be used for moderate to severe illness.

III. **Tularemia** is a systemic disease caused by *Francisella tularensis*. Important animal reservoirs include rabbits, hares, and ticks. Infection develops via tick bite, direct contact with infected tissues, inhalation of aerosolized organisms, ingestion of contaminated food or water, and bites of infected animals or mosquitoes. The South Central states are an endemic region. The average incubation period is 3–5 days. Ulceroglandular disease presents as an ulcer at the bite site and painful regional adenopathy. Glandular disease, typhoidal disease, and oculoglandular disease follow organism inoculation; primary pneumonic disease follows organism inhalation; and primary oropharyngeal disease follows organism ingestion.

A. **Diagnosis.** Acute and convalescent serologic studies or culture of *F. tularensis* from a lesion, bubo, or blood is diagnostic. For culture, the laboratory should be promptly notified that tularemia is suspected so that biohazard precautions are used.

B. **Treatment.** Streptomycin remains the drug of choice; 15–20 mg/kg IM qd in two divided doses for 7–14 days is effective. Gentamicin probably is equally effective. Oral alternatives include tetracycline (30 mg/kg PO loading dose, followed by 30 mg/kg PO in divided doses for 14 days), doxycycline (100 mg PO bid for 14 days), and perhaps ciprofloxacin, but relapse rates may be high with oral regimens.

IV. **Arboviral meningoencephalitis** is caused by multiple viral agents, resulting in endemic and epidemic disease in the United States (e.g., Eastern and Western equine encephalitis, LaCrosse encephalitis, St. Louis encephalitis). Infections usually occur in the summer months, and most are subclinical.

A. **Diagnosis** is often clinical. Definitive diagnosis can be established only with acute and convalescent serologic studies, except for Venezuelan equine encephalitis, which can be cultured from the pharynx or blood early in the illness.

B. **Treatment** is supportive.

V. **Cat-scratch disease** is a lymphadenopathy syndrome caused by *Bartonella henselae* after a cat-related exposure. Disease occurs worldwide, with most cases reported in children between August and January. An isolated skin lesion, followed by regional adenopathy with mild constitutional symptoms, is the most common presentation and occurs approximately 2 weeks after exposure. Head, neck, and axillary lymph nodes are involved most frequently. Symptoms resolve within 2–6 months. Atypical presentations include oculoglandular disease, encephalopathy, arthritis or arthropathy, and severe systemic disease.

A. **Diagnosis** is supported by a positive serologic workup for *B. henselae*.

B. Treatment with antibiotics might not hasten resolution of the clinical illness. Various regimens include RIF, ciprofloxacin, TMP/SMX, erythromycin, and azithromycin. Lymph node aspiration and drainage may provide symptomatic relief of suppurative lymphadenitis.

VI. Malaria is a systemic disease that is endemic to most of the tropical and subtropical world. *Plasmodium falciparum* malaria, the most severe form of the disease, is a potential medical emergency. Infection can occur year round. The onset of illness occurs within weeks to months of infection; with *Plasmodium vivax* and *Plasmodium ovale*, dormant hepatic forms might produce clinical disease 6–12 months after initial infection. Malaria is characterized by fever, chills, headache, myalgias, arthralgia, nausea, vomiting, or diarrhea. *P. falciparum* infections rarely present with periodic symptoms; *P. vivax* and *P. ovale* infections might present with symptoms at 48-hour intervals, and *Plasmodium malariae* might present with symptoms at 72-hour intervals.

A. Diagnosis. The diagnosis of malaria requires a heightened clinical suspicion when a febrile illness occurs in a patient who has recently visited an endemic area. Diagnosis is made by identification of the parasites in a blood smear stained with Giemsa stain.

B. Treatment. Chloroquine resistance in *P. falciparum* is common worldwide, except in Central America north of the Panama Canal, the Caribbean, and most countries in the Middle East. Sulfadoxine and pyrimethamine resistance occurs in Southeast Asia and the Amazon. Presumed chloroquine-resistant, mild to moderate *P. falciparum* malaria should be treated with quinine sulfate, 650 mg PO tid for 3 days, plus doxycycline, 100 mg PO bid for 7 days. Pyrimethamine, three tablets PO as a single dose, can be substituted for doxycycline outside of resistant areas. Severe *P. falciparum* infection requires parenteral therapy with quinidine gluconate, 10 mg/kg IV over 1–2 hours, followed by 0.02 mg/kg/minute as a continuous infusion, plus doxycycline, 100 mg PO or IV q12h. When the level of parasitemia is less than 1%, quinine sulfate can be substituted to complete a total of 3 days of quinidine and quinine. For *P. falciparum* parasitemias that exceed 10%, exchange transfusion should be considered. Mild to moderate *P. falciparum* malaria acquired in areas where chloroquine resistance does not occur can be treated with chloroquine, 600 mg base (or 1000 mg chloroquine phosphate) PO, followed in 6 hours by 300 mg base PO and an additional 300 mg base PO qd for 2 days. Non–*P. falciparum* malaria is less severe and usually responds to oral chloroquine. Because of dormant hepatic forms, patients with *P. vivax* or *P. ovale* infection should also be treated with primaquine, 26.3 mg salt (15 mg base) PO qd for 14 days, after the patient has been tested for glucose 6-phosphate dehydrogenase (G6PD) deficiency. G6PD-deficient patients can be treated with lower doses of primaquine over a longer time period.

C. Prophylaxis. Pretravel advice and appropriate chemoprophylaxis are essential. The choice of chemoprophylaxis depends on the types of resistance in the area of planned travel. Travelers to malaria-endemic areas may also need other prophylaxis or pretravel vaccination (e.g., yellow fever). Travelers should be referred to a travel clinic, or appropriate publications or experts should be consulted before pretravel recommendations are provided (see Centers for Disease Control at http://www.cdc.gov).

Human and Animal Bites

The need for rabies vaccination and immune globulin prophylaxis should be considered for all animal bites (see sec. **III.C**). Physical examination of the affected area should document the location and extent of injuries, range of motion, status of tendon and nerve function, local adenopathy, and presence of edema, warmth, erythema, and devitalized tissue.

I. **The general approach** to any bite first involves the obtaining of cultures from any visibly infected or moderate to severe bite wounds. Bite wounds should be copiously irrigated and débrided. An x-ray of the affected part should be considered when fracture is possible, when a foreign body may be present, when a bone or joint may have been penetrated, or when infection near a bone or joint is documented. Therapeutic antibiotic therapy should be administered for overtly infected wounds. Prophylactic antibiotic therapy (3–5 days) should be considered for wounds less than 8 hours old that are moderate to severe, involve crush injury, or exhibit edema; wounds that might involve a bone or joint or are adjacent to a prosthetic joint; hand wounds; cat bites; puncture wounds; and wounds in persons with underlying conditions that predispose them to more severe infection. Infected wounds and wounds older than 24 hours should not be closed; closure of other wounds is controversial. Tetanus booster should be given if none has been administered to the patient in the last 10 years. Wound elevation or immobilization should be provided for edematous wounds. Follow-up should be performed within 24–48 hours of the initial visit.

II. **Human bites,** particularly closed-fist bites, are more prone to infection and other complications than are other bites. Occlusive bites include those in which human teeth actually bite part of the body, whereas a closed-fist injury occurs when the metacarpophalangeal joint of one person's hand strikes the teeth of another person.

   A. **Bacteriology** reflects the normal aerobic and anaerobic oral flora of humans: viridans streptococci, staphylococci, *Bacteroides* species, *Corynebacterium* species, peptostreptococci, and *Eikenella corrodens*.

   B. **Treatment.** For occlusive bite wounds, amoxicillin/clavulanate (500 mg/125 mg PO tid or 875 mg/125 mg PO bid for 3–5 days) is effective as prophylaxis for uninfected wounds, but infected wounds generally require parenteral therapy (ampicillin/sulbactam, 1.5 g IV q6h; cefoxitin, 2 g IV q8h; or ticarcillin/clavulanate, 3.1 g IV q6h). Closed-fist bite injuries usually are infected and often require hospitalization for initial parenteral antibiotic therapy. Duration of therapeutic antibiotics is 1–2 weeks for cellulitis and 4–6 weeks for osteomyelitis.

III. **Animal bites**

   A. **Bacteriology** reflects the normal aerobic and anaerobic oral flora of specific animals. For dogs, the normal oral flora includes streptococci, staphylococci, and *Pasteurella multocida*. Dog bites are responsible for 80% of animal bites, but only 20% become infected. The normal oral flora of cats includes *P. multocida* and *S. aureus*. More than 80% of cat bites become infected.

   B. **Treatment.** Prophylactic antibiotic therapy with amoxicillin/clavulanate (500 mg/125 mg PO tid or 875 mg/125 mg PO bid for 3–5 days) should usually be administered, unless the bite is trivial and not cat related. For infected dog-bite wounds, amoxicillin/clavulanate, clindamycin plus ciprofloxacin (adults), clindamycin plus TMP/SMX (children), tetracycline, or cefuroxime axetil is effective. For infected cat-bite wounds, effective therapy includes amoxicillin/clavulanate, penicillin V (500 mg PO qid), oral doxycycline, or IV ceftriaxone. Duration of therapy is 1–2 weeks for cellulitis versus 4–6 weeks for osteomyelitis.

   C. **Rabies vaccination and immune globulin prophylaxis** (see also Appendix F). The need for such therapy should be determined after any animal bite. Because most domestic dogs have been vaccinated, individuals usually do not require rabies treatment after domestic dog bites. Endemic rabies is present in bats, foxes, skunks, raccoons, and other wild carnivores. Rates by species vary in different parts of the United States, although rabies is endemic in bats throughout the states. Rabies in wild rodents and lagomorphs (e.g., squirrels, rats, mice, rabbits, hares) is uncommon except in groundhogs.

      1. **Domestic dog and cat bites.** If the animal is healthy and available for 10 days of observation, no treatment is indicated unless the animal develops rabies. If the animal is rabid or suspected to be rabid, the

human diploid vaccine and rabies immune globulin should be administered (see Appendix F). If the animal's condition is unknown, the local health department should be contacted.

2. **Wild animal bites.** The need for vaccine is determined by the animal species and region of the country (*N Engl J Med* 329:1632, 1993). If rabies is endemic in the species involved, treatment is given (see Appendix F). If rabies is not endemic in the species involved but is endemic in other terrestrial animals in the area, treatment is given if the bite is from a wild carnivore or groundhog. If the bite is from some other species, the local health department should be consulted. If rabies is not endemic in any species in the area, treatment is withheld, or the local health department should be consulted.

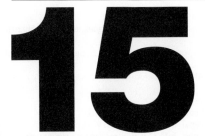

HIV Infection and AIDS

Woraphot Tantisiriwat
and Pablo Tebas

I. **HIV type 1** is a human retrovirus that infects lymphocytes and other cells that bear the CD4 surface protein, as well as a coreceptor belonging to the chemokine receptor family. Infection leads to lymphopenia and CD4 T-cell depletion, impaired cell-mediated immunity, and polyclonal B-cell activation. Over time, this immune dysfunction gives rise to **AIDS**, which is characterized by opportunistic infections (OIs) and malignancies. The time from onset of HIV infection to development of AIDS varies from months to years, with a median incubation period of 10 years. The virus is transmitted sexually or parenterally. Therapy for HIV infection and AIDS includes antiretroviral therapy, prophylaxis for and treatment of infections, and treatment of neoplasia.

II. **Before checking an individual's HIV serology,** the physician should obtain informed consent. Informed consent is required in most states and countries and is recommended always.

   A. **Serology.** HIV serology should be checked in the following persons:

   1. **Persons in high-risk categories,** including IV drug users, homosexual and bisexual men, hemophiliacs, sexual partners of the aforementioned patients, sexual partners of a known HIV patient, prostitutes and their sexual partners, persons with sexually transmitted diseases, persons who received blood products between 1977 and 1985, persons who have multiple sexual partners or who engage in unprotected intercourse, persons who consider themselves at risk, and patients with findings that are suggestive of HIV infection

   2. **Pregnant women**

   3. **Patients with active tuberculosis (TB)**

   4. **Hospitalized patients** between the ages of 15 and 54 years if the community seroprevalence rate exceeds 1% or AIDS cases number more than 1 per 1000 discharges

   5. **Donors of blood, semen, and organs**

   6. **Health care workers** who perform invasive procedures (depending on the policy of the institution in which they work)

   7. **Persons with occupational exposures** (e.g., needle-sticks) and source patients of the exposures

   B. **Methods and results.** Screening is performed with an enzyme-linked immunosorbent assay (ELISA). A positive screening test is confirmed by a repeat positive ELISA and a positive Western blot (presence of at least 2 of the following bands: p24, gp41, gp120/160). An isolated positive ELISA result should not be reported to the patient until this result is confirmed by a Western blot. An indeterminate test is one for which the ELISA is positive but the criteria for a positive Western blot are not fulfilled.

III. **Initial evaluation** of persons with a positive HIV test should include the following measures:

   A. **Complete history,** with emphasis on OIs and other complications

   B. **Psychological and psychiatric history.** Depression and other psychological problems are common and should be identified and treated as necessary.

C. Family and social support assessment

D. Contraception, educational issues, safer sex practices, and detoxification for drug abusers

E. Social worker referral and open discussions about aggressiveness of care when the disease advances

F. Complete physical examination

G. Laboratory tests

1. **CBC and routine chemistry**
2. **CD4 cell count** (normal range, 600–1500 cells/µl)
3. **Virologic markers.** Several quantitative HIV type 1 RNA viral load assays are currently in use, but the polymerase chain reaction (PCR) assay is the only one approved by the Food and Drug Administration. Regular PCR has a lower limit of detection of 400 viral copies/ml, whereas the newly developed ultrasensitive assay has a lower limit of detection of 40 copies/ml. The other two assays are a branched DNA (bDNA) assay and a nucleic acid sequence amplification assay. Regular PCR assay should be used for an initial visit.
4. **Tuberculin skin test**
5. **VDRL, *Toxoplasma* immunoglobulin G, and hepatitis B and C serologies**
6. **Cervical Papanicolaou smear**

H. Immunizations

1. **Pneumococcal vaccine.** Efficacy has not been clearly established in this population. Antibody responses are better when CD4 cell counts are greater than 350 cells/µl. Revaccination after 5 years should be considered.
2. **Hepatitis A and B virus (HAV and HBV).** HIV-infected patients are at higher risk of becoming chronic carriers of HBV after having an acute HBV infection. If antibodies against hepatitis B core and hepatitis B surface antigens are negative, HBV vaccination is indicated. Hepatitis C is very prevalent in this population (especially among IV drug abusers). Vaccination for HAV is recommended for homosexual males, food handlers, and patients who have chronic active hepatitis B or C and negative HAV antibodies.
3. **Influenza.** Influenza vaccination has been recommended in patients infected with HIV; vaccination may promote HIV replication and produce a transient increase in the viral load for up to 3 months after vaccination.

IV. Antiretroviral therapy should be individualized and closely monitored by measuring plasma HIV viral load. Reductions in plasma viremia correlate with increased CD4 cell counts and AIDS-free survival.

A. Indications for the initiation of **antiretroviral therapy** include the following.

1. **In the symptomatic patient** (with AIDS, thrush, or unexplained fever) therapy should be initiated regardless of the CD4 count or viral load.
2. **In the asymptomatic patient, if the CD4 count is less than 500 cells/µl** or the viral load is greater than 10,000 copies/ml by bDNA or 20,000 copies/ml by PCR, therapy should be offered.
3. **In the asymptomatic patient with CD4 count greater than 500 cells/µl** with a viral load less than 10,000 copies/ml by bDNA or less than 20,000 by PCR, therapy should be offered, although many experts would wait until the CD4 count is lower.

B. General principles for the treatment of HIV infection have been outlined (*2000 Guidelines for the Use of Antiretroviral Agents in HIV-Infected Adults and Adolescents*) (see http://hivatis.org).

1. Ongoing HIV replication leads to immune system damage and progression to AIDS.
2. Plasma HIV RNA levels indicate the magnitude of HIV replication and its associated rate of CD4 cell destruction, and CD4 cell counts indicate the extent of HIV-induced immune damage that has already been experienced.

3. Treatment decisions should be individualized by level of risk indicated by plasma HIV RNA levels and CD4 cell counts.

4. Complete suppression of HIV replication (measured by the ultrasensitive assay) should be the goal of therapy.

5. The most effective means of suppressing HIV replication is the simultaneous initiation of combination potent antiretroviral therapy.

6. Each drug should always be used according to optimum schedules and dosages.

7. Any change in antiretroviral therapy increases future therapeutic constraints and potential drug resistance.

8. Women should receive optimal antiretroviral therapy even if pregnant.

9. The same principles of antiretroviral therapy apply to HIV-infected children and adults.

10. Persons with acute primary HIV infections should be treated with potent antiretroviral therapy.

11. HIV-infected persons, even those with viral loads below detectable limits, should be considered infectious.

C. **Antiretroviral drugs.** Specific drug information is summarized in Tables 15-1, 15-2, and 15-3. Approved antiretroviral drugs are grouped into three categories:

1. **Nucleoside analog reverse transcriptase inhibitors (NRTIs)** constrain HIV replication by incorporation into the elongating strand of DNA, causing chain termination.

2. **Protease inhibitors (PIs)** are a very potent group of drugs that block the action of the viral protease required for protein processing late in the viral cycle. They are used in combination regimens. **All these drugs have important interactions with other medications, and concomitant medications should be reviewed carefully** (see **IV.H** and Table 15-4). Combinations of two PIs, especially with ritonavir, can decrease the dosage requirement of the other PIs.

3. **Nonnucleoside reverse transcriptase inhibitors (NNRTIs)** inhibit HIV by binding noncompetitively to the reverse transcriptase. Because onset of action is rapid, they may have a role in postexposure prophylaxis. A single dosage of nevirapine at the time of labor also prevents perinatal transmission.

D. **Initial therapy.** Antiretroviral therapy is usually started in the outpatient setting by a physician with expertise in the management of patients with HIV infection. Adherence is the key factor for success of antiretroviral therapy. Treatment should be individualized and adapted to the patient's lifestyle. Any treatment decision will influence future therapeutic options because of the possibility of drug cross-resistance. Potent antiretroviral therapy consists of either a combination of two NRTIs plus a PI or an NNRTI, or both, or two NRTIs plus two PIs. An alternative but possibly less potent regimen, especially in patients with high viral loads, is a combination of 3 NRTIs such as zidovudine + lamivudine + abacavir.

E. **Monitoring of therapy.** Plasma HIV RNA load is used for monitoring of therapy. The goal is to reduce the viral load levels below the detection limits. CD4 cell counts are checked to assess the immune status of the patient and to define the start of prophylactic therapy. After starting or changing antiretroviral therapy, viral load is checked after 4 weeks and the patient is reassessed to enhance adherence. When the ultrasensitive HIV RNA becomes undetectable and the patient is on a stable regimen, monitoring can be done every 3 months.

F. **Treatment failure** is defined as (1) less than a log (10-fold) reduction of the viral load after 4–6 weeks of starting a new antiretroviral regimen; (2) failure to reach undetectable viral load after 4–6 months of treatment; (3) detection of virus after initial complete suppression of viral load, which suggests development of resistance; or (4) persistent decline of CD4 cells or clinical deterioration. Confirmed treatment failure should prompt changes in antiretroviral

Table 15-1. Nucleoside analog reverse transcriptase inhibitors

	Zidovudine (ZDV, AZT)	Didanosine (ddI)	Zalcitabine (ddC)	Stavudine (d4T)	Lamivudine (3TC)	Abacavir (ABC)
Dosage	300 mg PO bid [Combivir (ZDV 300 mg + 3TC 150 mg) 1 tablet bid]	>60 kg: 200 mg PO bid <60 kg: 125 mg PO bid	0.75 mg PO tid	>60 kg: 40 mg PO bid <60 kg: 30 mg PO bid	150 mg PO bid <50 kg: 2 mg/kg bid	300 mg PO bid [Trizivir (ZDV 300 mg + 3TC 150 mg + ABC 600 mg) PO bid]
Food restrictions	No	Has to be taken on empty stomach	No	No	No	No
Common side effects	Bone marrow suppression, GI intolerance	Pancreatitis, peripheral neuropathy, diarrhea	Peripheral neuropathy, stomatitis	Peripheral neuropathy	Rare	Hypersensitivity reaction (flu-like symptoms, fever, rash, upper respiratory symptoms, GI intolerance)
Interactions with other antiretrovirals	Antagonist with d4T	Do not use with ddC, due to ↑ risk of neuropathy	Do not use with ddI, due to ↑ risk of neuropathy	Antagonist with ZDV	None	**Rechallenge after reaction can be fatal**
"Class" side effects	All nucleoside analogs have been associated with lactic acidosis syndrome, presumably related to mitochondrial toxicity					

Table 15-2. Nonnucleoside reverse transcriptase inhibitors*

	Nevirapine (NVP)	Delavirdine (DLV)	Efavirenz (EFV)
Dosage	200 mg PO qd for 2 wks, then 200 mg PO bid or 400 mg qd	400 mg PO tid	600 mg PO qhs
Food restrictions	No	No	Avoid taking after high-fat meals (level ↑ by 50%)
Common side effects	Hepatitis	Headaches	CNS symptoms (dizziness, somnolence, insomnia, abnormal dreams), false-positive cannabinoid test
"Class" side effects	Rash, ↑ AST, ↑ ALT, Stevens-Johnson syndrome		

ALT = alanine aminotransferase; AST = aspartate aminotransferase; ↑ = increases level of; ↓ = decreases level of.
*See Table 15-4 for interactions with other antiretrovirals.

therapy. In this situation at least two of the drugs should be substituted with others with no expected cross-resistance. HIV resistance testing may help determine a salvage regimen in the patients with prior antiretroviral experience. The importance of adherence should be stressed. Referral to an HIV specialist is highly recommended in this situation.

G. **HIV resistance testing** is done using two different types of assays: genotypic (in which the reverse transcriptase and the polymerase genes are sequenced using different techniques) and phenotypic (in which the behavior of HIV in vitro in the presence of antiretroviral drugs is examined). These tests are time consuming, expensive, and insensitive to the presence of minor variants.

H. **Drug interactions.** Antiretroviral medications, especially PIs, interact with multiple other medications that might increase the risk for toxicity. PIs and delavirdine are inhibitors and inducers of the p450 system. Interactions are frequent with other inhibitors of the p450 system, including macrolides (erythromycin, clarithromycin) and antifungals (ketoconazole, itraconazole), as well as inducers, such as rifamycins (rifampin, rifabutin) and anticonvulsants (phenobarbital, phenytoin, carbamazepine). Drugs with narrow therapeutic indexes that should be avoided or used with extreme caution include antihistaminics (loratadine is safe), antiarrhythmics (flecainide, encainide, quinidine), long-acting opiates (fentanyl, meperidine), long-acting benzodiazepines (midazolam, triazolam), warfarin, HMG-CoA reductase inhibitors (pravastatin is the safest), and oral contraceptives. The prokinetic agent cisapride also has potentially serious drug interactions with PIs and has been withdrawn from the U.S. market due to reports of fatal cardiac arrhythmias from interactions with a variety of drugs. Sildenafil concentrations are increased, and methadone and theophylline concentrations are decreased with concomitant administration of certain PIs. Grapefruit juice can increase levels of saquinavir and

Table 15-3. Protease inhibitors*

	Saquinavir	Ritonavir	Nelfinavir	Indinavir	Amprenavir	Lopinavir
Dosage	1200 mg PO tid (soft gel)	600 mg PO q12h	750 mg PO tid or 1250 mg PO bid	800 mg PO q8h	1200 mg PO bid	400 mg lopinavir in fixed combination with 100 mg ritonavir
Food restrictions	Take with food	Take with food	Take with food	No food Increase water ingestion	Take with food	Take with food
Common side effects	Headache, diarrhea	Nausea and vomiting, paresthesia, hepatitis, taste perversion, asthenia	Diarrhea	Nephrolithiasis, ↑ indirect bilirubin, headache	Rash, diarrhea, nausea	Diarrhea, hyperlipidemia
"Class" side effects	All protease inhibitors can produce increased bleeding in hemophilia, GI intolerance, and increased liver function tests, and all have been associated with metabolic abnormalities (although their etiologic role is still unclear), such as hyperglycemia and increases in triglycerides, cholesterol, and body fat redistribution.					

↑ = increases level of.
*See Table 15-4 for interactions with other antiretrovirals.

decrease levels of indinavir. See Table 15-4 for interactions with other antiretrovirals.

I. **Complications of antiretroviral therapy.** The prolonged use of antiretrovirals has been associated with long-term toxicities whose pathogenesis at this time is only partially understood. No controlled trials have been undertaken for the treatment of these complications.

1. **Lipodystrophy syndrome** is an alteration in body fat distribution. Changes consist of accumulation of visceral fat in the retroperitoneum and mesenterium and neck and pelvic areas, and/or depletion of subcutaneous fat. Fat accumulation and fat lipodystrophy are probably two distinct syndromes.

2. **Hyperlipidemia,** especially hypertriglyceridemia, is associated mainly with PIs (especially ritonavir). Improvement has been seen after treatment with atorvastatin and pravastatin and/or gemfibrozil. Changing the PIs to an alternative drug is another possibility.

3. **Hyperglycemia** has been occasionally associated with the use of PIs. Patients typically have peripheral insulin resistance and impaired glucose tolerance.

4. **Lactic acidosis** with liver steatosis is rarely associated with antiretroviral therapy (NRTIs) but can be fatal. The mechanism seems to be mitochondrial toxicity. Suspected drugs should be discontinued.

5. **Osteopenia and osteoporosis**

J. **Impact of potent antiretroviral therapy on OIs.** Potent antiretroviral therapy has decreased the incidence, changed the manifestations, and improved the outcome of OIs. A new clinical syndrome associated with the immune enhancement induced by potent antiretroviral therapy **(immune reconstitution syndrome)** has been described. Examples include paradoxical reactions with TB, localized *Mycobacterium avium* complex (MAC) adenitis, and CMV vitritis immediately after the initiation of potent antiretroviral therapy.

V. **Prophylaxis of OIs** can be divided into primary and secondary prophylaxis.

A. **Primary prophylaxis** is established before an episode of OI occurs. Institution of primary prophylaxis depends on the level of immunosuppression as judged by the patient's CD4 cell count. The following interventions are considered standards of care and should be applied in every patient (*MMWR Morb Mortal Wkly Rep* 48:RR-10, 1999):

1. *Pneumocystis carinii* **pneumonia (PCP) prophylaxis** should be initiated when the CD4 count is less than 200 cells/µl or if the patient has unexplained fever for more than 2 weeks or experiences an episode of oral candidiasis. Trimethoprim-sulfamethoxazole (TMP/SMX), 160 mg/ 800 mg [one double-strength (DS) tablet] PO once a day or three times a week, is the preferred regimen. If TMP/SMX is contraindicated, dapsone, 100 mg PO qd; atovaquone, 1500 mg PO qd; or inhaled pentamidine, 300 mg once a month, is an alternative.

2. **TB prophylaxis** should be given to patients with a positive purified protein derivative test (PPD; >5 mm of induration), a history of a previous untreated positive PPD, or recent contact with an active TB case. Isoniazid (INH), 300 mg PO qd, plus pyridoxine, 50 mg PO qd for 9 months, is the regimen of choice. Rifampin, 600 mg PO qd, with pyrazinamide, 20 mg/kg qd for 2 months, is an alternative. In INH-resistant TB, rifampin for 4 months is indicated.

3. **Anti-***Toxoplasma* **prophylaxis** is indicated for seropositive patients with CD4 cell counts less than 100 cells/µl. TMP/SMX DS once a day is the preferred regimen. A combination of dapsone, 50 mg PO qd, plus pyrimethamine, 50 mg PO weekly, and leucovorin, 25 mg PO weekly, is an alternative.

4. **MAC prophylaxis** is indicated if CD4 cell counts are less than 50 cells/µl and consists of azithromycin, 1200 mg PO weekly, or clarithromycin,

Table 15-4. Interactions between antiretrovirals

	Lopinavir (LPV)	Amprenavir (APV)	Nelfinavir (NFV)	Indinavir (IDV)	Ritonavir (RTV)	Saquinavir (SQV)	Efavirenz (EFV)	Delavirdine (DLV)	Nevirapine (NVP)
NVP	↓LPV (increase LPV to 533 mg PO bid)	Unknown	No change in dose required	↓IDV (increase IDV to 1000 mg PO tid)	No change in dose required	↓SQV (no clinical data)	↓EFV (no clinical data; use EFV 800 mg PO qd)	Unknown	
DLV	Unknown	Unknown	↑NFV (no change in dose required)	↑IDV (use IDV 600 mg PO tid)	↑RTV (reduce RTV to 400 mg PO bid)	↑SQV (no clinical data)	Unknown		
EFV	↓LPV (increase LPV to 533 mg PO bid)	↓APV (add RTV to APV)	↑NFV (no change in dose required)	↓IDV (increase IDV to 1000 mg PO tid)	↑RTV (no change in dose required)	↓SQV (do not use together)			
SQV	↑SQV (use regular dose of LPV and 800 mg PO bid of SQV)	↓SQV, ↓APV (do not use together)	↑SQV (use regular dose of NFV and 800 mg SQV PO tid)	Antagonistic; do not use together	↑SQV (use 400 mg PO bid of SQV and 400 mg PO bid RTV)				

RTV	Unknown	↑APV (use 100 mg PO bid of RTV and 600 mg PO bid of APV)	↑NFV (no clinical studies)	↑IDV (use RTV 100 mg PO bid and IDV 800 mg PO bid or RTV 400 mg PO bid and IDV 400 mg PO bid)
IDV	↑IDV (use IDV 800 mg PO bid)	↓IDV, ↑APV (no change in dose required)	↑IDV (use IDV 1200 mg PO bid)	
NFV	Unknown	↑APV (no clinical studies)		
APV	↑APV (use APV 750 mg PO bid)			
LPV				

↑ = increases level of; ↓ = decreases level of.

500 mg PO bid. Rifabutin, 300 mg PO qd, is an alternative, but its use may be limited by potential drug interactions.

  5. **Varicella-zoster virus (VZV) prophylaxis** is indicated if a significant exposure to chickenpox or shingles occurs and the patient does not have a history of chickenpox and is VZV seronegative. VZV immunoglobulin, 5 vials (1.25 ml each), should be given IM within 96 hours of exposure.

  6. **Primary prophylaxis is not routinely recommended** for the following OIs: recurrent bacterial pneumonia, mucosal candidiasis, cytomegalovirus (CMV) retinitis, cryptococcosis, and the endemic fungal infections such as histoplasmosis and coccidioidomycosis.

B. **Secondary prophylaxis** is instituted after an episode of infection has been adequately treated, as is addressed specifically in sec. **VI.** Most OIs in AIDS are incurable, and the patient usually requires lifelong therapy.

C. **Withdrawal of prophylaxis.** Recommendations suggest withdrawing primary PCP and MAC prophylaxis, and secondary CMV prophylaxis, if immune reconstitution has occurred (CD4 cell counts consistently above 150–200 cells/μl).

VI. **Management of specific infectious complications**
  A. **Viral infections**
    1. **CMV infections.** CMV retinitis occurs very frequently and accounts for 85% of CMV disease in patients with AIDS. CMV also can affect the GI tract, the lungs, and the CNS.
      a. **Treatment of CMV retinitis** can be local or systemic and is administered in two steps: induction and maintenance.
        (1) **Ganciclovir** is given at an induction dosage of 5 mg/kg IV q12h for 14–21 days and a maintenance dosage of 5 mg/kg IV q24h. Oral ganciclovir, 1 g tid, is an option for maintenance therapy in patients with limited non–sight-threatening lesions, but it has limited bioavailability and is expensive. The most common side effect of ganciclovir is myelotoxicity resulting in neutropenia, which may respond to granulocyte colony-stimulating factor therapy. An intraocular ganciclovir implant is effective but does not provide systemic CMV therapy.
        (2) **Foscarnet** is given at an induction dosage of 60 mg/kg IV q8h or 90 mg/kg IV q12h for 14–21 days, followed by a maintenance dosage of 90–120 mg/kg IV q24h indefinitely, unless immune reconstitution occurs (see sec. **V.C**). Nephrotoxicity is the major side effect; therefore, adequate hydration and electrolyte monitoring (including calcium) are required.
        (3) **Cidofovir** is effective using an induction dosage of 5 mg/kg IV weekly for 2 weeks, followed by a maintenance dosage of 5 mg/kg IV every 2 weeks. Probenecid (2 g PO 3 hours before and 1 g PO 2 and 8 hours after cidofovir is given) and saline hydration must be used to reduce the renal toxicity of cidofovir. Urinalysis and electrolytes should be monitored closely.
        (4) **Fomivirsen** is an antisense oligonucleotide given intraocularly 330 μg on days 1 and 15 and then monthly. It does not provide systemic therapy.
        (5) **Combination regimens** (ganciclovir and foscarnet) may be more effective than either drug alone, but together they are poorly tolerated.
      b. **For other invasive CMV disease,** the optimal therapy is with IV ganciclovir or IV foscarnet or a combination of both drugs in persons with prior anti-CMV therapy for at least 3–6 weeks. Foscarnet has the best cerebrospinal fluid penetration and is the drug of choice for CMV encephalitis and myelopathy. Maintenance therapy is indicated.
    2. **Other herpesvirus infections**
      a. **Herpes simplex virus infections** can be associated with large genital and perirectal lesions, esophagitis, proctitis, and pulmonary dis-

ease. Administration of acyclovir (400 mg PO tid), famciclovir (250 mg PO tid), or valacyclovir (500 mg PO tid) for 1 week usually is effective. For more severe disease, IV acyclovir, 5 mg/kg q8h, is recommended. Relapses are frequent, and acyclovir, 400 mg PO bid, may prevent their recurrence. Herpes simplex virus can become resistant to acyclovir, in which case foscarnet, 40 mg/kg IV q8h for 10–14 days, or one dose of cidofovir, 5 mg/kg IV, should be used.

   b. VZV may cause typical dermatomal lesions or disseminated infection. Acyclovir, 10 mg/kg IV q8h for 7–14 days, is recommended. For milder cases, administration of acyclovir (800 mg PO 5 times a day), famciclovir (500 mg PO tid), or valacyclovir (1 g PO tid) for 1 week usually is effective.

   c. Epstein-Barr virus infection is common in AIDS patients. It causes oral hairy leukoplakia, for which no treatment is required. It also is associated with primary CNS lymphoma in patients with advanced AIDS.

   d. Human herpesvirus 8 is the causative agent of Kaposi's sarcoma.

 3. JC virus is a papovavirus associated with progressive multifocal leukoencephalopathy (PML), which is characterized by mental status changes, weakness, and disorders of gait, with characteristic white matter lesions on MRI. Potent antiretroviral therapy has clearly improved survival of PML.

 4. Parvovirus B19. Chronic parvovirus infections can cause pure RBC aplasia. They can be treated with IV immunoglobulin, 0.4 g/kg IV qd for 10 days. Relapses are frequent.

 5. Chronic hepatitis B and C are frequent comorbidities that could be aggravated with the immune reconstitution associated with antiretroviral therapy. Studies are under way to address the treatment of these coinfections (see Chap. 18).

B. Bacterial infections. These are common in HIV-infected patients and often recur or follow atypical or aggressive courses. Intensive therapy generally is necessary, followed by chronic suppression.

 1. Bacillary angiomatosis is caused by *Bartonella henselae* and is characterized by multiple nodular, purplish lesions in the skin and other organs. Erythromycin, 500 mg PO q6h, is the drug of choice. Doxycycline, 100 mg PO bid, also is effective. Other macrolides and ciprofloxacin, 500 mg PO bid, are alternatives.

 2. *Campylobacter jejuni* can produce GI or disseminated infections in HIV-infected patients. Either erythromycin, 500 mg PO qid, or ciprofloxacin, 500 mg PO bid, is the drug of choice.

 3. *Rhodococcus equi* can produce pulmonary infections, which should be treated with vancomycin, 1 g IV q12h, followed by chronic suppression with erythromycin, 500 mg PO qid, plus rifampin, 600 mg PO qd, or with ciprofloxacin, 500 mg PO bid.

 4. *Salmonella* species produce recurrent bacteremia in AIDS patients. Antibacterial therapy should be based on susceptibility. Ceftriaxone (1 g IV qd), ampicillin (1 g IV q6h), TMP/SMX (one DS tablet PO bid), and ciprofloxacin (500 mg PO bid) are options, depending on the organisms' sensitivities.

 5. Bacterial pneumonias occur frequently in HIV-infected patients. If recurrent, they are AIDS defining. Usually, they are due to **Streptococcus pneumoniae** or **Haemophilus influenzae.** These pneumonias can have atypical presentations, especially in patients with advanced disease. Owing to the increasing frequency of antibiotic resistance, a third-generation cephalosporin such as ceftriaxone, 1 g IV qd, is the empiric drug of choice until susceptibilities are available. Gram-negative rods (especially *Pseudomonas aeruginosa*) may also produce pneumonia in advanced HIV disease.

6. **Syphilis** can have an atypical course in HIV-infected patients, and treatment failures are more frequent in this population. Benzathine penicillin, 2.4 million units IM one time for primary syphilis or weekly for 3 weeks for secondary or latent syphilis that is of more than 1 year's duration, is the regimen of choice. Doxycycline, 100 mg PO bid for 14 days, is an alternative. A spinal tap is recommended in HIV-infected patients with latent syphilis to rule out neurosyphilis. If neurosyphilis is present, penicillin G, 12–24 million units IV qd for 14 days, is the only reasonable choice. Therefore, allergic patients should be desensitized. Data regarding the use of ceftriaxone, 1–2 g IV qd for 14 days, are limited. Close monitoring and follow-up using the VDRL test at 3, 6, and 12 months are necessary in all cases. Persons with sustained VDRL should receive retreatment.

7. **Other sexually transmitted diseases** are treated as they would be in non–HIV-infected patients (see Chap. 14).

C. **Mycobacterial infections**

1. *Mycobacterium tuberculosis* (*MMWR Morb Mortal Wkly Rep* 47:RR-20, 1998) is especially frequent among HIV-infected patients, particularly among IV drug abusers. Primary as well as reactivated diseases occur. Clinical manifestations depend on the level of immunosuppression. Patients with higher CD4 cell counts tend to exhibit classic presentations, with apical cavitary disease. More immunosuppressed patients might demonstrate atypical presentations that may resemble disseminated primary infection, with diffuse or localized pulmonary infiltrates and hilar lymphadenopathy. Extrapulmonary dissemination is very common. For treatment recommendations see Chap. 14. Current recommendation suggests the substitution of rifabutin for rifampin in patients who are receiving concomitant antiretroviral therapy. The dosage for rifabutin should be reduced to 150 mg qd if the patient is receiving ritonavir, indinavir, nelfinavir, or amprenavir, whereas it should be increased to 450 mg qd when combined with nevirapine or efavirenz.

2. *Mycobacterium avium* complex infection is the most commonly occurring mycobacterial infection in AIDS patients, and it is responsible for significant morbidity in patients with advanced disease (CD4 cell count <100 cells/ml). Disseminated infection with fever, weight loss, and night sweats is the most frequent presentation. Anemia and an elevated alkaline phosphatase level are usual laboratory abnormalities. Initial therapy should include a macrolide (clarithromycin, 500 mg PO bid) and ethambutol (15 mg/kg PO qd). Rifabutin, 300 mg PO qd, or ciprofloxacin, 500 mg PO bid, can be added in severe cases.

3. *Mycobacterium kansasii* infection is frequent in HIV patients and should always be considered significant. Clinically, the infection appears similar to TB. A combination of rifampin (600 mg PO qd), ethambutol (15 mg/kg/day PO), and INH (300 mg PO qd) is recommended. Also recommended is consultation with an infectious disease specialist.

4. *Mycobacterium haemophilum* can produce skin lesions in AIDS patients. It requires treatment with a macrolide, rifampin, and two other active drugs.

D. **Fungal infections** (see Chap. 14)

1. **Candidiasis** (oral, esophageal, and vaginal infection) is common in the HIV-infected host. The severity of infection depends on the degree of a patient's immunosuppression. Oral and vaginal candidiasis usually respond to local therapy with troches or creams (nystatin or clotrimazole). For patients who do not respond or who have esophageal candidiasis, fluconazole, 100–200 mg PO qd, is the treatment of choice. Fluconazole-resistant candidiasis is increasingly recognized, especially in patients with advanced disease who have been receiving antifungal agents for prolonged periods. Itraconazole oral suspension (200 mg bid)

occasionally is effective. Many patients require amphotericin B, either as an oral suspension (100 mg/ml swish and swallow qid) or parenterally (see Chap. 13).

2. ***Cryptococcus neoformans*** is the most frequent cause of CNS fungal infection in patients with AIDS. Patients present with headaches and fever and may have mental status changes. Occasionally, the presentation is more subtle. Diagnosis is based on the lumbar puncture results and on the determination of latex cryptococcal antigen, which usually is positive in serum and cerebrospinal fluid. Cerebrospinal fluid opening pressure should always be measured to assess the possibility of elevated intracranial pressure. Initial treatment is with amphotericin B, 0.7 mg/kg/day IV, and 5-flucytosine, 25 mg/kg PO q6h for 2–3 weeks, followed by fluconazole, 400 mg PO qd for 8–10 weeks and then 200 mg PO qd indefinitely. The 5-flucytosine level should be monitored during therapy to avoid toxicity. A lipid preparation of amphotericin can be used in persons with renal insufficiency. Repeat lumbar punctures (removing ~30 ml CSF until the pressure is <20–25 cm H_2O) may be required to relieve elevated intracranial pressure. In persons who still continue to have persistent elevation of intracranial pressure, a temporary lumbar drain is indicated.

3. ***Histoplasma capsulatum*** infections occur often in AIDS patients who live in endemic areas such as the Mississippi and Ohio River Valleys. Such infection usually is disseminated at the time of diagnosis. Patients present with fever, hepatosplenomegaly, and weight loss. Pancytopenia is secondary to bone marrow involvement. Diagnosis is based on cultures. Urine *Histoplasma* antigen can also be used for diagnosis and to monitor treatment. Amphotericin B, 0.5 mg/kg IV qd for a total dose of 0.5–1.0 g, followed by itraconazole, 400 mg PO qd indefinitely, is the therapy of choice. Itraconazole absorption should be documented by a serum drug level.

4. ***Coccidioides immitis*** is another frequent infection in AIDS patients in endemic areas of the southwestern United States. Extensive disease with extrapulmonary spread is common. Amphotericin B therapy is indicated initially, followed by lifelong suppression with fluconazole, 400 mg PO qd, or itraconazole, 400 mg PO qd. Coccidioidal meningitis requires intracisternal or intraventricular therapy with amphotericin B. Fluconazole may also be effective.

5. **Aspergillosis** is increasing among HIV-infected patients, especially those who are neutropenic and those with advanced disease (fewer than 50 CD4 cells/µl). This infection can involve the lungs, the CNS, the heart, the kidneys, or the sinuses. Diagnosis requires biopsy of the tissue involved. Amphotericin B is the treatment of choice. Itraconazole also is active and may be indicated in some cases. Prognosis is poor.

E. **PCP** is the most common infection in patients with AIDS and is the leading cause of death in this population. Extrapulmonary disease has also been described, primarily in patients on inhaled pentamidine prophylaxis.

1. **TMP/SMX** is the treatment of choice. The dosage is 5 mg/kg of the TMP component IV q6–8h for severe cases, with a switch to oral therapy when the patient's condition improves. Total duration of therapy is 21 days. If no evidence of other infection is found, **prednisone** should be added if the patient has an arterial oxygen tension (PaO_2) of less than 70 mm Hg or an alveolar-arterial oxygen gradient [$P(A-a)O_2$] in excess of 35 mm Hg. The most frequently prescribed prednisone regimen is 40 mg PO bid on days 1–5, then 20 mg bid on days 6–10, and, finally, 20 mg qd on days 11–21.

2. **For patients who cannot receive TMP/SMX,** the following are alternatives.
   a. **For mild to moderately severe disease** [PaO_2 >70 mm Hg or $P(A-a)O_2$ <35 mm Hg]
      (1) **Trimethoprim,** 20 mg/kg/day PO, and dapsone, 100 mg PO qd. Glucose 6-phosphate dehydrogenase deficiency should be ruled out before dapsone is used.

      (2) **Clindamycin,** 600 mg IV or PO tid, plus **primaquine,** 15 mg PO qd. Glucose 6-phosphate dehydrogenase deficiency should be ruled out before primaquine is used.

      (3) **Atovaquone,** 750 mg PO tid. This drug should be administered with meals to increase absorption.

   b. For severe disease [PaO_2 <70 mm Hg or $P(A\text{-}a)O_2$ >35 mm Hg]

      (1) **Pentamidine,** 4 mg/kg IV qd, should be infused over 2 hours. Hypoglycemia or hyperglycemia is common, and monitoring of glucose and serum electrolytes (including calcium) is essential. Nephrotoxicity, hematologic toxicity, and hypotension also are frequent.

      (2) **Trimetrexate,** 45 mg/m^2 IV qd over 90 minutes, and leucovorin, 20 mg/m^2 IV or PO q6h, can be given.

      (3) **Prednisone** should be added (see sec. **VI.E.1**).

  3. Prophylaxis is indicated as described in sec. **V.A.1**.

F. Protozoal infections

  1. *Toxoplasma gondii* typically causes multiple CNS lesions and presents with encephalopathy and focal neurologic findings. Disease represents reactivation of previous infection, and the serologic workup usually is positive. The MRI scan is the best radiographic technique for diagnosis. Often, the diagnosis relies on response to empiric treatment, as seen by a reduction in the size of the mass lesions. **Sulfadiazine,** 25 mg/kg PO q6h, plus **pyrimethamine,** 100 mg PO on day 1 followed by 75 mg PO qd, is the therapy of choice. Leucovorin, 5–10 mg PO qd, should be added to prevent hematologic toxicity. For patients who are allergic to sulfonamides, clindamycin (600 mg IV or PO q8h) can be used instead of sulfadiazine. Doses are reduced after 3–6 weeks of therapy.

  2. Cryptosporidium produces chronic diarrhea in HIV-infected patients. Diagnosis is based on the visualization of the parasite in acid-fast staining of stool. **Paromomycin,** 500 mg PO tid or qid, occasionally is effective. Potent antiretroviral therapy has been reported to be effective.

  3. Cyclospora is very similar to Cryptosporidium and produces chronic diarrhea. **TMP/SMX,** one DS tablet PO bid for 7 days, usually is effective.

  4. *Isospora belli* produces chronic diarrhea. Treatment with **TMP/SMX,** one DS tablet PO qid for 10 days, followed by chronic suppression with TMP/SMX, one DS tablet PO qd, is effective.

  5. Microsporidia produce diarrhea and biliary tree disease in patients with advanced infection. Diagnosis is difficult and requires special staining of the stool. **Albendazole,** 400 mg PO bid, may be useful for *Enterocytozoon bieneusi* (90% of cases). **TMP/SMX** is effective for *Encephalitozoon intestinalis*, which can cause disseminated disease (10%).

  6. Strongyloides can produce disseminated infections in AIDS patients in endemic areas. **Thiabendazole,** 22 mg/kg (maximum, 1.5 g) PO qd for 2–3 days, is the drug of choice.

VII. Neoplasms associated with AIDS include Kaposi's sarcoma and Hodgkin's and non-Hodgkin's lymphoma.

  A. Kaposi's sarcoma is associated with human herpesvirus 8 infection. It commonly presents as skin lesions but can be disseminated. The GI tract and lung are the usual visceral organs involved. Potent antiretroviral therapy can regress Kaposi's sarcoma lesions. Local therapy can be with liquid nitrogen or intralesional injection of vinblastine. Systemic therapy involves chemotherapy (liposomal doxorubicin, paclitaxel, and liposomal daunorubicin), radiation, and interferon.

  B. Lymphoma associated with AIDS is primarily non-Hodgkin's lymphoma. Epstein-Barr virus appears to be the potential pathogen. Primary CNS lymphomas are common and can be multicentric; other potential extranodal sites of involvement include bone marrow, GI tract, and liver. Treatment involves chemotherapy and radiation.

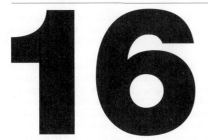

Transplant Medicine

Brent W. Miller
and Gary G. Singer

Transplantation has become widely accepted as a treatment for end-stage organ failure. A continued increase in the number of patients awaiting solid organ transplant is anticipated. It is beyond the scope of this chapter to cover the entire field of transplantation; hence, this chapter should serve as an introduction to the subject with a selection of pertinent references. Immunosuppressive medications, graft rejection, and selected long-term complications are emphasized. For indications and contraindications of heart, lung, kidney, and liver transplantations, see Chaps. 6, 10, 12, and 18, respectively (*N Engl J Med* 331:365, 1994; *N Engl J Med* 340:1081, 1999; *Surg Clin North Am* 78:679, 1998; *J Hepatol* 32:198, 2000).

Immunosuppressive Medications

Immunosuppressive medications are used to promote acceptance of a graft (induction therapy), to reverse episodes of acute rejection (rejection therapy), and to prevent rejection (maintenance therapy) (*JAMA* 278:1993, 1997; *Lancet* 353:1083, 1999). These agents are associated with immunosuppressive effects, immunodeficiency toxicity (e.g., infection and malignancy), and nonimmune toxicity (e.g., nephrotoxicity, diabetes mellitus, or neurotoxicity). Immunosuppressive medications should only be prescribed and administered by physicians and nurses who have appropriate knowledge and expertise.
 I. **Glucocorticoids** are immunosuppressive and anti-inflammatory. Their mechanisms of action include inhibition of cytokine transcription, induction of lymphocyte apoptosis, down-regulation of adhesion molecule and major histocompatibility complex expression, and modification of leukocyte trafficking. The side effects of chronic glucocorticoid therapy are well known (see Chap. 24). As a result of the associated morbidity, steroids are tapered rapidly in the immediate posttransplant period to achieve maintenance doses of 0.1 mg/kg or less. Some centers have opted for steroid withdrawal in stable patients following transplantation, despite an increased risk of acute rejection.
II. **Antiproliferative agents**
   A. **Azathioprine** is a purine analog that is metabolized by the liver to 6-mercaptopurine (active drug), which, in turn, is catabolized by xanthine oxidase. Azathioprine inhibits the synthesis of DNA and thereby suppresses the proliferation of activated lymphocytes. The major dose-limiting toxicity of this agent is myelosuppression, which is usually reversible after dose reduction or discontinuation of the drug.
   B. **Mycophenolate mofetil (MMF)** is converted to an active metabolite, mycophenolic acid (MPA). MPA inhibits the rate-limiting step in de novo purine synthesis. Because lymphocytes are relatively dependent on the de novo pathway for purine synthesis, lymphocyte proliferation is selectively inhibited by MPA. The major adverse effects of MMF are GI disturbances, includ-

ing nausea, diarrhea, and abdominal pain, and hematologic disturbances, namely, leukopenia and thrombocytopenia. Antacids that contain magnesium and aluminum interfere with the absorption of MMF and should not be given concurrently.

III. **Calcineurin inhibitors** bind to immunophilins (intracellular binding proteins). The calcineurin inhibitor–immunophilin complex inhibits a key phosphatase that is involved in transducing the signal from the T-cell receptor to the nucleus. The net effect is blockade of interleukin-2 and other cytokine transcription, leading to inhibition of T-lymphocyte activation and proliferation.

   A. **Cyclosporine A (CsA)** is a cyclic 11–amino acid peptide derived from a fungus. Its major nonimmune side effect is nephrotoxicity due to afferent arteriolar vasoconstriction. Angiotensin-converting enzyme inhibitors, volume depletion, and other nephrotoxins may potentiate this toxicity. Acute nephrotoxicity is reversible with dose reduction; chronic nephrotoxicity is generally irreversible. Other adverse effects include gingival hyperplasia, hirsutism, tremor, hypertension, glucose intolerance, hyperlipidemia, hyperkalemia, and rarely thrombotic thrombocytopenic purpura. CsA has a narrow therapeutic window, and doses are adjusted based on blood levels (recommended maintenance trough levels of 100–300 ng/ml and 2-hour peak levels <1200 ng/ml).

   B. **Tacrolimus (FK 506)** is a macrolide antibiotic and, like CsA, is nephrotoxic. Tacrolimus is more neurotoxic and diabetogenic than CsA, but it is associated with less hypertrichosis and gum hyperplasia. Tacrolimus dosing is based on trough blood levels (recommended maintenance levels of 5–15 ng/ml).

IV. **Biological agents**

   A. **Polyclonal antibodies**

   1. **Antithymocyte globulin (ATGAM)** is a polyclonal, horse antihuman thymocyte antibody. ATGAM depletes circulating T lymphocytes as a result of complement-mediated lysis and clearance of antibody-coated cells by the reticuloendothelial system. ATGAM also interferes with lymphocyte function by blocking and modulating the expression of cell surface molecules. The drug is usually infused over 4–6 hours through a central vein to avoid thrombophlebitis. The most common side effects are fever, chills, and arthralgias. Other important adverse effects include myelosuppression, serum sickness, and, rarely, anaphylaxis.

   2. **Thymoglobulin** is a polyclonal, rabbit antihuman thymocyte antibody. Its mode of administration and mechanism of action are similar to those of ATGAM, but the duration of lymphocyte depletion is more prolonged. Thymoglobulin has a side effect profile similar to that of ATGAM.

   B. **Monoclonal antibodies. OKT3** is a murine monoclonal antibody directed against the CD3ε chain associated with the T-cell receptor. It is administered as a bolus injection via a peripheral vein. OKT3 depletes CD3$^+$ T cells and modulates CD3 expression. The most common side effect is cytokine release syndrome, characterized by fever, chills, nausea, vomiting, diarrhea, myalgia, and, occasionally, hypotension and noncardiogenic pulmonary edema. Other side effects include encephalopathy, seizures, and aseptic meningitis.

V. **Newer immunosuppressive agents**

   A. **Sirolimus (rapamycin)** is a macrocyclic antibiotic produced by *Streptomyces hygroscopicus*. Sirolimus forms a complex with the same receptor-binding protein as tacrolimus; this complex inhibits the activation of a regulatory kinase, mammalian target of rapamycin, and thus prohibits T-cell progression from the G1 to the S phase of the cell cycle. Unlike the calcineurin inhibitors, sirolimus does not affect cytokine transcription but inhibits cytokine and growth factor–induced cell proliferation. The major adverse effects of this drug include hyperlipidemia and thrombocytopenia. Sirolimus is not nephrotoxic. The importance of therapeutic drug monitoring has not been established and continues to be studied.

   B. **Anti–interleukin-2 receptor monoclonal antibodies.** Daclizumab (humanized) and basiliximab (chimeric) are monoclonal antibodies that competi-

Table 16-1. Differential diagnosis of renal allograft dysfunction

<1 wk posttransplant	<3 mos posttransplant	>3 mos posttransplant
Acute tubular necrosis	Acute rejection	Prerenal azotemia
Hyperacute rejection	Cyclosporine toxicity	Cyclosporine toxicity
Accelerated rejection	Prerenal azotemia	Acute rejection
Obstruction	Obstruction	Obstruction
Urine leak	Infection	Recurrent renal disease
Vascular thrombosis	Interstitial nephritis	De novo renal disease
Atheroemboli	Recurrent renal disease	Renal artery stenosis

tively inhibit the alpha subunit of the interleukin-2 receptor (CD25) and thereby inhibit activation of T cells. Humanization and chimerization reduce the murine sequences of these genetically engineered antibodies, respectively. This results in antibodies with an extended half-life and minimizes the chances of developing human antimurine antibodies. These drugs are administered by a peripheral vein and are associated with few side effects.

VI. Important drug interactions are always a concern given the polypharmacy associated with transplant patients. The combination of allopurinol and azathioprine should be avoided or used cautiously due to the risk of profound myelosuppression. CsA is metabolized by cytochrome P-450 (3A4). Therefore, CsA levels are decreased by drugs that induce cytochrome P-450 activity, for example, rifampin, isoniazid, barbiturates, phenytoin, and carbamazepine. Conversely, CsA levels are increased by drugs that compete for cytochrome P-450, for example, verapamil, diltiazem, nicardipine, azole antifungals, erythromycin, and clarithromycin (see Appendix C). Similar effects are seen with tacrolimus and sirolimus. Tacrolimus and CsA should not be taken together because of the increased risk of severe nephrotoxicity. Lower doses of MMF should be used when either tacrolimus or sirolimus are taken concurrently. Concomitant administration of CsA and sirolimus may result in a twofold increase in sirolimus; to avoid this drug interaction, CsA and sirolimus should be dosed 4 hours apart.

Rejection

I. Acute rejection

  A. Kidney allograft rejection occurs in up to 30% of patients and is defined as an acute deterioration in renal function associated with specific pathologic changes. Most episodes of acute rejection occur in the first 6 months after transplantation. Late acute rejection (>1 year after transplantation) usually results from inadequate immunosuppression or patient noncompliance.

  1. **Manifestations** include an elevated serum creatinine, decreased urine output, increased edema, or worsening hypertension. Constitutional symptoms (fever, malaise, arthralgia, painful or swollen allograft) are uncommon in the cyclosporine era.

  2. **Differential diagnosis** varies with duration after transplantation (Table 16-1). Diagnosis of acute renal allograft rejection is made by renal biopsy after excluding prerenal azotemia via hydration and repeating laboratory tests, cyclosporine nephrotoxicity (trough and/or peak levels), infection (urinalysis and culture), and obstruction (renal ultrasound).

B. Lung transplant rejection occurs frequently and most commonly in the first few months after transplantation. The majority of patients have at least one episode of acute rejection. Multiple episodes of acute rejection predispose to the development of chronic rejection (bronchiolitis obliterans syndrome).

   1. Manifestations are nonspecific and include fever, dyspnea, and a nonproductive cough. The chest radiograph is usually unchanged, and, if it is abnormal (early), the findings are generally nondiagnostic (perihilar infiltrates, interstitial edema, pleural effusions). Pulmonary function testing is not diagnostic (specific), but a 10% or greater decline in forced vital capacity or forced expiratory volume in 1 second, or both, is usually clinically significant.

   2. Differential diagnosis. It is important to attempt to distinguish rejection from infection, because the treatments are markedly different.

   3. Diagnosis is generally made by fiberoptic bronchoscopy with bronchoalveolar lavage and transbronchial biopsies.

C. Heart transplant recipients have two to three episodes of acute rejection in the first year after transplantation and a 50–80% chance of having at least one rejection episode, most commonly in the first 6 months.

   1. Manifestations may include symptoms and signs of left ventricular dysfunction such as dyspnea, paroxysmal nocturnal dyspnea, orthopnea, syncope, palpitations, new gallops, and elevated jugular venous pressure, but many patients are asymptomatic. Acute rejection may also be associated with a variety of tachyarrhythmias, atrial more often than ventricular.

   2. Diagnosis is established by endomyocardial biopsy performed during routine surveillance or as prompted by symptoms. None of the noninvasive techniques has demonstrated sufficient sensitivity and specificity to replace the endomyocardial biopsy.

D. Liver transplant recipients commonly experience acute allograft rejection, with at least 60% having one episode. Acute rejection typically occurs within the first 3 months after transplant and often in the first 2 weeks after the operation.

   1. Manifestations may be absent or the patients may have signs and symptoms of liver failure, including fever, malaise, anorexia, abdominal pain, ascites, decreased bile output, elevated bilirubin, and/or transaminases.

   2. Differential diagnosis of early liver allograft dysfunction includes primary graft nonfunction, preservation injury, vascular thrombosis, biliary anastomotic leak, or stenosis. These should be excluded clinically or by Doppler ultrasonography. Late allograft dysfunction may be due to rejection, recurrent hepatitis B or C, cytomegalovirus (CMV) or Epstein-Barr virus infection, cholestasis, or drug toxicity.

   3. Diagnosis is made by liver biopsy after technical complications are excluded.

E. Treatment of acute allograft rejection depends on the histologic severity (grade). Mild rejection of heart and lung transplants is often left untreated. First-line therapy for acute rejection usually consists of either pulse methylprednisolone or high-dose prednisone, with a 60–80% response rate. Rejection that is more severe, recurrent, or refractory to glucocorticoid therapy is generally treated with antilymphocyte antibody preparations. Maintenance immunosuppressive agents are often added or substituted after an episode of acute rejection.

II. Chronic rejection is a slowly progressive, insidious decline in function of the allograft characterized by gradual vascular and ductal obliteration, parenchymal atrophy, and interstitial fibrosis. Diagnosis is often difficult and generally requires a biopsy. The process is mediated by immune and nonimmune factors. Chronic rejection or allograft dysfunction accounts for the vast majority of late graft losses and is the major obstacle to long-term graft survival. The manifestations of chronic rejection are unique to each organ system. To date, no effective therapy is available for established chronic rejection. Current investigational strategies are aimed at prevention.

Infectious Complications

Infectious complications can occur in either the allograft (often causing allograft dysfunction and possibly enhancing rejection) or in other organs as a consequence of the immunosuppressed state (*N Engl J Med* 338:1741, 1998).

I. **Time course.** Infections follow a typical course depending on the organ transplanted, the time from transplantation, and the net state of immunosuppression. During the first month after transplantation, infections related directly to the surgery and hospitalization predominate (wound infections, pneumonia, catheter-related bacteremia, and urinary tract infections). Opportunistic viral, parasitic, and bacterial infections occur during the next 6 months and after aggressive treatment of acute rejection episodes. Signs or symptoms of infection should be pursued aggressively, as infection is the second leading cause of death in transplant recipients.

II. **Etiology.** Several opportunistic infections should be considered in the transplant recipient (Table 16-2).

III. **Prevention**
   A. **Immunization.** Pneumococcal and hepatitis B vaccination should be given at the time of pretransplant evaluation. Influenza A vaccination should be administered yearly. Live vaccines should be avoided after transplantation.
   B. **Prophylaxis**
      1. Trimethoprim-sulfamethoxazole prevents urinary tract infections, *Pneumocystis carinii* pneumonia, and *Nocardia* infections. The optimal dose and duration of prophylaxis have not been determined.
      2. Acyclovir prevents reactivation of herpes simplex virus but is ineffective in CMV prophylaxis.
      3. Ganciclovir prevents CMV infection when administered to patients who are previously CMV seropositive or receive a CMV-positive organ, or both. CMV hyperimmune globulin or IV ganciclovir can also be used for this purpose.
      4. Fluconazole or ketoconazole can be given in patients with a high risk of systemic fungal infections or recurrent localized fungal infections. Both medications increase cyclosporine and tacrolimus levels (see Immunosuppressive Medications, sec. **VI**). Nystatin suspension or clotrimazole troches are used to prevent oropharyngeal candidiasis (thrush).

IV. **Diagnosis and treatment**
   A. **CMV infection** from reactivation of CMV in a seropositive recipient or new infection from a CMV-positive organ can lead to a wide range of presentations from a mild viral syndrome to allograft dysfunction, invasive disease in multiple organ systems, and even death. Because of the potential severity of disease, treatment is usually indicated in the transplant patient without tissue diagnosis of invasive disease. Shell-vial culture of the buffy coat is accurate only when plated within 24 hours of sample collection. Seroconversion with a positive immunoglobulin M titer or a fourfold increase in immunoglobulin M or immunoglobulin G titer suggests acute infection; however, many centers now use polymerase chain reaction–based diagnostic techniques. Treatment is with IV ganciclovir, 2.5–5.0 mg/kg bid (adjusted for renal function), for 3–4 weeks. Hyperimmune globulin is often used in combination with ganciclovir for patients with organ involvement. Foscarnet is a more toxic alternative. Prophylaxis during the highest incidence of severe CMV infection episodes (e.g., 3–6 months after transplantation in patients who are either seropositive or receive a seropositive organ) with oral ganciclovir

Table 16-2. Timing and etiology of posttransplant infections

Time period	Infectious complication	Etiology
<1 mo posttransplant	Nosocomial pneumonia, wound infection, urinary tract infection, catheter-related sepsis	Bacterial or fungal infections
1–6 mos posttransplant	Opportunistic infections	Cytomegalovirus
		Pneumocystis carinii
		Aspergillus spp.
		Toxoplasma gondii
		Listeria monocytogenes
		Varicella-zoster virus
	Reactivation of pre-existing infections	*Mycobacteria* spp.
		Endemic mycoses
>6 mos posttransplant	Community-acquired infections	Bacterial
	Chronic progressive infection	Hepatitis B
		Hepatitis C
		Cytomegalovirus
		Epstein-Barr virus
		Papillomavirus
	Opportunistic infections	*P. carinii*
		L. monocytogenes
		Nocardia asteroides
		Cryptococcus neoformans
		Aspergillus spp.

(1000 mg PO tid) has markedly reduced the incidence of life-threatening CMV infections.

B. Hepatitis B and C. Patients with active hepatitis or cirrhosis are not considered for nonhepatic transplantation. Immunosuppression increases viral replication in organ transplant recipients with either hepatitis B or C. **Hepatitis B** can recur as fulminant hepatic failure even in patients with no evidence of viral DNA replication before transplantation. In liver transplantation, the risk of recurrent hepatitis B virus infection can be reduced by the administration of hepatitis B immunoglobulin during and after transplantation. Experience with lamivudine therapy initiated before transplantation to lower viral load has shown decreased likelihood of recurrent hepatitis B virus. **Hepatitis C** typically progresses slowly in nonhepatic transplants, and the effect of immunosuppression remains to be determined on mortality due to liver disease. Treatment protocols for hepatitis C in the nonhepatic transplant population are not yet established. Hepatitis C nearly always recurs in liver transplant recipients whose original disease was due to hepatitis C. Therapy for recurrent hepatitis C virus with a combination of ribavirin and interferon results in histopathologic improvement of disease, although dosage and duration of therapy remain controversial.

C. Epstein-Barr virus plays a role in the development of posttransplant lymphoproliferative disease. This life-threatening lymphoma is treated by with-

drawal or reduction in immunosuppression and often aggressive chemotherapy (see Long-Term Complications of Transplantation).
D. The role of newly discovered **viral agents** such as HHV-6, HHV-7, HHV-8, and polyoma (BK) virus after transplantation remains to be established.
E. **Fungal and parasitic infections,** such as *Cryptococcus*, *Mucor*, aspergillosis, and *Candida* species, have increased mortality after transplantation and should be aggressively diagnosed and treated. The role of prophylaxis with oral fluconazole has not been established.

Long-Term Complications of Transplantation

I. **Cardiovascular complications**
A. **Hypertension** occurs in up to 80% of renal transplant patients and to a lesser degree in other solid organ transplant recipients. Blood pressure should be monitored and maintained below 140/90. Certain calcium channel blockers significantly increase CsA and tacrolimus levels (see Appendix C), and drug levels should be carefully monitored. Angiotensin-converting enzyme inhibitors should be avoided in the early posttransplant period because of the potential for increased nephrotoxicity when patients are receiving high doses of cyclosporine or tacrolimus. However, these agents may be renoprotective in the long term. When suspected, renal artery stenosis should be excluded.
B. **Coronary heart disease.** Graft atherosclerosis in cardiac allografts is partially immunologic in nature. Cardiac disease is the leading cause of death in renal transplant recipients and should be screened aggressively before transplantation, with aggressive modification of risk factors after transplantation.
II. **Endocrine and metabolic complications**
A. **Obesity** is a common problem in the late posttransplant period, with average weight gains in excess of 40 lb by 1 year. The approach should be multidisciplinary and include dietary and exercise counseling. Most medications that promote weight loss, however, impair blood pressure control.
B. **Hyperlipidemia** occurs in as many as 60% of solid organ transplant recipients. Elevated lipid levels may be related to medications (glucocorticoids, CsA, thiazides), comorbidity, and genetic factors. Hyperlipidemia is associated with cardiovascular disease and may also have a role in chronic allograft vasculopathy. Dietary intervention alone is often insufficient to achieve a therapeutic target, and treatment should follow the National Cholesterol Education Program guidelines.
C. **Diabetes mellitus.** Glucocorticoids, calcineurin inhibitors, and obesity all contribute to diabetes after transplantation. Tacrolimus may have a higher incidence of diabetes versus cyclosporine (approximately 20% vs. 5%, respectively). Patients should be screened with fasting plasma glucose levels as recommended by the American Diabetes Association.
D. **Bone disease.** Avascular necrosis and steroid-induced osteoporosis can be disabling, leading to multiple fractures and often requiring joint replacement. Bone densitometry at regular intervals monitors osteopenia, although cortical bone loss can occur rapidly within the first months of high-dose glucocorticoid therapy. Transplant recipients should be in positive calcium balance with calcium supplementation (calcium carbonate, 1000–1500 mg/day between meals or qhs). Vitamin D supplements, calcitonin, and bisphosphonates have been used in transplant recipients.
III. **Renal disease.** Chronic rejection is the leading cause of allograft loss in renal transplant recipients. Calcineurin inhibitor (CsA or tacrolimus) nephrotoxicity or recurrent native disease may also develop in these patients. Chronic

calcineurin inhibitor nephrotoxicity may also lead to chronic renal insufficiency and end-stage renal disease, requiring dialysis or transplantation in recipients of lung, heart, liver, or pancreas transplants.

IV. **Malignancy** occurs in transplant patients with an overall incidence that is threefold to fourfold higher than that seen in the general population (age matched). Some cancers occur at the same rate, whereas other neoplasms have a much higher frequency than normal. The spontaneous malignancies that occur most frequently in transplant recipients include cancers of the skin and lips, lymphoproliferative disease, bronchogenic carcinoma, Kaposi's sarcoma, uterine/cervical carcinoma, renal cell carcinoma, and anogenital neoplasms (*N Engl J Med* 323:1767, 1990).

A. **Skin and lip cancers** are the most common malignancies (40–50%) seen in transplant recipients, with an incidence 10–250 times that of the general population. Risk factors include immunosuppression, ultraviolet radiation, and human papillomavirus infection. These cancers develop at a younger age, and they are more aggressive in transplant patients than in the general population. Using protective clothing and sunscreens and avoiding sun exposure are recommended. Examination of the skin is the principal screening test, and early diagnosis offers the best prognosis.

B. **Posttransplant lymphoproliferative disease** accounts for one-fifth of all malignancies after transplantation, with an incidence of approximately 1%. This is 30- to 50-fold higher than in the general population. The majority of these neoplasms are large-cell non-Hodgkin's lymphomas of the B-cell type. Posttransplant lymphoproliferative disease results from Epstein-Barr virus–induced B-cell proliferation in the setting of chronic immunosuppression (especially antilymphocyte therapy). Diagnosis requires a high index of suspicion and a tissue biopsy. Treatment includes reduction or withdrawal of immunosuppression and chemotherapy.

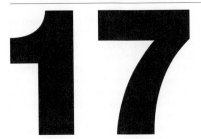

Gastrointestinal Diseases

Chandra Prakash

Gastrointestinal Bleeding

Overt GI bleeding presents with the passage of fresh or altered blood through the mouth [hematemesis, coffee-ground emesis, blood in nasogastric (NG) aspirate] or in the stool (melena, hematochezia, maroon stool). **Occult bleeding** refers to a positive fecal occult blood test (stool guaiac) or iron-deficiency anemia without visible blood in the stool. **Obscure bleeding** refers to GI blood loss of unknown origin that persists or recurs after negative initial endoscopic evaluation; obscure bleeding can be either overt or occult. The following segments refer primarily to overt bleeding.

I. **General considerations.** The initial evaluation is performed concurrently with resuscitative measures, regardless of the site of bleeding. History and physical examination are directed toward determining the anatomic level of bleeding, the quantity of blood lost, the etiology of bleeding, and precipitating factors.

A. **Initial evaluation**

1. **Intravascular volume and hemodynamic status.** Constant monitoring or frequent assessment of vital signs is necessary early in the evaluation, as a sudden increase in pulse rate or decrease in BP may be an early indication of recurrent or ongoing blood loss. If the baseline BP and pulse are within normal limits, sitting the patient up or having the patient stand may result in **orthostatic hemodynamic changes** (drop in systolic BP of >10 mm Hg, rise in pulse rate of >15 beats/minute). Orthostatic changes in pulse and BP are seen with loss of 10–20% of the circulatory volume; supine hypotension suggests a greater than 20% loss. Hypotension with a systolic blood pressure of less than 100 mm Hg or baseline tachycardia suggests significant hemodynamic compromise that requires urgent volume resuscitation.

2. **Laboratory evaluation.** At presentation, a complete blood count, coagulation parameters (prothrombin time, partial thromboplastin time, platelet count), blood group, and cross matching of 2–4 units of blood should be urgently performed. A chemistry profile including liver and renal function helps to stratify risk in case invasive intervention is required and may assist with differential diagnosis.

B. **Initial resuscitation**

1. **Restoration of intravascular volume.** Two large-bore IV lines with 14- to 18-gauge catheters or a central venous line should be established immediately in overt GI bleeding. Isotonic saline, lactated Ringer's solution, or 5% hetastarch can be initiated; patients in shock might require volume administration using pressure infusion devices or hand infused using large syringes and stopcocks. Blood should be used for volume replacement whenever possible and should be initiated as soon as it is evident that the patient's bleeding is massive, ongoing, or severe enough that colloid infusion alone is not adequate for tissue oxygenation. O-negative blood or simultaneous multiple-unit transfusion can be used in emer-

gent situations. **Packed RBC transfusion** should be continued until the patient's condition is hemodynamically stable and the hematocrit reaches 25% or greater; patients with cardiac or pulmonary disease may require transfusion to a hematocrit of 30% or greater. Vasopressors are generally not indicated, although transient IV pressor therapy is sometimes beneficial until enough volume is infused. The rate of volume infusion should be guided by the patient's condition and the rate and degree of volume loss.

2. **Correction of coagulopathy.** Discontinuation of the offending anticoagulant, if possible, followed by infusion of fresh frozen plasma (FFP), can be used to correct prolonged coagulation parameters. An initial infusion of 2–4 units of FFP can be supplemented with further infusion based on reassessment of the coagulation parameters. Protamine infusion (1 mg antagonizes ≈ 100 units of heparin) can be used for immediate reversal of anticoagulation from heparin infusion. Parenteral vitamin K (10 mg SC or IM) may be indicated for prolonged prothrombin time from warfarin therapy or hepatobiliary disease but takes several hours to days for adequate reversal; it should be repeated daily for a total of three doses in hepatobiliary disease. Platelet infusion may be indicated when the platelet count is less than $50,000/mm^3$.

3. **Airway protection.** Endotracheal intubation to prevent aspiration should be considered in situations in which diminished mental status (shock, hepatic encephalopathy), massive hematemesis, or active variceal hemorrhage is present.

II. History

A. **Degree of volume loss.** Estimates of amounts of blood loss can be inaccurate, as even a small quantity of blood can discolor water in a toilet bowl enough to suggest a larger volume of blood loss. In general, patients with lower GI bleeding have less hemodynamic compromise than those with upper GI bleeding.

B. **Level of bleeding.** Hematemesis or coffee-ground emesis ensures an upper GI source of blood loss, as does aspiration of blood or coffee grounds from an NG tube. Melena, a black sticky stool with a characteristic odor, indicates an upper source of blood loss, although small-bowel and sometimes right colonic bleeds can result in melena. Various shades of red blood are seen in the stool with distal small-bowel or colonic bleeding, depending on the rate of blood loss and colonic transit. Although patients with upper GI bleeding can also present with red blood in their stool, this is almost invariably associated with hemodynamic compromise and circulatory shock. Bleeding from the anorectal area typically results in bright blood coating the exterior of formed stool, sometimes associated with distal colonic symptoms (e.g., rectal urgency, straining with defecation).

C. **Etiology of bleeding.** Important points in the medical history include prior bleeding episodes, alcohol use, liver disease, coagulation disorders, and bleeding tendencies. Although not specific for this diagnosis, a history of emesis preceding upper GI bleeding may suggest a Mallory-Weiss tear. Nonsteroidal anti-inflammatory drugs (NSAIDs) and aspirin can result in mucosal damage anywhere in the GI tract. Hypotension and hypovolemic shock preceding the bleeding episode may suggest ischemic injury to the gut. Radiation therapy to the prostate or pelvis suggests radiation proctitis, and prior aortic graft surgery should bring to mind the possibility of an aortoenteric or aortocolonic fistula. Chronic constipation can result in stercoral (stool-induced) ulceration of the rectum and bleeding. A history of recent polypectomy may indicate postpolypectomy bleeding. Patients with chronic renal disease are prone to development of GI angiodysplasia; patients with hereditary hemorrhagic telangiectasias can have lesions in their GI tract that may be a source for blood loss.

D. **Precipitating factors.** In the presence of a potential source of blood loss in the GI tract, abnormalities in the coagulation mechanism from any cause can result in clinically evident bleeding. Medications that are known to affect the coagulation process include warfarin, heparin, aspirin, NSAIDs, and thrombolytic agents. Disorders of coagulation, such as liver disease, von Willebrand's disease, vitamin K deficiency, and disseminated intravascular coagulation, can also influence the course of GI bleeding (see Chap. 19).

III. Physical examination

    A. Color of stool. Direct examination of spontaneously passed stool or stool obtained during a digital rectal examination can provide important clues as to the level of bleeding (see sec. **II.B**).

    B. NG aspiration. An NG aspirate is useful in diagnosing upper GI bleeding in patients with a suggestive history and in ruling out upper GI bleeding in patients with red blood in their stool. In a small fraction of patients, a bleeding source in the duodenum can result in a negative NG aspirate. Hemoccult testing of a normal-appearing NG aspirate is of no clinical utility; the aspirate should be considered positive only if blood or dark particulate matter ("coffee grounds") is seen. Gastric lavage with water or saline may be useful in assessing the activity and severity of upper GI bleeding and in clearing the stomach of blood and clots before endoscopic examination. After a diagnosis of upper GI bleeding is made, the NG tube is not required further, as hemodynamic parameters and serial blood counts can be used to assess for continued bleeding, especially if endoscopy is to follow.

    C. Anoscopy/sigmoidoscopy. A digital rectal examination may identify a potential source of bleeding in the anorectum in addition to assessing the color of stool accurately. Anal fissures can result in extreme pain during a rectal examination and can typically be seen in the posterior midline on careful examination (see Other Gastrointestinal Disorders, sec. **VII.C**). Anoscopy may be useful in the detection of internal hemorrhoids. In an outpatient or emergency room setting, anoscopy and sigmoidoscopy may be useful in rapid diagnosis of the level of bleeding before patient triage. However, even if a potential source of bleeding is evident in this setting, subsequent endoscopic evaluation of the colon is the norm rather than the exception.

IV. Further evaluation and therapy. The level of bleeding, the acuity of blood loss, and the general comorbid illnesses of the patient should be considered in test selection.

    A. Esophagogastroduodenoscopy (EGD) can be performed at the patient's bedside and is the preferred method of investigation and therapy of upper GI bleeding. It is associated with high diagnostic accuracy, therapeutic capability, and low morbidity. It should be performed early in the clinical course, after the patient has received volume resuscitation and is hemodynamically stable. Although early diagnostic endoscopy does not reduce mortality, therapeutic endoscopy reduces transfusion requirements, need for surgery, and length of hospital stay (*N Engl J Med* 325:1142, 1991).

    B. Early **colonoscopy** after a rapid bowel purge is a relatively new concept. The yield of finding a potential bleeding source in the colon is thought to be greater if colonoscopy is performed within the initial 24 hours of presentation. The test is best performed in patients whose condition has clinically stabilized and who can tolerate an adequate bowel purge. Patients who are unable to drink adequate amounts of the balanced electrolyte solution can have an NG tube placed for infusion of the bowel purge. All patients with acute lower GI bleeding from an unknown source should eventually undergo endoscopic evaluation of the colon during the initial hospital stay, regardless of the initial mode of investigation.

    C. Tagged red blood cell (TRBC) scanning. RBCs labeled with technetium 99m remain in circulation for as long as 48 hours and extravasate into the bowel lumen with active bleeding. This extravasation can be detected as pooling of the radioactive tracer on scanning with a gamma camera. The pattern of peristaltic movement of the pooled tracer can help identify the potential site of bleeding. Bleeding rates as low as 0.1 ml/minute can be detected in research settings. A positive TRBC scan identifies a patient population that is more likely to require invasive intervention, with a higher in-hospital morbidity; a negative test may imply a better short-term prognosis. However, the scan is only positive 45% of the time. When positive, it is accurate in identification of the location of the bleeding source in 80% of cases. The false localization rate of approximately 20% precludes use of this test alone in directing surgical resection of the bleeding bowel segment. Therefore, the clinical utility of this test is for screening before arteriography, a more invasive test that requires a higher rate of bleeding.

D. **Arteriography** allows rapid localization and potential therapy of GI bleeding when bleeding rates exceed 0.5 ml/minute. Arteriography may also delineate the anatomy of the bleeding lesion and provide information regarding the etiology, especially bleeding diverticula or angiodysplasia; it is sometimes used in patients who are not actively bleeding, when a tumor blush or a late draining vein of an angiodysplasia may assist in localization of the bleeding source. In patients with upper GI bleeding, it is used most often when bleeding is so brisk that adequate endoscopy is impossible. In patients with small-bowel or lower GI bleeding, arteriography is the most common confirmatory test. Immediate or early extravasation demonstrated on TRBC scanning carries a greater likelihood of a positive arteriogram compared to delayed extravasation, hence the urgency in obtaining this test after a positive TRBC scan. In stable patients with recurrent, difficult-to-localize GI bleeding, infusion of anticoagulants (e.g., heparin) or thrombolytic agents (e.g., streptokinase) in addition to intra-arterial vasodilators during the procedure in a controlled fashion may increase the diagnostic yield of angiography. These provocative measures can be associated with excessive bleeding and should only be used in specialized centers in stable patients without comorbid illnesses. When an actively bleeding lesion is found during angiography, intra-arterial infusion of vasopressin can cause vasoconstriction and stop bleeding. Embolization of the bleeding artery is infrequently performed because of the risk of bowel infarction.

E. **Advanced procedures.** When radiologic evaluation suggests a jejunal bleeding source, or in recurrent (obscure) GI bleeding in which conventional endoscopy is unrevealing, enteroscopy to the jejunum can be performed using dedicated small-bowel enteroscopes. The distal ileum can be examined during colonoscopy after intubation of the ileocecal valve. When the risk of recurrent bleeding outweighs the risks of laparotomy, the entire small bowel can be examined endoscopically, with a surgeon manually threading bowel over an orally or rectally inserted endoscope; a potential bleeding source can be resected at the same operation if found.

F. **Surgery.** Emergent total colectomy may be required as a lifesaving maneuver for massive, unlocalized, lower GI bleeding; this should be preceded by emergent EGD to rule out a rapidly bleeding upper source whenever possible. Certain lesions (e.g., neoplasia, Meckel's diverticulum) require surgical resection for a cure. Splenectomy is curative in patients with bleeding from isolated gastric varices that result from splenic vein thrombosis. In situations in which bleeding is recurrent, transfusion requirements that exceed 4–6 units over 24 hours or 10 units overall, as well as more than two to three recurrent bleeding episodes from the same source, have been considered indications for surgery. The extent of comorbid medical conditions and the degree of bleeding also need to be factored in when considering surgery.

V. **Therapy of specific lesion**

A. **Peptic ulcer disease (PUD).** The use of high-dose proton pump inhibitors (PPIs; e.g., omeprazole, 40 mg PO bid) reduces the rate of recurrent bleeding and the need for surgery in patients with certain endoscopic stigmata of bleeding (nonbleeding visible vessels or adherent clots), but not for patients with arterial spurting or oozing (*N Engl J Med* 336:1054, 1997). However, this study did not use endoscopic therapy; therefore, the use of high-dose PPIs has documented utility only in patients who are awaiting endoscopic treatment or in those in whom endoscopy is contraindicated or postponed. Conventional oral doses of PPIs may suffice after endoscopic therapy has been administered. Therapeutic endoscopy offers the advantage of immediate treatment and should be implemented in all patients early in the hospital course (within 24 hours). Fluid resuscitation and hemodynamic stability are essential before endoscopy. Surgery may be required for intractable or recurrent bleeding, and a surgical consultation should be obtained early in severe bleeding with significant transfusion requirements or in recurrent bleeding after nonsurgical management. Angiotherapy may be a second option in patients who are considered poor surgical risks, wherein embolization of the bleeding artery can be performed. Risk factors for increased morbidity and mortality include age older than 60 years, more than one comorbid illness, blood loss of greater than 5 units, shock on admission, bright-red hematemesis with hypotension, coagulopathy, large (>2 cm) ulcers, recurrent hemorrhage (within 72 hours), and requirement for emergency surgery (see Peptic Ulcer Disease).

B. Variceal hemorrhage

   1. General measures. ICU admission and **endotracheal intubation** for airway protection should be considered in patients who are thought to be actively bleeding from varices. **Octreotide** infusion should be initiated immediately (50- to 100-µg bolus, followed by infusion at 25–50 µg/hour). Octreotide infusion has been shown to reduce portal pressures acutely with very few side effects, thereby improving the diagnostic yield and therapeutic success of subsequent endoscopy. **Vasopressin** (0.3 units/minute IV, followed by increments of 0.3 units/minute q30min until hemostasis is achieved, side effects develop, or the maximum dose of 0.9 units/minute is reached) is an alternative pharmacotherapeutic agent but is used less frequently because of significant complications (including myocardial ischemia and infarction, ventricular arrhythmias, cardiac arrest, mesenteric ischemia and infarction, and cutaneous ischemic necrosis). In patients with vascular disease or coronary artery disease, vasopressin should be used with caution in an ICU setting with cardiac monitoring. The infusion should be reduced or terminated if chest pain, abdominal pain, or arrhythmias develop. Concomitant infusion of **nitroglycerin** may reduce undesirable cardiovascular side effects of vasopressin therapy and may provide more effective control of bleeding. Nitroglycerin is administered only if the systolic BP is greater than 100 mm Hg, at a dose of 10 µg/minute IV, increased by 10 µg/minute q10–15min until the systolic BP falls to 100 mm Hg or a maximum dose of 400 µg/minute is reached.

   2. Esophageal varices

      a. Variceal ligation or **banding** is the endoscopic therapy of choice. It is effective in controlling active hemorrhage and achieves variceal eradication more rapidly, with lower rates of rebleeding and fewer complications than sclerotherapy. Complications of banding include superficial ulceration, dysphagia, transient chest discomfort, and, rarely, esophageal strictures.

      b. Sclerotherapy is also effective but is used less frequently because of complications (ulcerations, strictures, perforation, pleural effusions, adult respiratory distress syndrome, sepsis). Recurrent bleeding may be seen in up to 50% of patients but usually responds to repeat sclerotherapy. Fever may be seen in 40% of patients within the first 2 days of therapy; fever that lasts longer than 2 days should prompt investigation for bacteremia.

      c. Transjugular intrahepatic portosystemic shunt (TIPS) is a radiologic procedure wherein an expandable metal stent is placed between the hepatic veins and the portal vein to decompress the portal pressure. Indications include bleeding that is unresponsive to variceal ligation or sclerotherapy, or intractable bleeding. Encephalopathy may occur in up to 25% of patients but is usually controlled with medical therapy. Shunt stenosis is another significant complication; regular screening with duplex Doppler ultrasound is recommended.

d. **Shunt surgery** (portacaval or distal splenorenal shunt) should be considered in patients with good hepatic reserve if the patient (1) fails endoscopic or pharmacologic therapy, (2) is unable to return for follow-up visits, (3) is at high risk of death from recurrent bleeding because of cardiac disease or difficulty in obtaining blood products, or (4) lives far from medical care. Although bleeding may be controlled in 95% of cases, hospital death rates are high, and there is a significant incidence of postoperative encephalopathy, especially in higher grades of Child's classification (see Chap. 18).

e. **Balloon tamponade** has a very limited role in the therapy of variceal hemorrhage. It should only be used to temporize bleeding in situations in which more definitive therapy is available. Octreotide infusion and endoscopic therapy should have been attempted before balloon placement in all instances. The Sengstaken-Blakemore tube and the Minnesota tube have a gastric and esophageal balloon, whereas the Linton tube has a large-volume gastric balloon without an esophageal balloon. These tubes should be used according to the manufacturer's specific directions for placement, traction, and balloon volume. The following are general guidelines for the use of balloon tamponade: (1) **ICU admission** is mandatory, as is **endotracheal intubation.** (2) Modification of the Sengstaken-Blakemore tube by the placement of an NG tube above the esophageal balloon should be completed before insertion. This NG tube should be connected to intermittent suction to prevent aspiration of oropharyngeal secretions. This tube should be clearly labeled and not used for lavage. (3) Gastric balloon position should be confirmed by radiography before it is inflated. Inflating the gastric balloon in the esophagus can result in esophageal rupture. (4) Complications including mucosal ulceration and necrosis may occur, especially if large balloon volumes, high pressure, or traction are necessary to control bleeding. Balloon tamponade is associated with a high rate of major complications and mortality from tube displacement. Balloon pressure should be reduced intermittently, as stated in the manufacturer's instructions, and when bleeding has been controlled. The tube, with its balloon deflated, can be left in place so that pressure can be applied again if bleeding resumes. (5) Scissors must be kept at the patient's bedside to transect and withdraw the tube immediately if necessary.

3. **Gastric varices.** Octreotide infusion or other pharmacologic therapy should be initiated early as for esophageal variceal bleeding (see sec. **V.B.1**). Variceal ligation or banding is usually not successful in gastric variceal bleeding. Sclerotherapy can be attempted, but larger volumes of the sclerosant solution are generally required. Transjugular intrahepatic portosystemic shunt needs to be considered relatively early in the clinical course of gastric variceal bleeding, especially in the presence of portal hypertension. Assessment of the portal circulation with duplex Doppler ultrasound or portal venography is essential, as isolated gastric varices from splenic vein thrombosis can be effectively treated with splenectomy. If balloon tamponade is necessary, the Linton tube offers better control of bleeding than does the Sengstaken-Blakemore tube (see sec. **V.B.2.e**).

4. **Pharmacologic prophylaxis** with β-adrenergic antagonists has been shown to reduce portal pressure and lower the risk of recurrent bleeding. **Propranolol** and **nadolol** in doses sufficient to reduce the resting heart rate by 25% are effective prophylactic therapy for recurrent bleed-

Table 17-1. Dosage of acid-suppressive agents

Medication	Peptic ulcer disease	GERD	Parenteral therapy
Cimetidine*	300 mg qid 400 mg bid 800 mg qhs	400 mg qid 800 mg bid	300 mg q6h
Ranitidine*	150 mg bid 300 mg qhs	150–300 mg bid–qid	50 mg q8h
Famotidine*	20 mg bid 40 mg qhs	20–40 mg bid	20 mg q12h
Nizatidine*	150 mg bid 300 mg qhs	150 mg bid	—
Omeprazole	20 mg qd	20–40 mg qd–bid	—
Lansoprazole	15–30 mg qd	15–30 mg qd–bid	—
Rabeprazole	20 mg qd	20 mg qd–bid	—
Pantoprazole	20 mg qd	20–40 mg qd–bid	—

GERD = gastroesophageal reflux disease.
*Dosage adjustment required in renal insufficiency (see Appendix E).

ing as well as for primary prophylaxis, although no benefit in overall survival has been shown. Contraindications or side effects may limit their use. The addition of oral nitrates improves the therapeutic benefit of β-adrenergic antagonists.

  5. **Hepatic transplantation** in selected patients can reverse portal hypertension, thereby eliminating the risk of variceal bleeding.

C. **Angiodysplasia** can occur anywhere in the GI tract and can cause occult or overt GI bleeding. Renal failure and hereditary hemorrhagic telangiectasias are important predisposing factors. Actively bleeding angiodysplasias are best treated by endoscopic therapy (heater probe, laser or argon plasma coagulator), intra-arterial vasopressin, or embolization during angiography or surgical resection. Endoscopic ablation is recommended even when nonbleeding angiodysplasias are found in association with iron deficiency, especially if no other bleeding source is identified; however, frequently multiple lesions occur, and ablation may not be complete. Iron therapy and intermittent blood transfusions should be continued for several months as an initial approach to persistent anemia from angiodysplasia; if they are unsuccessful in maintaining blood counts, combination hormone therapy with estrogen and progesterone can be attempted (estradiol, 0.035–0.05 mg; norethisterone, 1 mg administered bid). Side effects are particularly troublesome for men and include sexual dysfunction, feminization, loss of libido, and gynecomastia; breast tenderness and vaginal bleeding can develop in women. A higher incidence of vascular thrombosis may be found in either sex.

D. **Stress ulcer** is encountered in the ICU setting, especially in patients who require mechanical ventilation for longer than 48 hours, with coagulopathy, sepsis, burns, or CNS processes. Prophylactic therapy should be administered in patients who are considered to be at increased risk. Histamine$_2$-receptor antagonists (H$_2$RAs) and sucralfate are effective in preventing severe bleeding. PPIs can also be used in standard doses (Table 17-1).

E. **Mallory-Weiss tear** is a mucosal tear at the gastroesophageal junction. Patients may have a history of retching or emesis followed by hematemesis.

Bleeding ceases spontaneously in almost all instances, and few patients require endoscopic or angiographic therapy. Acid suppression should be initiated for 1–2 weeks to promote healing.

F. Diverticulosis is a common finding at routine endoscopy, but bleeding develops in only approximately 5% of patients with diverticula. Spontaneous cessation of bleeding is seen in 80%, but recurrent bleeding may occur. Persistent or brisk bleeding may require intra-arterial vasopressin at angiography or even surgical resection (see Other Gastrointestinal Disorders, sec. **V**).

G. Aortoenteric fistula is an uncommon but lethal cause of GI bleeding. Most patients have a history of aortic graft surgery and present with bleeding months to years after surgery. The fistula is generally aortoduodenal but can be anywhere in the small bowel or colon. The classic presentation is a herald bleed hours to weeks before massive GI bleeding. Recognition of this condition is essential, as undiagnosed aortoenteric fistulas are uniformly fatal. Endoscopy with examination of the fourth portion of the duodenum should be performed immediately. Angiography or CT scanning may demonstrate leakage at the graft site, but a negative study does not exclude an aortoenteric fistula; surgery should not be delayed to perform such procedures if the index of suspicion is high.

H. Radiation proctitis/colitis can result months to years after exposure to radiation therapy. Typically, intermittent hematochezia results from aberrant superficial mucosal vasculature in the distal colon. Treatment consists of supportive measures and laser photocoagulation of the mucosal telangiectasias. Recurrence is common, and repeat sessions may be required. Use of aspirin and NSAIDs should be avoided if possible.

I. Hemorrhoids are the most common outpatient cause of hematochezia. Bleeding typically ceases spontaneously. Avoidance of constipation and dietary fiber supplements form the mainstay of supportive management (see Constipation, secs. **II.A** and **B**).

Esophageal Disease

I. Gastroesophageal reflux disease (GERD). The predominant symptom of GERD is heartburn, and response to a therapeutic trial of a PPI can be diagnostic (*Aliment Pharmacol Ther* 13:59, 1999). Early endoscopic evaluation is recommended for patients with **atypical symptoms** (cough, asthma, hoarseness, chest pain, aphthous ulcers, hiccups, dental erosions) and patients with **warning symptoms** of dysphagia, early satiety, weight loss, or bleeding. Patients with symptoms that are refractory to empiric acid suppression and those who require continuous medication for prolonged periods should also undergo endoscopy. Ambulatory pH monitoring is used to document or rule out GERD in patients with a negative endoscopy or those with atypical symptoms. **Complications** of GERD include ulceration, stricture formation, iron-deficiency anemia, and Barrett's epithelium. Endoscopic surveillance for Barrett's epithelium should be considered in patients with a symptom history that exceeds 5 years.

A. The basics of **lifestyle modification** include eating small meals; refraining from eating for 2–3 hours before lying down; elevating the head of the bed 6 in.; decreasing fat intake; decreasing intake of chocolate, coffee, cola, and alcohol; and smoking cessation. Medications such as calcium channel blockers, theophylline, sedatives/tranquilizers, anticholinergics, and alendronate may potentiate reflux and should be avoided if possible. Over-the-counter antacids and H_2RAs can be used prophylactically if necessary.

B. Medical therapy

1. H_2RAs. Standard doses of H_2RAs (cimetidine, 400 mg bid; ranitidine, 150 mg bid; famotidine, 20 mg bid; nizatidine, 150 mg bid) can result in symptomatic benefit in up to 60% of patients and endoscopic healing in

50%. Higher doses of H_2RAs (equivalent to ranitidine, 600 mg qd) improve the healing rate to 75% at a higher cost. Dosage adjustments are required in renal insufficiency.

2. **PPIs.** Omeprazole, 20 mg, and lansoprazole, 30 mg, PO qd have been demonstrated to be more effective than placebo or standard-dose H_2RA in symptomatic relief as well as endoscopic healing of GERD. Rabeprazole (20 mg PO qd) and pantoprazole (20 mg PO qd) have similar efficacy. Higher doses (omeprazole, 20–40 mg PO bid or equivalent) may be required in severe esophagitis. Continuous long-term therapy is safe and effective in maintaining remission of GERD symptoms. Breakthrough nocturnal symptoms can sometimes be treated by adding an H_2RA (ranitidine, 150–300 mg or equivalent) at bedtime. After initial response, maintenance therapy can be continued with H_2RAs for cost considerations if symptoms can be controlled with these agents.

3. **Prokinetic agents** may enhance the efficacy of H_2RAs and PPIs in providing symptomatic relief in GERD patients with poor esophageal clearance. Cisapride, a serotonin 5-hydoxytryptamine (5-HT_4)-receptor agonist that increases acetylcholine release in the myenteric plexus, has been withdrawn from the U.S. market because of the potential for serious cardiac arrhythmias in patients with a prolonged QT interval or in those who are receiving certain concomitant medications (see Appendix C). Alternative agents include bethanechol, a cholinergic agonist (25 mg half an hour before meals and at bedtime) and metoclopramide, a dopamine antagonist (10 mg half an hour before meals and at bedtime). Side effects include cholinergic symptoms (flushing, abdominal cramps, urinary frequency) and CNS effects (drowsiness, agitation, dyskinesias, tremor), respectively. Bethanechol is contraindicated in patients with ischemic heart disease, intestinal or urinary obstruction, and asthma. Metoclopramide rarely can be associated with irreversible tardive dyskinesia. Domperidone, another dopamine antagonist, has potentially fewer side effects, as it does not cross the blood-brain barrier, but it is not universally available.

C. **Surgery.** Indications for fundoplication include the need for continuous or increasing doses of medication in patients who are good surgical candidates or situations in which continuous PPI therapy is undesirable. Failure of medical therapy is sometimes considered an indication for surgery, especially in young individuals, but failures need careful evaluation to determine whether symptoms are indeed related to acid reflux. All patients who require aggressive long-term medical therapy should be offered the surgical option. Other indications include patient preference for surgery and noncompliance with medical therapy. The success rate of laparoscopic fundoplication in controlling GERD symptoms exceeds 90%, with fewer complications compared to the open technique.

II. **Infectious esophagitis** usually presents with odynophagia or dysphagia. It is seen most often with immunocompromised states, including AIDS, malignancy, and diabetes mellitus. Major pathogens include *Candida albicans*, herpes simplex virus (HSV), and cytomegalovirus (CMV). The presence of typical oral lesions (thrush, herpetic vesicles) may suggest an etiologic agent. Endoscopy with biopsy and brush cytology is often diagnostic. Symptomatic relief can be achieved with 2% viscous lidocaine swish and swallow (15 ml PO q3–4h prn) or sucralfate slurry (1 g PO qid). Concomitant acid suppression should also be administered.

A. *Candida* **esophagitis.** Mild disease can be treated with nystatin oral suspension, 400,000–600,000 units PO qid, or clotrimazole, 10-mg lozenges q6h for 2 weeks. Ketoconazole, 200 mg PO bid–qid or 400 mg PO qd, or fluconazole, 100 mg PO qd for 7 days, should be used in more severe disease. For unresponsive disease, a short course of parenteral amphotericin B (0.3–0.5 mg/kg/day) should be considered (see Chap. 15).

B. **HSV esophagitis.** In immunocompromised patients, HSV esophagitis can be treated with acyclovir, 5 mg/kg IV q8h for 7 days or 800 mg PO five times a day for 14 days. In healthy patients, this infection is usually self-limited, and treatment is supportive.

   C. CMV esophagitis. Ganciclovir may be effective for a variety of GI CMV infections in immunocompromised hosts (see Chap. 15).
III. Chemical esophagitis. Ingestion of caustics or medications such as oral potassium, doxycycline, quinidine, iron, NSAIDs, and aspirin can result in mucosal irritation and damage. Cautious early endoscopy is recommended to evaluate the extent and degree of mucosal damage in caustic ingestion; the procedure may have to be terminated if extensive damage is encountered. A second caustic agent to neutralize the first is contraindicated.
IV. Nonspecific ulceration. Nonspecific ulceration can be seen with medication, malignancy, or AIDS (idiopathic ulcer). Multiple biopsies, brushings, and culture specimens should be obtained at endoscopy. Idiopathic ulcer of AIDS may respond to oral steroid or thalidomide therapy. Concomitant acid suppression should always be administered.
V. Other esophageal disorders
   A. Achalasia is the most easily recognized motor disorder of the esophagus, characterized by failure of the lower esophageal sphincter (LES) to relax completely with swallowing and aperistalsis of the esophageal body. Presenting symptoms can include dysphagia, regurgitation, chest pain, weight loss, and aspiration pneumonia. Barium radiographs may demonstrate a typical appearance of a dilated intrathoracic esophagus with impaired emptying, an air-fluid level, absence of gastric air bubble, and tapering of the distal esophagus with the appearance of a bird's beak. Endoscopy may help exclude a stricture or neoplasia of the distal esophagus; the esophageal body may be dilated and contain food debris, whereas the LES, although pinpoint, typically allows passage of the endoscope into the stomach with minimal resistance. Achalasia is associated with a 0.15% risk of squamous cell cancer of the distal esophagus, a 33-fold higher risk relative to the nonachalasic population.
      1. Pharmacologic therapy consists of smooth-muscle relaxants such as nitrates or calcium channel blockers administered immediately before eating. On the whole, medications are not very effective and are only indicated as temporizing measures.
      2. Botulinum toxin injection into the LES at endoscopy can result in relief of achalasia symptoms that lasts several weeks to months and may be useful in elderly and frail patients who are poor surgical risks or as a bridge before more definitive therapy is undertaken. Some evidence has been found that botulinum toxin injection induces fibrosis in the region of the LES and makes subsequent surgery more cumbersome.
      3. Disruption of the circular muscle of the LES using **pneumatic dilation** can result in lasting reduction of LES pressure and hence symptomatic relief. Esophageal perforation is the most significant complication, commonly requiring prompt surgical repair, and occurs in 3–5% of instances. Gastroesophageal reflux can result, requiring lifelong acid suppression.
      4. A **surgical (Heller) myotomy** offers lasting relief and can now be performed laparoscopically with minimal complications. Surgical myotomy can result in gastroesophageal reflux, requiring lifelong acid suppression; laparoscopic myotomy typically is combined with an antireflux procedure.
   B. Diffuse esophageal spasm is a spastic disorder of esophageal peristalsis wherein primary peristaltic waves are present, but simultaneous, nonperistaltic contractions follow at least 30% of swallows. Concomitant incomplete LES relaxation may be present. The major symptoms are dysphagia and chest pain. Diagnosis is made after esophageal manometry; barium studies may show a beaded or "corkscrew" esophagus, sometimes with pseudodiverticula. Smooth-muscle relaxants including nitrates and calcium channel blockers may afford symptomatic relief. Low-dose tricyclic antidepressants (TCAs) can be effective for pain management, as they are for symptoms associated with other nonspecific spastic motor disorders of the esophagus.

Resistant cases may require empiric esophageal dilation, botulinum toxin injection, or even surgical myotomy, but these treatments are typically reserved for patients with severe dysphagia and regurgitation.

C. **Esophageal hypomotility** is typically idiopathic but can be associated with connective tissue diseases, Barrett's esophagus, and diabetes mellitus. Scleroderma can cause fibrosis that results in aperistalsis and atony of the distal esophagus and LES; the esophagus is involved in 75–85% of cases, with dysphagia and heartburn being the predominant symptoms. Acid suppression forms the mainstay of effective therapy. Promotility agents can be tried, although benefits may be minimal in advanced cases (see sec. **I.B.3** for cautions and contraindications).

Peptic Ulcer Disease

I. **General considerations.** The goals of therapy in PUD include relief of symptoms and prevention of recurrence and complications.

A. *Helicobacter pylori*, a spiral, gram-negative urease-producing bacillus, can be found in the stomach of approximately 99% of patients with duodenal ulcer and 70–80% of those with gastric ulcer. The presence of *H. pylori* can be ascertained by noninvasive methods (serum *H. pylori* antibody, carbon-labeled urea breath tests) or by endoscopic biopsy and rapid urease assay (CLO test), histopathology, or culture. Eradication of *H. pylori* requires antimicrobial therapy in addition to antisecretory medication (Table 17-2).

B. **NSAIDs and aspirin** can result in mucosal damage anywhere in the GI tract and are associated with an increased incidence of gastritis and PUD. Concomitant therapy with antisecretory agents may ameliorate dyspeptic symptoms in patients who have strong indications for continuation of NSAID therapy. **Misoprostol,** a synthetic prostaglandin E derivative (200 μg PO qid) can help prevent NSAID-related mucosal damage, but side effects (abdominal pain, diarrhea) can be limiting, especially in the elderly; **pregnancy should be excluded in women of reproductive age before administration. Cyclo-oxygenase-2 inhibitors** may cause less GI toxicity than traditional NSAIDS.

C. **Malignant ulcers.** Gastric ulcers can be malignant in approximately 5% of cases. The likelihood of malignancy is higher in solitary ulcers and ulcers located in the greater curvature of the stomach and in patients with chronic atrophic gastritis, pernicious anemia, gastric adenomatous polyps, and prior surgery for PUD. Endoscopic biopsy should be performed in all suspicious gastric ulcers. Follow-up EGD or upper GI series should be performed 8–12 weeks after initial diagnosis in suspicious lesions to document healing; repeat endoscopic biopsy or surgical management should be considered for nonhealing ulcers. Duodenal ulcers are almost never malignant, and therefore documentation of healing is unnecessary in the absence of symptoms.

D. **Zollinger-Ellison syndrome** is caused by a gastrin-secreting, non-beta islet cell tumor of the pancreas or duodenum. Multiple endocrine neoplasia type I is associated with this syndrome in 25% of patients. The resultant hypersecretion of gastric acid can cause multiple peptic ulcers in unusual locations, ulcers that fail to respond to standard medical therapy, or recurrent ulceration after surgical therapy. Diarrhea and gastroesophageal reflux symptoms are common. A fasting serum gastrin level while off acid suppression for at least 5 days serves as a screening test when this diagnosis is suspected; if it is elevated, a secretin stimulation test should be performed, wherein a 200-μg increment in gastrin level is seen after IV secretin in patients with gastrinomas. PPIs are generally required in higher doses than those used for PUD. Specialized nuclear medicine scans (octreotide scans) can be useful in localizing the neoplastic lesion for curative resection (*Ann Intern Med* 125:26, 1996).

Table 17-2. Regimens used for eradication of *Helicobacter pylori*[c]

Regimen	Dosage	Duration (days)	Eradication rate
Bismuth subsalicylate[a]	524 mg qid	14	>85%
Metronidazole	250 mg qid		
Tetracycline	500 mg qid		
Acid-suppressive agent	Standard dose		
Ranitidine bismuth subcitrate (Tritec)[a]	400 mg PO bid (14 days), then 1000 mg PO bid	28	77–82%
Clarithromycin	500 mg PO tid	14	
Clarithromycin[a]	500 mg PO bid	10–14	86–92%
Amoxicillin	1 g PO bid		
PPI[b]	bid		
Metronidazole	500 mg PO bid	10–14	87–91%
Clarithromycin	500 mg PO bid		
PPI	bid		
Metronidazole	500 mg PO bid	10–14	77–83%
Amoxicillin	1 g PO bid		
Omeprazole	20 mg PO bid		
Clarithromycin[a]	500 mg PO tid	14	70–80%
PPI	Standard dose		
Amoxicillin[a]	1 g PO tid	14	20–70%
PPI	Standard dose		

[a]U.S. Food and Drug Administration approved.
[b]PPI (protein pump inhibitor) = omeprazole, 20 mg, or lansoprazole, 30 mg.
[c]These doses are for patients with normal renal function (see Appendix E).

II. Treatment

A. Acid suppression. Multiple H_2RAs and PPIs are available for the therapy of PUD (see Table 17-1). For some agents, dosage intervals should be prolonged in the presence of renal insufficiency. Parenteral therapy should be reserved for patients who are unable to tolerate oral medication. Side effects are uncommon, but headache and mental status abnormalities (lethargy, confusion, depression, hallucinations) can result from H_2RA therapy. Rare hepatotoxicity, thrombocytopenia, and leukopenia have been observed with H_2RA. Cimetidine can impair metabolism of many drugs, including warfarin anticoagulants, theophylline, and phenytoin (see Appendix C).

B. Other agents. Sucralfate acts by coating the mucosal surface without blocking acid secretion and can be as effective as H_2RAs or high-dose antacids in healing duodenal ulcers. Side effects include constipation and reduction of bioavailability of certain drugs (e.g., cimetidine, digoxin, fluoroquinolones, phenytoin, and tetracycline) when administered concomitantly. **Antacids** are rarely used as primary therapy for PUD but can be useful as supplemental therapy for pain relief. The choice of antacid is determined by buffering capacity, formulation, and side effects. A typical dose is 30 ml of a high-potency liquid antacid, administered four to six times a day. Magnesium-containing antacids should be avoided in renal failure.

C. *H. pylori* **eradication.** Eradication of *H. pylori* promotes healing and markedly reduces recurrence of gastric and duodenal ulcers. Several antimicrobial and antisecretory agent regimens are available (see Table 17-2), and eradication is recommended in all *H. pylori*–infected patients with PUD.

D. Nonpharmacologic measures. Dietary modification should only include the avoidance of foods that are reproducibly associated with dyspeptic symptoms. Cigarette smoking is associated with an increased risk of peptic ulcer development, delayed healing, and recurrence; therefore, cessation of cigarette smoking should be encouraged in all instances. Alcohol in high concentrations can damage the gastric mucosal barrier, but no evidence exists to link alcohol with ulcer recurrence. NSAIDs and aspirin should be avoided if possible (see sec. **I.B**).

E. Surgery. Since the advent of improved medical therapies, the requirement for surgical therapy of PUD has declined dramatically. However, surgery is still occasionally required for intractable symptoms, GI bleeding, Zollinger-Ellison syndrome, and other complications of PUD. Surgical options vary depending on the location of the ulcer and the presence of associated complications. Significant morbidity can occur after surgical therapy for PUD, and adequate therapy requires a thorough understanding of the postsurgical complications.

1. **Abdominal symptoms.** Postoperative abdominal discomfort or vomiting after meals can be secondary to recurrent ulcer, afferent loop obstruction, bile reflux gastritis, gastric outlet obstruction, or stump carcinoma (a late complication). The **dumping syndrome** is caused by rapid gastric emptying of a large osmotic load into the small intestine and may be seen after gastroenteric anastomosis with or without subtotal gastrectomy, vagotomy, and pyloroplasty. Symptoms can be abdominal or vasomotor (palpitations, sweating, dizziness). Dietary modification to multiple small meals high in protein and low in refined carbohydrates can be beneficial; liquids with meals should be avoided. Anticholinergics, fiber supplements, and ephedrine may relieve the vasomotor symptoms. In refractory situations, SC administration of octreotide may be necessary. Mild diarrhea can be a common problem after vagotomy. Symptomatic measures are usually adequate (see Diarrhea, sec. **V**).

2. **Malabsorption.** Mild steatorrhea can occur as a result of decreased intestinal transit time and inadequate mixing of food with bile and pancreatic secretions. Bacterial overgrowth due to afferent loop stasis can also lead to steatorrhea (see Other Gastrointestinal Disorders, sec. **IV**).

3. **Anemia.** Deficiencies of folate, vitamin B_{12}, and iron can lead to anemia. In this population, postoperative iron-deficiency anemia is usually a result of dietary iron malabsorption, but blood loss from gastritis or recurrent ulcers may contribute.

III. Complications of PUD

A. GI bleeding (see Gastrointestinal Bleeding)

B. Gastric outlet obstruction is more likely to occur with ulcers that are close to the pyloric channel. Nausea and vomiting, sometimes several hours after meals, may occur. Plain abdominal radiographs often show a dilated stomach with an air-fluid level. NG suction should be maintained for 2–3 days to decompress the stomach, while repleting fluids and electrolytes intravenously. Although medical management may be temporarily effective, recurrence is common, and endoscopic balloon dilation or surgery is often necessary for definitive correction.

C. Perforation occurs in a small number of PUD patients and usually necessitates emergency surgery. Perforation may occur in the absence of previous symptoms of PUD. It may be asymptomatic in patients who are receiving glucocorticoids. A plain upright radiograph of the abdomen may demonstrate free air under the diaphragm.

D. Pancreatitis can result from penetration into the pancreas, most commonly seen with ulcers in the posterior wall of the duodenal bulb. The pain becomes severe and continuous, radiates to the back, and is no longer relieved by antisecretory therapy. Serum amylase may be elevated. CT scanning may be diagnostic. These patients frequently require surgery.

Inflammatory Bowel Disease

Ulcerative colitis (UC) is an idiopathic chronic inflammatory disease of the colon and rectum, characterized by mucosal inflammation and typically presenting with bloody diarrhea. Rectal involvement is almost universal. Patients with disease that is refractory to medical therapy or with complications (toxic megacolon, neoplasia) often require surgery; total proctocolectomy can be curative. In contrast to UC, **Crohn's disease** can affect any part of the tubular GI tract and is characterized by inflammation that involves deeper layers of the colonic wall in addition to mucosal disease. Common presenting symptoms include nonbloody diarrhea, abdominal pain, and weight loss. Fistulas, strictures, and abscesses can occur as complications. Bowel resection may be required for obstruction or refractory disease but does not afford a cure.

I. **Anti-inflammatory agents**

A. **5-Aminosalicylate (ASA) compounds.** Drugs that deliver 5-aminosalicylate typically to the bowel mucosa constitute first-line therapy in UC and Crohn's disease. The choice of agent depends on the site of disease activity.

1. **Sulfasalazine** reaches the colon intact, where it is metabolized to 5-ASA and a sulfapyridine moiety. It is therefore used for colonic disease (UC and Crohn's disease limited to the colon), either as initial therapy (0.5 g PO bid, increased to 0.5–1.5 g PO qid) or to maintain remission (1 g PO bid–qid). Adverse effects are mainly caused by the sulfapyridine moiety and include headache, nausea, vomiting, and abdominal pain; a reduction in dose may be beneficial. Hypersensitivity reactions are less common and include skin rash, fever, agranulocytosis, hepatotoxicity, and aplastic anemia. Reversible reduction in sperm counts can be seen in males. Paradoxic exacerbation of colitis is a rare adverse effect. Folic acid supplementation is recommended, as sulfasalazine impairs folate absorption.

2. **Newer 5-ASA preparations** lack the sulfa moiety of sulfasalazine and are associated with fewer side effects. **Mesalamine** (5-ASA) is available in several formulations. An oral preparation released at pH greater than 7 (Asacol, 800–1600 mg PO tid) is useful in UC as well as ileocecal/colonic Crohn's disease. A second preparation with time- and pH-dependent release of the active ingredient throughout the GI tract (Pentasa, 0.5–1.0 g PO qid) is useful in diffuse Crohn's disease that also affects the small bowel; it can be used in UC as well. Rare hypersensitivity reactions occur and include pneumonitis, pancreatitis, hepatitis, and nephritis. Mesalamine preparations can be used for initiation and maintenance therapy. **Olsalazine** is a 5-ASA dimer that is cleaved by bacteria in the colon and can be used in UC and Crohn's colitis. Diarrhea is a major side effect and can limit its use.

B. **Glucocorticoids** are beneficial in achieving remission of active disease in UC and Crohn's disease. They are not recommended for mild disease; they can be used concurrently with other anti-inflammatory agents in moderate to severe disease, especially with flare-ups of disease activity. Extracolonic manifestations of inflammatory bowel disease (IBD; ocular lesions, skin disease, and peripheral arthritis) also respond to glucocorticoids. A typical starting oral dose of prednisone is 40–60 mg given once a day in the morning. Depending on response, the dose can be reduced by 10 mg every 5–10 days and tapered off in 3–6 weeks. In severe disease or in patients who cannot tolerate oral medication, IV administration (methylprednisolone, 20–40 mg qd–bid, or equivalent) may be necessary for brief periods; higher doses may be necessary in refractory disease. Glucocorticoids are not recommended for maintenance therapy, and alternatives should be sought for the patient who appears dependent on these medications. **Glucocorticoids should not be prescribed before ruling out an infectious process and should never be initiated for the first time over the telephone.**

C. **Immunosuppressive agents. 6-Mercaptopurine,** a purine analog, and **azathioprine,** its S-imidazole precursor, cause preferential suppression of T-cell activation and antigen recognition. They are used orally in doses of 1.0–1.5 mg/kg body weight qd. Both agents have more favorable side effect profiles than do glucocorticoids and are used as steroid-sparing agents in severe or refractory IBD. Response may be delayed for up to 1–2 months. Side effects include reversible bone marrow suppression, pancreatitis, and allergic reactions. **Methotrexate** (25 mg IM weekly) has also been used as a steroid-sparing agent. Side effects include hepatic fibrosis, bone marrow suppression, alopecia, pneumonitis, allergic reactions, and teratogenicity. IV **cyclosporine** has been used in refractory cases of UC and Crohn's disease, as well as in fistulous Crohn's disease; however, the benefit is temporary. Side effects include nephrotoxicity, hepatotoxicity, hypertrichosis, seizures, and lymphoproliferative disorders.

D. **Antibiotics.** Metronidazole (250–500 mg PO tid) can be used as an alternate first-line agent or adjunctive therapy in mild to moderate Crohn's disease. Peripheral neuropathy is a concern with long-term use. Ciprofloxacin (500 mg PO bid) has also been used in Crohn's disease. The two agents can be used concurrently in perianal Crohn's disease for prolonged periods with good results. An alternative agent that is sometimes used is sulfamethoxazole-trimethoprim.

E. **Infliximab** is a monoclonal antibody against tumor necrosis factor-alpha that induces inflammatory cell lysis by binding to tumor necrosis factor receptors on the cell surface. Infliximab is approved for fistulous Crohn's disease (up to 3 IV infusions of 5 mg/kg every 4–6 weeks) as well as inflammatory-type Crohn's disease (single infusion of 5 mg/kg). Side effects are minor and short lived.

F. **Local therapy.** UC that is limited to the rectum or distal left colon can be treated effectively with 5-ASA and/or glucocorticoid enemas or suppositories administered once to twice a day; concurrent systemic therapy may be required in severe cases. Symptomatic benefit may be achieved in perianal Crohn's disease with sitz baths, analgesic, and hydrocortisone creams and local heat, in addition to systemic anti-inflammatory agents and antibiotics.

II. **Supportive therapy**

A. **Antidiarrheal agents** may be useful as adjunctive therapy in selected patients with mild exacerbations or postresection diarrhea. They are contraindicated in severe exacerbations and toxic megacolon.

B. **Diet and nutrition.** For patients whose disease is in remission, no specific dietary restrictions are necessary. A low-roughage diet often provides symptomatic relief in patients with mild to moderate disease. Elemental diets have been used in acute phases of the diseases, especially Crohn's disease, but are unpalatable and disliked by patients. Total parenteral nutrition and bowel rest may be required in severe disease, for nutritional maintenance and symptom relief while waiting for the effects of medical treatment, or as a bridge to surgery. Patients with Crohn's ileitis or ileocolonic resection may need vitamin B_{12} supplementation. Specific oral replacement of calcium, magnesium, folate, iron, vitamins A and D, and other micronutrients may be necessary in patients with small-bowel Crohn's disease (see Chap. 2). Extensive small-bowel Crohn's disease and ileal resection may also predispose to calcium oxalate nephrolithiasis; this is treated with a low-fat, low-oxalate, high-calcium diet.

III. Surgery in IBD is generally reserved for patients with fistulas, obstruction, abscess, perforation, or bleeding, and rarely for medically refractory disease and neoplastic transformation. Surgery in IBD should be performed by experienced surgeons who are well versed in the diseases (see sec. **IV**).

IV. Special considerations

A. Ulcerative colitis. In patients with colitis that lasts longer than 8–10 years, annual colonoscopic surveillance for neoplasia with four quadrant mucosal biopsies every 5–10 cm is recommended. Histopathologic evidence of any grade of dysplasia is an indication for total colectomy.

B. Crohn's disease. The most common indications for surgery in Crohn's disease are bowel obstruction, strictures, fistulas, and inflammatory masses. Recurrence close to the resected margins is common after bowel resection. Efforts should be made to avoid multiple resections in Crohn's disease because of the risk of short-bowel syndrome. Immunosuppressive agents should be discontinued before surgery and reinstituted if necessary during the postoperative period. Metronidazole, ciprofloxacin, oral immunosuppressive agents, and infliximab are useful in the medical management of fistulous and perianal disease.

C. Fulminant colitis and **toxic megacolon.** Acute fulminant colitis presents as severe diarrhea with abdominal pain, bleeding, fever, sepsis, electrolyte disturbances, and dehydration. Toxic megacolon occurs in 1–2% of patients with UC; the colon becomes atonic and modestly dilates, but systemic toxicity is the dominant feature. Patients should be kept NPO, with NG suction if there is evidence of small-bowel ileus. Dehydration and electrolyte disturbances should be treated vigorously. Anticholinergic and opioid medication should be discontinued. Intensive medical therapy with IV corticosteroids (hydrocortisone, 100 mg IV q6h or equivalent) and broad-spectrum antimicrobials should be initiated. Deterioration or lack of improvement despite 7–10 days of intensive medical management, evidence of bowel perforation, or peritoneal signs are indications for urgent total colectomy.

D. Intestinal obstruction. Stricture formation can result in intestinal obstruction in Crohn's disease. Presentation may resemble a flare, and a careful history, physical examination, and imaging studies are essential for diagnosis. NG tube decompression, parenteral hydration, and bowel rest may resolve minor episodes, but surgery may be necessary. Stricturoplasty is an accepted procedure for focal tight strictures; biopsies should be obtained to rule out cancer at stricture sites. Patients with intermittent obstructive symptoms should avoid highly indigestible foods such as nuts, pits, hulls, skins, seeds, and pulps that may precipitate obstruction.

Functional Gastrointestinal Disorders

I. General considerations. Functional GI disorders constitute the presence of abdominal symptoms in the absence of a demonstrable organic disease process. Symptoms can arise from any part of the luminal gut. Irritable bowel syndrome (IBS), primarily characterized by abdominal pain linked to altered bowel habits, is the best-recognized functional bowel disease and the most commonly diagnosed GI illness. Clinical evaluation and investigation should be directed toward prudently excluding organic processes in the involved area of the gut while initiating therapeutic trials when functional symptoms are suspected.

II. Therapy is dependent on the nature and severity of symptoms and the degree of functional impairment.

A. Nonspecific measures. Patient education, reassurance, and help with diet and lifestyle modification are key to an effective physician-patient relationship. The psychosocial contribution to symptom exacerbation should be determined, as its management may be sufficient for many patients. Low-dose tricyclic antidepressants (TCAs) (e.g., amitriptyline, nortriptyline, imipramine, doxepin: 25–100 mg qhs) have neuromodulatory and analgesic properties that are independent of their psychotropic effects and can be beneficial, especially in pain-predominant functional GI disorders. Selective serotonin-reuptake inhibitors (e.g., fluoxetine, 20 mg; paroxetine, 20 mg; sertraline, 50 mg) are less effective but have better side effect profiles (see Chap. 1).

B. **Functional esophageal symptoms** can coexist with GERD as well as disorders of affect, including anxiety and depression. Patients with functional chest pain and heartburn may have symptomatic relief from standard-dose PPI therapy with or without concomitant low-dose TCAs.

C. **Nonulcer dyspepsia.** The benefit of empiric *H. pylori* eradication remains unconfirmed but is likely small. If this organism is identified during the workup, eradication is recommended at least to reduce the likelihood of future PUD episodes. Acid suppression and low-dose TCA therapy can be attempted.

D. **Functional nausea and vomiting** consist of intermittent or persistent symptoms in the absence of a structural or organic etiology. Antiemetic agents and low-dose TCAs form the mainstay of therapy. Anecdotal evidence suggests that patients with cyclic vomiting syndrome (stereotypic episodes of vigorous vomiting with asymptomatic intervals between episodes) may also benefit from sumatriptan (25–50 mg PO, 5–10 mg transnasally, or 6 mg SC at the beginning of an episode), especially if it is administered during a prodrome or early in the episode.

E. **Sphincter of Oddi dysfunction.** Patients with biliary-type pain in association with at least two of the following benefit from sphincterotomy: (1) a dilated common bile duct, (2) slow drainage (>45 minutes) of contrast from the biliary tree during endoscopic retrograde cholangiopancreatography (ERCP), and (3) abnormal liver function tests on two separate occasions. If only one of the three features is present in addition to biliary-type pain, sphincter of Oddi manometry is indicated, with sphincterotomy only if basal sphincter pressures are greater than 40 mm Hg. Medical therapy with anticholinergic agents, calcium channel blockers, or low-dose TCAs is recommended for patients with only biliary-type pain without objective evidence of biliary pathology. Pancreatic duct correlates of sphincter of Oddi dysfunction have also been identified.

F. **Irritable bowel syndrome.** When pain and bloating are the predominant symptoms, antispasmodic or anticholinergic medications (hyoscyamine, 0.125–0.25 mg PO/sublingual up to qid; dicyclomine, 10–20 mg PO qid) or low-dose TCAs (see sec. **II.A**) are recommended. Constipation-predominant IBS may benefit from increased dietary fiber (25 g/day) supplemented with laxatives prn. Newer 5-HT$_4$–receptor agonists (prucalopride, tegaserod) may be useful for the constipation associated with IBS. Loperamide (2–4 mg, up to qid/prn) can reduce stool frequency, urgency, and fecal incontinence.

Acute Intestinal Pseudo-Obstruction (Ileus)

I. **General considerations.** Acute intestinal pseudo-obstruction or ileus consists of intestinal dilatation with other clinical features of obstruction without a mechanical explanation. Predisposing causes include virtually any medical insult, particularly life-threatening systemic diseases, infection, vascular insufficiency, surgery, and electrolyte abnormalities. Colonic dilatation in the presence of a competent ileocecal valve is termed **Ogilvie's syndrome** or acute colonic pseudo-obstruction and is particularly worrisome because of the potential for cecal rupture. A careful history and physical examination are important initial steps in assessing for peritoneal signs and other evidence of a primary intra-abdominal inflammatory process or mechanical obstruction that may require surgical attention. Conventional laboratory studies help assess for electrolyte abnormalities or intra-abdominal infectious/inflammatory processes. An obstructive series (supine and upright abdominal x-rays with a chest x-ray) determines the distribution of intestinal gas and assesses for the presence of free intraperitoneal air. Additional imaging studies, including CT scanning, contrast enema, or small-bowel series, may be required.

II. Therapy

A. General measures. Basic supportive measures consist of nothing by mouth, fluid replacement, and correction of electrolyte imbalances. Prompt antimicrobial therapy is indicated adrenergic agonists, if an infectious process is suspected. Medications that slow GI motility (adrenergic agonists, TCAs, sedatives, narcotic analgesics) should be withdrawn or doses reduced. Temporary total parenteral nutrition may be required in protracted cases. The ambulatory patient is encouraged to remain active and to undertake short walks.

B. Decompression. Intermittent NG suction prevents swallowed air from passing distally. In protracted cases, gastric decompression, either using an NG tube or a percutaneous endoscopic gastrotomy tube, eliminates upper GI secretions and decreases vomiting and gastric distension. Rectal tubes help decompress the distal colon; more proximal colonic distension may necessitate **colonoscopic decompression,** especially when the cecal diameter approaches 9–10 cm. A flexible decompression tube can be left in the proximal colon during colonoscopy. Turning the patient from side to side may potentiate the benefit of colonoscopic decompression.

C. Surgery. Surgical consultation is required when the clinical picture is worrisome for mechanical obstruction or if peritoneal signs are present. Cecostomy is rarely required when colonoscopic decompression fails in acute colonic distension. Surgical exploration is reserved for acute cases with peritoneal signs, ischemic bowel changes, or other evidence for perforation.

D. Medications. Neostigmine (2 mg IV administered slowly over 3–5 minutes) is beneficial in selected patients with acute colonic distension (*N Engl J Med* 341:137, 1999). The drug can induce rapid re-establishment of colonic tone and is contraindicated if mechanical obstruction remains in the differential diagnosis. Side effects include abdominal pain, excessive salivation, symptomatic bradycardia, and syncope. A trial of neostigmine may be warranted before colonoscopic decompression in patients without contraindications. Erythromycin (200 mg IV) acts as a motilin agonist and stimulates upper gut motility; it has been used with some success in refractory postoperative ileus. Guanethidine, bethanechol, and metoclopramide have all been used with mixed results.

Pancreaticobiliary Disorders

I. Acute pancreatitis. The most common causes are alcohol and gallstone disease. Less common causes include abdominal trauma, hypercalcemia, hypertriglyceridemia, and a variety of drugs; post-ERCP pancreatitis occurs in 5–10% of patients undergoing ERCP. The morbidity and mortality associated with acute pancreatitis are higher when necrosis is present, especially if the necrotic area is also infected; therefore, dual-phase CT scanning is useful in the initial evaluation of severe acute pancreatitis. The Ranson criteria (Table 17-3) provide useful prognostic information.

A. Therapy is largely supportive. Specific therapy is reserved for complications.

Table 17-3. Ranson criteria for severity assessment in acute pancreatitis*

	Alcoholic pancreatitis	Nonalcoholic pancreatitis
On admission		
Age	>55 yrs	>70 yrs
WBC count	>16,000/μl	>18,000/μl
Blood glucose	>200 mg/dl	>220 mg/dl
LDH	>350 IU/L	>400 IU/L
AST	>250 units/L	>440 units/L
During the first 48 hrs of admission		
Fall in hematocrit	>10%	>10%
Serum calcium	<8 mg/dl	<8 mg/dl
Base deficit	>4.0 mEq/L	>5.0 mEq/L
Increase in blood urea	>5 mg/dl	>2 mg/dl
Fluid sequestration	>6 L	>6 L
Arterial PO_2	<60 mm Hg	<60 mm Hg

AST = aspartate aminotransferase; LDH = lactic dehydrogenase; PO_2 = oxygen tension.
*The presence of three or more criteria indicates severe pancreatitis.

1. Aggressive **volume repletion** with IV fluids must be undertaken, with careful monitoring of fluid balance and awareness of the potential for significant fluid sequestration within the abdomen. Serum electrolytes, calcium, and glucose levels should be monitored and supplemented as necessary.
2. **Narcotic analgesics** are usually necessary for pain relief. Meperidine is the most commonly used agent, as it has the least effect on the sphincter of Oddi; however, it is contraindicated in renal failure. Morphine and pentazocine should be avoided if possible. Patient-controlled analgesia may be necessary for adequate relief of pain.
3. Patients should receive **nothing by mouth** until they are free of pain and nausea. NG suction is reserved for patients with ileus or protracted nausea and vomiting and is not required routinely.
4. Urgent **ERCP and biliary sphincterotomy** within 72 hours of presentation can improve the outcome of severe gallstone pancreatitis. This is thought to result from reduced biliary sepsis rather than being a true improvement of pancreatic inflammation.
5. **Acid suppression** may be necessary in severely ill patients with risk factors for stress ulcer bleeding (see Gastrointestinal Bleeding, sec. **V.D**).

B. **Complications**
   1. **Necrotizing pancreatitis** represents a severe form of acute pancreatitis, usually identified on dynamic dual-phase CT scanning with IV contrast. The presence of radiologically identified pancreatic necrosis increases the morbidity and mortality of acute pancreatitis. Increasing abdominal pain, marked leukocytosis, and bacteremia suggest infected pancreatic necrosis that requires surgical débridement. CT-guided percutaneous aspiration for Gram stain and culture can confirm the diagnosis of infected necrosis.
   2. The presence of **pseudocysts** is suggested by persistent pain or hyperamylasemia. Complications include infection, hemorrhage, rupture (pancreatic ascites), and obstruction of adjacent structures. Generally, asymptomatic nonenlarging pseudocysts of less than 6 cm can be fol-

lowed clinically with serial imaging studies. Decompression of symptomatic or complicated pseudocysts can be performed by percutaneous, endoscopic, or surgical techniques.

3. **Infection.** Potential sources of fever include pancreatic necrosis, abscess, infected pseudocyst, cholangitis, and aspiration pneumonia. Cultures should be obtained, and broad-spectrum antimicrobials that are appropriate for bowel flora should be administered (see Chap. 14). In the absence of fever or other clinical evidence for infection, prophylactic antimicrobial therapy has no clear role in acute pancreatitis.

4. **Pulmonary complications.** Atelectasis, pleural effusion, pneumonia, and acute respiratory distress syndrome can develop in severely ill patients (see Chap. 9).

5. **Renal failure.** Severe intravascular volume depletion or acute tubular necrosis can cause renal failure (see Chap. 12).

II. **Gallstone disease**

A. **Asymptomatic cholelithiasis** is a common incidental finding for which no specific therapy is generally necessary. **Symptomatic cholelithiasis** may present as biliary colic, which is a constant pain lasting for hours, located in the right upper quadrant, radiating to the back or right shoulder, and sometimes associated with nausea or vomiting. Other complications of gallstones include acute cholecystitis, acute pancreatitis, cholangitis, and gallbladder cancer.

1. **Cholecystectomy** is the therapy of choice for symptomatic gallstone disease. Laparoscopic cholecystectomy compares favorably with the open procedure, with lower morbidity, shorter hospital stay, and better cosmetic results.

2. **Medical therapy** might be prudent in a small select group of patients with cholesterol stones who have uncomplicated biliary colic or who are at high risk of complications from surgical therapy. Such patients may qualify for prolonged medical therapy with ursodeoxycholic acid, 8–10 mg/kg/day PO in two to three divided doses. Selection criteria include small radiolucent stones (<20 mm in diameter) that float in a functioning gallbladder, as judged by oral cholecystography. The dissolution rate of stones ranges from 25% to 50% after 2 years of therapy. Side effects include diarrhea and reversible elevation in serum transaminase levels.

3. **Other nonsurgical therapies** include percutaneous instillation of contact solvents such as methyl-tertiary-butyl ether into the gallbladder and extracorporeal shock-wave lithotripsy combined with oral bile acid dissolution therapy. Experience with these therapies is limited, and neither is definitive as the gallbladder remains in place.

B. **Acute cholecystitis** is caused most often by obstruction of the cystic duct by gallstones, but acalculous cholecystitis can occur in severely ill, hospitalized patients. Ultrasound scans have a high degree of accuracy in diagnosis; a hydroxy iminodiacetic acid (HIDA) scan can demonstrate nonfilling of the gallbladder in difficult cases. Cholecystectomy is the mainstay of treatment. Supportive measures include IV fluid resuscitation and broad-spectrum antimicrobial agents, especially in the event of complications such as sepsis, perforation, peritonitis, abscess, or empyema formation. Percutaneous cholecystotomy and decompression of the gallbladder can be performed under fluoroscopy in severely ill patients who are not surgical candidates.

C. **Choledocholithiasis.** In patients who have undergone cholecystectomy, retained common bile duct stones can complicate the postoperative course. Common bile duct obstruction, jaundice, biliary colic, cholangitis, or pancreatitis can result. ERCP with sphincterotomy and stone extraction is curative.

D. Patients with **acute ascending cholangitis** present with right upper quadrant pain, fever with chills, and jaundice (Charcot's triad), usually in the setting of biliary obstruction (choledocholithiasis, neoplasia, sclerosing cholangitis, biliary stent occlusion). Elderly patients may lack abdominal symptoms. Cholangitis represents a medical emergency with high morbidity and mortality if biliary decompression is not performed urgently. The patient's condition should be stabilized with IV fluids and broad-spectrum antibiotics (see Chap. 14). Drainage of the biliary tree can be performed through the endoscopic (ERCP with sphincterotomy) or percutaneous approach under fluoroscopic guidance.

III. Chronic pancreatitis is commonly seen with chronic alcohol abuse. A plain abdominal radiograph may demonstrate a calcified pancreas.

    A. Pain management is critical in chronic pancreatitis. Narcotic analgesics are frequently required, and narcotic dependence is common. In patients with mild to moderate exocrine insufficiency, the addition of oral pancreatic enzyme supplements may be beneficial for pain control. Patients with pancreatic duct obstruction from stones, strictures, or papillary stenosis may benefit from ERCP and sphincterotomy. Intractable pain may necessitate celiac ganglion block or even surgery.

    B. Exocrine insufficiency typically manifests as weight loss and steatorrhea. In the presence of steatorrhea, a serum trypsinogen level of less than 10 ng/ml is diagnostic of chronic pancreatitis. Most patients can be managed with a low-fat diet (<50 g/day) and pancreatic enzyme supplements. Non–enteric-coated pancrelipase preparations (Viokase or Cotazym, 2–4 tablets with each meal) are administered with acid suppression to prevent degradation by gastric acid. Enteric-coated preparations (Pancrease or Creon, 1–2 capsules with meals) are stable at acid pH and should not be given with concomitant acid suppression. Fat-soluble vitamin supplementation may be necessary.

    C. Endocrine insufficiency may result from destruction of islet cells. The resultant diabetes mellitus is characteristically brittle, as glucagon-producing islet cells are also destroyed. Insulin therapy is generally required (see Chap. 22).

Other Gastrointestinal Disorders

I. Gastroparesis can result from chronic disorders (diabetes mellitus, scleroderma, intestinal pseudo-obstruction, previous gastric surgery) or, less frequently, from acute metabolic derangements (hypokalemia, hypercalcemia, hypocalcemia, hyperglycemia) or medications (narcotic analgesics, anticholinergic agents, chemotherapeutic agents). Mechanical obstruction should always be excluded. Symptoms include nausea, bloating, and vomiting, often hours after a meal. A gastric emptying study consists of gamma-camera scanning after a radiolabeled meal and can confirm the diagnosis. Patients should avoid high-fat, high-fiber meals; high-calorie liquid iso-osmotic meals may be beneficial in refractory situations. Underlying metabolic derangements should be corrected. **Prokinetic agents** have been used with varying degrees of success. Metoclopramide (10 mg PO qid half an hour before meals) has variable efficacy, and side effects (drowsiness, tardive dyskinesia) may be limiting. Erythromycin (250 mg PO tid or 200 mg IV) also stimulates gastric motility. Intermittent nausea and vomiting in patients with gastroparesis may also respond to treatment for functional nausea and vomiting (see Functional Gastrointestinal Disorders, sec. **II.D**).

II. Patients with **celiac sprue** are sensitive to gluten, a group of proteins that are present in wheat, barley, and rye. This results in malabsorption of dietary nutrients by the abnormal small-bowel mucosa and prompt improvement when compliant with a gluten-free diet. Noninvasive tests include antigliadin and antiendomysial antibodies, but biopsy revealing severe blunting or complete absence of villi is the gold standard for diagnosis. Secondary lactase deficiency may coexist. Patients may require iron, folate, calcium, and vitamin supplements. Corticosteroids (prednisone, 10–20 mg/day) may be required in refractory cases, although the most common cause of refractory disease is dietary indiscretion. If symptoms persist despite strict dietary restriction, radiologic and endoscopic evaluation of the small bowel should be performed to rule out **small-bowel lymphoma.**

III. **Lactose intolerance** results from selective deficiency of lactase in the intestinal brush border. Undigested lactose in the intestinal lumen results in osmotic diarrhea, abdominal cramps, and flatulence. Symptoms are associated with ingestion of dairy products. Temporary lactase deficiency may result from bacterial or viral enteritis. Avoidance of dairy products is usually sufficient for diagnosis and treatment. Lactose tolerance and hydrogen breath tests can be used for diagnosis in difficult cases. Lactase supplements (2–4 tablets or capsules with each lactose meal) can also be used for treatment.

IV. **Bacterial overgrowth** of the small intestine can result from any condition that causes intestinal stasis (small-bowel diverticulosis, afferent loop obstruction, scleroderma, intestinal pseudo-obstruction, strictures, adhesions). Deconjugation of bile salts by the bacteria causes fat malabsorption. The bacteria also may compete for dietary vitamin B_{12}, causing anemia. Diagnosis is suspected by history and radiography and can be confirmed using breath tests and culture of small-bowel aspirate obtained at endoscopy. Broad-spectrum antimicrobials (tetracycline, 250 mg PO qid; amoxicillin/clavulanate, 250–500 mg PO tid; ciprofloxacin, 250 mg PO bid) can be used in 2-week courses intermittently. Vitamin supplementation may be necessary (see Chap. 2). Surgical correction of the predisposing disorder may be indicated.

V. **Diverticulosis** is asymptomatic and does not require any specific treatment other than increased dietary fiber. **Diverticular bleeding** can be profuse and may require invasive measures, including angiography, intra-arterial vasopressin infusion, or surgery for control (see Gastrointestinal Bleeding, sec. **V.F**). **Diverticulitis** results from microperforation of a diverticulum and resultant extracolonic or intramural inflammation. Typical presenting symptoms include left lower quadrant abdominal pain, fevers and chills, and alteration of bowel habits, usually associated with an elevated WBC count. Imaging studies [CT scanning, sodium diatrizoate (Hypaque) enema] are useful in confirming the diagnosis. Hospital admission, bowel rest, IV fluids, and antimicrobial agents are typically required in the majority of patients. Mild cases can be managed in the outpatient setting with a low-residue diet and oral antibiotics (e.g., ciprofloxacin, 500 mg PO bid, and metronidazole, 500 mg PO tid for 10–14 days). Broad-spectrum IV antimicrobials that are appropriate for intra-abdominal infection are advisable for hospitalized patients. Surgical consultation should be obtained early, as operative intervention may be necessary should complications arise.

VI. **Acute mesenteric ischemia** results from arterial (or rarely venous) compromise to the superior mesenteric circulation. Emboli are the most common cause, although **nonocclusive mesenteric ischemia** from vasoconstriction can also give rise to the disorder. Patients present during the ischemic episode with abdominal pain, but physical examination and imaging studies may be unremarkable until infarction has occurred. As a result, diagnosis is late and mortality is high. Angiography should be urgently performed if the diagnosis is suspected. Treatment is essentially surgical. **Ischemic colitis** is more common and manifests typically as transient bleeding in most cases; severe insults can lead to stricture formation, gangrene, and perforation. Symptoms are nonspecific and can follow a hypotensive event. Vasculitis, sickle cell disease, vasospasm, and marathon running can also predispose to ischemic colitis. Characteristic "thumbprinting" may be seen on plain x-rays of the abdomen. Colonoscopy may reveal mucosal ulceration, edema, and bleeding; evidence of gangrene or necrosis is an indication for surgical intervention. In the absence of peritoneal signs or evidence of gangrene or perforation, expectant management with fluid and electrolyte repletion, broad-spectrum antimicrobials, and maintenance of an adequate blood pressure usually suffices.

VII. Anorectal disorders

　　A. Thrombosed external hemorrhoids present as acutely painful, tense, bluish lumps covered with skin in the anal area. The thrombosed hemorrhoid can be surgically excised under local anesthesia for relief of severe pain. In less severe cases, oral analgesics, sitz baths (sitting in a tub of warm water), stool softeners, and topical ointments (see sec. **VII.B**) may provide symptomatic relief.

　　B. Internal hemorrhoids commonly present with either bleeding or a prolapsing mass with straining. Bulk-forming agents such as fiber supplements are useful in preventing straining at defecation. Sitz baths and Tucks pads (cotton soaked in witch hazel) may provide symptomatic relief. Ointments and suppositories that contain topical analgesics, emollients, astringents, and hydrocortisone [e.g., Anusol-HC Suppositories, 1 per rectum (PR) bid for 7–10 days] can also be used to decrease inflammation. Hemorrhoidectomy or band ligation can be curative.

　　C. Anal fissures present with acute onset of pain during defecation and are often caused by passage of hard stool. Anoscopy reveals an elliptical tear in the skin of the anus, usually in the posterior midline. Acute fissures generally heal in 2–3 weeks with the use of stool softeners, oral or topical analgesics, and sitz baths. Topical nitroglycerin ointment, 0.2%, applied three times a day may be beneficial (*Dis Colon Rectum* 42:1000, 1999). Chronic fissures often require surgical therapy.

　　D. Perirectal abscess commonly presents as a painful induration in the perianal area. Patients with IBD and immunocompromised states are particularly susceptible. Prompt drainage is essential to avoid the serious morbidity associated with delayed treatment. Antimicrobials directed against bowel flora (metronidazole, 500 mg PO tid, and ciprofloxacin, 500 mg PO bid) should be administered in patients with significant inflammation, systemic toxicity, or immunocompromised states.

Dysphagia and Odynophagia

Oropharyngeal dysphagia (difficulty in transferring food from the mouth to the esophagus, often associated with symptoms of nasopharyngeal regurgitation and pulmonary aspiration) needs to be distinguished from esophageal dysphagia, characterized by the sensation of difficulty in passage of food down the esophagus. Dysphagia for solids suggests an obstructive process in the esophagus. Progressive symptoms are typically seen with neoplasia or peptic strictures; webs and rings result in intermittent symptoms. Dysphagia for solids and for liquids suggests a motility disorder, for example, achalasia or esophageal spasm. Acute onset of dysphagia, usually in temporal relationship to a meal, suggests food impaction.

I. General considerations. Patients with oropharyngeal dysphagia may demonstrate signs of a neurologic disorder on examination. Assessment is initiated with barium videofluoroscopy or a modified barium swallow. Esophageal dysphagia of insidious onset is characteristically investigated with a barium swallow; however, rings and webs may not be visualized unless a solid bolus is used. Endoscopy is also a suitable initial test for esophageal dysphagia because of its biopsy and treatment capabilities. Esophageal manometry can characterize esophageal motor disorders when other studies are normal or suggest a motility disorder. Acute esophageal obstruction is best investigated with endoscopy.

II. Therapy

　　A. Dysphagia. Benign structural lesions including webs and rings can be dilated using rigid dilators with resolution of dysphagia. Recurrences are common but usually respond to repeat dilation. Esophageal stent placement can alleviate dysphagia in inoperable neoplasia. Endoscopic retrieval of an obstructing food bolus can result in dramatic resolution of acute dysphagia from food impaction. Glucagon (2- to 4-mg IV bolus) can be attempted but is frequently unsuccessful; sublingual nitroglycerin can also be given, but meat tenderizer should not be administered. Subsequent esophageal dilation or manometry, or both, should be scheduled and acid suppression prescribed.

B. Odynophagia generally responds to specific therapy of the causative lesion (see Esophageal Disease). Concomitant acid suppression and viscous lidocaine swish-and-swallow solutions may afford additional symptomatic relief.

Nausea and Vomiting

Nausea and vomiting may result from systemic illnesses, CNS disorders, and primary GI disorders, and as side effects of medications. Vomiting that occurs during or immediately after a meal can result from a pyloric channel ulcer or from functional disorders. Vomiting within 30–60 minutes after a meal suggests gastric or duodenal pathology, whereas delayed vomiting after a meal with undigested food from a previous meal can suggest gastric outlet obstruction or gastroparesis. **Bowel obstruction and pregnancy should be ruled out.** The patient's medication list should be scrutinized.

I. Nonspecific measures. Oral intake should be withheld or limited to clear liquids. Many patients with self-limited illnesses require no further therapy. NG decompression and IV fluids may be required for patients with bowel obstruction or protracted nausea and vomiting of any etiology.

II. Pharmacotherapy

A. Phenothiazines and related agents. Prochlorperazine, 5–10 mg PO tid–qid, 10 mg IM or IV q6h, or 25 mg PR bid; promethazine, 12.5–25.0 mg PO, IM, or PR q4–6h; trimethobenzamide, 250 mg PO tid–qid, 200 mg IM tid–qid, or 200 mg PR tid–qid; and triethylperazine, 10 mg PO, IM, or PR qd–tid are effective. Drowsiness is a common side effect, and acute dystonic reactions may occur.

B. Dopamine antagonists include metoclopramide (10 mg PO 30 minutes before meals and at bedtime), a prokinetic agent that also has central antiemetic effects. IV metoclopramide is used in nausea and vomiting associated with chemotherapy (see Chap. 21). Drowsiness and extrapyramidal reactions may occur.

C. Ondansetron, 32 mg IV infused over 15 minutes beginning 30 minutes before chemotherapy or 0.15 mg/kg IV q4h for three doses, is effective in chemotherapy-associated emesis. It can also be used in emesis that is refractory to other medications. Constipation may occur (see Chap. 21).

D. Other prokinetic agents are generally not recommended for acute nausea and emesis. In chronic cases in which dysmotility of the upper GI tract is thought to play a significant role, metoclopramide, 5–10 mg PO before meals and at bedtime, can be tried, keeping in mind the cautions associated with the use of this medication (see Esophageal Disease, sec. **I.B.3**). Domperidone may be an alternative agent but is not universally available.

Diarrhea

I. General considerations. Empiric therapy of diarrhea is used as a temporizing measure while diagnostic testing is being conducted, when specific therapy of the etiology fails to provide symptomatic benefit, and when diagnostic testing fails to identify a cause.

II. **Acute diarrhea.** Infectious agents, toxins, and drugs are the major causes of acute diarrhea. IBD may also present with acute diarrhea. In hospitalized patients, pseudomembranous colitis, antibiotic- or drug-associated diarrhea, and fecal impaction should be considered. Stool cultures, *Clostridium difficile* toxin assay, fecal leukocytes, stool ova and parasite examination, and flexible sigmoidoscopy may be warranted in patients with severe, prolonged, or atypical symptoms. Patients in whom diarrhea develops after bone marrow transplantation should be investigated for graft-versus-host disease (see Chap. 21).

A. **Bacterial and viral infections.** Bacterial infections with *Escherichia coli*, *Shigella*, *Salmonella*, *Campylobacter*, and *Yersinia* species, and viral enteritis, constitute the most common causes of acute diarrhea. Most cases are self-limiting and do not require antimicrobial therapy. Empiric antibiotic therapy is only recommended in patients with moderate to severe disease and associated systemic symptoms, while stool cultures are incubating. Fluoroquinolones (ciprofloxacin, 500 mg PO bid for 3 days, or norfloxacin, 400 mg PO bid for 3 days) and trimethoprim-sulfamethoxazole (160 mg/800 mg PO bid for 5 days) can be used.

B. **Pseudomembranous colitis** is usually seen in the setting of antimicrobial therapy and is caused by toxins produced by *C. difficile*. Metronidazole (250–500 mg PO tid, IV if not tolerated PO, for 7–14 days) is the treatment of choice. Vancomycin (125 mg PO qid, IV if enteral administration is not possible) is reserved for resistant cases or intolerance to metronidazole. Relapses are common and may require longer courses of treatment. *Saccharomycetes boulardii* (500 mg PO bid for 4 weeks) can be used as an adjunct to antibiotic therapy in refractory cases and to prevent relapse. Cholestyramine (1 g PO tid–qid) is a bile salt binding resin that may be useful in decreasing diarrhea in refractory cases. It should be administered at least 2 hours after antibiotics to ensure that the antibiotic is absorbed.

C. **Parasitic infections. Amebiasis** may cause acute diarrhea, especially in travelers to areas with poor sanitation and in homosexual men. Demonstration of trophozoites or cysts of *Entamoeba histolytica* in the stool, or a serum antibody test, confirms the diagnosis. Treatment of symptomatic disease is metronidazole, 750 mg PO tid or 500 mg IV q8h for 5–10 days. This should be followed by paromomycin, 500 mg PO tid for 7 days, or iodoquinol, 650 mg PO tid for 20 days, to eliminate cysts. **Giardiasis** is confirmed by identification of *Giardia lamblia* trophozoites in the stool, in duodenal aspirate, or in small-bowel biopsy specimens. A stool immunofluorescence assay is also available for rapid diagnosis. Therapy consists of metronidazole, 250 mg PO tid for 5–7 days, or tinidazole, 2-g single dose. Quinacrine, 100 mg PO tid for 7 days, is an alternative agent. More prolonged therapy may be necessary in the immunocompromised patient.

D. **Diarrhea related to medication use.** Common offending agents include laxatives, antacids, cardiac medications (e.g., digitalis, quinidine), colchicine, and antimicrobial agents. Symptoms usually respond to discontinuation of the offending agent.

III. **Chronic diarrhea** is defined as the production of loose stools with or without increased stool frequency for more than 4 weeks. A careful history and thorough physical examination can complement routine laboratory tests. Stool should be tested for ova and parasites in the appropriate clinical setting. Further investigation is performed to classify diarrhea into one of the following categories: watery diarrhea (secretory or osmotic), inflammatory diarrhea, or fatty diarrhea (steatorrhea). The **fecal osmotic gap** is calculated as $290 - 2([Na^+] + [K^+])$ in watery stools. Secretory processes typically have stool osmotic gaps of less than 50 mOsm/kg, whereas osmotic diarrheas have gaps of greater than 125 mOsm/kg. A positive fecal occult blood test or fecal leukocyte test suggests inflammatory diarrhea. Steatorrhea is traditionally diagnosed by demonstration of fat excretion in stool of greater than 7 g/day in a 72-hour stool collection while the patient is on a 100-g/day fat diet. Because compliance is an issue with this method, Sudan staining of a stool specimen can be performed instead; greater than 100 fat globules per high-power field is suggestive of steatorrhea. Laxative screening should be performed in any patient with chronic diarrhea that remains undiagnosed.

IV. Diarrhea in HIV disease. Opportunistic agents, including *Cryptosporidium*, *Microsporidium*, CMV, *Mycobacterium avium* complex, and *Mycobacterium tuberculosis*, may cause diarrhea in patients with advanced HIV and should be looked for specifically. Venereal infections (syphilis, gonorrhea, chlamydiosis, HSV infection) as well as other nonvenereal infections (amebiasis, giardiasis, salmonellosis, shigellosis) may also cause diarrhea. Other causes of diarrhea in this population include intestinal lymphoma and Kaposi's sarcoma. Stool studies (ova and parasites, culture), endoscopic biopsies, and serologic testing may assist diagnosis. The most likely cause of undiagnosed diarrhea is missed pathogens; however, drugs, antibiotics, HIV acting as a pathogen, autonomic disturbance, and abnormal intestinal motility may also contribute to diarrhea. Management consists of specific therapy if pathogens are identified; symptomatic measures may be of benefit in idiopathic cases.

V. Symptomatic therapy. Adequate hydration is an essential part of the therapy of diarrheal disease (see Chap. 2). IV hydration is required in severe cases. Long-term IV fluids or parenteral nutrition is sometimes necessary in refractory diarrhea. Opiates (loperamide, 2–4 mg up to 4 times a day; tincture of opium; belladonna; and opium capsules) are the most effective nonspecific antidiarrheal agents. Octreotide (100–200 μg bid–qid prn) can be of benefit as a second-line agent in some cases. Bile acid–binding resins (e.g., cholestyramine, 1 g up to qid) are beneficial in bile acid–induced diarrhea.

Constipation

I. General considerations. The acuity of onset of constipation is critical in the initial assessment. A recent change in bowel habits may indicate an organic disorder, whereas constipation of several years' duration is more likely due to a functional disorder. Medication (e.g., calcium blockers, opiates, anticholinergics, iron supplements, barium sulfate) and systemic disease (e.g., diabetes mellitus, hypothyroidism, systemic sclerosis, myotonic dystrophy) may also contribute to the etiology of constipation. Other predisposing factors include lack of exercise, disorders that cause pain on defecation (e.g., anal fissures, thrombosed external hemorrhoids), and prolonged immobilization. Endoscopy and barium studies help to rule out structural disease, particularly in older individuals. Colonic transit studies, anorectal manometry, and defecography are reserved for resistant cases without an organic explanation.

II. Therapy. Treatment of underlying disease and correction of predisposing conditions are important initial steps in the treatment of constipation. Regular exercise and adequate fluid intake are other nonspecific measures that may be of benefit.

    A. Fiber supplementation. An increase in dietary fiber intake to 20–30 g/day may be beneficial in many adults with constipation. Fecal impactions should be resolved before fiber supplementation is initiated. A fiber supplement such as wheat bran or psyllium with water two to four times a day can be initiated; fluid intake should be increased with these preparations. Transient bloating often occurs.

    B. Laxatives

        1. Emollient laxatives consist of docusate salts and mineral oil. Docusate sodium, 50–200 mg PO qd, and docusate calcium, 240 mg PO qd, allow water and fat to penetrate the fecal mass. Mineral oil (15–45 ml PO q6–

8h) can be given orally or by enema. Tracheobronchial aspiration of mineral oil can result in lipoid pneumonia.

2. **Stimulant cathartics** such as castor oil, 15 ml PO, stimulate intestinal secretion and increase intestinal motility. Anthraquinones (cascara, 5 ml PO qd; senna, 1 tablet PO qd–qid) stimulate the colon by increasing fluid and water accumulation in the proximal colon. Chronic use can result in benign staining of the colonic mucosa (melanosis coli) and colonic atony from smooth-muscle atrophy and damage to the myenteric plexus. Bisacodyl (10–15 mg PO qhs, 10-mg rectal suppositories) is structurally similar to phenolphthalein and stimulates colonic peristalsis.

3. **Osmotic cathartics** include nonabsorbable salts or carbohydrates that cause water retention in the lumen of the colon. Magnesium salts include milk of magnesia (15–30 ml q8–12h) and magnesium citrate (200 ml PO); they should be avoided in renal failure. Lactulose (15–30 ml PO bid–qid) can cause bloating as a side effect. Polyethylene glycol solution is often used as a bowel-cleansing agent before colonoscopy; smaller doses of a powder form (Miralax) can be used regularly or intermittently for constipation. Nonabsorbable phosphate (phosphosoda, 2 doses of 1.5 oz with 500 ml water 8 hours apart) can also be used for bowel cleansing and for refractory constipation. Phosphosoda can result in severe dehydration and should be used with caution in elderly individuals; it is contraindicated in renal failure.

C. **Enemas.** Sodium biphosphate (Fleet) enemas (1–2 rectally prn) can be used for mild to moderate constipation and for bowel cleansing before sigmoidoscopy. However, these should be avoided in patients with renal failure because of the risk of developing hyperphosphatemia and subsequent hypocalcemia. Tap water enemas (1 L) are also useful for bowel cleansing. Oil-based enemas (cottonseed colace, Hypaque) are reserved for refractory cases.

D. **Other agents.** Newer 5-HT_4–receptor agonists (prucalopride, tegaserod) may be of benefit for some patients with functional constipation.

18

Liver Diseases

Raj Satyanarayana and
Mauricio Lisker-Melman

Evaluation of Liver Function

Liver disease is classified on the basis of duration of abnormalities as acute (<6 months) or chronic (>6 months).

I. **Laboratory evaluation**

A. **Serum enzymes.** Hepatic disorders associated predominantly with elevation in aminotransferases are referred to as **hepatocellular;** hepatic disorders with predominant elevation in alkaline phosphatase (AP) are referred to as **cholestatic.**

1. Elevation of **serum aminotransferases** [aspartate aminotransferase (AST; SGOT) and alanine aminotransferase (ALT; SGPT)] indicates hepatocellular injury and necrosis. Markedly elevated levels (>1000 units/L) typically occur with acute hepatocellular injury (e.g., viral, drug-induced, or ischemic), whereas mild to moderate elevation may be seen in a variety of conditions (e.g., acute or chronic hepatocellular injury, infiltrative diseases, biliary obstruction). The ratio of serum AST to ALT is typically greater than 2 in alcoholic liver disease. In viral hepatitis, this ratio is characteristically less than 1.

2. **AP** is an enzyme that is present in a variety of body tissues (bone, intestine, kidney, leukocytes, liver, and placenta). The concomitant elevation of other hepatic enzymes [e.g., gamma-glutamyl transpeptidase (GGT) or 5'-nucleotidase] is used in establishing the hepatic origin of AP. Serum AP level is often elevated in biliary obstruction, space-occupying lesions, infiltrative disorders, and conditions that cause intrahepatic cholestasis (primary biliary cirrhosis, primary sclerosing cholangitis, drug-induced cholestasis). The degree of elevation of AP does not differentiate the site or cause of cholestasis.

3. **5'-Nucleotidase** is comparable to AP in sensitivity in detecting biliary obstruction, cholestasis, and infiltrative hepatobiliary diseases.

4. **GGT** is an enzyme present in a variety of tissues. Increases in GGT and AP tend to occur in similar hepatic diseases. GGT may be elevated in individuals who ingest barbiturates, phenytoin, or alcohol even when other liver enzyme and bilirubin levels are normal.

B. **Excretory products**

1. **Bilirubin** is a degradation product of hemoglobin and nonerythroid hemoproteins (e.g., cytochrome, catalase). Total serum bilirubin is composed of conjugated (direct) and unconjugated (indirect) fractions. Unconjugated hyperbilirubinemia occurs as a result of **excessive bilirubin production** (neonatal or physiologic jaundice, hemolysis and hemolytic anemias, ineffective erythropoiesis, and resorption of hematomas), **reduced hepatic bilirubin uptake** (Gilbert's syndrome and drugs such as rifampin and probenecid), or **impaired bilirubin con-**

jugation (Gilbert's or Crigler-Najjar syndromes). Elevation of conjugated and unconjugated fractions occurs in Dubin-Johnson and Rotor's syndromes and in conditions associated with **intrahepatic** (from hepatocellular, canalicular, or ductular damage) and **extrahepatic** (from mechanical obstruction) **cholestasis.**

2. **Bile acids** are produced in the liver and are secreted into bile where they are required for lipid digestion and absorption. Elevated levels of serum bile acids are specific but not sensitive markers of hepatobiliary disease. Levels of individual bile acids are not useful in the differential diagnosis of liver disorders.

3. **Serum ammonia** levels are often elevated in hepatic encephalopathy. However, absolute levels do not correlate with clinical findings or grade of encephalopathy.

C. **Synthetic products**

1. **Serum albumin** concentration is frequently decreased in chronic liver disease. However, chronic inflammation, expanded plasma volume, and GI and renal losses may also lead to hypoalbuminemia. Because the half-life of albumin is relatively long (≈ 20 days), serum levels may be normal in acute liver disease.

2. Several important proteins that are involved in hemostasis and fibrinolysis [coagulation factors (except factor VIII, which is produced by the liver and endothelium), α_2-antiplasmin, antithrombin, heparin cofactor II, high-molecular-weight kininogen, prekallikrein, protein C, and protein S] are synthesized by the liver. The synthesis of factors II, VII, IX, and X and proteins C and S depends on the presence of vitamin K. The adequacy of hepatic synthetic function can be estimated by the **prothrombin time (PT)** (see Chap. 19). PT prolongation may result from impaired coagulation factor synthesis or vitamin K deficiency. Normalization of PT after administration of vitamin K indicates vitamin K deficiency. In **fulminant hepatic failure** (see Miscellaneous Disorders), the level of factor V (half-life, 2 hours) predicts outcome.

3. Other synthetic products whose levels may be measured in specific liver diseases are α_1**-antitrypsin, alpha-fetoprotein, and ceruloplasmin.**

4. **Cholesterol** is synthesized in the liver. Patients with advanced liver disease may have very low cholesterol levels. However, in primary biliary cirrhosis, levels of serum cholesterol may be markedly elevated.

II. **Radiographic evaluation**

A. **Ultrasonography** is used to screen for dilation of the biliary tree and to detect gallstones and cholecystitis in patients with right-sided abdominal pain associated with abnormal liver blood tests. It can detect and characterize liver masses, abscesses, and cysts. Color-flow Doppler ultrasonography can assess patency and direction of blood flow in the portal and hepatic veins. Ultrasonography is the diagnostic modality of choice for hepatocellular carcinoma screening.

B. **Helical CT** scan with IV contrast is useful in the evaluation of parenchymal liver disease, has the added feature of contrast enhancement to define space-occupying lesions (e.g., abscess and tumor), and allows calculation of liver volume.

C. **MRI** offers similar information as the CT scan but visualizes vessels without the use of IV contrast. It is useful in the diagnosis of benign masses such as **focal nodular hyperplasia** and **hemangioma.** MRI should not be performed in individuals with cochlear implants, cardiac pacemakers and defibrillators, intracoronary stents, aneurysm clips, and certain metallic objects.

D. **Percutaneous transhepatic cholangiography and endoscopic retrograde cholangiopancreatography (ERCP)** involve the instillation of contrast into the biliary tree and are most useful after preliminary determination of biliary tree abnormalities by ultrasonography, CT, or MRI. The risk of acute pancreatitis following ERCP is at least 5%. **Magnetic resonance cholangio-**

pancreatography (MRCP) provides an alternative noninvasive diagnostic modality for visualizing the bile ducts. However, therapeutic intervention is not possible with MRCP.

E. **Technetium-99m RBC scan** is helpful in confirming hepatic hemangioma.

F. **Positron emission tomography** is an emerging modality that uses differences in metabolism among normal, inflammatory, and malignant tissues.

III. **Pathologic evaluation.** Percutaneous liver biopsy can be performed with or without ultrasonographic guidance. In the presence of coagulopathy or thrombocytopenia, it can be obtained by the transjugular route. Biopsy of masses that are suspicious for carcinoma is usually performed with ultrasonography/CT guidance. Liver biopsy is generally safe and can be performed as an outpatient procedure with observation for 4–6 hours after biopsy. Bleeding, pain, and injury to neighboring organs are possible complications.

Viral Hepatitis

I. The hepatotropic viruses include **hepatitis A (HAV), hepatitis B (HBV), hepatitis C (HCV), hepatitis D (HDV), hepatitis E (HEV),** and **hepatitis G** (Tables 18-1 and 18-2). **Acute viral hepatitis** is a major public health problem with approximately 300,000 cases reported annually in the United States. HAV and HEV (fecal-oral route of transmission) infections have no chronic form. In contrast, HBV, HCV, and HDV (parenteral route of transmission) infections may progress to chronic hepatitis and cirrhosis. **Chronic viral hepatitis** is defined as the presence of persistent liver inflammation for at least 6 months. Histopathologic classification of chronic viral hepatitis is based on etiology, grade, and stage. Grading and staging are measures of the severity of the necroinflammatory process and scarring, respectively.

A. **HAV** infection is usually transmitted via the fecal-oral route; large-scale outbreaks due to contamination of food and drinking water can occur. Sexual transmission and parenteral transmission may occur, although the period of viremia is brief. The period of greatest infectivity is during the 2 weeks before the onset of clinical illness; however, fecal shedding continues for 2–3 weeks after the onset of symptoms. The diagnosis of HAV is made by detection of **anti-HAV [immunoglobulin M (IgM)] antibody.** Liver biopsy is usually not necessary for diagnosis. **Anti-HAV [immunoglobulin G (IgG)] antibody** develops after recovery or immunization and provides lifelong immunity.

B. **HBV** infection is transmitted by parenteral routes (e.g., needle-stick injury, injection-drug use, transfusion, sexual contact, and from mother to infant). Although blood is the most effective vehicle for transmission, HBV is present in other body fluids (e.g., saliva and semen). Therefore, patients with HBV infection should avoid intimate contact (e.g., sharing razors and toothbrushes, unprotected sex) with nonimmune individuals. Immunity may develop after natural infection or immunization with HBV vaccine. HBV is a DNA virus that contains a number of antigens that elicit a corresponding antibody response. **Hepatitis B surface antigen (HB$_s$Ag)** is detectable in serum in acute and chronic HBV infection and disappears after clearance of the virus. **Hepatitis B core antigen (HB$_c$Ag)** is not found in serum but can be detected within liver cells by immunoperoxidase staining during active viral replication. **Hepatitis B$_e$ antigen (HB$_e$Ag)** appears shortly after HB$_s$Ag, and its persistence is indicative of active viral replication and a high degree of infectivity. Antibody against HB$_s$Ag **(anti-HB$_s$)** appears after the disappearance of HB$_s$Ag and after vaccination. Anti-HB$_s$ confers immunity (except in rare cases of chronic HBV infection, when very low titers of heterotypic anti-HB$_s$ are detectable). IgM antibody against HB$_c$Ag **(anti-HB$_c$IgM)** usually is present in acute infection but occasionally can be detected during periods of high viral replication in chronic disease. **Anti-HB$_c$ IgG** is detectable in

Table 18-1. Clinical and epidemiologic features of hepatotropic viruses

Organism	Hepatitis A	Hepatitis B	Hepatitis C	Hepatitis D	Hepatitis E
Incubation	2–6 wks	1–6 mos	2 wks–6 mos	1–6 mos	3–6 wks
Transmission	Fecal-oral	Blood	Blood	Blood	Fecal-oral
		Sexual contact	Sexual contact	Sexual contact	
		Perinatal contact	Perinatal contact		
Risk groups	Residents of and travelers to endemic regions	Injection-drug users	Injection-drug users	Any person with hepatitis B virus	Residents of and travelers to endemic regions
	Children and care-givers in day care centers	Multiple sexual partners	Health care workers	Injection-drug users	
		Men having sex with men	Transfusion recipients		
		Asians and native Alaskans			
		Infants born to infected mothers			
		Health care workers			
		Transfusion recipients			
Sequelae					
Fulminant failure	0.1–2.0%	<1%	<1%	Varies by geo-graphical region	1–2%
					15–20% in pregnant women
Carrier state	No	Yes	Yes	Yes	No
Chronic hepatitis	No	Yes	Yes	Yes	No
Cirrhosis	No	Yes	Yes	Yes	No

Table 18-2. Viral hepatitis serologies

Hepatitis	Acute	Chronic	Recovered/latent	Vaccinated
HAV	Anti-HAV IgM+	NA	Anti-HAV (total) +	Anti-HAV (total) +
HBV	Anti-HB$_c$ IgM+ HB$_e$Ag+ HB$_s$Ag+ HBV DNA+	Anti-HB$_c$ (total) + HB$_e$Ag± Anti-HB$_e$ ±[a] HB$_s$Ag+ HBV DNA±	Anti-HB$_c$ (total) + HB$_e$Ag− Anti-HB$_e$ ± HB$_s$Ag− HBV DNA− Anti-HB$_s$ +	Anti-HB$_s$ +
HCV	All tests possibly negative HCV RNA+ Anti-HCV Ab+ in 8–10 wks	Anti-HCV Ab+ HCV RNA+ RIBA+	Anti-HCV Ab+ HCV RNA−[b] RIBA+	NA
HDV	Anti-HDV (IgM) HD Ag+[c]	Anti-HDV (total) +	Anti-HDV (total) +[c]	See text (sec. **II.A.3**)
HEV	Available from CDC and research-specialty laboratories	NA	Available from CDC and research-specialty laboratories	NA

Ab = antibody; CDC = Centers for Disease Control and Prevention; HAV = hepatitis A virus; HB$_c$ = hepatitis B core antigen; HB$_e$Ag = hepatitis B$_e$ antigen; HB$_s$Ag = hepatitis B surface antigen; HBV = hepatitis B virus; HCV = hepatitis C virus; HDV = hepatitis D virus; HEV = hepatitis E virus; IgM = immunoglobulin M; NA = not applicable; RIBA = recombinant immunoblot assay.

[a]HB$_e$Ag is present during periods of high replication along with HBV DNA. Anti-HB$_e$ is present during periods of low replication when HB$_e$Ag and HBV DNA are undetectable.

[b]Negative HCV RNA results should be interpreted with caution. There are differences in thresholds for detection among assays and among laboratories.

[c]Markers of HBV infection are also present, because HDV cannot replicate in the absence of HBV.

chronic infection and, in association with anti-HB$_s$, after recovery. Rarely, patients with isolated anti-HB$_c$ can reactivate HBV in the setting of immunosuppression (e.g., transplantation). Antibody against HB$_e$Ag **(anti-HB$_e$)** usually indicates low-level replication. Detection of HBV viral DNA **(HBV DNA)** in serum provides a measure of active replication.

C. **HCV** is most commonly transmitted parenterally (e.g., transfusion, injection drug use). It may be transmitted sexually and from mother to offspring, although at a much lower frequency than HBV. The average risk of HCV transmission after a needle-stick injury is estimated at 1.8%. HCV has an incubation period of 2 weeks to 6 months. The screening test that is most widely used to detect antibody to HCV virus is performed by the **enzyme-linked immunosorbent assay (ELISA)** technique. The antibody may be undetectable for 8 weeks after infection, and acute HCV infection is usually subclinical. The antibody does not confer immunity. Chronic hepatitis develops in more than 80% of infected individuals. ELISA has a sensitivity of 97%; however, the positive predictive value in a low-risk population is only 25%. **Recombinant immunoblot assay (RIBA)** offers greater specificity and is particularly useful in low-risk individuals. **Polymerase chain reaction (PCR)** tests detect HCV RNA in blood as early as 1–2 weeks after infection. **Qualitative** (reported as positive or negative) and **quantitative** (estimate of viral load) PCR assays use different techniques for amplification that have not been standardized and have different thresholds for detection. Nevertheless, assays that use the same technique can be helpful in gauging response to treatment. Tests to detect **HCV genotype** are commercially available. HCV genotype influences response to treatment.

D. **HDV** is found throughout the world. It is endemic to the Mediterranean basin, the Middle East, and portions of South America. Outside these areas, infections occur primarily in individuals who have received transfusions or injection-drug users. HDV requires the presence of HBV for infection and replication. Clinical forms of presentation are **coinfection** (simultaneous acquisition with HBV infection) and **superinfection** (acute HDV infection in chronic HBV infection). Chronic hepatitis occurs more often after superinfection. Diagnosis is made by finding HDV RNA or HDV antigen in serum or liver and by detecting antibody to HDV antigen.

E. **HEV** has been implicated in epidemics in India, Southeast Asia, Africa, and Mexico. Reported cases in the United States have been in travelers to endemic areas. Transmission closely resembles that of HAV. HEV diagnostic testing (antibody against HEV, IgM, and IgG) is available through the hepatitis branch of the Centers for Disease Control. HEV is associated with high fatality in pregnant women.

F. **Hepatitis G** is an RNA virus similar to HCV that is frequently detected in patients with chronic liver disease; however, causality has not been proved.

G. **Non A-E hepatitis** is the exclusionary category of hepatotropic viruses that remains when serologic tests for other viruses are negative.

II. **Prophylaxis**
   A. **Pre-exposure prophylaxis** (see Appendix F)
      1. **HAV**
         a. **Pre-exposure prophylaxis** with **HAV vaccine** should be given to travelers to endemic areas, men who have sex with men, illegal drug users, persons who have high occupational risk for infection (research personnel working with HAV or HAV-infected primates), and persons who have clotting factor disorders. The course of HAV infection may be more severe in individuals with chronic liver disease; hence, immunization against HAV is advisable in this population. In the United States, children residing in areas where the incidence of hepatitis A is twice the national average should be vaccinated.

  b. Vaccination should occur at least 4 weeks before travel to an endemic area. For individuals who require immediate protection, the first dose of HAV vaccine can be administered concomitantly with **immune globulin (IG)** 0.02 ml/kg at different anatomic injection sites.

  c. Travelers who are allergic to a vaccine component or who elect not to undergo vaccination should receive a single dose of IG (0.02 ml/kg if the desired duration of protection is <2 months or 0.06 ml/kg if the desired duration is 2–5 months). The dose should be repeated if the travel period exceeds 5 months.

2. HBV

  a. Pre-exposure prophylaxis with **HBV vaccine** should be considered in individuals with multiple anticipated transfusions (e.g., transplant recipients, clotting factor deficiencies), patients with chronic renal failure (who are receiving or are likely to receive hemodialysis), health care workers, injection drug users, household and heterosexual contacts of HB_sAg carriers, homosexual individuals, residents and employees of institutions for the mentally retarded, travelers (>6 m) to hyperendemic regions, and natives of Alaska and the Pacific islands.

  b. Many countries have included HBV vaccination (20 μg at 0, 1, and 6 months) in their infant or adult immunization programs. The Centers for Disease Control has recommended a universal vaccination program for infants and sexually active adolescents in the United States.

  c. Prevaccination screening for previous exposure or infection is recommended in the high-risk groups to avoid vaccinating recovered individuals or those with chronic infection.

  d. For patients who require rapid immunity, the dosage schedule can be escalated to 0, 1, and 2 months, but a follow-up booster at 6 months is required for long-lasting immunity.

  e. Additional doses, higher doses, or revaccination can be considered in nonresponders and hyporesponders (anti-HB_s <10 mIU/ml) to elicit protective levels of immunity. Booster doses may be needed in immunosuppressed individuals in whom anti-HB_s levels fall below 10 mIU/ml on annual testing.

3. Pre-exposure prophylaxis for HCV and HEV is not available. Individuals succesfully vaccinated against HBV are protected against HDV.

B. Postexposure prophylaxis (see Appendix F)

1. HAV

  a. Postexposure prophylaxis for HAV with IG (0.02 ml/kg) should be given within 2 weeks of the last exposure to unvaccinated individuals.

  b. Household and sexual contacts and persons who have shared illegal drugs with a person who has serologically confirmed acute HAV should receive IG and the first dose of vaccine at different anatomic sites.

  c. IG should be administered to all previously unvaccinated staff and attendees of day care centers if one or more cases of HAV are recognized in children or employees or if cases are recognized in two or more households of center attendees. HAV vaccine can be administered at the same time as IG.

  d. If a food handler is diagnosed with HAV, IG should be administered to other food handlers at the same establishment and to patrons who can be identified and treated within 2 weeks of exposure.

2. HBV

  a. Infants born to HB_sAg-positive mothers should receive both HBV vaccine and **hepatitis B immune globulin (HBIG)** 0.5 ml within 12 hours of birth. Immunized infants should be tested at approximately 12 months of age for HB_sAg, anti-HB_s, and anti-HB_c. The presence of HB_sAg indicates the infant is actively infected. The presence of anti-HB_s and anti-HB_c suggests that infection occurred but was probably modified by immunoprophylaxis and that immunity is likely to be prolonged. The presence of anti-HB$_s$ alone is indicative of vaccine-induced immunity.

b. Susceptible sexual partners of individuals with acute HBV and victims of needle-stick injury (with HBV contamination) should receive HBIG (0.04–0.07 ml/kg) and the first dose of HBV vaccine at different sites on the body as soon as possible (preferably within 48 hours but no more than 7 days following exposure). A second dose of HBIG can be administered 30 days after exposure.

c. Postexposure prophylaxis with HBIG should be used after liver transplantation for end-stage liver disease that results from HBV (see Liver Transplantation).

III. Management of viral hepatitis

A. Acute viral hepatitis. Management is supportive and generally occurs in the ambulatory clinic setting. Serum liver enzymes (AST and ALT), hepatic synthetic function (albumin and PT), bilirubin, and the appropriate serologic tests (see sec. I and Table 18-2) should be monitored to assess recovery. Symptomatic treatment of nausea and vomiting is recommended. Rarely, patients require hospitalization for dehydration. Alcohol should be avoided. In a small group of patients (see Table 18-1), fulminant hepatic failure ensues, as reflected by alteration in mental status (hepatic encephalopathy) and prolongation of PT (unresponsive to vitamin K supplementation). Such patients should be monitored in an ICU and urgently referred for liver transplantation (see Liver Transplantation).

B. Chronic viral hepatitis is defined as the presence of persistent liver inflammation for at least 6 months and is associated with HBV, HCV, and HDV infections (see Table 18-1).

1. Treatment for chronic HBV is **interferon (IFN) alpha-2b,** 5 million units SC qd or 10 million units SC three times a week for 16 weeks. This results in a sustained loss of viral replication (disappearance of HBV DNA and HB$_e$Ag and appearance of anti-HB$_e$) and biochemical and histologic remission in approximately one-third of patients. Loss of HB$_s$Ag occurs in approximately 10%. Current U.S. Food and Drug Administration guidelines restrict the use of IFN for chronic HBV to patients with active viral replication and elevated serum ALT who have no evidence of decompensated liver disease (i.e., no history of variceal bleeding, ascites, or encephalopathy). Side effects of IFN include flu-like symptoms, leukopenia and thrombocytopenia, emotional lability, mood disorders, and disorders of thyroid function (hypo- or hyperthyroidism). Rarely, patients may have suicidal ideation that mandates cessation of therapy and psychiatric consultation. Several nucleoside analogs have an inhibitory effect on HBV replication. **Lamivudine** (100 mg PO qd) is similarly effective and is better tolerated than IFN. Unresolved issues with lamivudine include duration of therapy and emergence of resistant mutant strains. **Famciclovir** and **adefovir dipivoxil** appear safe and are being tested in clinical trials. Coinfection with HDV makes successful treatment less likely.

2. Treatment of chronic HCV consists of a combination of **IFN** (3 million units SC 3 times per week) and **ribavirin** (1200 mg/day or 1000 mg/day for body weight <70 kg in 2 divided doses) administered for 12 months. Sustained response (defined as normalization of serum ALT and clearance of HCV RNA from serum 6 months after completion of treatment) is observed in 30–60% of patients. Therapy is appropriate only in selected patients, owing to significant toxicity and side effects. Additional toxicity from ribavirin includes reversible hemolysis and teratogenicity. Contraindications to treatment with ribavirin include myocardial ischemia and chronic renal failure. These patients may receive monotherapy with IFN, 3 million units SC for 12–24 months. **Pegylated IFN** (IFN attached to polyethylene glycol to prolong half-life) alone or in combination with ribavirin is currently undergoing clinical trials to determine efficacy.

3. **Liver transplantation** may be indicated in advanced disease, but disease recurrence has been documented in HBV, HCV, and HDV (see Chap. 16).

Toxic and Drug-Related Liver Disease

Chemical agents that damage the liver include **intrinsic** (true or predictable) **hepatotoxins** (e.g., carbon tetrachloride and phosphorus) and **idiosyncratic** (unpredictable) **hepatotoxins** (e.g., isoniazid).

I. **Idiosyncratic hepatotoxicity** may be mediated by immunologic (hypersensitivity) or metabolic mechanisms.

   A. **Hypersensitivity reactions** are characterized by clinical (fever, rash, and/or eosinophilia) and histologic (eosinophilic or granulomatous inflammation) features of hypersensitivity and occur after a sensitization period of 1–5 weeks. Repeat challenge with the same agent leads to prompt recurrence of the reaction. Examples include sulfonamides, dapsone, and sulindac.

   B. **Metabolic idiosyncratic hepatotoxicity** occurs in susceptible patients as a result of altered drug clearance or accelerated production of hepatotoxic metabolites (e.g., isoniazid and methyldopa).

II. **Management of hepatotoxicity** includes cessation of exposure to the offending drug and institution of supportive measures. An attempt to remove the agent from the GI tract should be made in most cases of acute toxic ingestion using lavage or cathartics (see Chap. 26). No specific therapy is available in most cases.

III. **Alcoholic liver disease** is a significant medical and socioeconomic problem. Although **ethyl alcohol** exerts a direct toxic effect on the liver, significant liver damage develops in only 10–20% of chronic alcoholics. Thus, additional factors (e.g., genetic, nutritional, environmental) may be important in the pathogenesis of alcoholic liver disease. The spectrum of alcoholic liver disease is broad, and a single patient may be affected by more than one of the following conditions. Potentially dangerous interactions may occur between alcohol and a variety of medications including sedative-hypnotics, anticoagulants, and acetaminophen, even in the absence of alcoholic liver disease, because of shared metabolic pathways.

   A. **Fatty liver** is the most commonly observed abnormality in alcoholics. Patients are usually asymptomatic. Clinical findings include hepatomegaly and mild liver enzyme abnormalities. The disorder is reversible if alcohol intake is stopped and an adequate diet is consumed.

   B. **Alcoholic hepatitis** may be clinically silent or severe enough to lead to the rapid development of hepatic failure and death. Clinical features include fever, upper abdominal pain, anorexia, nausea, vomiting, and weight loss. In patients with underlying cirrhosis, manifestations of portal hypertension may predominate. Laboratory tests typically demonstrate elevation in serum aminotransferases (with AST characteristically higher than ALT) and AP. Hyperbilirubinemia and prolongation of PT may be seen. Although clinical presentation is helpful, liver biopsy is required for diagnosis. Features associated with a poor prognosis include prolongation of the PT that does not normalize with vitamin K, a markedly elevated total bilirubin, leukocytosis, and renal failure.

   C. **Alcoholic (Laënnec's) cirrhosis** is a common cause of cirrhosis and hepatocellular carcinoma worldwide.

   D. **Therapy for alcoholic liver disease** includes abstinence from alcohol and nutritional support. Treatment of acute alcoholic hepatitis with corticosteroids is controversial.

IV. **Acetaminophen** may cause significant hepatocellular injury in accidental or intentional overdose. Toxic potentiation of alcohol in combination with even therapeutic doses of acetaminophen has been demonstrated to cause significant hepatocellular injury. Management of acetaminophen overdose is a medical emergency (see Chap. 26). Observation for signs of **fulminant hepatic failure** is necessary (see Complications of Hepatic Insufficiency).

Cholestatic Liver Disease

Cholestatic liver disease is characterized by elevation predominantly in serum AP and bilirubin, although serum bilirubin may be normal until late in the course of illness.

I. **Primary biliary cirrhosis (PBC)** is a cholestatic disorder of unknown etiology that most often affects middle-aged women and progresses along a path of increasingly severe histologic damage **(florid bile duct lesion, ductular proliferation, scarring, and, cirrhosis).** The course is highly variable, and patients may be asymptomatic for many years. Fatigue and pruritus are often the most troublesome symptoms. Typical features include elevated levels of AP, cholesterol, IgM, and bile acids; **antimitochondrial antibodies** are present in more than 90% of patients. Treatment includes control of pruritus, management of steatorrhea, and symptom-specific therapy. No curative therapy is available. **Ursodeoxycholic acid** (15 mg/kg PO qhs or in three divided doses) improves liver function test abnormalities and appears to delay progression of disease. Hepatic transplantation may be necessary in advanced disease (see Liver Transplantation).

II. **Primary sclerosing cholangitis (PSC)** is an idiopathic cholestatic disorder characterized by inflammation, fibrosis, and eventual obliteration of the extrahepatic and intrahepatic bile ducts. Most patients are middle-aged men, and the disorder is frequently associated with inflammatory bowel disease (IBD; 70% with ulcerative colitis). PSC should be considered in individuals with IBD who have increased levels of AP even in the absence of symptoms of hepatobiliary disease. It is confirmed by demonstration of strictures or irregularity of the intrahepatic and extrahepatic bile ducts by ERCP or MRCP. Liver biopsy is helpful in the diagnosis of small-duct PSC, in the exclusion of other diseases, and in the staging of disease. Clinical manifestations typically include intermittent episodes of jaundice, hepatomegaly, pruritus, weight loss, and fatigue. Patients are at risk for development of ascending **bacterial cholangitis** and **cholangiocarcinoma.** No specific therapy has proved successful. Colectomy does not affect the course of PSC associated with ulcerative colitis. Episodes of cholangitis should be managed with IV antibiotics and with dilatation and placement of stents across dominant strictures. Patients with advanced disease or recurrent cholangitis should be referred for liver transplantation (see Liver Transplantation).

III. **Granulomatous hepatitis** presents primarily as a cholestatic disorder. Patients typically have fever and elevated liver enzyme levels (particularly AP) and may have hepatosplenomegaly. The differential diagnosis includes infections (e.g., syphilis, mycobacterial, fungal, and rickettsial diseases), sarcoidosis, drug-induced injury, and idiopathic causes. Specific therapy is directed at the underlying cause. If the clinical suspicion for tuberculosis is high, an empiric trial of antituberculous therapy may be warranted despite negative mycobacterial cultures.

IV. **Complications of cholestatic liver disease**
  A. **Nutritional deficiencies** result from fat malabsorption. In patients with steatorrhea, a low-fat diet (40–60 g/day) may be helpful. **Fat-soluble vitamin deficiency** (vitamins A, D, E, K) is often present in advanced disease and

especially in patients with steatorrhea. Fat-soluble vitamin replacement can be accomplished by water-soluble preparations of **vitamin A,** 5000–10,000 IU PO qd; **vitamin K,** 5–10 mg PO qd; and **vitamin E,** 100 IU PO qd. Vitamin D deficiency can be corrected by **25-hydroxyvitamin D₃ (25-cholecalciferol),** 20–50 µg PO three to five times a week. Serum levels of vitamin A and 25-cholecalciferol should be monitored to assess the adequacy of replacement therapy and avoid toxicity. Zinc deficiency may occur in some patients and is corrected with **zinc sulfate,** 220 mg PO daily (50 mg elemental zinc) for 4 weeks (see Chap. 2).

B. **Osteoporosis and osteomalacia** can occur in patients with cholestatic liver disease. Bone mineral density should be measured in all patients at the time of diagnosis. Treatment of bone disease includes exercise, oral calcium supplementation (1.0–1.5 g/day), estrogen replacement in postmenopausal women, and vitamin D supplementation in patients with deficiency.

C. **Pruritus** is best treated with **cholestyramine,** a bile acid sequestrant resin. The dose is one packet (4 g) mixed with water before and after the morning meal, with additional doses before lunch and dinner to control symptoms. Cholestyramine should not be given concurrently with vitamins or other medications as it may impair absorption. **Antihistamines** (diphenhydramine or doxepin, 25 mg PO qhs) and petrolatum may provide symptomatic relief. **Rifampin** (300–600 mg/day) is reserved for intractable pruritus.

Metabolic Liver Disease

A number of treatable metabolic disorders present with hepatocellular dysfunction, including Wilson's disease and hereditary hemochromatosis. Other rare disorders include glycogen storage disease, phospholipidoses, and α_1-antitrypsin deficiency.

I. **Wilson's disease** (incidence, 1 in 30,000) is an inherited (autosomal recessive) disorder (ATP7B gene on chromosome 13) that results in progressive copper overload. The average age at presentation of liver dysfunction is 10–15 years; neuropsychiatric disorders can manifest later. Patients may rarely present with fulminant hepatic failure. The diagnosis is suggested by a Kayser-Fleischer ring on slit lamp examination of the eyes, elevated serum free copper level (>25 mg/dl), a low serum ceruloplasmin level (<20 mg/dl), and an elevated 24-hour urinary copper level (>100 µg). The diagnosis is made by measuring **hepatic copper level** (>250 µg/g dry weight) on biopsy. Treatment is with copper-chelating agents (penicillamine or trientine and zinc salts). Liver transplantation is necessary in patients in whom fulminant hepatic failure develops or in those with progressive dysfunction despite chelation therapy (see Liver Transplantation).

II. **Hereditary hemochromatosis** (incidence, 1 in 200 to 1 in 800) is a common inherited (autosomal recessive) disorder of iron overload that is usually not diagnosed until middle age (40–60 years). It may present with slate-colored skin, diabetes, cardiomyopathy, arthritis, hypogonadism, or hepatic dysfunction. The diagnosis is suggested by elevated serum ferritin levels (>300 ng/ml in men, >200 ng/ml in women) and high transferrin saturation (>55% in men, >45% in women) and is confirmed by measurement of **hepatic iron concentration (HIC)** and calculation of **hepatic iron index (HII).** HIC is often reported in µg/g dry weight. Dividing by 56 (the atomic weight of iron) allows HIC to be expressed in µmol/g. HII is calculated by dividing HIC (µmol/g) by age in years. An HIC of greater than 4000 µg/g dry weight and an HII of greater than 1.9 are diagnostic of hemochromatosis. Tests are available for detection of the most common mutations (C282Y and H63D). First-degree relatives should be screened if the mutation is detected in the proband or if they have a high serum ferritin level or transferrin saturation, or both. Therapy consists of phlebotomy (500 ml whole blood per week) until iron depletion is confirmed by mild anemia, and ferritin levels are below 50 ng/ml, or transferrin saturation is less than 30%. Thereafter, maintenance phlebotomy of 1–2 units of blood three to four times a year is continued for life. Genetic counseling is important. Patients with cirrhosis are at increased risk for the development of hepatocellular carcinoma despite therapy. The survival rate in appropriately treated noncirrhotic patients is identical to that of the general population.

III. α_1-**Antitrypsin deficiency** (incidence, 1 in 1600) may present with pulmonary, hepatic, or pancreatic manifestations. Clinically significant liver disease develops in 10–15% of patients with the PiZZ phenotype during the first 20 years of life. The diagnosis is suggested by a low serum α_1-antitrypsin level and is confirmed by liver biopsy. No specific medical therapy for the hepatic disease is available, but transplantation is curative.

Miscellaneous Disorders

I. **Vascular diseases** of the liver can be due to impaired arterial or venous blood flow. The portal vein and the hepatic artery provide two-thirds and one-third of hepatic blood flow, respectively.

A. **Ischemic hepatitis** results from liver hypoperfusion. Clinical circumstances include severe blood loss, severe burns, cardiac failure, heat stroke, and sepsis. Characteristic features include the rapid rise and fall in levels of serum AST, ALT, and lactic dehydrogenase accompanied by midzonal and centrilobular necrosis on liver biopsy. Prognosis is determined by the rapid and effective treatment of the underlying cause.

B. **Budd-Chiari syndrome** results from hepatic venous outflow obstruction. Etiologies include webs in the suprahepatic inferior vena cava, hypercoagulable states, myeloproliferative disorders (50% of cases), tumors, estrogen use, pregnancy, and paroxysmal nocturnal hemoglobinuria. Approximately 20% of cases are idiopathic. Patients may present with an acute, subacute, or chronic illness characterized by ascites, hepatomegaly, and right upper quadrant abdominal pain. Serum to ascites albumin gradient is greater than 1.1 g/dl, and serum albumin, bilirubin, AST, ALT, and PT are mildly abnormal. Hepatic venography establishes the diagnosis. Nonsurgical management [anticoagulants, thrombolytics, diuretics, angioplasty, stents, transjugular intrahepatic portosystemic shunt (TIPS)], surgical decompressive procedures, and liver transplantation are the main therapeutic options.

C. **Veno-occlusive disease (VOD)** refers to obliteration of terminal hepatic venules within the liver and consequent sinusoidal engorgement and necrosis of hepatocytes in the centrilobular region of the hepatic acinus. It is seen in bone marrow transplant recipients who have received total body irradiation and high-dose chemotherapy (see Chap. 21), in renal transplant recipients who are immunosuppressed with azathioprine, and in association with ingestion of Jamaican bush teas. Diagnosis is based on the triad of **hepatomegaly, weight gain ($\geq$2-5% of baseline body weight), and hyperbilirubinemia (>2mg/dl),** occurring generally within 3 weeks after transplantation. The severity of VOD varies from mild reversible disease to severe disease with multiorgan failure. Chemotherapeutic drugs and radiation therapy affect the incidence and severity of VOD. Reported mortality ranges from 0 to 67%. Treatment is supportive as the disease is self-limited in the majority of patients.

D. Portal vein thrombosis in adults is seen in a variety of clinical settings, including abdominal trauma, cirrhosis, hypercoagulable states, intra-abdominal infections, pancreatitis, and after portocaval shunt surgery or splenectomy. It can manifest with variceal hemorrhage or ascites. Portosystemic shunts may be beneficial.

II. Hepatic abscess may be either pyogenic or amebic.

   A. Pyogenic abscess can result from hematogenous infection, spread from intra-abdominal infection or ascending infection from the biliary tract. Approximately 20% of cases are cryptogenic in origin. Clinical features include fever, chills, weight loss, and abdominal pain from tender hepatomegaly. About one-half of the patients are jaundiced. Laboratory studies may demonstrate leukocytosis and elevated AP. Diagnosis is confirmed by CT or ultrasonography. More than half the patients have positive blood cultures at the time of presentation. Attempts should be made to collect culture material before initiating broad-spectrum antibiotic therapy. Treatment includes a prolonged course of antibiotic therapy, and, in select cases, percutaneous or surgical drainage. Repeat imaging is recommended to document resolution.

   B. Amebic liver abscess should be considered in patients from endemic areas. Diagnosis requires a high index of clinical suspicion. Specific serologic tests such as indirect hemagglutination are helpful in establishing the diagnosis in low-prevalence areas. Amebic abscesses are treated with metronidazole or chloroquine.

III. Autoimmune hepatitis is characterized by the presence of clinical symptoms, elevated levels of serum aminotransferases, circulating autoantibodies (antinuclear antibody, smooth-muscle antibody, and liver-kidney microsomal antibody), and hypergammaglobulinemia. It occurs most often in women (10–30 years and late middle age) and frequently presents with cirrhosis. In approximately 30% of cases, the presentation is acute and similar to viral hepatitis. Extrahepatic manifestations (arthritis, skin rashes, thyroiditis) are common. Patients may present in fulminant hepatic failure or with asymptomatic elevation of serum ALT. Diagnosis requires the presence of characteristic histology (plasmacytic inflammation of the portal triads with interface hepatitis), autoimmune markers, and the absence of virologic markers. Therapy is initiated with either (1) prednisone alone (40–60 mg/ day), or (2) a combination of prednisone (40–60 mg/day) and azathioprine (1–2 mg/kg/day). Prednisone is tapered with biochemical and clinical improvement to a maintenance dose of 5–10 mg/day. Histologic remission occurs in as many as 80% of patients. Relapses occur in at least 50% after cessation of therapy, and some patients require lifelong low-dose therapy. Liver transplantation should be considered in patients with end-stage disease (see Liver Transplantation).

IV. Nonalcoholic steatohepatitis (NASH) is often identified by the presence of elevated liver-associated enzymes (ALT) on routine blood testing. The diagnosis is confirmed by liver biopsy (histologic findings are similar to those of alcoholic hepatitis) and exclusion of alcohol abuse by history. Conditions associated with NASH include obesity, diabetes, hyperlipidemia, and certain drugs such as amiodarone. Therapy should be directed at the underlying condition. Controversy persists regarding the pathogenesis and natural history of NASH. Liver transplantation should be considered in patients with end-stage liver disease (see Liver Transplantation).

V. Hepatocellular carcinoma (hepatoma) frequently occurs in patients with cirrhosis, especially in association with viral hepatitis (HBV or HCV), alcoholic cirrhosis, α_1-antitrypsin deficiency, and hemochromatosis. It can be multifocal. Early diagnosis is essential as surgical resection and liver transplantation can provide long-term survival. Alternative therapy for unresectable tumors includes percutaneous alcohol injection, arterial chemoembolization, or radiofrequency ablation. Patients with cirrhosis should therefore be monitored

Table 18-3. Grading system for hepatic encephalopathy

Grade	Level of consciousness	Personality and intellect	Neurologic abnormalities	EEG abnormalities
0	Normal	Normal	Normal	Normal
1	Inverted sleep pattern, restless	Forgetful, mild confusion, agitation, irritable	Tremor, apraxia, incoordination, impaired hand-writing	Slowing triphasic waves
2	Lethargic, slow responses	Disorientation for time, amnesia, decreased inhibitions, inappropriate behavior	Asterixis, dysarthria, hypoactive reflexes	Slowing triphasic waves
3	Somnolent but can be aroused, confused	Disorientation for place, aggressive	Asterixis, hyperactive reflexes, Babinski's sign, muscle rigidity	Slowing triphasic waves
4	Coma	Nil	Decerebrate	Slow delta activity

Source: From NC Gitlin. Hepatic Encephalopathy. In: D Zakim, TD Boyer, eds. *Hepatology,* 3rd ed. Philadelphia: Saunders, 1996, with permission.

for hepatocellular carcinoma by periodic measurement of **serum alpha-fetoprotein level** and radiologic imaging (CT or ultrasonography).

Complications of Hepatic Insufficiency

VI. **Fulminant hepatic failure** is defined as onset of hepatic encephalopathy within 8 weeks of initial symptoms of liver disease in an otherwise healthy individual. Acetaminophen hepatotoxicity and viral hepatitis are the most common causes of fulminant hepatic failure. Other causes are autoimmune hepatitis, drug and toxin exposure, ischemia, acute fatty liver of pregnancy, Wilson's disease, and Reye's syndrome. Manifestations of fulminant hepatic failure include encephalopathy, worsening jaundice, GI bleeding, sepsis, coagulopathy, hypoglycemia, renal failure, and electrolyte abnormalities. Supportive therapy in the ICU setting (in cooperation with a hepatology-liver transplant team) is essential. Blood glucose and fluid and electrolyte status should be monitored carefully. Vitamin supplements (including vitamin K) and stress ulcer prophylaxis should be given. Fresh frozen plasma and blood should be administered when evidence of active hemorrhage is found. In patients with signs that are suggestive of elevated intracranial pressure (see Chap. 26) or grade III or IV hepatic encephalopathy (Table 18-3), an intracranial pressure monitor should be placed. Mortality exceeds 80% in patients with grade IV encephalopathy. Death often results from progressive liver failure, GI bleeding, cerebral edema, sepsis, or arrhythmia. Transplantation should be urgently considered in cases of fulminant hepatic failure (see Liver Transplantation).

VII. **Hepatic encephalopathy** is the syndrome of disordered consciousness and altered neuromuscular activity that is seen in patients with acute or chronic hepatocellular failure or portosystemic shunting. The pathogenesis of hepatic encephalopathy is controversial, and numerous mediators have been implicated.

A. **Precipitating factors** include azotemia; use of a tranquilizer, opioid, or sedative-hypnotic medication; GI hemorrhage; hypokalemia and alkalosis (diuretics and diarrhea); constipation; infection; high-protein diet; progressive hepatocellular dysfunction; and, portosystemic shunts (surgical and following TIPS).

B. **Grading** of hepatic encephalopathy (see Table 18-3)

C. **Treatment** should be initiated promptly.

   1. Precipitating factors should be identified and corrected if possible.

   2. The rationale and benefit of dietary protein restriction are controversial. Once the patient is able to eat, a diet containing 30–40 g protein per day is initiated. Protein intake is gradually increased and titrated to correct encephalopathy. Special diets (vegetable protein or branched-chain amino acid–enriched) may be beneficial in patients with encephalopathy that is refractory to usual measures.

   3. Medical therapies include **nonabsorbable disaccharides** (lactulose, lactitol, and lactose in lactase-deficient patients), neomycin, and metronidazole. The initial dose of lactulose is 15–45 ml PO bid–qid. Maintenance dose should be adjusted to produce three to five soft stools per day. Oral lactulose should not be given to patients with an ileus or possible bowel obstruction. **Lactulose enemas** (prepared by the addition of 300 ml lactulose to 700 ml distilled water) can be administered. **Neomycin** (1 g q6h) can be given by mouth or as a retention enema (1% solution in 100–200 ml isotonic saline). Approximately 1–3% of the administered dose of neomycin is absorbed, with the attendant risk of ototoxicity and nephrotoxicity. The risk of toxicity is increased in patients with renal insufficiency. Because lactulose is as effective as neomycin, it is preferred for initial and maintenance therapy. Combination therapy with lactulose and neomycin should be considered in cases that are refractory to either agent alone. **Metronidazole** (250 mg PO q8h) is useful for short-term therapy when neomycin is unavailable or poorly tolerated. Long-term metronidazole is not recommended owing to toxicity.

VIII. **Portal hypertension** frequently complicates cirrhosis and presents with ascites, GI bleeding, and splenomegaly. GI bleeding most often results from varices (esophageal and gastric). Other sources of bleeding include duodenal and rectal varices, hemorrhoids and portal hypertensive gastropathy and colopathy. The cause of bleeding is generally determined by endoscopy (see Chap. 17 for diagnosis and treatment). Causes of portal hypertension in patients without cirrhosis include idiopathic portal hypertension, schistosomiasis, congenital hepatic fibrosis, sarcoidosis, cystic fibrosis, arteriovenous fistulas, splenic and portal vein thrombosis, myeloproliferative diseases, nodular regenerative hyperplasia, and focal nodular hyperplasia.

IX. **Ascites** is the abnormal (>25 ml) accumulation of fluid within the peritoneal cavity. It is a common manifestation of decompensation in cirrhosis. It is a consequence of portal hypertension, decreased plasma oncotic pressure, and avid sodium retention by the kidneys. In cirrhosis, the ascitic fluid has a low albumin concentration and low opsonic activity.

A. **Serum to ascites albumin gradient (SAAG)** that is greater than 1.1 g/dl indicates portal hypertension–related ascites (97% specificity). SAAG less than 1.1 g/dl is found in nephrotic syndrome, peritoneal carcinomatosis, serositis, tuberculosis, and biliary and pancreatic ascites.

B. **Management**

   1. **Dietary salt restriction** (2 g salt or 88 mmol Na^+ per day) should be initiated and continued thereafter unless the renal ability to excrete

sodium spontaneously improves. In selected cases, it may be necessary to restrict sodium intake further. The use of potassium-containing salt substitutes can lead to serious hyperkalemia. Routine water restriction is not necessary. If dilutional hyponatremia (serum Na^+ <125 mmol/L) occurs, fluid restriction to 1000–1500 ml/day usually suffices.

2. **Diuretic therapy** can be initiated along with salt restriction. The goal of diuretic therapy should be a daily weight loss of no more than 1.0 kg in patients with edema and approximately 0.5 kg in patients without edema until ascites is adequately controlled. Diuretics should not be administered to individuals with an increasing serum creatinine level. **Spironolactone** (100 mg PO in a single daily dose with food) is the diuretic of choice. The daily dose can be increased by 100 mg every 7–10 days until satisfactory weight loss, a maximum dose of 400 mg, or side effects occur. Hyperkalemia and gynecomastia are common side effects. Amiloride or triamterene (potassium-sparing diuretics) are substitutes that can be used in patients in whom painful gynecomastia develops from spironolactone. Loop diuretics such as furosemide (20–40 mg, increasing to 160 mg PO qd) or bumetanide can be added when a 200-mg dose of spironolactone fails to initiate a diuresis. Patients should be observed closely for signs of dehydration, electrolyte disturbances, encephalopathy, muscle cramps, and renal insufficiency.

3. **Paracentesis** should be performed for diagnosis [e.g., new-onset ascites, suspicion of malignant ascites, or spontaneous bacterial peritonitis (SBP)] or as a therapeutic maneuver when tense ascites causes significant discomfort or respiratory compromise. Diagnostic testing should include fluid cell and differential counts, albumin, total protein, lactic dehydrogenase, glucose, and culture. Amylase and triglyceride measurement, cytology, and mycobacterial smear/culture should be performed to confirm specific diagnoses. **Bleeding** and **intestinal perforation** are possible complications. Rarely, rapid large-volume paracentesis may lead to circulatory collapse, encephalopathy, and renal failure. Concomitant administration of IV colloid (5–8 g albumin/L ascites removed) can be used to minimize these complications.

4. **TIPS** has proved effective in the management of refractory ascites. Complications include shunt occlusion, bleeding, infection, cardiopulmonary compromise, and hepatic encephalopathy.

X. **SBP** is an infectious complication of portal hypertension–related ascites. Its occurrence is related to low protein level and impaired opsonic activity in ascitic fluid.

A. **Clinical manifestations** include abdominal pain and distension, fever, decreased bowel sounds, and worsening of hepatic encephalopathy; however, the disease may be present in the absence of specific clinical signs. Therefore, cirrhotic patients with ascites and evidence of any clinical deterioration should undergo diagnostic paracentesis to exclude SBP.

B. **The diagnosis is likely when the ascitic fluid contains more than 250 neutrophils per μl.** Gram stain reveals the organism in only 10–20% of samples. A positive culture confirms the diagnosis. **Cultures are more likely to be positive when 10 ml ascitic fluid is inoculated into two blood culture bottles at the bedside.** The most common organisms are *Escherichia coli*, *Klebsiella*, and *Streptococcus pneumoniae*. Blood cultures are positive in approximately one-half of cases with SBP. Polymicrobial infection is uncommon and should lead to the suspicion of secondary bacterial peritonitis.

C. In suspected cases without bacteremia, empiric antibiotic therapy with a third-generation cephalosporin (e.g., ceftriaxone, 2 g IV qd or cefotaxime, 1–2 g IV q4–8h depending on renal function; see Appendix E) is appropriate for 5 days. Paracentesis should be repeated if no clinical improvement occurs in 48–72 hours, especially if the initial ascitic fluid culture was negative.

Table 18-4. Diagnostic criteria of hepatorenal syndrome

Major criteria

Low glomerular filtration rate, as indicated by serum creatinine >1.5 mg/dl or 24-hr creatinine clearance <40 ml/min

Absence of shock, ongoing bacterial infection, fluid losses, and current treatment with nephrotoxic drugs

No sustained improvement in renal function (decrease in serum creatinine to 1.5 mg/dl or increase in creatinine clearance to 40 ml/min) after diuretic withdrawal and expansion of plasma volume with 1.5 L of a plasma expander

Proteinuria <500 mg/day and no ultrasonographic evidence of obstructive uropathy or parenchymal renal disease

Additional criteria

Urine volume <500 ml/day

Urine sodium <10 mEq/L

Urine osmolality greater than plasma osmolality

Urine RBCs <50/high-power field

Serum sodium concentration <130 mEq/L

Note: All major criteria must be present for the diagnosis of hepatorenal syndrome. Additional criteria are not necessary for the diagnosis but provide supportive evidence.
Source: From V Arroyo, P Gines, AL Gerbes, et al. Definition and diagnostic criteria of refractory ascites and hepatorenal syndrome in cirrhosis. International Ascites Club. *Hepatology* 23:164, 1996, with permission.

    D. Norfloxacin (400 mg PO qd) reduces the frequency of recurrent episodes of SBP but does not improve survival.
  XI. Coagulopathy occurs as a result of impaired hepatic synthesis of coagulation factors and thrombocytopenia. Vitamin K deficiency can be corrected by parenteral administration of 10 mg/day for 3 consecutive days. Transfusion of fresh frozen plasma and platelets should be reserved for patients with active bleeding or for those who are undergoing invasive procedures (see Chap. 19).
  XII. Hepatorenal syndrome (HRS) is characterized by impairment in renal function in the setting of acute or, more commonly, chronic liver disease. Major and minor diagnostic criteria are summarized in Table 18-4. **Type I** HRS progresses rapidly and is characterized by doubling of the initial serum creatinine to greater than 2.5 mg/dl or a 50% reduction of the initial 24-hour creatinine clearance to less than 20 ml/minute in less than 2 weeks. **Type II** HRS progresses more slowly but relentlessly and often clinically manifests as diuretic-resistant ascites. No clear or established treatments are available for HRS. Prognosis without transplantation is poor.

Liver Transplantation

The severity of chronic liver disease is often graded on the basis of **Child-Turcotte-Pugh (CTP)** classification (Table 18-5). The need for liver transplantation in chronic liver disease is determined by CTP class.
  I. Indications
    A. In patients with fulminant hepatic failure and signs of advanced encephalopathy (grade III or IV; see Table 18-3), marked coagulopathy (PT >20 seconds), or hypoglycemia, liver transplantation is the accepted therapy.

Table 18-5. Child-Turcotte-Pugh scoring system to assess severity of liver disease

Clinical and biochemical measurements	Points scored for increasing abnormality		
	1	2	3
Albumin (g/dl)	>3.5	2.8–3.5	<2.8
Bilirubin (mg/dl)	1–2	2–3	>3
For cholestatic diseases: bilirubin (mg/dl)	<4	4–10	>10
PT (secs prolonged)*	1–4	4–6	>6
or			
INR*	<1.7	1.7–2.3	>2.3
Ascites	Absent	Slight	Moderate
Encephalopathy (grade)	None	1 and 2	3 and 4

*Prothrombin time (PT) or international normalized ratio (INR) may be used for scoring.

Class	Total points
A	5, 6
B	7–9
C	10–15

> **B.** Timing of liver transplantation in patients with chronic liver disease is a complex issue. Patients should be evaluated for transplantation when they have a decline in hepatic synthetic or excretory functions, ascites, hepatic encephalopathy (CTP class B or C), or other complications such as ascending cholangitis, SBP, HRS, and hepatocellular carcinoma. Patients with cholestatic liver disease can be transplanted for disabling intractable pruritus.

II. Contraindications. Contraindications to liver transplantation include severe and uncontrolled extrahepatic infection, HIV infection, advanced cardiac or pulmonary disease, extrahepatic malignancy, multiorgan failure, and unresolved psychosocial and medical noncompliance issues.

III. Recurrent disease. Certain forms of liver disease (especially viral hepatitis) recur after transplantation (see Chap. 16).

> **A. Recurrent HBV** can be prevented by the administration of HBIG during and after transplantation. Lamivudine (100 mg PO qd) initiated before transplantation to lower viral load reduces the likelihood of recurrent HBV.

> **B.** Treatment of recurrent HCV with a combination of ribavirin and IFN is under investigation.

IV. The number of transplants performed is limited by the availability of organs. Improvements in surgical technique have resulted in successful **split liver and live donor (partial liver) transplants.** Immunosuppressive, infectious, and long-term complications are discussed in Chap. 16.

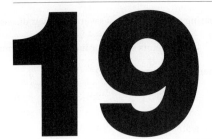

Disorders of Hemostasis

Amir Tabatabai

Evaluation of Patients with Hemostatic Disorders

I. **Normal hemostasis** involves the cessation of blood loss from damaged vessels.
   A. **Primary hemostasis** is an immediate (seconds to minutes) but unstable response to injury. Platelets and von Willebrand's factor (vWF) form a primary plug, and blood vessels constrict, limiting flow.
   B. **Secondary hemostasis (coagulation)** is a slower process (minutes to hours) but results in a definitive fibrin clot. The revised theory of coagulation proposes a single pathway, as opposed to the traditional intrinsic and extrinsic pathways, in which the contact factors, including factor XII, high-molecular-weight kininogen, and prekallikrein, are not required. However, it is still useful to refer to the classic definition of these pathways when interpreting studies of coalulation (i.e., prothrombin time, activated partial thrombin time) (Fig. 19-1). Coagulation is initiated when tissue injury exposes tissue factor to factor VIIa. The tissue factor–VIIa complex activates factor X, but this activation is rapidly dampened by tissue factor pathway inhibitor. Therefore, for coagulation to proceed, activation of factor IX by the tissue factor–VIIa complex is critical. Generation of thrombin results in feedback activation of factors V, VIII, and XI, and the end result is the formation of a fibrin clot (*Annu Rev Med* 46:103, 1995).
   C. **History and physical examination.** The severity of a bleeding disorder can be estimated from the duration and severity of bleeding (especially the requirement for blood product transfusion) in response to hemostatic challenge (e.g., dental extraction, trauma, pregnancy, and surgery). Pertinent medical history (e.g., liver disease, malabsorption, or HIV infection) may guide the workup. Family history of thrombosis or bleeding should be documented. Use of medications [e.g., aspirin, nonsteroidal anti-inflammatory drugs (NSAIDs), anticoagulants, oral contraceptives, and antibiotics] should be noted. Habits relevant to hemostasis include excessive use of alcohol and the amount of vitamins K and C in the diet. On **physical examination,** problems with primary hemostasis are suggested by spontaneous mucous membrane bleeding. This condition may manifest as focal areas (<2 mm) of SC bleeding that do not blanch with pressure, called **petechiae;** larger patches (<1 cm), designated **purpura;** or extensive areas of bruising (>1 cm), called **ecchymoses.** Petechiae typically present in areas subjected to increased hydrostatic force such as dependent regions or the periorbital area following coughing or vomiting. Disorders of secondary hemostasis usually produce deep ecchymoses, hematomas, hemarthroses, or delayed bleeding after trauma or surgery.
II. **Laboratory evaluation** of patients with suspected hemostatic disorders should be guided by the history and physical examination. Initial studies may include platelet count, bleeding time, prothrombin time (PT), activated partial thromboplastin time (aPTT), and a peripheral smear. If a detailed bleeding

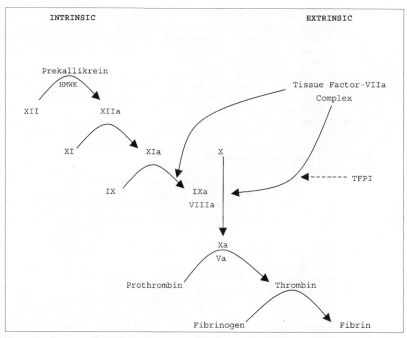

Fig. 19-1. Coagulation cascade. Solid arrows indicate activation, and dotted arrow represents inhibition. (HMWK = high-molecular-weight kininogen; TFPI = tissue factor pathway inhibitor.) (Modified from GJ Broze Jr. Tissue factor pathway inhibitor and the revised theory of coagulation. *Annu Rev Med* 46:103, 1995.)

history is negative, preoperative screening should include only a PT, aPTT, and platelet count.

A. Tests of primary hemostasis

1. The **platelet count** is determined by automated cell counters, but abnormal counts must be verified manually. Pseudothrombocytopenia is caused by platelet clumping due to ethylenediaminetetra-acetic acid (EDTA), and, in this case, the platelet count should be repeated using blood collected in citrated tubes.

2. The **bleeding time** is neither a good preoperative screening test for asymptomatic patients nor a global test of hemostasis. It is most helpful in the absence of overt thrombocytopenia in implicating platelet dysfunction as the cause of symptoms, suggesting a primary hemostatic disorder. This test should not be performed after aspirin use or in the setting of severe thrombocytopenia (<20,000/μl). A prolonged bleeding time may indicate a problem with platelet function or capillary integrity. Generally, bleeding time is not prolonged by disorders of secondary hemostasis.

3. A **von Willebrand's disease (vWD) screen** is appropriate in the setting of a positive bleeding history with a normal platelet count and prolonged bleeding time. Because the phenotype is variable and the screening tests are relatively insensitive, one negative workup does not exclude vWD. If the clinical suspicion is high, repeated testing is appropriate (see Inherited Bleeding Disorders, sec. **II**).

   a. **vWF antigen (vWF:Ag)** is a measure of circulating vWF protein by immunoassay.

b. **vWF activity (vWF:RCo)** is a functional assay of the ability of vWF in patient plasma to agglutinate platelets in vitro in the presence of ristocetin. A variety of conditions may increase (e.g., oral contraceptives, pregnancy, liver disease) or decrease (e.g., hypothyroidism, type O blood) vWF:RCo and vWF:Ag.

c. **Factor VIII activity (VIII:C)** is assayed after mixing the sample with factor VIII–deficient plasma. Because vWF stabilizes factor VIII in plasma, loss of vWF protein or mutations at the factor VIII binding site lead to a decrease in VIII:C.

4. **Platelet function** studies such as secretion and aggregation in response to agonists can implicate platelet dysfunction as a cause of bleeding but rarely are indicated in the initial evaluation of patients.

B. **Tests of secondary hemostasis**

1. The **aPTT** is the time required for clot formation after activation of anti-coagulated (i.e., citrated) blood with calcium, phospholipid, and a negatively charged surface, such as kaolin. This test is prolonged by deficiencies of factors that are collectively known as the "intrinsic pathway" (high-molecular-weight kininogen, prekallikrein, factor XII, factor XI, factor IX, and factor VIII) and, to a lesser extent, members of the "common pathway" (factor V, factor X, prothrombin, and fibrinogen). Factor levels must be reduced to the range of 25–40% of normal activity to prolong the aPTT. Heparin prolongs the aPTT by facilitating the antithrombin III (ATIII)-mediated inactivation of thrombin.

2. The **PT** is the time required for clot formation after the addition of thromboplastin (tissue factor and lipid) and calcium to anticoagulated blood. This test is sensitive to deficiencies in factor VII, the prothrombinase complex, and fibrinogen. The result is highly dependent on the quality of thromboplastin used. The **international normalized ratio (INR)** has evolved to allow comparison of PT assays performed in laboratories using different thromboplastin reagents. The formula is as follows:

$$INR = (patient\ PT/control\ PT)^{ISI}$$

where ISI (international sensitivity index) is a measure of thromboplastin sensitivity. The lower the ISI (i.e., the closer to one), the more sensitive is the thromboplastin. The INR is used to monitor warfarin therapy under steady-state conditions (i.e., not at the onset of warfarin therapy). It is not useful to evaluate liver disease or disseminated intravascular coagulation (DIC).

3. **Thrombin time** measures time to clot formation after addition of thrombin to anticoagulated blood. It is sensitive to quantitative and qualitative deficiencies of fibrinogen and to interference by heparin, fibrin degradation products, and paraproteins. Heparin can be neutralized by the addition of protamine sulfate to the sample.

4. **Mixing studies** should be performed in the initial workup of a prolonged coagulation test. A prolonged PT or aPTT may represent either a factor deficiency or the presence of an inhibitor. If the test plasma is mixed 1:1 with normal plasma, deficient factors will be restored to at least 50% of normal levels, sufficient to normalize the clotting assay, whereas inhibitors typically will remain in excess, and therefore, the prolonged assay will not correct. If a prolonged assay does correct in a 1:1 mix, specific factor assays should be performed to identify the deficient factor (Table 19-1). If mixing studies fail to correct a prolonged coagulation assay, confirmatory testing for the **lupus anticoagulant** or specific factor inhibitors should be conducted.

5. **Inhibitors** are antibodies that interfere with coagulation assays. Specific antibodies to factors such as VIII and IX are acquired by hemophiliacs who are treated with infusion of factor concentrates or occur spontaneously in untreated individuals. They cause true in vivo factor deficiency. The **lupus anticoagulant** prolongs the aPTT and occasionally the PT by

Table 19-1. Factor deficiencies that cause prolonged prothrombin time (PT) or activated partial thromboplastin time (aPTT)

Abnormal assay	Suspected factor deficiency
aPTT	XI, IX, XII, or VIII
PT	VII vs. multiple factors
PT and aPTT	II, V, X, or fibrinogen vs. multiple factors

reacting with the phospholipid used in the assays. It does not cause in vivo factor deficiency (see Thromboembolic Disorders, sec. **I.B.1**). The presence of the lupus anticoagulant can be confirmed with the dilute Russell's viper venom test or a phospholipid neutralization assay.

6. A **disseminated intravascular coagulation (DIC) screen** should be ordered in patients with a typical clinical presentation (see Acquired Coagulation Disorders, sec. **III**). Because of the dynamic nature of DIC, serial assays may be necessary to establish a diagnosis. This is especially helpful in distinguishing DIC from liver failure. A falling platelet count and rising aPTT and PT are typical. Fibrinogen is typically consumed, although this is variable. Microangiopathic features on the peripheral smear are also not consistently present. The most sensitive finding is elevation of fibrin degradation products or the cross-linked fragment, D-dimer.

7. **Factor XIII deficiency** will be missed by the standard screening assays. Diagnosis of this rare disorder requires a specific assay (e.g., clot urea stability).

C. **Evaluation for hypercoagulability** in patients with a history of **venous thrombosis** is individualized based on age, site of thrombosis, family history, and clinical and laboratory findings (see Thromboembolic Disorders, sec. **I.A** and **B**). Screening tests for **inherited** thrombophilia include ATIII activity, protein C level and activity, protein S level (free and total) and activity, fasting homocysteine level, fibrinogen (Clauss method), activated protein C (APC) resistance (functional assay for factor V Leiden mutation), and prothrombin 20210A mutation, which causes elevated prothrombin levels. Some assays are unreliable in certain clinical situations. ATIII assays should not be performed during heparin therapy; protein C and S measurements should be obtained before warfarin is administered. Acute thrombosis, oral contraceptives, and liver disease may lower the levels of all three proteins, whereas pregnancy lowers just protein C and S levels. Nephrotic syndrome leads to a reduction in free protein S and ATIII levels and elevation of protein C and total protein S levels. If fasting homocysteine levels are normal, a methionine challenge test can be performed if hyperhomocysteinemia is suspected. The workup of **acquired** hypercoagulability should include an assay for antiphospholipid antibody (see Thromboembolic Disorders, sec. **I.B.1**) If unexplained cytopenias are present, paroxysmal nocturnal hemoglobinuria should be ruled out by flow cytometric analysis of peripheral blood. Evaluation of **arterial thrombosis** is generally similar but may include serum protein electrophoresis to rule out hyperviscosity syndrome, lipoprotein(a) in premature coronary artery disease, cryoglobulins, and antinuclear antibody in vasculitis.

Platelet Disorders

I. **Thrombocytopenia** exists when the platelet count is less than 150,000/μl. Usually, increased bleeding is not attributable to thrombocytopenia until the count drops below 50,000/μl. The risk of spontaneous life-threatening (e.g., CNS, GI) bleeding increases significantly at counts below 20,000/μl and substantially at counts below 10,000/μl. A helpful diagnostic strategy is to differentiate disorders of marrow production from conditions that result in increased platelet use or sequestration. Generally, a bone marrow examination is used to help in this distinction. In general, thrombocytopenic patients should not be subjected to invasive procedures. Agents such as aspirin, NSAIDs, and anticoagulants that further impair hemostasis are relatively contraindicated. Nursing precautions include avoidance of IM injections and nasotracheal suction.

A. Underproduction of platelets is suggested by a reduced number of mega-karyocytes in a bone marrow biopsy.

1. **Viral suppression** of megakaryocytes with a variety of human viral pathogens, including HIV, may cause thrombocytopenia. Platelet recovery is spontaneous after clearance of the viral infection.

2. **Marrow infiltration (myelophthisis)** by tumors, storage diseases, or infectious agents may interfere with normal platelet production. The diagnosis is made by examination of a bone marrow biopsy and culture of an aspirate, if indicated clinically. The peripheral smear may reveal leukoerythroblastic features such as nucleated RBCs and immature myeloid forms. Treatment is directed toward the underlying cause of the marrow infiltration.

3. **Drug-induced** thrombocytopenia commonly is iatrogenic (e.g., following chemotherapy or radiotherapy). Ethanol is also a common and potent inhibitor of thrombopoiesis. Chemotherapy-induced thrombocytopenia can be treated with recombinant **interleukin-11** (50 μg/kg/day) SC. Side effects include fluid retention and atrial fibrillation.

4. **Vitamin B$_{12}$ and folate deficiency** may cause thrombocytopenia, which resolves with appropriate supplementation.

B. Increased destruction of platelets may be due to consumption or immunologic clearance.

1. **Immune thrombocytopenia** is caused by antibodies [usually immunoglobulin G (IgG)] binding to platelet surface antigens, resulting in their clearance by the reticuloendothelial system.

   a. **Immune thrombocytopenic purpura (ITP)** in adults, unlike children, is a chronic disorder. It is caused by production of antiplatelet autoantibodies.

      (1) **The diagnosis** of ITP is suggested by an isolated thrombocytopenia in the absence of other causes. In adults, typically it presents as mild mucocutaneous bleeding that develops over several weeks. Asymptomatic cases may be detected on a routine CBC. Serologic tests for antiplatelet antibodies generally are not helpful. Testing for HIV, systemic lupus erythematosus (SLE), antiphospholipid antibody, or thyroid disorders can be done based on history and physical examination. Bone marrow biopsy should be performed to exclude myelodysplastic syndrome in the elderly (age >60).

      (2) **Treatment** is initiated with glucocorticoids (prednisone, 1 mg/kg PO qd). Patients with life-threatening hemorrhage or severe thrombocytopenia (<10,000/μl) should be hospitalized and emergently treated with parenteral glucocorticoids (methylprednisolone, 1–2 g IV qd for 3 days), IV immune globulin (IVIG, 1 g/kg IV qd for 2 days), and platelet transfusions, as needed. Despite a slow steroid taper (over 3–6 months), many patients with chronic ITP require additional therapy to maintain a platelet count of more than 30,000/μl; therefore, intermittent steroids, IVIG, or anti-Rh(D) may be necessary. Anti-Rh(D) can only be used in Rh(D)-positive patients who have intact spleens. Splenectomy can salvage two-thirds of refractory patients. Pneumococcal, meningococcal, and *Haemophilus influenzae* type B vaccines should be administered at

least 2 weeks before splenectomy. Patients who relapse after splenectomy initially should receive a trial of glucocorticoids and can be
safely managed chronically on low daily (5–10 mg) or alternate-day
doses of prednisone. Radionuclide imaging occasionally identifies
an accessory spleen as the cause of relapse. Other salvage therapies, including danazol, vincristine, azathioprine, or cyclophosphamide, are of unproved benefit but are occasionally used in
refractory cases (*Blood* 88:3, 1996).

(3) ITP during pregnancy may be difficult to distinguish from gestational thrombocytopenia (see sec. **I.B.3**). IVIG is initial therapy with
platelet counts of less than 10,000/µl during the first trimester or
less than 30,000/µl during the second or third trimester. Steroids
have also been used. Approximately 5–20% of neonates who are
born to these mothers have severe thrombocytopenia, raising the
concern of intracranial hemorrhage during vaginal delivery. Invasive fetal blood sampling generally is not recommended. No consensus governs cesarean versus vaginal delivery (*Blood* 88:3, 1996).

b. Posttransfusion purpura is a rare syndrome characterized by the
formation of alloantibodies, most commonly against the platelet surface antigen PL^{A1} in PL^{A1}-negative patients who receive blood or
platelet transfusions from PL^{A1}-positive donors. It occurs most commonly in multiparous women who are transfused for the first time.
Thrombocytopenia occurs within 1 week and is usually severe. Treatment is with IVIG or plasmapheresis. Platelet transfusions from random donors are not helpful because they are rapidly destroyed, as the
vast majority of the population is PL^{A1} positive. Blood products that
are PL^{A1} negative can be used but are difficult to procure.

c. HIV-associated thrombocytopenia is usually multifactorial (e.g.,
splenomegaly, infections, or medications). In addition, ITP is a frequent complication of HIV and may be the presenting symptom. It
responds to standard ITP therapy. Decreased thrombopoiesis can be
a direct result of HIV and generally improves with antiretroviral
therapy. Thrombotic thrombocytopenic purpura (TTP) is also found
more frequently in HIV-infected patients and is treated using standard approaches (see sec. **I.B.2**).

d. Drug-induced immune thrombocytopenia is seen with a variety of
commonly prescribed medications. Anti-platelet IgG may be detectable
after the addition of the drug to the patient's serum, but the sensitivity
of this assay is variable with different drugs. If drug-induced thrombocytopenia is suspected, only essential medications should be continued. IVIG can be administered if thrombocytopenia is life threatening.

e. Heparin-induced thrombocytopenia (HIT) is a hypercoagulable
state associated with venous or arterial (cerebral or limb) thrombosis. Skin necrosis in patients who receive SC heparin may be a sign
of HIT. It is mediated by an immunoglobulin, usually IgG, that tar-
gets the complex between heparin and platelet factor 4 (PF4). HIT
usually develops 5 or more days after heparin exposure, but patients
with previous exposure may develop HIT within 2 days. It rarely
develops after 2 weeks of heparin use. Mild decreases in platelet
counts in patients who are receiving heparin are more common, are
not immune mediated, usually develop within 4 days, and may
resolve despite continuing heparin. Typically, HIT produces modest
reductions in platelet counts to 50,000–100,000/µl. The incidence of
HIT is approximately 2% with adjusted-dose unfractionated heparin
and even lower with prophylactic-dose unfractionated heparin and
low-molecular-weight heparin (LMWH).

(1) The diagnosis is suggested by a drop in platelet count by greater
than 50% or to a level of less than 100,000/µl during heparin

therapy by any route (including heparin flushes) in the absence of other causes of thrombocytopenia. The diagnosis needs to be confirmed by laboratory testing. Two types of assays are available: **functional** (platelet aggregometry or serotonin release assay) and **antigenic** (enzyme-linked immunosorbent assay for heparin-PF4 complex). Neither is 100% sensitive, and therefore they can complement each other.

- **(2) Therapy** starts with stopping all heparin use (including heparin-coated lines) once the diagnosis is suspected. **Recombinant hirudin (lepirudin), argatroban,** and **danaparoid** have been used successfully in HIT (see Anticoagulants, secs. **IV, V,** and **VI**). Danaparoid, however, has the small potential risk of in vivo cross reactivity with the HIT antibody (in vitro cross reactivity is 10%). LMWH should be avoided. Warfarin is not effective in the early therapy of HIT, and, more importantly, it must be discontinued if it was started a few days before the diagnosis of HIT, because it has been associated with limb gangrene in this setting. If clinical suspicion is high, empiric treatment should not be delayed while waiting for laboratory confirmation. Patients with HIT with new or pre-existing thrombosis should be anticoagulated with lepirudin, argatroban, or danaparoid. Thrombocytopenia should not be regarded as a contraindication to anticoagulation, unless the patient is bleeding. Patients with HIT and isolated thrombocytopenia (no new or pre-existing thrombosis) should also be considered for at least several days of anticoagulation, until thrombocytopenia resolves. Doppler ultrasound of the lower extremities can be considered to exclude deep venous thrombosis (DVT; the most common complication), because thrombosis develops in up to 30% of patients with HIT. If long-term anticoagulation is necessary, parenteral therapy should overlap warfarin until steady-state INR is achieved. In general, warfarin should not be started until several days after the cessation of heparin and the resolution of thrombocytopenia (*Thromb Haemost* 79:1, 1998).

2. **Thrombotic thrombocytopenic purpura** is a systemic disorder characterized by platelet aggregation in the microcirculation. The complete clinical pentad, which is present in fewer than 30% of cases, includes consumptive thrombocytopenia, microangiopathic hemolytic anemia, fever, renal dysfunction, and fluctuating neurologic deficits. Thrombocytopenia and microangiopathic hemolytic anemia are sufficient to make the diagnosis in the absence of other causes. The **hemolytic-uremic syndrome** may share a common pathogenesis with TTP, but its systemic manifestations are limited to the kidney. The etiology is obscure, although TTP occurs postpartum and in pregnancy (see sec. **I.B.3**) and has been associated with HIV and toxigenic strains of *Shigella* and *Escherichia coli*. TTP also can be drug induced (e.g., mitomycin-C, cyclosporin A, ticlopidine) or can occur after bone marrow transplantation. Hereditary forms also exist. Even though the etiology of TTP remains obscure, it has been shown that patients with TTP have elevated levels of high-molecular-weight multimers of vWF due to a deficiency of vWF-cleaving protease. (*N Engl J Med* 339:1578, 1998).

   a. **Laboratory evaluation** reveals intravascular hemolysis (anemia, low haptoglobin, elevated lactate dehydrogenase, and indirect bilirubin), thrombocytopenia, and renal insufficiency. The peripheral smear reveals schistocytes. Coagulation studies usually are normal. A commercial assay for vWF-cleaving protease is under development. Differential diagnosis includes DIC, malignant hypertension, and vasculitis.

   b. **Treatment** of TTP is critical, as it is a medical emergency that requires immediate hospitalization, usually in an ICU. **Plasma exchange** (1.0

plasma volume qd) is the mainstay of therapy. Remission rates are as high as 90% when plasma exchange is initiated without delay. The addition of **glucocorticoids** (methylprednisolone, 200 mg IV qd) has become standard practice. **Antiplatelet agents** (aspirin, 325 mg PO qd, and dipyridamole, 100 mg PO q6h) are included in some regimens, but additional benefit is not conclusive (*N Engl J Med* 325:393, 1991). RBCs should be given as needed. Platelet transfusions, however, are relatively contraindicated because of the increased risk of clinical deterioration. The end point of therapy is not well defined, but plasma exchange should be continued for at least 5 days or for 2 days after normalization of the platelet count and lactate dehydrogenase, resolution of neurologic signs, and improvement in microangiopathy. Schistocytes may persist for several weeks into a durable remission. Renal failure may be slower to improve, and persistent azotemia does not necessarily indicate treatment failure. Patients who do not respond generally receive a trial of plasma exchange with cryosupernatant in place of fresh frozen plasma (FFP). Relapse occurs most commonly within a month. Patients with relapsing TTP may enjoy long remissions with intermittent plasma exchange. **Splenectomy** may salvage some patients with TTP that is refractory to plasma exchange or may reduce the frequency of relapses in patients who experience recurrent episodes (*Semin Hematol* 34:159, 1997).

3. **Gestational thrombocytopenia** is a common (5–10%) finding in the third trimester. However, thrombocytopenia can be seen in **preeclampsia** (in 15–20% of cases), **eclampsia** (in 40–50% of cases), or **HELLP** syndrome (**h**emolysis, **e**levated **l**iver enzymes, **l**ow **p**latelets). All clinical signs, including thrombocytopenia, usually resolve promptly after delivery. Plasma exchange is typically not effective in eclampsia but is indicated in severely affected patients. The differential diagnosis of low platelet counts in pregnancy includes DIC, ITP, and TTP. TTP in the peripartum period may be indistinguishable from eclampsia, and its management is similar to that of the nonpregnant patient (*Semin Hematol* 34:159, 1997).

4. **Hypersplenism** is a syndrome characterized by splenomegaly and sequestration of up to 90% of circulating platelets. A variety of disorders may result in splenomegaly, but most produce only a modest decrease in the platelet count. Treatment is directed toward the underlying condition. Splenectomy is a consideration if the cause of splenomegaly is not remediable, if the splenomegaly is symptomatic, or as a diagnostic procedure in idiopathic splenomegaly.

II. Thrombocytosis

A. **Reactive thrombocytosis** is a rise in platelet count to more than 500,000/μl in response to splenectomy or conditions such as iron deficiency, chronic infectious or inflammatory conditions, and malignancy. Patients with this condition apparently do not have an increased risk of bleeding or thrombosis. No specific therapy is required except for correction of the underlying disorder.

B. **Essential thrombocythemia (ET)**, like the other chronic myeloproliferative disorders (e.g., chronic myelogenous leukemia, polycythemia vera), is a clonal disorder of hematopoietic stem cells.

1. **Diagnosis and clinical features.** ET is a diagnosis of exclusion in a patient who has a platelet count of more than 600,000/μl with no cause for reactive thrombocytosis and absence of the Philadelphia chromosome on bone marrow cytogenetic analysis. ET slightly predisposes to bleeding (mucosal) and thrombosis (most often arterial) with equal tendency.

2. **Management.** Daily aspirin (81–325 mg PO qd) is safe, but its additional benefit to cytoreduction is unclear. Cytoreduction to a target platelet count of 400,000/μl can be achieved with anagrelide or hydroxyurea. Interferon-alpha can be used in pregnancy or during childbearing years. Patients with age greater than 60 or prior thrombosis require

cytoreduction. Those with age less than 60, absence of prior thrombosis or cardiovascular risk factors, and platelet counts of less than 1.5 million/μl can be observed. Asymptomatic patients with platelet counts greater than 1.5 million/μl may be observed only if they lack cardiovascular risk factors (http://hematology.org/education/hematology99.html). Acute thrombosis is managed best with platelet pheresis in combination with aspirin. Platelet transfusion is appropriate for life-threatening hemorrhage because ET platelets often are dysfunctional.

III. **Qualitative platelet disorders** are suggested by a prolonged bleeding time in the face of a normal platelet count. Acquired defects are vastly more prevalent than hereditary disorders.

A. **Acquired defects** in platelet function generally cause less severe hemostatic problems than do the inherited disorders. In fact, patients with isolated platelet dysfunction may not bleed abnormally unless superimposed coagulation defects are present.

1. **Drug-induced** platelet dysfunction is exceedingly common because of the prevalence of aspirin use. A single low dose of **aspirin** (81 mg PO) irreversibly inhibits the entire circulating platelet pool. This effect gradually diminishes over 7 days, the time required for biosynthesis of a new cohort of platelets. All other **NSAIDs** reversibly inhibit platelet function only during their half-lives in plasma. Numerous other drugs (including beta-lactam antibiotics) cause platelet dysfunction in vitro but do not increase the risk of bleeding. **Ethanol** causes platelet dysfunction and may synergize with aspirin to prolong the bleeding time. **Ticlopidine** also inhibits platelet function but can cause neutropenia. **Clopidogrel** is an alternative, as it causes less neutropenia. Because of its prolonged half-life, ticlopidine should be withheld beginning 10 days before elective invasive procedures. Patients on aspirin who are undergoing elective procedures should avoid taking the drug for 5 days before surgery. The risk of significant bleeding in most patients who are receiving aspirin and require urgent surgery (excluding ophthalmic surgery and neurosurgery) probably is too low to warrant any delay (*N Engl J Med* 324:27, 1991). The bleeding time is not predictive of postoperative bleeding. Platelet transfusion compensates completely for aspirin-induced platelet dysfunction and should be reserved for patients with significant bleeding.

2. **Uremia** causes platelet dysfunction in vitro but is associated variably with clinical bleeding. A confounding variable is that anemia, itself a result of renal failure, independently prolongs the bleeding time. No reliable prospective means can identify patients who are at risk of spontaneous or iatrogenic bleeding; therefore, treatment should be reserved for individuals who bleed. **Dialysis** should be considered for bleeding patients. **RBC transfusion** to maintain a hematocrit of at least 30% improves hemostasis. **Desmopressin** [diamino-8-D-arginine vasopressin (DDAVP)] may be significantly beneficial for up to 4 hours (0.3 μg/kg in 50 ml normal saline IV over 30 minutes); the same dose can be given SC q12–24h in less than 1.5 ml/injection site. Alternatively, the high-concentration 1.5-mg/ml nasal preparation can be administered, one spray in each nostril q24h. Tachyphylaxis develops after repeated dosing. Hyponatremia may result from the antidiuretic effect of DDAVP. Conjugated **estrogens** (0.6 mg/kg IV qd for 5 days) may improve platelet function for up to 2 weeks. Transfused platelets acquire the uremic defect rapidly but may have transient utility in actively bleeding patients.

3. **Myeloproliferative disorders** may predispose to thrombosis but are associated also with acquired platelet dysfunction that may lead to bleeding. Asymptomatic patients with even markedly elevated platelet counts should not receive treatment specifically directed at lowering the bleeding risk. Patients with a bleeding history may benefit from control of the platelet count.

B. **Inherited disorders** of platelet function are rare. They include defects in the functions of platelets, either secretory (e.g., storage pool disease) or adhesive (e.g., Bernard-Soulier syndrome). Patients with these disorders are managed conservatively, with platelet transfusions reserved for significant bleeding.

IV. **Platelet transfusion guidelines**

A. **Platelet products.** A unit of platelets is the amount recovered from a single donor, either by apheresis or by isolation from whole blood. In patients with thrombocytopenia resulting from a pure platelet production problem, transfusion of either one single-donor apheresis unit or six random-donor units results in an increment in the platelet count of approximately 30,000/µl. However, because of the lower risk of alloimmunization, single-donor units are the product of choice in patients who are expected to be heavily transfused. Platelets are infused IV over 30 minutes; premedication is unnecessary. Many of the risks and complications of RBC transfusion (see Chap. 20) apply to platelet transfusion as well.

B. **Transfusion threshold.** Asymptomatic outpatients should be transfused for platelet counts less than 20,000/µl (10,000/µl for inpatients). Prophylactic transfusion is reasonable for patients with counts of 10,000–20,000/µl if a minor invasive procedure is performed or if a coagulopathy also is present. If a major invasive procedure is performed, a 50,000/µl threshold should be used. High-risk surgery (e.g., neurosurgery, ophthalmic surgery, cardiopulmonary bypass) may warrant prophylactic transfusion to keep the platelet count greater than 100,000/µl. Platelet transfusion thresholds change if there is evidence of bleeding. For minor mucosal bleeding (minor epistaxis, occult GI bleeding, petechiae), the count should be maintained at more than 20,000/µl. In the event of major bleeding (postoperative, CNS bleeding), a level of 100,000/µl should be used. Unless the platelet half-life is shortened severely, as in sepsis, fever, or alloimmunization, no rationale mandates checking counts and transfusing more frequently than every 24 hours.

C. **Platelet refractoriness** is due to alloantibodies that develop in multiply transfused patients. It can be documented by measuring the platelet count before and 60 minutes after transfusion. An increment of less than 5000/µl after one apheresis unit or six random-donor units is an indication of refractoriness. Use of single-donor platelets, HLA-matched platelets, ABO-identical platelets, platelets from family members, or IVIG may decrease refractoriness.

Inherited Bleeding Disorders

I. **Hemophilia.** The X-linked forms, hemophilia A and B, account for 99% of cases and are caused by deficiencies in factors VIII and IX, respectively. One unit/ml represents the amount of factor VIII or IX activity (100%) in 1 ml normal pooled plasma. Normal factor VIII and IX activity levels are 50–150% (0.5–1.5 units/ml).

A. **Hemophilia A (classic hemophilia)** represents 85% of cases. The clinical phenotype is dictated by the factor VIII level: severe (<1% activity), moderate (1–5% activity), and mild (>5% activity). Severe hemophiliacs have spontaneous bleeding episodes two to four times per month, on average. Mild hemophiliacs may require intervention only after trauma or surgery. Moderate hemophiliacs have an intermediate phenotype. The clinical manifestations are typical of a coagulation disorder (hemarthroses, hematomas, delayed posttraumatic and postoperative bleeding). Repeated bleeding into a "target" joint can cause chronic synovitis and hemophilic arthropathy.

1. **Primary therapy** is factor replacement and should be directed by a hematologist who is experienced in treating hemophilia. The choice of therapeutic agent depends on the patient's starting factor VIII level and the

type and severity of hemorrhage. A good rule of thumb is that factor VIII levels increase 2% for every 1 unit/kg factor VIII concentrate infused, regardless of type of product. Thus, 50 units/kg IV bolus raises factor VIII levels to 100%. This dosage can be followed by 25 units/kg IV bolus q12h. To stop most mild bleeds, 30–50% of normal factor levels is necessary. Home therapy with factor replacement allows outpatient therapy of minor bleeds. One to three doses of factor usually suffice. Moderate to severe hemorrhages require 50–100% of normal levels, and several days of hospitalization may be required, with daily monitoring of factor levels. Treatment of a hemophiliac with suspected bleeding should never be delayed while awaiting results of diagnostic studies (*Hematol Oncol Clin North Am* 12:1315, 1998). Purity of product refers to the concentration of factor. Most high-purity products are either plasma derived or recombinant. Plasma-derived products are virally deactivated either by pasteurization or by solvent/detergent treatment. The latter does not eradicate parvovirus or hepatitis A. The recombinant products are the most expensive and are associated with a greater risk of inducing low-titer inhibitor formation. They should be reserved for use in HIV-seronegative and hepatitis C virus–seronegative or previously untreated patients.

2. **Inhibitors.** These IgG antibodies to factor VIII develop in deficient patients treated with factor concentrates. Inhibitors reduce the efficacy of therapy by accelerating the clearance of infused factor. The standard measure of inhibitor strength is the Bethesda unit (BU); 1 BU/ml is the reciprocal of the patient plasma dilution that depletes the factor level by 50% after a 2-hour incubation in vitro. Low responders have minimal anamnesis (recall) on repeat exposure to factor VIII and have low inhibitor titers (<5 BU). High responders produce rapid amnestic response and usually have higher titers. Treatment of bleeding patients with factor VIII inhibitors depends on the severity of hemorrhage because a Bethesda assay may not be immediately available. **Life- or limb-threatening bleeding** should be treated with 100 units/kg of porcine factor VIII (Hyate-C) IV bolus followed by 4 units/kg/hour IV. Less severe bleeds can be treated with 100 units/kg IV bolus of human factor VIII followed by an infusion of 10 units/kg/hour. If clinical and laboratory parameters (bleeding, aPTT, factor VIII level drawn 10 minutes after a bolus) do not improve, a 100- to 200-unit/kg bolus of porcine factor VIII should be given followed by an infusion of 10 units/kg/hour. If there is still no response, prothrombin complex concentrates (PCC) at 100 units/kg IV q12h or activated PCC at 50–75 units/kg IV q12h are given; however, they carry the risk of thrombosis and DIC. Alternatively, recombinant factor VIIa (NovoSeven) at 90 µg/kg IV bolus q2–3h can be used. Patients who continue to bleed despite these measures should undergo plasmapheresis followed by repeated infusions of human or porcine factor VIII. With minor bleeds, if there is time to measure BU, and if the BU is <5, then DDAVP 0.3 µg/kg IV can be given. If there is no response, human or porcine factor VIII can be given as above.

3. **Ancillary therapy** includes the use of **DDAVP** and **epsilon-aminocaproic acid.** DDAVP transiently raises factor VIII levels fourfold (see Platelet Disorders, sec. **III.A.2**) and can be used every 12 hours in minor hemorrhage in mild type A hemophiliacs. The factor VIII level should be assayed before and 60 minutes after administration of DDAVP to document an adequate increment. Tachyphylaxis often develops after several doses. The antifibrinolytic agent epsilon-aminocaproic acid can be given PO or IV as an adjunct during dental surgery or in spontaneous oral mucosal bleeds (100 mg/kg loading dose, up to 10 g, then 50 mg/kg up to 5 g q6h for 2–7 days), but it **is contraindicated in genitourinary bleeds** (because of the risk of ureteral occlusion). Aspirin and other NSAIDs should be avoided because they increase the risk of bleeding.

B. In hemophilia B the clinical manifestations and principles of therapy are similar to those of hemophilia A. The severity is a function of factor IX levels. DDAVP does not play a role in hemophilia B therapy. A variety of purified factor IX preparations are available; intermediate-purity preparations should not be used. Because of differences in pharmacokinetics, the initial bolus of factor IX should be 100 units/kg IV, followed by 50 units/kg IV q24h. Inhibitors develop less frequently in hemophilia B and are managed with PCC or activated PCC.

II. **von Willebrand's disease** is the most common inherited bleeding disorder (1% of population). The spectrum of disease is heterogenous. Most forms are autosomal dominant. vWF has two important functions: to facilitate adherence of platelets to injured vessel walls and to stabilize factor VIII in plasma. The characteristic clinical finding is mucocutaneous bleeding, such as epistaxis, menorrhagia, GI bleeding, and easy bruising. Trauma, surgery, or dental extractions may result in life-threatening bleeding in severely affected patients. Many patients with mild disease remain undiagnosed.

A. **Classification** follows a revised nomenclature for vWD that recognizes three main types: type 1 vWD, partial quantitative deficiency; type 2 vWD, qualitative deficiency; and type 3 vWD, severe quantitative deficiency (see Evaluation of Patients with Hemostatic Disorders, sec. **II.A.3**). Type 1 accounts for 70–80% of cases, and vWF:Ag and vWF:RCo are proportionally low. In most subtypes of type 2 vWD, VIII:C is normal, whereas vWF:RCo is decreased out of proportion to vWF:Ag. In type 3 vWD, levels of vWF:Ag are almost undetectable.

B. **Management** consists of raising vWF:RCo and factor VIII levels to normal.

1. **Minor bleeding** in type 1 vWD usually responds to DDAVP. DDAVP may also be useful in some patients with type 2 vWD; however, it is not useful in type 3 vWD (see Platelet Disorders, sec. **III.A.2**). Oral contraceptives may be useful for menorrhagia. vWF:RCo levels of greater than 50% for up to 3 days are sufficient for most minor bleeds.

2. **Major bleeding** or **surgical prophylaxis** requires plasma product infusion (Alphanate, Humate-P, or Koate) q8–12h to raise vWF:RCo levels to 100% initially and above 50% for 5–10 days. In general, 50 IU vWF:RCo/kg raises the vWF activity level to 100%. Humate-P is the plasma product richest in high-molecular-weight vWF multimers. Cryoprecipitate contains significant amounts of vWF and factor VIII but carries the risk of viral transmission. Type 1 vWD patients who are undergoing minor procedures can receive DDAVP 1 hour before surgery and q12–24h for 2–3 days postoperatively, but for more extensive surgery plasma products should be administered. In type 3 vWD, factor VIII:C level should also be monitored and kept therapeutic.

Acquired Coagulation Disorders

I. **Vitamin K deficiency** can be caused by malabsorption states or poor dietary intake combined with antibiotic-associated loss of intestinal bacterial production. Warfarin induces an iatrogenic functional state of vitamin K deficiency by interfering with conversion to its active (reduced) state. Vitamin K is required by hepatocytes to complete synthesis (gamma-carboxylation) of clotting factors (II, VII, IX, X) and the natural anticoagulant proteins C and S. Manifestations of vitamin K deficiency are bleeding and prolongation of the PT out of proportion to the aPTT.

A. **Fresh frozen plasma** is given for acute bleeds or before invasive procedures at a usual starting dose of two units (400–450 ml). Repeat measurement of the PT and aPTT after infusion are necessary to determine the need for further infusions. A starting dose of up to 10–15 ml/kg may be needed with severe bleeding and significant PT prolongation. Because factor VII has a half-life of 6 hours, the PT may become prolonged sooner than the aPTT after infusion.

B. **Vitamin K replacement** is administered to bleeding or asymptomatic patients with a prolonged PT but may take up to several days to normalize the PT. The IM route should be avoided. Oral replacement (phytonadione, 10–20 mg PO qd) is well absorbed. Parenteral replacement is available (phytonadione solution, 10 mg SC or IV over 20 minutes qd for 3 days), although the IV preparation occasionally causes severe allergic reactions.

II. **Liver disease** can alter hemostasis profoundly by reducing synthesis of most clotting factors and by causing hypersplenism (leading to thrombocytopenia) and cholestasis (which impairs vitamin K absorption).

A. **Vitamin K** is appropriate for asymptomatic, mild prolongation of the PT. This therapy does not always reverse the coagulopathy, as a hepatic synthetic defect more often is the culprit.

B. **Fresh frozen plasma** is appropriate if coagulation parameters are abnormal (PT or aPTT greater than one and a half times control) in the setting of bleeding or the need for an invasive procedure.

C. **Cryoprecipitate,** 1.5 bags for every 10 kg body weight, can be given IV to correct severe hypofibrinogenemia (<100 mg/dl) if there is bleeding or the need for invasive procedures. This should be followed by periodic measurement of a fibrinogen level.

D. **Platelet transfusions** are indicated for bleeding in the setting of thrombocytopenia or for counts of less than 20,000/μl.

III. **DIC** is seen in a variety of systemic illnesses, including sepsis, trauma, burns, shock, vascular disease, liver disease, obstetric disasters, and malignancies (notably, acute promyelocytic leukemia). It is characterized by the inappropriate coexistence of enhanced fibrin production and fibrinolysis. Laboratory abnormalities usually exist out of proportion to clinical evidence of overt bleeding or thrombosis. The best approach for resolving DIC is to correct the underlying illness. Hematologic treatment is largely supportive, consisting of administration of FFP, cryoprecipitate, and platelets (see secs. I and II). The fear that administration of plasma products "fuels the fire of DIC" is unfounded. The use of heparin to prevent thrombosis in DIC is controversial. Adjusted-dose **heparin** (see Anticoagulants, sec. I.A) is appropriate therapy for large-vessel thrombosis in DIC.

IV. **Acquired inhibitors of coagulation** appear in hemophiliacs treated with factor concentrates or may also occur spontaneously in the postpartum period, in association with an underlying immunologic disease (e.g., SLE) or in otherwise normal individuals. Inhibitors against specific clotting factors tend to cause bleeding and are recognized by the failure of a prolonged coagulation assay to correct in a 1:1 mix with normal plasma. In contrast, nonspecific inhibitors (e.g., the lupus anticoagulant) tend to cause thrombosis (see Thromboembolic Disorders, sec. I.B.1). The most common specific inhibitor is directed against factor VIII. Patients with acquired factor VIII inhibitors are managed in the same manner as are hemophiliacs with acquired alloantibodies to factor VIII (see Inherited Bleeding Disorders, sec. I.A.2). Long-term therapy includes immunosuppression with steroids and cyclophosphamide to decrease production of the autoantibody. Acquired inhibitors of vWF and other coagulation factors are much less common.

Thromboembolic Disorders

I. **Predisposing conditions** are identified in more than half of patients with thromboses.

A. **Inherited** thrombophilic disorders are suggested by a history of thrombosis at a young age, a positive family history of thrombosis, recurrent thrombosis, or thrombosis in unusual anatomic locations (see Evaluation of Patients with Hemostatic Disorders, sec. **II.C**). The most common mutation is factor V Leiden, which causes activated protein C (APC) resistance. Mutations that affect proteins C, S, or ATIII are 10 times less common. The annual risk of thrombosis in patients who are heterozygous for any of these four mutations is 1–2%.

1. **Acute thromboembolism** in patients with inherited thrombophilia is managed in the same manner as is idiopathic thromboembolism (see sec. **III.B.2**), with a few important caveats. Patients with protein C deficiency may experience coumarin-induced skin necrosis, caused by depletion of protein C levels before other vitamin K–dependent clotting factors are depleted. To avoid this complication, optimal management of these patients may begin with full heparin anticoagulation, followed by gradual warfarin loading (2 mg qd for 3 days, then increments of 2–3 mg each day until the target INR is reached).

2. **Prophylaxis** against thromboembolism in patients with an inherited predisposition includes avoiding additional risk factors for thrombosis such as smoking and estrogen-containing oral contraceptives. Asymptomatic carriers of any of these mutations should receive adjusted-dose heparin or warfarin when immobilized during surgery or prolonged illness. Infusion of ATIII concentrate (50 units/kg) should be considered before major surgery in deficient patients.

3. **Hyperhomocysteinemia** should be treated with folate alone or in combination with vitamins B_{12} and B_6.

B. **Acquired** states of hypercoagulability are seen in association with chronic medical illnesses (CHF, diabetes mellitus, obesity, nephrotic syndrome), estrogen use, immobilization, the postoperative and postpartum periods, and paroxysmal nocturnal hemoglobinuria. Thrombosis associated with malignancy may be disease related (e.g., Trousseau's syndrome) or treatment related (e.g., mitomycin, L-asparaginase).

1. **Antiphospholipid antibody syndrome** can present with arterial or venous thrombosis, thrombocytopenia, or recurrent fetal loss. It is caused by autoantibodies that react with negatively charged phospholipids and can be detected by two assays, **lupus anticoagulant** (clot-based assay) or **anticardiolipin antibody** (immunoassay). Both assays must be performed, as neither is 100% sensitive. The aPTT is frequently slightly elevated but does not predispose to bleeding and is not a sensitive screening test. The lifetime probability of thrombosis is approximately 40%. At least 10% of patients with SLE have evidence of lupus anticoagulants; however, most patients with lupus anticoagulants do not have SLE.

2. **Therapy** for an isolated asymptomatic antiphospholipid antibody is not warranted. Acute thrombosis is treated with heparin, although the inability to follow the aPTT is problematic; therefore, anti-Xa activity can be measured. Subsequent therapy is with long-term (i.e., years) warfarin, unless resolution of autoantibody is shown on at least two different occasions several months apart. Intensive-dose warfarin (INR, 3.0–3.5) is more effective than standard-dose warfarin (INR, 2.0–3.0); however, the risk of bleeding is higher, and, therefore, patients with comorbid conditions (history of GI bleeding and stroke, renal insufficiency, anemia) or age older than 65 years may not be suitable candidates for intensive anticoagulation. Regardless, most experts agree that an INR of at least 2.5 is necessary. Thrombocytopenia is treated similarly to ITP, with prednisone or IVIG. Antiphospholipid antibodies may appear transiently in association with some infections and medications but apparently do not pose an increased risk of thrombosis in these settings. Women with recurrent fetal loss have been managed successfully through pregnancy with aspirin, prednisone, and heparin, alone or in combination (*Adv Rheumatol* 81:151, 1997).

II. **Arterial thrombosis** can be due to atherosclerosis, vasculitis, or an underlying hypercoagulable state (see Evaluation of Patients with Hemostatic Disorders, sec. **II.C**). Acute peripheral arterial thromboemboli generally require anticoagulation with heparin, followed by a definitive procedure (see Chaps. 5 and 25 for management).

III. **Venous thromboembolism** may result from stasis, hypercoagulability, or trauma to venous endothelial surfaces.

   A. **Superficial thrombophlebitis** is common, especially in varicose veins, and may be the presenting sign of a hypercoagulable disorder. Treatment includes elevation, heat, NSAIDs, and compression stockings. Most resolve within a few weeks with symptomatic therapy. Anticoagulation and venous stripping can be considered, especially for recurrent cases, but standard of care is not established (*Angiology* 50:523, 1999).

   B. **Deep venous thrombosis** presents with swelling, pain, or erythema of the affected extremity. It most commonly occurs in the lower limbs, and half will cause pulmonary emboli in the absence of treatment.

      1. **Diagnosis** is most commonly made by compression ultrasonography (>90% sensitive); however, this does not visualize pelvic vessels and is less sensitive (50%) for calf vein thrombosis. Venography is the gold standard and can be considered if clinical suspicion is high, although it does carry a 5% risk of inducing phlebitis. Diagnosis should not be made on clinical grounds alone.

      2. **Therapy** reduces mortality, morbidity, and rate of recurrence.

         a. **Inpatient** treatment of proximal vein thrombosis begins with heparin, administered either by continuous IV infusion or by intermittent SC injection. LMWH can be used in place of unfractionated heparin. Warfarin (adjusted to INR of 2.0–3.0) should be started after achievement of a therapeutic aPTT. Heparin can be discontinued 48 hours after the INR has been therapeutic. In patients with an absolute contraindication to anticoagulation, or pulmonary embolism that occurs despite anticoagulation, **inferior vena cava filter** placement is indicated. Bed rest is not necessary, but leg elevation is helpful. Knee-high compression stockings provide comfort and reduce the incidence of **postphlebitic syndrome.** Selected patients with massive ileofemoral thrombosis should be considered for thrombolytic therapy, as it reduces the incidence of postphlebitic syndrome [*Chest* 114(Suppl):571S, 1998].

         b. **Outpatient** treatment with LMWH is safe in selected patients. Those with major bleeding risk, renal failure, compliance issues, or other comorbid conditions require inpatient anticoagulation.

         c. **Duration** of therapy is an evolving area and is individualized. High-risk patients (recurrent thrombosis, malignancy, antiphospholipid antibody, or multiple genetic defects) are anticoagulated long-term (i.e., years). Moderate-risk patients (APC resistance, idiopathic thrombosis without provocation, deficiencies of proteins C or S or antithrombin) are anticoagulated for 6 months and receive **prophylaxis** during surgery, prolonged immobilization, and pregnancy, using adjusted-dose heparin or warfarin. However, they can be considered for lifelong anticoagulation if the first thrombotic event was life threatening. Low-risk individuals (no known defects and DVT after major provocation) require at least 3 months of therapy.

      3. **Complications** include pulmonary embolism (see Chap. 10) and **postphlebitic syndrome** (see sec. **III.B.2**). The latter results in chronic swelling, pain, and skin ulceration due to venous stasis that results from incompetent venous valves. Compression stockings and leg elevation may alleviate symptoms.

      4. **Calf vein thrombosis** is not dangerous unless it extends proximally (20% within 2 weeks of presentation). High-risk (e.g., previous thrombosis) or symptomatic patients should be anticoagulated. Others can be

Table 19-2. Low-molecular-weight heparins (LMWHs) used in venous thromboembolism

LMWH	Prophylatic	Therapeutic[a]
Enoxaparin	30 mg q12h[b,c] or 40 mg q24h[d]	1 mg/kg q12h or 1.5 mg/kg q24h
Ardeparin	50 U/kg q12h[e]	130 U/kg q12h
Dalteparin	2500 U q24h[f] or 5000 U q24h[c,d]	100 U/kg q12h or 200 U/kg q24h

Note: Doses are in mg or anti-Xa units SC up to 100 kg body weight. Adjustments in dosing should be made for patients with renal insufficiency.
[a]Twice-daily dosing may be more effective, especially with malignancy and morbid obesity.
[b]Start 12–24 hrs after orthopedic or high-risk general surgery (see Thromboembolic Disorders, sec. **III.C.2**).
[c]High-risk medical patients (e.g., prior deep venous thrombosis, malignancy).
[d]Start 10–12 hrs before orthopedic or high-risk general surgery.
[e]Start 12–24 hrs after orthopedic surgery.
[f]Start 1–2 hrs before moderate-risk surgery (or use enoxaparin, 20 mg q24h).
Source: Data from GP Clagett, FA Anderson Jr, W Geerts, et al. Prevention of venous thromboembolism. *Chest* 114:531S, 1998.

observed with serial compression ultrasonography for 2 weeks (*N Engl J Med* 335:1816, 1996).

5. **Upper extremity thrombosis** is primarily caused by indwelling venous catheters or pacemaker wires, with embolization occurring in 20% of cases. Anatomic causes such as a cervical rib should be considered. Treatment includes elevation, warm compresses, and removal of the indwelling line if no longer needed. Oral anticoagulation is indicated for at least 3 months (even when the catheter is removed); however, many clinicians anticoagulate for as long as the catheter is in place (*Lancet* 349:1188, 1997).

C. **DVT prophylaxis** decreases the incidence of pulmonary embolism and venous thrombosis.

1. **In nonsurgical patients** with stroke or myocardial infarction, LMWH or low-dose unfractionated heparin (LDUH) can be used (see Anticoagulants, secs. **I** and **II**). Elastic stockings and pneumatic compression boots (PCB) can be used if there is a bleeding risk. Medical ICU patients should have DVT prophylaxis as part of their routine admission orders (*N Engl J Med* 341:797, 1999). General medical patients should receive prophylaxis in the presence of risk factors (immobility, malignancy, etc.), especially those with CHF or pneumonia. A once-daily LMWH or warfarin (1 mg) can be used to prevent upper extremity thrombosis in patients with long-term central vein catheters.

2. **In general surgical patients** pharmacologic prophylaxis (LMWH or LDUH) is as effective as PCB, and combining both may give better protection, especially in high-risk general surgery patients (major surgery with age >60 years or age 40–60 years with additional risk factors). Moderate-risk general surgery patients (age 40–60 without risk factors with major surgery or with additional risk factors and having minor surgery) require either pharmacologic or mechanical methods of prophylaxis. Low-risk general surgery patients (age <40, no risk factors) require early ambulation only. **Orthopedic surgery** patients can receive LMWH (Table 19-2), danaparoid, PCB, or warfarin (INR, 2–3; initiate on day of operation). In **neurosurgical** patients PCB with or without elastic stockings can be used; however, LMWH and LDUH may also be acceptable. Prophylaxis should continue until patients are fully ambula-

Table 19-3. Weight-based heparin dosing

Initial therapy[a]	
Bolus	60–80 units/kg[b]
Infusion	14–18 units/kg/hr
Adjustments[c]	
aPTT <40	2000 units IV bolus; increase infusion by 2 units/kg/hr
aPTT 40–44	Increase infusion by 1 unit/kg/hr
aPTT 45–70	No change
aPTT 71–80	Decrease infusion by 1 unit/kg/hr
aPTT 81–90	Hold for 0.5 hr; decrease infusion by 2 units/kg/hr
aPTT >90	Hold for 1 hr; decrease infusion by 3 units/kg/hr

aPTT = activated partial thromboplastin time.
Note: Target aPTT can vary among hospitals depending on reagents and instruments used.
[a]Round all doses to nearest 100 units.
[b]Maximum, 5000 units.
[c]Draw aPTT 6 hours after any bolus or change in infusion rate.
Source: Barnes-Jewish Hospital Pharmacy, St. Louis, MO.

tory, and in orthopedic patients the trend is to give prophylaxis for up to 2–3 weeks after discharge [*Chest* 114(Suppl):531S, 1998].

Anticoagulants

Anticoagulants have relatively narrow therapeutic windows. They are relatively contraindicated in patients with inherited bleeding diatheses and anatomic lesions who are at risk for bleeding (e.g., active GI bleeding, trauma, cerebrovascular accident, pericarditis, surgical wounds) and in noncompliant patients.

 I. **Unfractionated heparin** is derived from porcine or bovine intestinal mucosa. It catalyzes the inactivation of thrombin and factor Xa by ATIII. Factor VIIa is unaffected. Therefore, heparin administration at usual doses prolongs the thrombin time and aPTT, but generally not the PT.

 A. **Administration.** Heparin must be given parenterally. Its onset of action is immediate by the IV route and within 20–60 minutes by the SC route; its half-life is 60 minutes. Clearance is prolonged in liver or renal failure. The standard dosage for DVT prophylaxis is 5000 units SC q12h, but in high-risk patients (e.g., malignancy, prior DVT) it is given q8h. No laboratory monitoring is necessary with SC dosing. Therapeutic doses typically are given IV. Weight-based dosing most reliably provides rapid prolongation of the aPTT into the therapeutic range (*Ann Intern Med* 119:874, 1993). Table 19-3 provides dosing guidelines; however, the target aPTT can vary among hospitals depending on reagents and instruments used. Alternatively, the total daily IV dose can be converted to two divided doses SC q12h, with the aPTT measured at the midpoint between the doses.

 B. **Complications.** Bleeding occurs in 5–10% of patients, although fatal hemorrhage attributable to heparin is seen in fewer than 1%. Concomitant use of antiplatelet agents increases the risk of bleeding and should be avoided if possible. Stools should be monitored for signs of occult blood loss before and during heparin use. GI bleeding is a relative contraindication to heparin administration and warrants investigation for an underlying anatomic abnormality. Mild bleeding can be addressed by discontinuing heparin, as its anticoagulant effect will resolve within hours. Heparin can be reversed rapidly by infusion of **protamine sulfate** (reserved for major bleeding because of risk of anaphylaxis to protamine). Protamine is administered IV over 10 minutes at a dose of 1 mg/100 units circulating heparin, up to a maximum dose of 250 mg. If heparin is given as an IV infusion, the protamine dose should be calculated to neutralize half of the hourly heparin dose. Daily surveillance for thrombocytopenia is warranted when heparin is given by any route (see Platelet Disorders, sec. **I.B.1.e**). Osteoporosis is a significant complication of long-term heparin use (>1 month).

II. **Low-molecular-weight heparin** preparations (see Table 19-2) contain the smaller fractions (mean molecular weight, 4000–5000 daltons) of the more heterogeneous native heparin molecule (mean molecular weight, 15,000 daltons). Administration is by SC route. Adjustments in dosing LMWH should be made for patients with renal insufficiency. LMWH inactivates factor Xa to a greater extent than it does thrombin. Therefore, the aPTT and thrombin time are affected minimally by typical therapeutic doses. Laboratory monitoring can be achieved with anti-Xa units, but because of the more predictable anticoagulation response and the trend toward a lower incidence of bleeding compared to standard heparin, laboratory monitoring is not required. Monitoring of anti-Xa activity should be considered in renal failure and pregnancy and in obese patients, with a therapeutic range of 0.4–0.8 units/ml. The incidence of osteoporosis is lower than that of unfractionated heparin. **Protamine** (1 mg for every 100 anti-Xa units of dalteparin or 1 mg for every mg of enoxaparin) can partially reverse (up to 60%) anticoagulation. Patients who receive any dose of LMWH should **avoid spinal punctures or epidurals,** if possible, because of the risk of spinal hematomas.

III. **Warfarin** inhibits conversion of vitamin K to its active form. Consequently, administration of warfarin leads to depletion of the vitamin K–dependent clotting factors (II, VII, IX, and X) in addition to proteins C and S.

A. **Administration.** Warfarin is well absorbed orally but requires 4–5 days before a full anticoagulant effect is achieved. For this reason, if a patient needs acute anticoagulation, heparin should be overlapped with warfarin for the first 4–5 days. Its half-life is 36–42 hours. Warfarin should be started at 5 mg PO qd and then adjusted to the target INR. For most indications, an INR in the 2.0–3.0 range is adequate. Patients with mechanical valves require a higher intensity of anticoagulation (INR, 2.5–3.5). Patients who are receiving chronic therapy should discontinue warfarin 4–5 days before elective surgery. If ongoing anticoagulation is needed, heparin can be substituted until immediately before surgery. Important drug interactions exist (see Appendix C).

B. **Complications.** Bleeding occurs in 5% of patients in the therapeutic range. Minor bleeding or an asymptomatic elevation of the INR should be managed by holding or reducing warfarin therapy until the INR returns to the appropriate value. Marked elevation of the INR (>5) in asymptomatic patients can be corrected partially with low-dose **vitamin K** (1.0–2.5 mg PO) without jeopardizing anticoagulant control. Higher doses of vitamin K (3–5 mg PO) can be given if the INR is greater than 9.0 in asymptomatic patients. Serious bleeds should be treated with IV vitamin K (10 mg) by slow IV infusion and FFP. Coumarin-induced skin necrosis is a rare complication. **Warfarin is contraindicated in the first trimester of pregnancy because of teratogenicity** but is safe for infants of nursing mothers [*Chest* 114(Suppl):445S, 1998].

IV. **Lepirudin (recombinant hirudin)** is a thrombin-specific inhibitor that is used in the treatment of **HIT** (see Platelet Disorders, sec. **I.B.1.e**). It has a half-life of 1.5 hours and is renally cleared (see Table 19-4 for dose adjustments in renal insufficiency). No antidote is available. The prophylactic dose is 0.1 mg/kg/hour IV, and the therapeutic dose is 0.4 mg/kg (up to 110 kg body weight) IV bolus followed by 0.15 mg/kg/hour (up to 110 kg) IV infusion. It is monitored using the aPTT (1.5–2.5 times normal), which can be checked 4 hours after dose adjustments. Increments in the infusion rate by 20% are made for subtherapeutic levels. Infusion should be stopped for 2 hours for supratherapeutic levels and the rate decreased by 50%, as recommended by the manufacturer. Patients who are

Table 19-4. Lepirudin infusion rates in renal impairment

Creatinine clearance (ml/min)	Serum creatinine (mg/dl)	Adjusted infusion rate (mg/kg/hr)
45–60	1.6–2.0	0.075
30–44	2.1–3.0	0.045
15–29	3.1–6.0	0.0225
<15	>6.0	Avoid or stop infusion

Source: Barnes-Jewish Hospital Pharmacy, St. Louis, MO.

receiving three-times-weekly hemodialysis can be bolused with 0.1–0.2 mg/kg IV before dialysis. Of note, however, some dialysis filters remove lepirudin. Patients on continuous venovenous hemodialysis can receive a continuous IV infusion starting at 0.005 mg/kg/hour [*Thromb Haemost* 82(Suppl):457, 1999]. Lepirudin can also increase the PT, which must be taken into account when interpreting INRs of patients who are taking warfarin.

V. **Danaparoid** is a heparinoid prepared from porcine intestinal mucosa from which heparin has been removed. Active components are heparan sulfate, dermatan sulfate, and chondroitin sulfate. Danaparoid mainly facilitates factor Xa inactivation by antithrombin, and dosing is in anti-Xa units. It is approved for use in postoperative DVT prophylaxis but has been also used in **HIT**. However, cross reactivity with antiheparin antibodies has been observed. The half-life is 24 hours, and no antidote is available. The prophylactic dosage is 750 units given SC twice a day. The therapeutic dose is 2500 units (1250 units if <55 kg, 3750 units if >90 kg) IV bolus followed by a step-down maintenance infusion (400 units/hour for 4 hours, 300 units/hour for 4 hours, then 150–200 units/hour). Danaparoid cannot be monitored with an aPTT; rather, anti-Xa activity is measured (target, 0.5–0.8 units/ml for therapeutic level). Active venous thrombosis can also be treated with 1500 units IV bolus followed by 1500 units SC bid (http://www.hematology.org). Clearance is by the renal route, and experience in renal failure is limited. Patients who are on alternate-day hemodialysis can receive 3750 units IV before the first and second dialysis and 3000 units before the third (decrease dose by 20% if <55 kg), and the anti-Xa level should be less than 0.3 units/ml predialysis; otherwise the dose should be reduced. Danaparoid has been used safely in several pregnancies [*Thromb Haemost* 82(Suppl):457, 1999].

VI. **Argatroban** is a synthetic thrombin inhibitor that is approved for both prevention and treatment of thrombosis in **HIT**. Therapy is initiated with an intravenous infusion of 2.0 µg/kg/minute; an aPTT should be obtained 2 hours later. The infusion rate is adjusted to achieve a steady-state aPTT of 1.5–3.0 times normal (maximum, 100 seconds). No antidote is available; however, the half-life is less than 1 hour. Dose adjustments are necessary in hepatic dysfunction. The INR is also affected; therefore, when warfarin is coadministered, argatroban can be discontinued when the INR is greater than 4. The INR should then be measured again within 4–6 hours, and if it is subtherapeutic, argatroban should be resumed and the procedure repeated daily until a therapeutic INR is achieved off argatroban. Its effect on the INR is less predictable at doses higher than 2.0 µg/kg/minute; therefore, for these patients, the dose should be temporarily reduced to 2.0 µg/kg/minute, and 4–6 hours later an INR measured and the process described above followed.

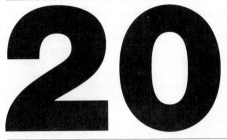

Anemia and Transfusion Therapy

Morey A. Blinder

Approach to the Patient with Anemia

Anemia is a commonly encountered clinical condition that is caused by an acquired or hereditary abnormality of the RBC or its precursors or may be a manifestation of an underlying nonhematologic disorder. Anemia is defined as a decrease in the circulating RBC mass; the usual criteria are a hemoglobin (Hb) of less than 12 g/dl [hematocrit (Hct) <36%] in women and less than 14 g/dl (Hct <41%) in men.

I. **Clinical manifestations** of anemia vary depending on the etiology, degree, and rapidity of onset. Other underlying disorders such as cardiopulmonary disease may contribute to the severity of symptoms. Severe anemia may be well tolerated if it develops gradually, but, generally, patients with a Hb of less than 7 g/dl have symptoms of tissue hypoxia (fatigue, headache, dyspnea, lightheadedness, angina). Pallor, visual impairment, syncope, and tachycardia may signal anemic hypovolemia, which requires immediate attention.

II. **History and physical examination.** The acute or chronic onset of the anemia should be assessed, and clues to any underlying systemic process should be sought. One must look for a family history of anemia, drug exposure (including ethanol), or blood loss. Physical findings that aid in diagnosis include lymphadenopathy, hepatic or splenic enlargement, jaundice, bone tenderness, neurologic symptoms, and evidence of blood in the feces.

III. **Laboratory evaluation** should always include the Hb and Hct, reticulocyte count, mean corpuscular volume (MCV), and an examination of the peripheral blood smear.

A. **The Hb and Hct** serve as an estimate of the RBC mass, but their interpretation must take into consideration the volume status of the patient. Immediately after acute blood loss, the Hb will be normal because compensatory mechanisms have not had time to restore normal plasma volume.

B. **The reticulocyte count** reflects the rate of production of RBCs and is an indicator of the bone marrow response to the anemia. The reticulocyte count is usually reported as reticulocytes/100 RBCs (% reticulocytes), but newer methods in determining the reticulocyte count may also report an absolute number:

Absolute reticulocyte count = $(\% \text{ reticulocytes}/100) \times \text{RBC count}$

An increase of reticulocytes to greater than 100,000/mm^3 suggests a hyperproliferative bone marrow.

C. **The MCV** is often used in classifying anemia (microcytic, normocytic, and macrocytic for anemia with low, normal, and high MCV, respectively). Proper use of the MCV in establishing a diagnosis depends on examination of the peripheral smear for the following reasons: (1) Small and large cells may be present simultaneously, resulting in a normal MCV; (2) reticulocytes are larger than mature RBCs and will raise the MCV; and (3) abnormal cells may be present in numbers that are too small to affect the MCV.

D. **Examination of a well-prepared peripheral blood smear** is mandatory. RBC morphology is best evaluated in a portion of the smear where the RBCs are nearly touching one another. Heterogeneity in RBC size (anisocytosis) and shape (poikilocytosis) may be seen. Specific morphologic abnormalities should be sought, as well as any abnormalities in the WBCs or platelets.

E. **Additional testing** to establish an exact diagnosis should be guided by the initial findings, and, whenever possible, some tests [peripheral smear, glucose 6-phosphate dehydrogenase (G6PD) level, Hb analysis] should be performed before blood transfusions.

IV. **Classification of anemias.** Typically, anemia is characterized by the MCV and reticulocyte count. Anemia with a low reticulocyte count suggests impaired RBC production or ineffective erythropoiesis. An increased reticulocyte count is associated with loss or destruction of RBCs. Determination of the MCV and an examination of the peripheral smear often suggest a single diagnosis or a limited number of diagnoses that can be investigated with specific tests. Anemia may be multifactorial in origin (e.g., alcoholism with GI bleeding, nutritional deficiencies, and liver disease). Evaluation of anemia also requires consideration of the WBC and platelet count, because bicytopenia or pancytopenia often suggests other causes.

Anemias Associated with Decreased Red Blood Cell Production

I. **Iron-deficiency anemia** is a common disorder worldwide. In the United States, most cases are caused by menstrual blood loss and increased iron requirements of pregnancy. In the absence of menstrual bleeding, GI blood loss is the presumed etiology in most patients; appropriate radiographic and endoscopic procedures should be performed to identify a source and to exclude occult malignancy. Decreased iron absorption (celiac disease, postgastrectomy) or increased iron requirements (lactation, infancy) may also lead to iron deficiency. Complete evaluation of iron deficiency requires identification of the cause.

A. **History and physical examination.** Evidence for a source of blood loss (melena, menorrhagia) should be sought. In severe iron-deficiency anemia, a history of pica (consumption of substances such as ice, starch, or clay) may be obtained. Splenomegaly, koilonychia ("spoon nail"), and the Plummer-Vinson syndrome (glossitis, dysphagia, and esophageal webs) are rare findings.

B. **Laboratory results.** The MCV is usually normal in early iron deficiency. As the Hct falls below 30%, anisocytosis increases and hypochromic microcytic cells appear, followed by a decrease in the MCV. Other findings on the peripheral smear include "pencil cells" and occasional target cells. The platelet count may be increased. Diagnosis requires the documentation of low iron stores, which can usually be accomplished indirectly by measuring serum ferritin.

1. **A serum ferritin level** of less than 10 ng/ml in women or 20 ng/ml in men is indicative of low iron stores. Ferritin is an acute-phase reactant, so that normal levels may be seen in inflammatory states, liver disease, or malignancy despite low iron stores. A serum ferritin level of greater than 200 ng/ml generally indicates adequate iron stores regardless of other underlying conditions. **Serum iron** is usually low (<50 µg/dl), and **total iron-binding capacity** is increased (>420 µg/dl) in iron deficiency, but these values may fluctuate in a number of common clinical conditions and hence are less reliable indicators of iron stores than the serum ferritin.

2. **A bone marrow biopsy** that shows absent staining for iron is the definitive test for establishing iron deficiency and is helpful when the serum ferritin level fails to confirm a diagnosis. Alternatively, a **therapeutic**

challenge with supplemental iron can help determine which anemias are iron responsive.

C. **Therapy** of iron-deficiency anemia requires repleting iron stores with supplemental oral or parenteral iron; normal dietary intake only meets daily losses. With therapy, the reticulocyte count will peak in 5–10 days, and the Hb will rise over 1–2 months. The most common cause of poor response to therapy is noncompliance; other causes, such as poor absorption, continued blood loss, or a multifactorial anemia, must also be considered.

1. **Oral therapy** with ferrous sulfate, 325 mg PO tid (65 mg elemental iron), taken between meals to maximize absorption, usually corrects the anemia and repletes iron stores (as determined by normalization of the serum ferritin) over approximately 6 months. Concomitant use of antacids is an underappreciated cause of an impaired response to oral iron. GI side effects, such as constipation, cramping, diarrhea, or nausea, develop in approximately 25% of patients. These side effects can be decreased by initially administering the drug with meals or once a day and increasing the dose as tolerated. Ferrous gluconate and fumarate at a similar dose are well-tolerated alternative therapies. Polysaccharide iron complex (Niferex) that contains 150 mg elemental iron is as effective as other preparations and seems to have fewer GI side effects. Sustained-release or enteric-coated preparations dissolve poorly and generally should not be recommended. Concomitant administration of vitamin C has been used to maintain the iron in the reduced state and improve absorption.

2. **Parenteral iron therapy** may be useful in patients with (1) poor absorption (e.g., inflammatory bowel disease, malabsorption), (2) very high iron requirements that cannot be met with oral supplementation (e.g., ongoing bleeding), or (3) intolerance of oral preparations. The following formula can be used to approximate the amount of iron that is required to restore the Hb to normal levels and replenish the iron stores:

$$\text{Iron (mg)} = 0.3 \times \text{body weight (lb)} \times (100 - \{[\text{Hb (g/dl)}/14.8] \times 100\})$$

Most patients require 1000–2000 mg iron to correct the deficit. Iron dextran and sodium ferric gluconate are the available parenteral agents. Iron dextran can be administered IM or IV. A single dose of IV iron dextran (diluted in 250–500 ml normal saline and infused at 6 mg/minute) has been used with few complications and is the generally preferred route (*J Lab Clin Med* 111:566, 1988). IM and IV therapy of iron dextran may rarely be complicated by anaphylaxis, and a 0.5-ml IM or IV test dose should be administered 1 hour before therapy is initiated. Delayed reactions to IV iron, such as arthralgia, myalgia, fever, pruritus, and lymphadenopathy, may be seen within 3 days of therapy and usually resolve spontaneously or after treatment with nonsteroidal anti-inflammatory agents. A typical IM dosing schedule is 1 ml (50 mg) into each buttock per week until the total dose is administered. Extravasation into SC tissue may cause staining of the skin; this can be avoided by injecting with a Z-track technique. Local pain and muscle necrosis may also occur. Ferric gluconate has become available as an alternative to iron dextran and can be used in patients who have an adverse reaction to iron dextran. The recommended dosage is 125 mg diluted in 100 ml normal saline infused IV over 1 hour, repeated as needed to achieve the target dose. A 25-mg test dose diluted in 50 ml normal saline and administered over 1 hour is recommended.

II. **The thalassemias** are a heterogeneous group of inherited disorders characterized by underproduction of either the alpha- or beta-globin chains of the Hb molecule. Thalassemia occurs in persons of Mediterranean, African, Middle Eastern, Indian, and Asian descent. In beta-thalassemia, there is a reduced production of beta-globin chains with normal amounts of alpha-globin production. The excess alpha-globin chains form insoluble tetramers in the RBCs, resulting in membrane damage, ineffective erythropoiesis, and hemolytic anemia. In alpha-thalassemia, the beta-tetramers that form are more soluble, and thus the clinical severity is milder. A family history of microcytosis or microcytic anemia may aid in the diagnosis. Splenomegaly and bone abnormalities caused by the expanded marrow are common in more severe forms of thalassemia. A microcytic anemia with hypochromic cells with poikilocytosis, target cells and nucleated RBCs may be present on the peripheral smear. Hb analysis may aid in the diagnosis.

A. **Alpha-thalassemia.** Clinically apparent alpha-thalassemia occurs with a deletion or mutation of three alpha-globin genes, resulting in hemoglobin H (HbH) disease, which is characterized by splenomegaly, chronic hemolytic anemia, and the presence of beta-globin tetramers. A loss of all four alpha-globin genes causes hydrops fetalis. Treatment of HbH disease rarely requires transfusion or splenectomy, but oxidant drugs similar to those that exacerbate G6PD deficiency should be avoided because increased hemolysis may occur.

B. **Beta-thalassemia.** Production of beta-globin chains may be reduced or absent from each allele and are described as beta$^+$-thalassemia or beta°-thalassemia, respectively. Beta-thalassemia is commonly classified by the severity of anemia; many genotypes exist for each phenotype. **Thalassemia minor (trait)** is caused by diminished or absent beta-globin chain synthesis from one gene. Patients are asymptomatic with a hypochromic microcytic anemia (Hb >10 g/dl). **Thalassemia intermedia** is usually associated with dysfunction of both beta-globin genes. Clinical severity is intermediate (Hb 7–10 g/dl), and patients are usually not transfusion dependent. **Thalassemia major** (Cooley's anemia) is caused by severe dysfunction of both beta-globin genes. Anemia is severe, and RBC transfusions are required to sustain life. **Treatment** is centered on RBC transfusions that are adequate to sustain life, improve exercise tolerance, and prevent skeletal abnormalities. In severe forms of thalassemia, the transfusions result in tissue iron overload, which may cause CHF, hepatic dysfunction, glucose intolerance, and secondary hypogonadism due to deposition of iron in the hypothalamus. Iron chelation therapy with deferoxamine mesylate may prevent these complications (see sec. **II.B.3**).

1. **Transfusions.** A Hb of greater than 9 g/dl prevents skeletal deformities and can usually be achieved with 1 unit of RBCs every 2–3 weeks or 2 units every month (see Transfusion Therapy).

2. **Splenectomy** removes the primary site of extravascular hemolysis and should be considered if RBC transfusion requirements increase and exceed one and a half times the previous levels. It should not be performed if the patient is younger than 5–6 years because of the risk of sepsis. To decrease the risk of postsplenectomy sepsis, immunization against *Pneumococcus*, *Haemophilus influenzae,* and *Neisseria meningitidis* should be administered at least 2 weeks before surgery if this was not done previously.

3. **Iron chelation therapy** with deferoxamine mesylate, 50–100 mg/kg/day, is usually administered by continuous SC infusion for 10–12 hours/day beginning in childhood when the iron burden has reached approximately 50 units. Once clinical organ deterioration has begun, it may not be reversible. Therapy may be complicated by local irritation at the injection site, and pruritus and hypotension may occur if the drug is infused too rapidly. Continuous IV infusion of deferoxamine through an indwelling venous catheter at the same dosage and schedule can also be used (*Am J Hematol* 41:61, 1992). Although iron chelation therapy is generally safe, long-term side effects, particularly with high-dose therapy, include optic neuropathy, sensorineural hearing loss, and increased risk of infection. Patients who are receiving deferoxamine should have baseline and yearly vision and hearing examinations.

4. **Bone marrow transplant (BMT)** should be considered in young patients with thalassemia major who have human leukocyte antigen (HLA)-identical related donors.

III. **Myelodysplastic syndrome (MDS)** is an acquired clonal disorder of hematopoietic stem cells that is classified according to morphologic findings on the peripheral smear and bone marrow biopsy: (1) refractory anemia, (2) refractory anemia with ringed sideroblasts, (3) refractory anemia with excess blasts, (4) refractory anemia with excess blasts in transformation, and (5) chronic myelomonocytic leukemia. MDS may be idiopathic or secondary to radiation, chemotherapy, or toxin exposure. Presentations range from mild cytopenias without symptoms to severe pancytopenia. Progression to marrow failure or acute leukemia commonly occurs. **Sideroblastic anemias** are a heterogeneous group of acquired or hereditary disorders characterized by abnormal RBC iron metabolism. Causes of acquired sideroblastic anemia include drugs (Table 20-1), lead toxicity, malignancy, chronic inflammation, and infection.

- A. **Laboratory results.** The MCV is usually normal or slightly elevated in MDS but may be microcytic in some patients with acquired sideroblastic anemia. Serum ferritin levels are normal or elevated. The diagnosis is established by demonstrating abnormal hematopoietic cells in the bone marrow.
- B. **Therapy** of MDS is supportive and rarely curative. Myelosuppressive drugs should be stopped, and nutritional deficiencies should be corrected. **Deferoxamine mesylate** (see sec. II.B.3) should be considered in patients with a good prognosis after 50–100 units of RBCs have been transfused.
    1. **Pyridoxine,** 50–200 mg PO qd, can be tried empirically, although the response rate is low and usually occurs in patients with refractory anemia with ringed sideroblasts.
    2. **Erythropoietin (Epo),** 100–300 units/kg SC three times a week, may be useful in decreasing RBC transfusion requirements in approximately 20% of patients and is more likely to be effective when the serum Epo level is below 200 mU/ml. **Granulocyte colony-stimulating factor,** 1–5 µg/kg SC qd, is likely to result in improved neutrophil counts in patients with neutropenias. The simultaneous use of both growth factors may have a synergistic effect on the erythroid response *(Blood* 87:4076, 1996).
    3. **Chemotherapy** is not usually of benefit for MDS but is frequently attempted in patients in reasonable health; initiating treatment after progression to acute leukemia has a low complete response rate. **BMT** should be considered in patients younger than 50 years of age who have an HLA-identical sibling.
- IV. **The megaloblastic anemias** are a group of disorders associated with altered morphology of hematopoietic cells and other rapidly dividing cells because of abnormalities in DNA synthesis. Almost all cases are because of folic acid or vitamin B_{12} deficiency. **Folic acid deficiency** may develop within a few months, and common causes include (1) decreased intake (alcoholism), (2) malabsorption, and (3) increased utilization (hemolytic anemia, pregnancy). In addition, some drugs (ethanol, trimethoprim, pyrimethamine, methotrexate, sulfasalazine, oral contraceptives, and anticonvulsants) may lead to a perturbed folate metabolism. **Vitamin B_{12} deficiency** takes years to develop because very little of the body's store is used each day. Causes of vitamin B_{12} deficiency include (1) pernicious anemia, (2) gastrectomy, (3) pancreatic insufficiency, (4) GI bacterial overgrowth, (5) ileitis or ileal resection, and (6) intestinal parasites.
    - A. **History and physical examination.** Symptoms are primarily attributable to anemia, although glossitis, jaundice, and splenomegaly may be present. Vitamin B_{12} deficiency may cause decreased vibratory and positional sense, ataxia, paresthesias, confusion, and dementia. Neurologic complications may occur in the absence of anemia and may not resolve completely despite adequate treatment. Folic acid deficiency does not result in neurologic disease.
    - B. **Laboratory results.** A macrocytic anemia is usually present, and leukopenia and thrombocytopenia may occur. The peripheral smear may show anisocytosis, poikilocytosis, and macro-ovalocytes; hypersegmented neutrophils (containing ≥5 nuclear lobes) are common. Lactate dehydrogenase (LDH) and indirect bilirubin are typically elevated, reflecting ineffective erythropoiesis and premature destruction of RBCs.

Table 20-1. Drugs that can induce RBC disorders

Sideroblastic anemia	Aplastic anemia[a]	Hemolytic episode in G6PD deficiency	Immune hemolytic anemia		
			Autoantibody	Hapten	Immune complex[b]
Chloramphenicol	Acetazolamide	Dapsone	α-Methyldopa	Akfluor 25%	Amphotericin B
Cycloserine	Antineoplastic agents	Furazolidone	Cephalosporins	Cephalosporins	Antazoline
Ethanol	Carbamazepine	Methylene blue	Diclofenac	Penicillins	Cephalosporins
Isoniazid	Chloramphenicol	Nalidixic acid	Ibuprofen	Tetracycline	Chlorpropamide
Pyrazinamide	Gold salts	Nitrofurantoin	Interferon-alpha	Tolbutamide	Diclofenac
	Hydantoins	Phenazopyridine	L-Dopa		Diethylstilbestrol
	Penicillamine	Primaquine	Mefenamic acid		Doxepine
	Phenylbutazone	Sulfacetamide	Procainamide		Hydrochlorothiazide
	Quinacrine	Sulfamethoxazole	Teniposide		Isoniazid
		Sulfanilamide	Thioridazine		p-Aminosalicylic acid
		Sulfapyridine	Tolmetin		Probenecid
					Quinidine
					Quinine
					Rifampin
					Sulfonamides
					Thiopental
					Tolmetin

G6PD = glucose-6-phosphate dehydrogenase.
[a]Drugs with more than 30 cases reported; many other drugs rarely are associated with aplastic anemia and are considered low-risk.
[b]Some sources list the mechanism for many of these drugs as unknown.
Source: Data compiled from multiple sources. Agents listed are available in the United States.

1. **Serum vitamin B$_{12}$ and RBC folate levels** should be measured. RBC folate is a more accurate indicator of body folate stores than serum folate, particularly if measured after folate therapy or improved nutrition has been initiated.
2. **Serum methylmalonic acid and homocysteine (HC)** may be useful when the vitamin B$_{12}$ or folate level is equivocal. Methylmalonic acid and HC are elevated in vitamin B$_{12}$ deficiency; only HC is elevated in folic acid deficiency.
3. **A Schilling test** may be useful in the diagnosis of pernicious anemia due to vitamin B$_{12}$ deficiency but rarely affects the therapeutic approach. Detecting **antibodies to intrinsic factor** is specific for the diagnosis of pernicious anemia.
4. **Bone marrow biopsy** may be necessary to rule out MDS and hematologic malignancy; these disorders may present with findings similar to those of megaloblastic anemia on peripheral smear.

C. **Therapy** is directed toward replacing the deficient factor. Symptomatic hypokalemia may occur within 48 hours of initiating therapy, and supplemental potassium may be needed. Blood transfusions are rarely required and may be associated with volume overload when used for these disorders. With therapy, the reticulocytosis should begin within 1 week, followed by a rising Hb over 6–8 weeks. Coexisting iron deficiency is present in one-third of patients and is a common cause for an incomplete response to therapy.

1. **Folic acid** can be administered at 1 mg PO qd until the deficiency is corrected. High doses of folic acid (5 mg PO qd) may be needed in patients with malabsorption syndromes.
2. **Vitamin B$_{12}$** deficiency is corrected by administering cyanocobalamin. A typical schedule is 1 mg IM qd for 7 days, then weekly for 1–2 months or until normalization of the Hb occurs. Long-term therapy is 1 mg/month.

V. **Anemia of chronic renal insufficiency** is attributed primarily to decreased endogenous Epo production and may occur as the creatinine clearance declines below approximately 50 ml/minute.

A. **Laboratory results.** The Hct is usually 20–30%, and the MCV is normal. On peripheral smear the RBCs are normochromic, with the occasional presence of echinocytes (burr cells) or acanthocytes (spur cells).

B. **Treatment** of anemia of chronic renal insufficiency has been revolutionized by the availability of recombinant human Epo. Therapy is indicated in predialysis and dialysis patients who are symptomatic. Objective benefits of reversing the anemia include enhanced exercise capacity, improved cognitive function, elimination of RBC transfusions, and reduction of iron overload. Subjective benefits include increased energy, enhanced appetite, better sleep patterns, and improved sexual activity.

1. **Administration of Epo** can be IV (hemodialysis patients) or SC (predialysis or peritoneal dialysis patients). More than 97% of patients increase their Hct by 10 points or to a level greater than 32% within 12 weeks of therapy. A typical initial dosage is 50–100 units/kg three times a week until the Hct reaches 32%; the average maintenance dosage is 75 units/kg three times a week. Approximately 10% of patients need more than 200 units/kg three times a week. It may be possible to give SC therapy less often than IV to maintain the Hct, and the SC route appears to have better pharmacokinetics, resulting in lower doses required.
2. **Adverse reactions** to Epo therapy are uncommon. Hypertension may develop or worsen in some patients while the Hct is increasing. Seizures may occur, although the etiology is not well characterized.
3. **Suboptimal responses** may occur with coexisting iron deficiency; thus, many patients benefit from IV iron supplementation. Chronic inflammatory conditions and acute or chronic bleeding affect the response to Epo as well. Hemodialysis patients may also suffer from aluminum intoxication, which blunts the response to Epo. Secondary hyper-

parathyroidism that causes bone marrow fibrosis and relative Epo resistance may also occur.

VI. **Anemia of chronic disease** often develops in patients with long-standing inflammatory diseases, malignancy, autoimmune disorders, and chronic infection. Abnormalities in iron metabolism, Epo production, anclin response to endogenous Epo, as well as humoral inhibition of erythropoiesis have all been implicated in the pathogenesis.

A. **Laboratory results.** A normocytic normochromic anemia is typical. The peripheral smear is usually normal, although microcytes may be present. **Ferritin** is generally normal but may be elevated because it is an acute-phase reactant. No laboratory test is diagnostic for the anemia of chronic disease.

B. **Treatment** is directed at the underlying cause and at eliminating exacerbating factors such as nutritional deficiencies and marrow-suppressive drugs. Doses of Epo that are effective are higher than those reported in renal anemia. A variety of doses and schedules have been reported and vary from 150 to 1500 units/kg/week. If no response has been observed at 900 units/kg/week, further escalation is unlikely to be effective. Treatment should only be considered in patients with symptoms of severe anemia or a Hb of less than 10 g/dl.

C. **Anemia in cancer patients** who are receiving chemotherapy may be successfully prevented and treated with Epo at dosages of 100–150 units/kg three times a week. In anemic patients with myeloma or non-Hodgkin's lymphoma, a dosage of 200 units/kg/week is usually effective in those with residual marrow function (as indicated by a normal platelet count), whereas a dosage of 500 units/kg/week is recommended in patients with a hypoproliferative anemia (*Blood* 89:4248, 1997).

VII. **Anemia associated with HIV infection** is common. In many cases dysplasia similar to that seen in MDS is found on bone marrow examination. Treatment with Epo at weekly doses of 24,000–48,000 units should be considered in symptomatic anemic patients with a serum Epo level of less than 500 mU/ml. Certain situations warrant specific mention.

A. *Mycobacterium avium* **complex** infections are frequently associated with severe anemia, and this may occur in the absence of other cytopenias. This diagnosis should be considered in patients in whom new-onset or worsening anemia develops. The treatment of *M. avium* complex is described in Chap. 15.

B. **Parvovirus B19** should be considered in HIV-infected patients with transfusion-dependent anemia and a low reticulocyte count. Antiparvovirus antibodies, which develop in immunocompetent patients and provide long-term immunity, are typically not elevated in HIV-infected patients. Treatment with IV immune globulin (IVIG; 0.4 g/kg IV qd for 5–10 days) typically results in erythropoietic recovery. Relapses have occurred between 2 and 6 months and can be successfully managed with intermittent IVIG at an empiric maintenance dose of 0.4 g/kg IV for 1 day given every 4 weeks (*Ann Intern Med* 113:926, 1990).

C. **Zidovudine** induces a macrocytic anemia in all treated patients. Epo (100–200 units/kg SC 3 times/week) improves the Hct in patients with an endogenous Epo level of ≤500 mU/ml. RBC transfusion requirements are decreased by approximately one-half, and up to 40% of patients become transfusion independent. No hematologic benefit occurs if the serum Epo level is ≥500 mU/ml (*Ann Intern Med* 117:739, 1992).

VIII. **Pancytopenia** may occur in a variety of situations, including MDS, acute leukemia, HIV infection, and infiltration of the marrow with tumor or granuloma. In immunocompromised patients, pancytopenia is frequently due to immunosuppressive agents or viral infection. A bone marrow examination is frequently required to establish the diagnosis. **Aplastic anemia** is an acquired abnormality of bone marrow stem cells that may present with pancytopenia. Most cases are idiopathic, although approximately 20% are associated with drug or chemical exposure (see Table 20-1) and another 10% are associated with viral illnesses [e.g., viral hepatitis, Epstein-Barr virus, cytomegalovirus

(CMV)]. Presenting symptoms are usually due to anemia or thrombocytopenia, although some patients present with fever and leukopenia. **Therapy** for aplastic anemia is supportive and potentially curative. Any suspected offending drugs should be discontinued and exacerbating factors corrected.

A. **Early referral** to a center experienced in managing aplastic anemia is recommended. When feasible, BMT from an HLA-identical sibling is generally recommended and has achieved a long-term survival of 60–70%. **Immunosuppressive treatment** with cyclosporine, glucocorticoids, and antithymocyte globulin should be considered in patients who do not undergo a BMT.

B. **Transfusions** with RBCs should be kept to a minimum. Prophylactic platelet transfusions are generally recommended if the platelet count is below 10,000/μl. Transfusion with blood products from family members should be avoided while BMT is being considered.

C. **Infection.** Patients should be instructed to seek medical attention immediately in the event of fever over 38.5°C. Fevers with neutropenia require a diagnostic and empiric antimicrobial regimen similar to that used in patients with chemotherapy-induced myelosuppression (see Chap. 21).

Anemias Associated with Increased Red Blood Cell Loss or Destruction

Anemias associated with increased erythropoiesis (i.e., an elevated reticulocyte count) are caused by bleeding or destruction of RBCs (hemolysis) and may exceed the capacity of normal bone marrow to correct the Hct. Typically, the bilirubin and LDH are normal in the bleeding patient and elevated in the patient with hemolysis.

I. **Bleeding is much more common than hemolysis.** Hidden sites of bleeding (retroperitoneum, fractured hip) may result in laboratory findings that are similar to those seen with a hemolytic process. All patients with suspected hemolysis should have a direct antiglobulin test (DAT, or direct Coombs' test). This test detects the presence of immunoglobulin G (IgG) and the third component of complement (C3) on the surface of RBCs and usually differentiates between immune and nonimmune causes of hemolysis. Treatment of the bleeding patient is discussed in Transfusion Therapy.

II. **Hemolytic anemias** are characterized by the predominant site of hemolysis.

A. **Intravascular hemolysis** may present with fever, chills, tachycardia, and backache. Serum haptoglobin levels decrease markedly, as this protein binds and removes Hb from the plasma. If hemolysis is severe, free Hb can be measured in the plasma and urine. Renal failure may develop with hemoglobinuria.

B. **Extravascular hemolysis** is characterized by RBC destruction in the reticuloendothelial system, primarily the spleen. Jaundice and splenomegaly may be present. Haptoglobin levels are normal or slightly reduced.

III. **Sickle cell disease** includes homozygous sickle cell anemia (HbSS) and other sickling syndromes with double-heterozygous conditions (HbS-beta thalassemia, HbSC). These disorders are associated with structurally abnormal Hb molecules that polymerize under reduced oxygen conditions. The clinical features are a consequence of a chronic hemolytic anemia and vaso-occlusive ischemic tissue injury. **Sickle cell trait** occurs in individuals who are heterozygous for HbS. A monograph on sickle cell disease is available and provides useful guidelines (National Institutes of Health publication No. 95-2117 at www.nhlbi.nih.gov/health/prof/blood/sickle).

A. **Clinical manifestations** of sickle cell disease vary widely. Treatment is determined by the specific complications that occur. Individuals with sickle cell trait are usually healthy but appear to have an increased risk of sudden death with rigorous exercise.

B. Laboratory results. The Hb ranges from 5 to 10 g/dl in sickle cell anemia, and the MCV may be slightly elevated due to the increased reticulocyte count. Chronic neutrophilia (10,000–20,000/mm^3) is often present, and the platelet count may be increased. The peripheral smear will show the classic distorted sickle-shaped erythrocytes. Howell-Jolly bodies may be seen because of functional asplenism, which usually occurs by the age of 10 years. Target cells may be present, particularly in HbS–beta-thalassemia and HbSC. Hb analysis distinguishes HbSS from sickle cell trait and other abnormal Hbs.

C. Prevention and health maintenance

1. **Dehydration and hypoxia** should be avoided because they may precipitate or exacerbate sickling. Intense exercise, activities at high altitude, and flying in unpressurized aircraft should be strongly discouraged.

2. **Folic acid,** 1 mg PO qd, should be administered to patients with sickle cell disease because of chronic hemolysis.

3. **Antimicrobial prophylaxis** with penicillin VK, 125 mg PO bid up to age 3 years, then 250 mg PO bid until 5 years, is effective in reducing the risk of infection. Patients who are allergic to penicillin should receive erythromycin, 10 mg/kg PO bid. In most patients, antimicrobial prophylaxis should be discontinued after 5 years of age (*J Pediatr* 127:685, 1995).

4. **Immunizations** against the usual childhood illnesses should be given to children with sickle cell disease. After 2 years of age, a polyvalent pneumococcal vaccine should be administered. Hepatitis B vaccine is recommended for hepatitis B surface antibody–negative patients. Yearly influenza vaccine is recommended.

5. **Regular yearly ophthalmologic examinations** are recommended in adults because of a high incidence of proliferative retinopathy leading to vitreous hemorrhage and retinal detachment. Laser photocoagulation is effective in preventing these complications.

6. **Surgery and anesthesia.** Local and regional anesthesia can be used without special precautions. With general anesthesia, measures to avoid volume depletion, hypoxia, and hypernatremia are crucial. For major surgery, RBC transfusions to increase the Hb concentration to 10 g/dl seem to be as effective as more aggressive transfusion regimens in most circumstances (*N Engl J Med* 333:206, 1995).

D. Infections in adults typically occur in tissues that are susceptible to vaso-occlusive infarcts (bone, kidney, lung). Treatment of osteomyelitis should be directed by culture of biopsied tissue. *Staphylococcus, Salmonella,* and enteric organisms are most common. Urinary tract infections should be treated based on the culture data. Pneumonia is most likely to be caused by *Mycoplasma, Staphylococcus aureus,* or *H. influenzae* and must be distinguished from acute chest syndrome (see sec. **III.F.2**). In patients with indwelling venous access devices, infection with *Staphylococcus* is common.

E. Complications of chronic hemolysis

1. **Aplastic crisis** is characterized by a sudden decrease in Hb and reticulocyte count. This crisis is usually a complication of infection with parvovirus B19. Transfusion with RBCs is the mainstay of therapy, and most patients recover in 10–14 days. Patients who are suspected of having a parvovirus infection should be in respiratory isolation to prevent exposure to other susceptible patients and pregnant women.

2. **Cholelithiasis,** primarily with bilirubin stones, is present in more than 50% of adult patients. Acute cholecystitis should be treated medically, and cholecystectomy should be performed when the attack subsides. Elective cholecystectomy for asymptomatic gallstones is controversial.

F. Acute vaso-occlusive complications

1. **Vaso-occlusive pain crises** are the most common manifestation of sickle cell disease. Pain is typically in the back, ribs, and limbs and lasts

for 5–7 days. The pattern of pain is usually consistent in any one patient from crisis to crisis. A deviation from the pattern may suggest another diagnosis such as cholecystitis. Precipitating factors such as an infection should be excluded. Many painful episodes are managed on an outpatient basis with PO fluids (3–4 L/day) and analgesia. Patients who require parenteral opioids, who cannot consume adequate PO fluids, or in whom another complication is suspected (infection, acute chest syndrome) require hospital admission. Morphine (0.3–0.6 mg/kg PO q4h or 0.1–0.15 mg/kg IV q3–4h) is the drug of choice for moderate or severe pain. Supplemental oxygen does not benefit acute pain crisis unless hypoxia is present. **RBC transfusions do not change the immediate course of an acute pain crisis.** Some patients do not require significant amounts of analgesic therapy between crises, although opioids may be required by others. Patients who experience severe recurrent pain crisis that requires frequent medical intervention may benefit from chronic partial exchange transfusions or treatment with hydroxyurea (see sec. **III.H.2**).

2. **Acute chest syndrome** is associated with chest pain, pulmonary infiltrates, leukocytosis, and hypoxia and is indistinguishable from pneumonia. The most frequently identified pathogens are *Chlamydia pneumoniae*, *Mycoplasma* species, respiratory syncytial virus, and *S. aureus*. Initial management should include hospitalization, administration of supplemental oxygen to correct hypoxia, adequate analgesia, and empiric coverage with antimicrobials. Transfusion of RBCs is recommended in most cases, and exchange transfusion should be considered in patients with multiple-lobe involvement, worsening disease, or hypoxemia (arterial oxygen tension <60 mm Hg) (*N Engl J Med* 342:1859, 2000).

3. **Splenic sequestration crisis** is associated with sudden splenomegaly due to pooling of blood into the spleen, hypovolemic shock, and sudden death. Hemodynamic support and RBC transfusions are usually required. This complication generally occurs in patients with an intact spleen, such as infants with HbSS or adults with HbSC or HbS–beta$^+$-thalassemia.

4. **Priapism** refers to painful erection from vaso-occlusion, which may respond to hydration and analgesics. Transfusions and surgical drainage should be considered for acute events that last longer than 24 hours. Permanent impotence can occur.

G. Chronic organ damage

1. **Osteonecrosis** of the femoral and humeral heads may cause considerable morbidity in approximately 10% of patients. Treatment consists of local heat, analgesics, and avoidance of weight bearing. Hip and shoulder arthroplasty may be effective in decreasing symptoms and improving function and should be considered.

2. **Stroke** occurs most commonly in children younger than 10 years and is usually caused by cerebral infarction. Without treatment approximately two-thirds of patients will experience recurrent stroke. Long-term transfusions to maintain the HbS concentration at less than 50% for a minimum of 5 years reduce the incidence of recurrence.

3. **Leg ulcers** should be treated with rest, leg elevation, and intensive local care. Wet-to-dry dressings should be applied every 4–6 hours to débride the ulcer. Local care with moist occlusive dressings and control of edema with leg elevation, Ace wraps, and careful diuresis are usually helpful. An Unna's boot (zinc oxide–impregnated bandage), changed weekly for 3–4 weeks, can be used for nonhealing or more extensive ulcers. Otherwise, long-term transfusions, split-thickness skin grafts, and free-flap grafts may be necessary.

4. **Renal tubular defects** caused by sickling in the anoxic hyperosmolar environment of the renal medulla may lead to isosthenuria (inability to

concentrate urine) and hematuria in sickle cell disease and sickle cell trait. These conditions predispose patients to dehydration, which increases the risk of vaso-occlusive events.

H. Treatment

1. **RBC transfusions** are indicated for patients with strokes, transient ischemic attacks, acute chest syndrome, and priapism that is unresponsive to supportive care, and in preparation for general anesthesia. Guidelines for chronic transfusions should be followed (see Transfusion Therapy).

2. **Hydroxyurea** (15–35 mg/kg PO qd) has been shown to increase levels of fetal Hb and decrease the incidence of vaso-occlusive pain episodes by approximately 50% in adults with sickle cell anemia (*N Engl J Med* 332:1317, 1995).

IV. Glucose 6-phosphate dehydrogenase deficiency is the most common of the hereditary RBC enzyme deficiencies. It is a sex-linked disorder that typically affects men. The enzyme deficiency results in RBCs that are more susceptible to oxidant stress than normal RBCs, leading to chronic or episodic hemolysis.

A. Classification. A mild form of the deficiency occurs in approximately 10% of African-American men and is characterized by hemolytic episodes that are triggered by infections or drug exposure (see Table 20-1). A more severe enzyme deficiency, such as the Mediterranean variety, results in hemolysis when susceptible individuals are exposed to fava beans. The most severe type causes a chronic, hereditary, nonspherocytic hemolytic anemia in the absence of an inciting cause.

B. Laboratory results. The peripheral smear shows "bite cells"; RBC inclusions **(Heinz bodies)** are seen with special stains. Measurement of enzyme levels usually establishes the diagnosis. However, senescent RBCs contain less G6PD and are more easily destroyed than younger cells so that after a hemolytic episode, the G6PD level may be normal, reflecting the younger population of cells in the circulation.

C. Treatment consists of adequate hydration to protect renal function during hemolysis, avoidance of precipitating factors, and, if necessary, RBC transfusion.

V. Autoimmune hemolytic anemia (AIHA) is caused by antibodies to RBCs. In warm AIHA, antibodies interact best with RBCs at 37°C, whereas in cold AIHA, antibodies are most active at lower temperatures. The DAT is often positive in both forms of AIHA.

A. Warm antibody AIHA is usually caused by an IgG autoantibody. It may be idiopathic or associated with an underlying malignancy (lymphoma, chronic lymphocytic leukemia), collagen vascular disorder, or drugs (see Table 20-1).

1. **Clinical presentation** may include weakness, jaundice, and splenomegaly. Severe hemolysis may be associated with fever, chest pain, syncope, symptoms of CHF, and hemoglobinuria.

2. **Laboratory findings** include a decrease in haptoglobin, an increase in LDH, and a positive DAT for IgG. The peripheral smear shows spherocytes.

3. **Therapy** should be directed at identifying and treating any underlying cause. In most cases the hemolysis should be treated with glucocorticoids or splenectomy, or both. The approach to treatment is similar to that of immune thrombocytopenic purpura (see Chap. 19). **RBC transfusions** are occasionally necessary in severe cases and pose a special problem. The conventional cross-matching procedure is difficult because autoantibodies are commonly present in the serum so that alloantibodies may escape detection, posing a risk of hemolysis. Treatment with folic acid is also recommended.

B. Cold antibody AIHA is associated with episodic cold-induced hemolysis and vaso-occlusive events resulting in cyanosis of the ears, nose, fingers, and toes. When transfusions are indicated, the blood should be warmed to 37°C to prevent exacerbation of hemolysis. **Cold agglutinin disease** is the most common syndrome. It may be chronic and caused by a paraprotein (lymphoma, Waldenström's macroglobulinemia) in approximately one-half of cases or acute and transient, secondary to an infection (*Mycoplasma*, mononucleosis). Immunoglobulin M (IgM) and C3 are found on the RBCs (the DAT identifies only the presence of C3). Hemolysis is extravascular. Treatment is directed at the underlying disease; the acute form usually requires only supportive measures.

VI. Drug-induced hemolytic anemia may be caused by any of three distinct mechanisms. In all cases, treatment consists of discontinuing the offending agent. Medications known to cause these effects are listed in Table 20-1.

   A. Drug-induced autoantibodies present similarly to warm antibody AIHA. The DAT is positive for IgG, and the anemia gradually resolves after discontinuation of the drug.

   B. Haptens form when a drug (usually an antimicrobial) coats RBC membranes, forming a new antigenic determinant. If antibodies against the drug are present and the patient receives the drug (particularly at high doses), a DAT-positive hemolytic anemia may result.

   C. Immune complexes. IgM (occasionally IgG) antibodies may develop against a drug and form a drug-antibody complex that adheres to RBCs. Because the antibody involved is usually an IgM, the DAT will be positive only for C3.

VII. Microangiopathic hemolytic anemia is a syndrome of traumatic intravascular hemolysis that is thought to be caused by deposition of fibrin strands in the lumen of small blood vessels. It may be seen in disseminated intravascular coagulation (DIC), thrombotic thrombocytopenic purpura, hemolytic-uremic syndrome, severe hypertension, vasculitis, eclampsia, and some disseminated malignancies. The peripheral smear shows schistocytes (fragmented RBCs) and frequently thrombocytopenia. Management of DIC, thrombotic thrombocytopenic purpura, and hemolytic-uremic syndrome is described in Chap. 19. **Traumatic (macroangiopathic) hemolytic anemia** refers to intravascular hemolysis that is most commonly associated with a malfunctioning prosthetic aortic valve. Porcine valves or valves in the mitral position are not as likely to cause significant hemolysis. The peripheral smear shows schistocytes, and therapy involves correction of the mechanical abnormality.

Transfusion Therapy

Advances in collection, preparation, and administration have allowed transfusion of blood components to become useful in a wide variety of clinical situations. However, blood products are a limited resource, and their administration exposes the patient to the risk of a number of adverse effects, some of which may be life threatening. **The benefits and risks of transfusion therapy must be carefully weighed in each situation.** In each case, the indications for transfusion should be recorded in the medical record. It is generally agreed that, if possible, informed consent should be obtained for the administration of all blood products. In elective surgery, this may require informing the patient several weeks in advance of the procedure so that the options of autologous donation and directed donation can be explored.

   I. RBC transfusion is indicated to increase the oxygen-carrying capacity of blood in anemic patients when the anemia is responsible for poor tissue oxygenation. Adequate tissue oxygenation can usually be attained with a Hb of 7–8 g/dl in a normovolemic patient. One unit of RBCs increases the Hb by 1 g/dl in the average adult. Patient age, cause and severity of anemia, and coexisting disorders such as cardiopulmonary disease must be considered when determining the need for transfusion. If the cause of anemia is easily treatable (e.g., iron or folic acid deficiency) and no cerebrovascular or cardiopulmonary compromise is present, it is preferable to avoid transfusions. RBCs should not be used as volume expanders, to enhance wound healing, or to improve general "well-being" if symptoms are not related to anemia. Many options are available to the responsible physician regarding the preparation and administration of blood (e.g., types of filter, flow rates), and these should be detailed in the medical orders.

II. Preparation and administration of RBCs

A. The type and screen procedure tests the recipient's RBCs for the A, B, and D (Rh) antigen and also screens the recipient's serum for antibodies against other RBC antigens. **Cross matching** tests the patient's serum for antibodies against antigens on the donor's RBCs and is performed before a specific unit of blood is dispensed for a patient.

B. Leukocyte-depleting (Leukopoor) filters remove 99.9% of WBCs from blood products and are recommended in the following circumstances: (1) in patients who have had one or more nonhemolytic febrile transfusion reactions that were not responsive to acetaminophen and diphenhydramine, (2) in patients who are undergoing RBC exchange transfusions, (3) in patients in whom cross-match incompatibilities are identified, and (4) to prevent CMV infection in patients who require CMV-negative blood products that are not available. Leukocyte-depleting filters may also be helpful to decrease the risk of platelet alloimmunization (*Ann Intern Med* 117:151, 1992).

C. Irradiation of blood products eliminates immunologically competent lymphocytes and is recommended for immunocompromised bone marrow or organ transplant recipients or for any patient who is receiving directed donations from HLA-matched donors or first-degree relatives.

D. Washed RBCs should be considered in patients in whom plasma proteins may cause a serious reaction [e.g., immunoglobulin A (IgA)-deficient recipients or patients with paroxysmal nocturnal hemoglobinuria].

E. CMV-negative blood products are indicated in immunocompromised bone marrow or organ transplant recipients who are CMV antibody negative.

F. Premedication with acetaminophen and diphenhydramine, 25–50 mg PO or IV, is recommended in all patients who are receiving RBC transfusion. Occasionally, glucocorticoids (e.g., hydrocortisone, 50–100 mg IV) are also of benefit in patients with previous nonhemolytic reactions.

G. Administration. Patient and blood product identification procedures must be carefully followed to avoid mishandling errors. The IV catheter should be at least 18 gauge to allow adequate flow. All blood products that are not leukocyte depleted should be administered through a 170- to 260-μm "standard" filter to prevent infusion of macroaggregates, fibrin, and debris. Only 0.9% NaCl should be used with blood components to prevent cell lysis. Patients should be observed for the first 5–10 minutes of each transfusion for adverse side effects and at regular intervals thereafter. Each unit of blood should be administered within 4 hours.

III. Risks are incurred with all blood component therapy. Patient concerns are primarily focused on transfusion-associated viral infections.

A. Infection. Current testing for viral infections includes HIV-1, HIV-2, human T-lymphotropic virus type-1 (HTLV-1), hepatitis B virus, and hepatitis C virus. The risk of transfusion-associated transmission of HIV-1, HIV-2, and HTLV-1 from screened blood is estimated to be 1 in 500,000. Estimates of hepatitis B and hepatitis C virus transmission are approximately 1 in 100,000. Viral infections occur when donors are in the seronegative window period, allowing the infection to escape detection. CMV transmission from RBC and platelet transfusion is an important risk in immunocompromised patients. CMV-negative blood products are recommended, but leukocyte-depleting filters seem to be effective in decreasing the risk. Bacterial transmission may occur, and the risk increases with prolonged storage time; *Yersinia* is most frequently described with RBC transfusions.

B. Hemolytic transfusion reactions

1. Acute hemolytic reactions are usually caused by preformed antibodies in the recipient and are characterized by intravascular hemolysis of the transfused RBCs soon after the administration of the incompatible blood.

Fever, chills, back pain, chest pain, nausea, vomiting, and symptoms related to hypotension may develop. Acute renal failure with hemoglobinuria may occur. In the unconscious patient, hypotension or hemoglobinuria may be the only manifestation. If a hemolytic transfusion reaction is suspected, the transfusion should be stopped immediately and all IV tubing should be replaced. Clotted and ethylenediaminetetra-acetic acid (EDTA)–treated samples of the patient's blood should be delivered to the blood bank along with the remainder of the suspected unit for repeat of the cross match. Serum bilirubin and tests for DIC should be obtained, and the plasma and freshly voided urine should be examined for free Hb. Management includes preservation of intravascular volume and protection of renal function. Urine output should be maintained at 100 ml/hour or greater with the use of IV fluids and diuretics or mannitol, if necessary. The excretion of free Hb can be aided by alkalinization of the urine. Sodium bicarbonate can be added to IV fluids to increase the urinary pH to 7.5 or greater.

2. **Delayed hemolytic transfusion reactions** may occur within 3–4 weeks after transfusion and are caused by either a primary or anamnestic antibody response to specific RBC antigens. Usually the Hb and Hct fall and the bilirubin increases. While hemolysis is ongoing, the DAT may be positive, resulting in confusion with AIHA. Delayed hemolytic transfusion reaction may at times be severe; these cases should be treated similarly to acute hemolytic reactions.

C. **Nonhemolytic febrile transfusion reactions** are characterized by fevers, chills, urticaria, pruritus, and respiratory distress and are usually seen in previously transfused patients or multiparous women. Antibodies against donor plasma proteins or leukocyte antigens are thought to be the cause. Treatment of symptoms with acetaminophen for fever and diphenhydramine, 25–50 mg PO or IV, is usually sufficient. Rarely, epinephrine or glucocorticoids are required. Meperidine, 25–50 mg IV, is effective in preventing shaking chills. Some patients may require premedication with acetaminophen and diphenhydramine, or leukocyte-depleting filters to prevent recurrence with subsequent transfusions. **Anaphylactic reactions** may be seen in patients with IgA deficiency who receive IgA-containing blood products and develop anti-IgA antibodies.

D. **Volume overload** with signs of CHF may be seen when patients with cardiovascular compromise are transfused with RBCs. Slowing the rate of transfusion and judicious use of diuretics help prevent this complication.

E. **Transfusion-related acute lung injury (TRALI)** is indistinguishable from adult respiratory distress syndrome and occurs within 4 hours of a transfusion. Antileukocyte antibodies are frequently identified in the donor's serum, causing dyspnea, hypotension, fever, chills, and hypoxemia. A number of patients require ventilatory assistance. Despite clinical or radiographic findings that suggest edema, available data indicate that diuretics have no role and may be detrimental.

F. **Transfusion-associated graft-versus-host disease** is usually seen in immunocompromised patients and is thought to result from the infusion of immunocompetent T lymphocytes. This entity has been reported in immunocompetent patients who share an HLA haplotype with HLA-homozygous blood donors (usually a relative or members of inbred populations). Rash, elevated liver function tests, and severe pancytopenia are seen. The mortality is greater than 80%. Irradiation of blood products prevents this disease (see sec. II.C). Because the chances of shared HLA haplotypes with a random blood donor are extremely low, irradiation of nonrelated blood products is not indicated for the immunocompetent patient.

G. **Posttransfusion purpura** is a rare syndrome of severe thrombocytopenia and purpura or bleeding that starts 7–10 days after exposure to blood products that contain platelets. The disorder is described in Chap. 19.

IV. **Adverse effects due to massive transfusion.** Administration of blood products greater than the normal blood volume of the patient in a 24-hour period **(massive transfusion)** may be associated with several additional complications.
  A. **Hypothermia** caused by rapid infusion of chilled blood may cause cardiac dysrhythmias. A blood-warming device can prevent this problem.
  B. **Citrate intoxication** occurs in patients with hepatic dysfunction and can cause hypocalcemia, resulting in paresthesias, tetany, hypotension, and decreased cardiac output. On rare occasions the patient may require calcium gluconate, 10 ml of a 10% solution IV. Calcium should never be added directly to the transfusion product because it may cause the blood to clot.
  C. **Acidemia and hyperkalemia** may occur. Hyperkalemia is not usually significant unless the patient was hyperkalemic before transfusion (e.g., because of renal failure or muscle injury). Twenty-four hours after massive transfusion, hypokalemia may occur as RBCs become more metabolically active and take up potassium from the plasma.
  D. **Bleeding complications** from dilution of platelets and plasma coagulation factors may be seen during massive transfusion. Correction of platelet and coagulation factor deficiencies should be based on clinical findings and laboratory monitoring rather than an empiric formula.
V. **Long-term RBC transfusion therapy** is indicated in a variety of diseases. These patients likely will require either premedication or leukocyte-depleting filters to prevent nonhemolytic febrile reactions. Transfusion burdens in excess of approximately 50 units of RBCs require consideration of iron chelation therapy (see Anemias Associated with Decreased Red Blood Cell Production). Consideration should also be given to performing an expanded RBC antigen panel to determine RBC phenotypic matches and decrease the risk of RBC alloimmunization and delayed hemolytic transfusion reactions.
VI. **Emergency RBC transfusions** should be used only in situations in which massive blood loss has resulted in cardiovascular compromise. Volume expansion with normal saline should be attempted initially. Blood typing can be performed in 10 minutes and cross matching within 30 minutes in emergency situations. If unmatched blood must be used, it should be group O/Rh-negative type that has been previously screened for reactive antibodies. At the first sign of a transfusion reaction, the infusion should be stopped.
VII. **Approach to patients who are unwilling or unable to receive RBC transfusions.** The treatment of acute or severe anemia in which transfusions are not an option (i.e., patient refusal) raises difficult issues for the health care team. Understanding and documentation of any ethical or religious preferences and the patient's beliefs (e.g., Jehovah's Witness) along with early consultation with any liaison groups help to avoid confrontation and delay in therapy. Management includes reducing blood loss by phlebotomy and obtaining necessary testing in pediatric tubes. Hemorrhagic losses, particularly related to surgical blood loss, should be pursued aggressively. Blood production can be maximized with Epo, 100–300 units/kg SC daily for several days, then three times per week. An increase in Hb of 1–2 g/dl over about a week is generally observed. IV iron therapy may also be beneficial (see Anemias Associated with Decreased Red Blood Cell Production, sec. **I.C.2**).

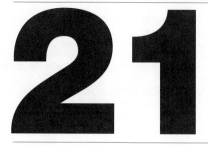

Medical Management of Malignant Disease

Joanne E. Mortimer
and Randy Brown

Approach to the Cancer Patient

I. **General.** Before chemotherapy or radiation therapy is initiated, all patients should have a diagnosis of cancer based on tissue pathology, and, if possible, a clinical, biochemical, or radiographic marker of disease should be identified to assess the results of therapy.

A. **Stage and grade of tumor.** Stage is a clinical or pathologic assessment of tumor spread. The major roles of staging are to determine local and regional disease amenable to surgical and radiation therapy and to define the optimal therapy and prognosis in subsets of patients. The **grade** of a tumor defines its retention of characteristics compared to the cell of origin and is designated as low, moderate, or high as the tissue loses its normal appearance.

B. **Therapy. Induction** is the chemotherapy used to achieve a complete remission. **Consolidation chemotherapy** is administered to patients who initially respond to treatment. **Maintenance therapy** refers to low-dose, outpatient treatment used to prolong remissions; its use has proved effective in a few malignancies. **Adjuvant chemotherapy** is given after complete surgical or radiologic eradication of a primary malignancy to eliminate any presumed but unmeasurable metastatic disease.

C. **Response to treatment** can be defined either by clinical or pathologic criteria. A **complete response** (or remission) is achieved when all evidence of malignancy is eradicated. A **partial response** is defined as a decrease in tumor mass by more than 50%.

D. **Palliative care and pain therapy.** Pain is present at diagnosis in 5–10% of patients with localized cancer and 60–90% of patients with metastases. Improved oral analgesics, use of indwelling venous access devices, development of home nursing care agencies, and public acceptance of the hospice philosophy now allow patients to receive a large portion of their palliative treatment out of the hospital. Successful treatment of the underlying disease usually provides relief of pain. Painful foci of disease that is refractory to systemic intervention can be controlled with local radiation therapy, regional nerve block, or an ablative surgical procedure. In many situations, however, analgesics are necessary (see Chap. 1). Nonopioid analgesics should be used initially, followed by opioid analgesics as needed. Medication administered on a prescribed schedule is more effective in maintaining analgesia than that taken intermittently once pain has developed. **Sustained-release morphine** (30–60 mg PO q8–12h) or **long-acting oxycodone** (10–40 mg PO q8–12h) is particularly effective in the management of chronic pain. An immediate-release preparation (such as morphine or oxycodone) should be administered PO q2–3h for "breakthrough pain" until adequate analgesia has been achieved with long-acting preparations. Occasionally, infusions of morphine, 3–5 mg/hour IV, increased by 2–4 mg/hour as needed, are necessary. When a morphine drip is used, the patient must be monitored for respiratory depression, and **naloxone,** 2 ampules IV (0.4 mg/

ampule), should be available at the patient's bedside. Under supervision, morphine drips can be used in the home setting. Although tolerance and physical dependency can develop with long-term narcotic administration, drug abuse and psychological dependency seldom occur in the setting of chronic pain from cancer. **These concerns should not compromise the patient's ability to achieve adequate analgesia.**

II. Therapy of selected solid tumors. Recommendations regarding specific chemotherapeutic regimens are beyond the scope of this chapter. This section defines guidelines for a treatment plan, but consultation with an oncologist should be obtained before drug and dosage are selected.

A. Breast cancer

1. **Approach to an undiagnosed lump in the breast.** Breast cancer will develop in approximately 11% of women in the United States. A breast lump in a premenopausal woman is less likely to be cancerous than a breast lump in a postmenopausal woman. In a younger woman, a mass should be observed for 1 month to identify any cyclic changes that suggest benign disease. If the mass is still present, bilateral mammography should be performed. The accuracy of mammography to diagnose cancer in pre- and postmenopausal women is approximately 90%. Estrogen receptor (ER) and progesterone receptor levels and her-2 analysis (by gene amplification or protein expression) should be measured with all newly diagnosed breast cancers.

2. **Surgical options.** Treatment is focused on local control and the risk of systemic spread. Local control with **tylectomy** (lumpectomy and axillary lymph node dissection) is as effective as a modified radical mastectomy. An axillary lymph node dissection should be included because it provides prognostic information and is of therapeutic value.

3. **Adjuvant chemotherapy.** The presence or absence of axillary lymph node metastases is the most important prognostic factor in breast cancer. All women with axillary nodal involvement should receive adjuvant therapy. Women with node-negative breast cancer should also be considered for adjuvant therapy if the tumor is greater than 1 cm, is ER negative, or has overexpression of her-2. Chemotherapy should be considered in patients who are premenopausal, have cancers that are ER negative, or overexpress her-2. Tamoxifen, 20 mg/day for 5 years, is recommended for all ER-positive breast cancers (*J Natl Cancer Inst* 90:1601, 1998). In selected women with axillary nodal involvement, radiation therapy to the axilla may provide an additional survival advantage.

4. **Metastatic disease.** Menopausal status, hormone receptor status, her-2 expression, and sites of metastatic disease dictate initial treatment. ER-negative breast cancer, lymphangitic lung disease, or liver metastasis seldom responds to hormonal manipulation and should be treated with chemotherapy. In other metastatic sites, ER-positive disease is treated with hormonal manipulation. Premenopausal women are initially treated with tamoxifen and a luteinizing hormone–releasing hormone (LHRH) agonist; postmenopausal women should receive a hormonal agent such as tamoxifen or an aromatase inhibitor. If the disease responds to hormonal therapy, subsequent disease progression may respond to other hormonal agents. Chemotherapy should be considered if there is no response to initial hormonal therapy or if there is progression during subsequent hormonal manipulations. In her-2 overexpressing cancers, the addition of the humanized antibody trastuzumab (see Chemotherapy, sec. **III.H.1.a**) to first-line chemotherapy produces an improvement in survival compared to chemotherapy alone. In women with more than one osteolytic metastasis, the monthly administration of pamidronate, 90 mg IV, produces an improvement in quality of life, greater response to therapy, fewer extravertbral fractures, and possibly a prolongation in survival (*J Clin Oncol* 16:3890, 1998).

5. **Inflammatory and unresectable cancers.** Inflammatory breast cancer manifests as "peau d'orange" changes or erythema involving more than one-third of the chest wall. Because of the high likelihood of metastases at diagnosis, these patients and patients with inoperable primary breast cancers are initially treated with chemotherapy. Subsequently, surgery and radiation therapies are used for maximal local control.

6. **Radiation therapy** is indicated for patients treated with tylectomy and for some patients with axillary lymph node involvement. It is also used for palliation of painful or obstructing metastatic lesions.

B. **GI malignancies** commonly present with vague symptoms and are often advanced at the time of diagnosis.

1. **Esophageal cancers** are either squamous cell (associated with cigarette smoking and alcohol use) or adenocarcinoma (arising in Barrett's esophagus). Surgical resection of the esophagus is recommended in small primary tumors and in selected patients after chemoradiation. Local control of unresectable cancers can be achieved with combined chemotherapy and radiation therapy (*N Engl J Med* 335:462, 1996). Palliation of obstructive symptoms can be accomplished by radiation therapy, dilatation, prosthetic tube placement, or laser therapy.

2. **Gastric cancer** is usually adenocarcinoma and can be cured with surgery in the rare patient with localized disease. Chemotherapy has been ineffective as adjuvant therapy. Locally advanced but unresectable cancers may benefit from concomitant chemotherapy and radiation therapy. Chemotherapy may offer palliation for metastatic disease.

3. **Colon and rectal** adenocarcinomas are primarily treated by surgical resection. A prolonged survival in patients with colon cancer and regional lymph node involvement is seen with administration of postoperative 5-fluorouracil (FU) and levamisole for 12 months or FU and leucovorin (LV) for 6 months (*Ann Intern Med* 122:321, 1995). Rectal cancer that arises below the peritoneal reflection commonly recurs locally after surgery alone; postoperative radiation therapy and FU are recommended. FU is the mainstay of treatment for metastatic colon or rectal cancer, with a response rate of 20%. The addition of LV results in higher response rates but does not clearly prolong survival compared to FU alone. In metastatic disease, the addition of irinotecan to FU/LV produces a higher likelihood of response but no survival advantage. Selected patients with metastases confined to the liver may be candidates for liver resection (*J Clin Oncol* 15:938, 1997). In all patients who are undergoing surgical resection of colon or rectal cancer, a preoperative **carcinoembryonic antigen (CEA)** level should be measured. A persistently elevated or increasing level may indicate residual or recurrent tumor.

4. **Anal cancer.** Chemotherapy with concurrent radiation therapy appears to result in a higher cure rate than surgical resection and usually preserves the anal sphincter and fecal continence (*Cancer* 76:1731, 1995). Surgical resection should be used only as salvage therapy.

C. **Genitourinary malignancies**

1. **Bladder cancer** in the United States is usually a transitional cell carcinoma. A variety of chemical carcinogens, including those in cigarette smoke, have been implicated. Unifocal tumors confined to the mucosa should be managed with cystoscopy and transurethral resection or fulguration, repeated at approximately 3-month intervals; multifocal mucosal disease is treated with intravesicular bacillus Calmette-Guérin, thiotepa, or mitomycin-C. Locally invasive cancers should be resected. Adjuvant chemotherapy improves survival when regional lymph node involvement is confirmed in the cystectomy specimen. In metastatic or recurrent disease, the highest response rates are seen with cisplatin-containing regimens.

2. **Prostate cancer.** Local control of the primary lesion can be achieved with either prostatectomy or radiation therapy. Prostate-specific antigen

is useful as a marker for recurrence, bulk of disease, and response to therapy, and may detect asymptomatic early-stage disease. In patients with metastatic disease, bilateral orchiectomy, LHRH analogs with or without an antiandrogen produce tumor regression in approximately 85% of cases for a median of 18–24 months. Disease that has relapsed after hormonal therapy may respond to withdrawal of that antiandrogen (*Urol Clin North Am* 24:421, 1997). Anthracyclines, taxanes, vinblastine, and estramustine may be of palliative value in hormone-refractory disease. Anemia and bone pain dominate the advanced phases of this disease and are best relieved with transfusions, growth factors, and palliative radiation therapy (see Complications of Cancer, sec. **II**).

3. **Renal cell cancer** is treated by surgical resection, which may be curative if disease is localized; no effective adjuvant therapy is available. In metastatic disease, progestational agents (e.g., medroxyprogesterone) produce tumor regression in fewer than 15% of patients. Chemotherapy, interferon-alpha, and interleukin-2 have reported response rates of 15–30%.

4. **Cancer of the testis** is one of the most curable malignancies when treated with chemotherapy. The patient who is suspected of having cancer of the testis should only have tissue obtained through an inguinal orchiectomy because a transscrotal incision facilitates tumor spread to the inguinal lymph nodes. The initial evaluation should include a serum alpha-fetoprotein and beta subunit of human chorionic gonadotropin, a CT scan of the abdomen and pelvis, and possibly a lymphangiogram. Most patients with seminoma should be treated with radiation therapy. In nonseminomatous germ cell cancer, a retroperitoneal lymph node dissection should be performed for staging, except in the instance of bulky abdominal disease or pulmonary metastasis. If microscopic disease is identified at surgery, two alternatives are acceptable: two cycles of postoperative chemotherapy or observation until relapse occurs followed by institution of chemotherapy. With gross metastatic disease, cisplatin-based chemotherapy is curative in most germ cell cancers. If tumor markers normalize after chemotherapy but a radiographic mass persists, exploratory surgery should be performed. The lesion will prove to be residual cancer in approximately one-third of the patients. Patients with residual cancer should receive additional chemotherapy (*J Clin Oncol* 8:1777, 1990).

D. **Gynecologic malignancies**

1. **Cervical cancer.** The recognized risk factors are multiparity, multiple sexual partners, and human papillomavirus. Carcinoma in situ and superficial disease can be treated by endocervical cone biopsy. Microinvasive disease is treated with an abdominal hysterectomy. Advanced local disease (invasion of the cervix or local extension) is initially treated with surgery. The addition of chemotherapy to radiation therapy postoperatively is associated with an improved survival (*N Engl J Med* 340:1154, 1999). Inoperable cancer can be controlled with radiation therapy. Metastatic disease is treated with cisplatin-based chemotherapy.

2. **Ovarian cancer** is primarily a disease of postmenopausal women. Because symptoms are uncommon with localized disease, most patients present with advanced local disease, malignant ascites, or peritoneal metastases. Surgical staging and treatment include an abdominal hysterectomy, bilateral oophorectomy, lymph node sampling, omentectomy, peritoneal cytology, and removal of all gross tumor. If the tumor is localized to the ovary, the surgery may be curative and further treatment is not routinely recommended. However, if microscopic foci of cancer are identified, chemotherapy is administered postoperatively. The serum marker **CA-125**, though not specific, is elevated in more than 80% of women with epithelial ovarian cancer and is a sensitive indicator of response. After a response is achieved, a "second-look laparotomy" is

performed to restage and remove residual tumor. Approximately one-third of the patients who are in pathologic complete remission after a second-look laparotomy are cured. Those patients who have residual cancer should receive additional chemotherapy.

3. **Endometrial cancer** risks include obesity, nulliparity, polycystic ovaries, and the use of unopposed estrogens (including tamoxifen). Patients generally present with vaginal bleeding. Surgery and radiation therapy are often curative.

E. **Head and neck cancer** is usually a squamous cell cancer. It may arise in a variety of sites, each of which has a different natural history. Early lesions can be cured with surgery, radiation therapy, or both. Despite aggressive surgical and radiation therapy, approximately 65% of patients with head and neck cancer have uncontrolled local disease. Chemotherapy added to radiation therapy improves the survival in patients with nasopharyngeal cancers and selected patients with other primary disease sites (*J Natl Cancer Inst* 91:2081, 1999). Chemotherapy is used for treatment of disseminated disease and produces high response rates with a modest improvement in survival.

F. **Lung cancer** is the most common cause of cancer death in the United States and is the most preventable given its relationship to cigarette smoking. Treatment is based on the histology and stage of the disease. Whenever possible, surgical resection should be attempted for non–small-cell lung cancer because it affords the best chance of cure. Small-cell and non–small-cell lung cancers are treated according to whether disease is limited (confined to one hemithorax and ipsilateral regional lymph nodes) or extensive stage.

1. **Small-cell lung cancer** is often responsible for a variety of paraneoplastic syndromes (see Complications of Cancer, sec. II). In limited disease, combination chemotherapy results in an 85–90% response rate, a median survival of 12–18 months, and a cure in 5–15% of patients. In extensive disease, the median survival is 8–9 months, but cures are rare. For patients who achieve a complete remission with chemotherapy, **prophylactic whole-brain radiation therapy** has been shown to improve the overall survival and decrease the risk of CNS metastases (*N Engl J Med* 341:476, 1999). Radiation therapy to the chest as consolidation therapy may improve survival in limited disease but is not recommended in extensive disease except for palliation of local symptoms.

2. **Non–small-cell lung cancer** survival rates after resection are not improved with adjuvant chemotherapy or radiation therapy. Radiation therapy is the conventional treatment for unresectable disease that is confined to the lung and regional lymph nodes. The use of chemotherapy before or concurrent with radiation may improve survival in patients with a good performance status. In patients with metastatic disease, cisplatin-based combination chemotherapy may modestly improve survival.

G. **Malignant melanoma** should be considered in any changing or enlarging nevus, and suspicious lesions should be removed by excisional biopsy. Subsequently, a wide local excision is performed to remove possible vertical and radial spread of tumor. Deeper invasion is associated with a worse prognosis. High-dose interferon prolongs the survival of selected high-risk resected patients (*J Clin Oncol* 14:7, 1996). Systemic disease may respond to dacarbazine, interferon-alpha, or interleukin-2 in 10–30% of patients.

H. **Sarcomas** are tumors that arise from mesenchymal tissue and occur most commonly in soft tissue or bone. Initial evaluation should include a CT scan of the chest, because hematogenous spread to the lungs is common.

1. **The prognosis for soft-tissue sarcoma** is primarily determined by tumor grade and not by the cell of origin. Surgical resection should be performed when feasible and may be curative. In low-grade tumors, local and regional recurrence is most common, and adjuvant radiation therapy may be of benefit. High-grade tumors often recur systemically, but no advantage to the routine use of adjuvant chemotherapy has been

demonstrated. In metastatic disease, doxorubicin, ifosfamide, and dacarbazine produce responses in 40–55% of patients.

2. **Osteogenic sarcomas** are treated with surgical resection followed by adjuvant chemotherapy for 1 year. Treatment of isolated pulmonary metastasis by surgical resection is associated with long-term survival.

3. **Kaposi's sarcoma** in an immunocompetent patient is generally a low-grade lesion of the lower extremities that is readily treated with local radiation therapy or vinblastine. When Kaposi's sarcoma complicates organ transplantation or AIDS, it is more aggressive and may arise in visceral sites. Liposomal doxorubicin alone is as effective as combination chemotherapy for palliation (*J Clin Oncol* 14:2353, 1996).

I. **Cancer with an unknown primary site.** Approximately 5% of cancer patients present with symptoms of metastatic disease, but no primary tumor site is identifiable on physical examination, routine laboratory studies, and chest radiography. The histopathologic cell type and the site of the metastasis should direct a search for the primary tumor. Immunohistochemical stains may identify specific tissue antigens that help to define the origin of the tumor and guide subsequent therapy. **In general, systemic therapy is only helpful if the primary site is identified;** chemotherapeutic regimens do not improve survival when compared to palliative therapy. Two potentially curative circumstances are described below.

1. **Cervical adenopathy suggests cancer of the lung, breast, head and neck, or lymphoma.** In this case, initial evaluation usually includes panendoscopy (nasendoscopy, laryngopharyngoscopy, bronchoscopy, and esophagoscopy) and biopsy of any suspicious lesion before excision of the lymph node. If squamous cell carcinoma is identified, the patient is presumed to have primary head and neck cancer, and radiation therapy may be curative.

2. **Midline mass in the mediastinum or retroperitoneum.** In both sexes, a midline mass in the mediastinum or retroperitoneum may be an extragonadal germ cell cancer. Elevations in alpha-fetoprotein or the beta subunit of human chorionic gonadotropin further suggest this diagnosis. This neoplasm is potentially curable (see sec. **II.C.4**).

III. **Therapy of hematologic tumors**

A. **Lymphoma** is usually diagnosed by biopsy of an enlarged lymph node.

1. **Staging** of Hodgkin's disease and non-Hodgkin's lymphoma is organized into four categories.

a. **Stage I** is disease localized to a single lymph node or group.

b. **Stage II** is disease involving more than one lymph node group but confined to one side of the diaphragm.

c. **Stage III** is disease in the lymph nodes or the spleen and occurs on both sides of the diaphragm.

d. **Stage IV** is disease involving the liver, lung, skin, or marrow.

e. **B symptoms** include fever above 38.5°C, night sweats that require a change in clothes, or a 10% weight loss over 6 months. These symptoms suggest bulky disease and a worse prognosis.

2. **Hodgkin's disease** usually presents with cervical adenopathy and spreads in a predictable manner along lymph node groups. Treatment is based on the presenting stage of the disease; the cell type is relatively unimportant in the natural history and prognosis. Initial evaluation includes a CT scan of the abdomen and pelvis, bilateral bone marrow biopsies, and lymphangiography to determine the clinical stage of the disease. Exploratory laparotomy with splenectomy and liver biopsy is performed if the findings will change the disease stage and treatment. **Stage IA and IIA** disease are treated with radiation therapy unless a mediastinal mass that exceeds one-third of the chest width is present, in which case chemotherapy is included. **Stage IIIA** disease can be treated either by radiation therapy or chemotherapy, whereas all **stage IV**

patients should receive combination chemotherapy. When **B symptoms** are present, chemotherapy is recommended regardless of the stage.

3. **Non-Hodgkin's lymphoma** is classified as low, intermediate, or high grade based on the histologic type. Staging evaluation is the same as for Hodgkin's disease, but non-Hodgkin's lymphoma has a less predictable pattern of spread. Advanced-stage disease (stage III or IV) is very common and can usually be diagnosed by CT scans or bone marrow biopsy so that exploratory laparotomy and lymphangiography are rarely necessary.

   a. **Low-grade lymphoma** often involves the bone marrow at diagnosis, but the disease has an indolent course. Because this tumor is not curable with standard chemotherapy, treatment can be delayed until the patient is symptomatic ("watch and wait"). Radiation therapy or an alkylating agent (e.g., cyclophosphamide) is used to ameliorate symptoms. Radiation therapy may produce a long-term complete remission in stage I or II disease. Rituximab is a humanized monoclonal antibody that recognizes the CD20 antigen that is expressed by most indolent lymphomas (see Chemotherapy, sec. **III.H.1.b**). This agent produces objective response in approximately 50% of patients with follicular lymphoma without the usual toxicities of chemotherapy.

   b. **Intermediate-grade lymphoma** has a more aggressive course, usually does not involve the bone marrow at diagnosis, and can be cured with chemotherapy. Complete response rates exceed 80%. Features associated with a lower likelihood of cure include an elevated lactate dehydrogenase, stage III/IV disease, age older than 60 years, more than one extranodal site, and poor performance status.

   c. **High-grade lymphoma (Burkitt's, lymphoblastic)** includes the most aggressive subtypes and has a high frequency of CNS and bone marrow involvement. Cerebrospinal fluid (CSF) cytology should be included as part of the initial evaluation. Combination chemotherapy is the mainstay of treatment and should include CNS prophylaxis if the CSF is cytologically free of tumor. If tumor cells are seen in the CSF, additional therapy may be indicated (see Complications of Cancer, sec. **I.B**). Prophylaxis to prevent **tumor lysis syndrome** (see Complications of Treatment, sec. **I.F**) should be performed before induction chemotherapy.

B. **Acute leukemias** may present with manifestations of cytopenias, including fatigue and dyspnea (anemia), cutaneous or mucosal hemorrhage (thrombocytopenia), and fever/infection (neutropenia). Patients may also present with leukemic infiltration of organs, manifested as lymphadenopathy, splenomegaly (more common in acute lymphocytic leukemia), gingival hyperplasia, and skin nodules (more common in acute myeloid leukemia). Leukemic blasts are usually present in the blood. Bone marrow aspiration/biopsy is performed to establish the diagnosis and often shows nearly complete replacement by blasts. Flow cytometry and cytogenetics must be performed on the bone marrow aspirate for classification and to provide prognostic information.

   1. **Acute myeloid leukemia (AML)** constitutes approximately 80% of adult acute leukemia. Approximately 50–80% of patients achieve complete remission with induction chemotherapy that includes cytarabine (cytosine arabinoside; ara-C) and daunorubicin. Consolidation is given with at least one additional cycle of chemotherapy, which is typically ara-C at a dose of 10–30 times that used for induction (high-dose ara-C). High-dose ara-C consolidation results in cure in approximately 30–40% of patients younger than 60 years. Pretreatment factors associated with a low (<10%) chance for cure include preceding myelodysplastic syndrome; prior exposure to radiation, benzene, or chemotherapy; and adverse cytogenetic abnormalities. For these high-risk patients, allogeneic stem cell transplant in first remission increases the likelihood of cure. Acute promyelocytic leukemia (APL) is characterized by a chromosomal translocation [t(15;17)] that

results in a hybrid protein (pml-rar). Treatment with oral tretinoin (*all-trans* retinoic acid) results in complete remission in greater than 90% of patients. Following consolidation chemotherapy approximately 75% of patients are cured.

2. **Acute lymphocytic leukemia (ALL)** is predominantly a disease of child-hood, with 25% of all cases occurring in patients over the age of 15 years. For adults, induction and consolidation involve treatment with multiple chemotherapeutic agents over a period of approximately 6 months fol-lowed by at least 18 months of lower-dose maintenance chemotherapy. To prevent CNS relapse, patients receive intrathecal (IT) chemotherapy and either cranial radiation or CNS penetrating chemotherapy. Approxi-mately 60–80% of adults achieve complete remission, with about 30–40% being cured; increasing age, higher WBC, and longer time to remission are associated with reduced survival. Cytogenetics are crucial in deter-mining prognosis, and allogeneic stem cell transplantation should be con-sidered in patients with a poor prognosis in first remission.

C. **Chronic lymphocytic leukemia (CLL)** usually presents with lymphocytosis, lymphadenopathy, and splenomegaly. Malignant cells resemble mature lym-phocytes. Treatment is similar to that for **low-grade lymphoma** (see sec. **III.A.3.a**) except that fludarabine appears to be more active than alkylating agents. Median survival is approximately 6–8 years with anemia and throm-bocytopenia associated with shortened survival. As in low-grade lymphoma, patients are treated for control of symptoms or cytopenia. Because CLL is accompanied by immunodeficiency, life-threatening infections may occur. Therefore, febrile patients must be evaluated carefully. Immune hemolytic anemia or immune thrombocytopenia may develop as a complication of CLL. Treatment of these conditions is with glucocorticoids (e.g., prednisone, 1 mg/kg PO qd) or chemotherapy, or both. CLL may transform to an inter-mediate- or high-grade lymphoma (Richter's transformation).

D. **Chronic myelogenous leukemia (CML)** presents with leukocytosis and a left shift, usually with splenomegaly. Thrombocytosis, basophilia, and eosinophilia are also common. The diagnosis is confirmed by demonstration of the **Philadel-phia chromosome** (t9:22), which results in production of a hybrid protein (bcr-abl). During stable phase, leukocytosis, thrombocytosis, and splenomegaly can be controlled for several years with oral hydroxyurea, and most patients are asymptomatic. However, acute leukemic transformation (blast phase) is inevi-table and unpredictable, with a median time to transformation of 5–7 years. Blast phase is highly resistant to treatment and is usually fatal. For younger patients (40–50 years old) with human leukocyte antigen (HLA)-identical sib-lings, allogeneic stem cell transplantation in stable phase within 1 year of diag-nosis is the treatment of choice, resulting in a 50–70% likelihood of cure. For older patients and for those without an HLA-identical sibling, options include unrelated donor transplant or therapy with interferon-alpha. The latter agent delays blast phase in some patients. STI571 is an investigational agent that was designed to specifically inhibit the bcr-abl tyrosine kinase. This medication is orally administered and has far fewer toxicities than interferon. Further, STI571 appears to be more active than interferon, although long-term follow-up is not available. U.S. Food and Drug Administration approval is pending.

E. **Hairy-cell leukemia** represents 2–3% of all adult leukemias. Clinical presen-tation includes splenomegaly, pancytopenia, and infection. Patients are at increased risk for bacterial, viral, and fungal infections and have a unique susceptibility to atypical mycobacterial infections. Bone marrow biopsy reveals infiltration by cells that have prominent cytoplasmic projections. A single 7-day course of chlorodeoxyadenosine produces remission in over 90% of patients. Although this drug is not curative, 5-year progression-free sur-vival exceeds 50%.

F. **Multiple myeloma** is a malignant plasma cell disorder that is usually accom-panied by a serum or urine paraprotein, or both. Presenting manifestations may include hypercalcemia, anemia, lytic bone lesions with bone pain, and acute renal failure. The initial evaluation should include a radiographic bone survey, bone marrow aspiration and biopsy, serum and urine protein electrophoresis, β_2-microglobulin, and quantitative immunoglobulins. Treatment generally includes a combination of an oral alkylating agent (i.e., melphalan) and prednisone or vincristine/doxorubicin/dexamethasone. Local radiation therapy should be used to relieve painful bone lesions, and pamidronate, 90 mg IV/month, decreases skeletal complications. After induction chemotherapy, consolidation with high-dose therapy and autologous stem cell transplant improves survival (see Hematopoietic Stem Cell Transplantation).

Complications of Cancer

I. **Complications related to tumor mass**
   A. **Brain metastasis.** Patients with parenchymal brain metastasis may present with headache, mental status changes, weakness, or focal neurologic deficits. Papilledema is observed in only 25% of patients. In patients with malignancy, a CT scan of the head showing one or more round, contrast-enhancing lesions surrounded by edema is usually sufficient for the diagnosis. If cancer has not been diagnosed previously, tissue should be obtained from the brain lesion or a more accessible site before radiation therapy is initiated. Therapy with dexamethasone, 10 mg IV or PO, is initiated to decrease cerebral edema and should be continued at a dosage of 4–6 mg PO q6h throughout the course of radiation therapy, or longer if symptoms related to edema persist. Subsequent therapy depends on the number and location of the brain lesions as well as the prognosis of the underlying cancer. Patients with a chemotherapy-responsive neoplasm and a solitary accessible lesion should be considered for surgical resection. All patients who have not received prior radiation therapy should receive whole-brain radiation therapy.
   B. **Meningeal carcinomatosis** should be suspected in a cancer patient with headache or cranial neuropathies. This pattern of spread is most often seen with lung or breast cancer, melanoma, or lymphoma; the diagnosis is confirmed by cytology of the CSF. In general, a CT scan of the head is performed to rule out parenchymal metastases or hydrocephalus before a lumbar puncture is performed. Local radiation therapy or intrathecal (IT) chemotherapy may provide temporary relief of symptoms (see Chemotherapy, sec. **II.C**). Meningeal lymphoma may respond to IV ara-C.
   C. **Spinal cord compression** is most commonly caused by hematogenous spread of cancer to the vertebral bodies followed by expansion into the spinal canal or ischemia of the spinal cord. The most common malignancies that cause spinal cord compression are breast, lung, and prostate cancer, but the diagnosis should be considered in any patient with cancer who complains of back pain. Evaluation and therapy are discussed in Chap. 25.
   D. **Superior vena cava obstruction** is most commonly caused by cancers such as lymphoma or lung cancer that arise in or spread to the mediastinum. The compressed superior vena cava leads to swelling of the face or trunk, chest pain, cough, or shortness of breath. Dilated superficial veins of the chest, neck, or sublingual area suggest an engorged collateral circulation. The presence of a mass determined by chest radiograph or CT scan usually confirms the diagnosis. Because collateral veins develop, the cerebral circulation is not significantly affected, but a mediastinal mass may compromise the airway. If the histologic origin of the obstruction is unknown, tissue can be obtained for diagnosis via bronchoscopy or mediastinoscopy. Therapy is directed at the underlying disease. Chemotherapy should be administered through a vein

that is not obstructed by the lesion. Neoplasms that are not responsive to chemotherapy are treated with radiation therapy (*J Clin Oncol* 2:961, 1984).

E. Malignant effusions

1. **Malignant pericardial effusion** commonly results from cancer of the breast or lung. In some patients, the initial presentation is acute cardiovascular collapse from cardiac tamponade, requiring emergency pericardiocentesis. After cardiovascular stabilization, some patients may improve with treatment if the tumor is chemotherapy sensitive. When the pericardial effusion is a complication of uncontrolled disease, palliation can be achieved by pericardiocentesis with sclerosis; the effusion should be completely drained, followed by instillation of 30–60 mg bleomycin through the drainage catheter, which is subsequently clamped for 10 minutes and then withdrawn (*Int J Cardiol* 16:155, 1987). Subxiphoid pericardotomy can be performed in patients whose effusions do not respond to other treatment (*JAMA* 257:1088, 1987).

2. **Malignant pleural effusion** develops as a result of pleural invasion by tumor or obstruction of lymphatic drainage. When systemic control is not feasible and reaccumulation of fluid occurs rapidly after drainage, removal of the fluid followed by instillation of a sclerosing agent into the pleural space is recommended. Resistant effusions can be controlled with pleurectomy.

3. **Malignant ascites** is most commonly caused by peritoneal carcinomatosis and is best controlled by systemic chemotherapy. Therapeutic paracenteses can provide symptomatic relief. Intraperitoneal instillation of chemotherapy has been used but is not routinely recommended.

F. Bone metastases may result in spontaneous fracture. Prophylactic surgical pinning and radiation therapy may be indicated. Bisphosphonates may also protect against skeletal complications from myeloma and breast cancer (*N Engl J Med* 334:488, 1996).

II. Paraneoplastic syndromes are complications of malignancy that are not directly caused by a tumor mass effect and are presumed to be mediated by either secreted tumor products or the development of autoantibodies. Paraneoplastic syndromes can affect virtually every organ system, and in most cases, successful treatment of the underlying malignancy eliminates these effects.

A. Metabolic complications

1. **Hypercalcemia** is the most common metabolic complication in malignancy and can cause mental status changes, GI discomfort, and constipation. Acute and chronic management of hypercalcemia is discussed in Chap. 3.

2. **Syndrome of inappropriate antidiuretic hormone (SIADH)** should be considered in a euvolemic cancer patient with unexplained hyponatremia. Although a variety of neoplasms have been described in association with SIADH, small-cell lung cancer is most often responsible. If chemotherapy is ineffective, radiation therapy may decrease the tumor mass and relieve symptoms (see Chap. 3).

3. **Cancer cachexia** refers to the clinical syndrome of anorexia, distortion of taste perception, and loss of muscle mass. The asthenic appearance of patients is more often related to tumor type than to tumor burden. Megestrol acetate, 160 mg PO qd, has been used as an appetite stimulant and results in weight gain in some patients (*J Natl Cancer Inst* 89:1763, 1997).

B. Neuromuscular complications

1. **Polymyositis and dermatomyositis.** Dermatomyositis, more often than polymyositis, has been associated with a variety of malignancies, including non–small-cell lung, colon, ovarian, and prostate cancer. In some patients, successful treatment of the underlying malignancy has resulted in resolution of the symptoms. An exhaustive search for a malignancy is not recommended because a primary malignancy will be found in fewer than 20% of patients (*N Engl J Med* 326:363, 1992) (see Chap. 24).

2. **Lambert-Eaton myasthenic syndrome** is characterized by proximal muscle weakness, decreased or absent deep tendon reflexes, and autonomic dysfunction. Electromyography using high-frequency nerve stimulation may show posttetanic potentiation. Small-cell lung cancer is most often associated with this syndrome, and effective chemotherapy may result in improvement. Worsening symptoms have been reported with the use of calcium channel antagonists; these agents are contraindicated in this syndrome (*N Engl J Med* 321:1567, 1989).

C. **Hematologic complications.** While cytopenias occur more often as a complication of treatment or marrow involvement with cancer, elevated counts may be explained by paraneoplastic syndromes (see Complications of Treatment, sec. **I.B**).

1. **Erythrocytosis** is a rare complication of hepatoma, renal cell cancer, and benign tumors of the kidney, uterus, and cerebellum. Debulking the tumor with surgery or radiation therapy generally results in resolution of the erythrocytosis. Occasionally, therapeutic phlebotomy is indicated.

2. **Granulocytosis** (leukemoid reaction), in the absence of infection, occurs in cancer that arises in the stomach, lung, pancreas, brain, and lymphoma. Because the neutrophils are mature and seldom exceed $100,000/mm^3$, complications are rare and intervention is unnecessary.

3. **Thrombocytosis** in patients with cancer may be caused by splenectomy, iron deficiency, acute hemorrhage, or inflammation; treatment is not usually necessary.

4. **Thromboembolic complications.** Mucin-secreting adenocarcinomas of the GI tract and lung cancer have been associated with a "hypercoagulable state," resulting in recurrent venous and arterial thromboembolism. Nonbacterial thrombotic (marantic) endocarditis, usually involving the mitral valve, may also occur. Heparin anticoagulation or low-molecular-weight heparin should be instituted, as well as treatment of the underlying cancer. Long-term warfarin with a target international normalized ratio of 2–3 or daily low-molecular-weight heparin is recommended to prevent subsequent thrombi (*Ann Intern Med* 130:800, 1999). In many patients, biochemical evidence of disseminated intravascular coagulation coexists with thromboemboli (see Chap. 17).

D. **Glomerular injury** resulting in renal failure has been observed as a paraneoplastic syndrome. Minimal change disease is often associated with lymphoma, especially Hodgkin's disease; membranous glomerulonephritis is more often seen with solid tumors. The process can be reversed with treatment of the underlying cancer (see Chap. 12).

E. **Clubbing of the fingers** and **hypertrophic osteoarthropathy** (polyarthritis and periostitis of long bones) are most often observed in non–small-cell lung cancer but are also seen with lesions that are metastatic to the mediastinum. Some improvement in the osteoarthropathy can be achieved with nonsteroidal anti-inflammatory drugs, but definitive therapy requires treatment of the underlying malignancy.

F. **Fever** may accompany lymphoma, renal cell cancer, and hepatic metastasis. Once an infectious etiology for the fever has been excluded, nonsteroidal anti-inflammatory drugs (e.g., ibuprofen, 400 mg PO qid, or indomethacin, 25–50 mg PO tid) may provide symptomatic relief.

Chemotherapy

I. **Administration of chemotherapeutic drugs.** The dosage of chemotherapy is usually based on body surface area (Table 21-1); for some agents, dosage is determined by body weight and should be adjusted when changes in body

Table 21-1. Doses and common toxicities of antineoplastic agents

Agent	Dose range-schedule	N & V	Mucositis	Diarrhea	Days to nadir	Myelosup-pression	Other toxicity or cautions
Antimetabolites							
Capecitabine	1250 mg/m² PO q12h × 14 days/off 7 days	+	+	++	7–14	+	Hand-foot syndrome
Cytarabine (cytosine arabin-oside; Ara-C)	20 mg/m² IV infusion × 14–21 days	0	0	+	10–14	+++	—
	100–200 mg/m² IV qd × 5–7 days	++	+	++	10–14	+++	—
	1.5–3 g/m² IV q12h × 3–6 days	+++	+	++	10–14	+++	Cerebellar dysfunction, conjunctivitis
Fludarabine	15–30 mg/m² qd × 5 days	+	0	0	7–14	+++	Neurotoxicity
5-Fluorouracil	350–450 mg/m² IV × 5 days	0	+	+	7–14	++	—
	200–1000 mg/m² infusion × 5 days	0	+++	+++	7–14	+	Phlebitis, cerebellar symptoms
	20 mg/m² qd × 28–56 days	0	+	+	—	—	Hand-foot syndrome
	With leucovorin	0	+	+++	7–14	+	Hand-foot syndrome
Gemcitabine	1 g/m² q1wk × 3 doses every 4 wks	+	0	0	—	++	Peripheral edema
Methotrexate	10–60 mg/m² IV q1–3wk	+	++	++	7–14	++	Dermatitis, interstitial nephritis, pneumonitis; modify dose for renal dysfunction
With leucovorin	>1.5 g IV qd × 1 wk	+++	+++	+++	7–14	+++	Modify dose with effusions
Pentostatin (2-deoxycofor-mycin)	4 mg/m² IV q2wk	+	0	0	7	+	Erythema, lethargy, renal failure

Drug	Dose				Nadir		Toxicity/Comments
6-Mercaptopurine	75–100 mg/m² PO qd	+	0	0	7–14	++	Hepatotoxicity; modify dose for renal dysfunction, allopurinol
Thioguanine	100 mg/m² PO qd 1–4 days	+	+	0	10–30	++	Modify dose for renal dysfunction
Cladribine (2-chlorodeoxyadenosine)	0.09 mg/kg/day IV × 7 days	+	0	0	7–14	+++	—
Alkylating agents							
Busulfan	2–4 mg/m² PO qd	0	0	0	14–28	++	Hyperpigmentation Addison-like syndrome, pulmonary fibrosis
Chlorambucil	6–14 mg PO qd	0	0	0	10–14	++	—
Cyclophosphamide	60–150 mg/m² PO qd × 14 days	+	0	0	10–12	++	Interstitial pneumonitis, hemorrhagic cystitis
	500–1500 mg/m² IV every 21 days	++	+	0	7–14	++	Hemorrhagic cystitis
	120–200 mg/kg IV × 2–4 doses for BMT	+++	+++	+++	7–14	+++	Cardiomyopathy
Dacarbazine (DTIC)	150–250 mg/m² IV qd × 5 days every 21–28 days	+++	0	0	—	—	Flu-like symptoms; modify dose for renal dysfunction
Altretamine (hexamethylmelamine)	260 mg/m²/day PO × 14–21 days	++	0	0	21–28	+	Peripheral neuropathy
Ifosfamide	800–1500 mg/m² IV qd × 3–5 days every 21–28 days	+++	0	0	7–10	+++	Encephalopathy, hemorrhagic cystitis, administer with mesna (bladder protection)
Mechlorethamine	8 mg/m² IV every 28 days	+++	+	+	7–14	++	Rash; vesicant
Melphalan	4–8 mg/m² PO qd × 4 days	0	0	0	10–14	++	—
Thiotepa	Up to 1.25 g/m² IV with BMT	++	+++	+++	7–14	+++	Rash
Nitrosoureas							
Carmustine (BCNU)	60–100 mg/m² IV qd × 3 days	+++	0	0	28–35	++	Interstitial pneumonia

(continued)

Table 21-1. (continued)

Agent	Dose range-schedule	N & V	Mucositis	Diarrhea	Days to nadir	Myelosuppression	Other toxicity or cautions
Lomustine (CCNU)	130 mg/m² PO × 1 day	+	0	0	21–42	++	—
Tumor antimicrobials							
Bleomycin	10–20 mg/m² SC every wk	0	0	0	—	—	Erythroderma, interstitial pneumonitis, modify dose for renal dysfunction, test dose
Dactinomycin	0.4–1.0 mg/m² IV every wk	++	++	0	14–21	++	Rash
Daunorubicin	45–60 mg/m² IV qd × 3 days	++	+	+	7–14	+++	Vesicant; cardiotoxicity; modify dose for renal and hepatic dysfunction
Doxorubicin	10–60 mg/m² IV every 7–28 days	++	+	+	7–14	+++	Vesicant; cardiotoxicity; modify dose for renal and hepatic dysfunction
Idarubicin	12 mg/m² IV qd × 3 days	++	+	+	7–14	+++	Vesicant; cardiotoxicity; modify dose for renal and hepatic dysfunction
Mitomycin-C	10–20 mg/m² IV q4–6wk	+	+	0	21–28	++	Vesicant; hemolytic-uremic syndrome
Mitoxantrone	10–30 mg/m² IV every 21–28 days	+	+	+	7–14	++	Cardiotoxicity
Streptozocin	500 mg/m² IV qd × 5 days or 1000–1500 mg/m² IV qwk	+++	0	0	—	—	Glycosuria, nephrotoxicity
Plant alkaloids							
Etoposide	50–200 mg/m² PO or IV qd × 5 days	0	0	0	10–14	++	—
Vinblastine	5–10 mg/m² IV q1–4 wk	+	+	0	4–10	++	Vesicant; neuropathy (especially obstipation); modify dose for hepatic dysfunction

Agent	Dose			Nadir (d)		Comments
Vincristine	1–2 mg IV q1–4 wk	0	0	—	—	Vesicant; neuropathy (especially sensory); modify dose for hepatic dysfunction
Vinorelbine	30 mg/m² IV every wk	+	0	—	—	Pain at infusion site; neuropathy
Paclitaxel (Taxol)	135–250 mg/m² every 21 days	+	0	10–14	++	Premedicate with steroids to avoid anaphylactoid reaction; neuropathy; dose modification for hepatic dysfunction
Docetaxel (Taxotere)	60–100 mg/m² every 21 days	+	0	10–14	++	Decadron starting 1 day pretreatment qd ×5 to avoid third spacing of fluids; modify dose in hepatic dysfunction
Other agents						
Carboplatin	200–360 mg/m² IV every 21–28 days	++	0	14–28	++	Modify dose with renal failure
Cisplatin	20–120 mg/m² IV qd ×1–5 days	+++	0	—	—	Peripheral neuropathy; nephropathy; ototoxicity
Hydroxyurea	500–2000 mg PO qd	0	0	7–10	++	Atrophic skin
L-Asparaginase	1000–10,000 IU SC qd ×3 days	0	0	—	—	Coagulopathy, pancreatitis, hypersensitivity reactions
Procarbazine	100–200 mg/m² PO qd ×7–14 days	+	0	7–10	++	Rash, encephalopathy
Topotecan	1.5 mg/m² IV qd ×5 days every 21 days	++	+	10–14	+++	Modify dose for renal dysfunction
Irinotecan	125 mg/m² every week for 4 wks	++	+++	7–10	+++	Diarrhea controlled with atropine in first 24 hours, then with loperamide; asthenia, fever, abdominal pain common

0 = none; + = mild; ++ = moderate; +++ = severe; BMT = bone marrow transplant; N & V = nausea and vomiting.

weight occur. An assessment of the patient disease status, determination of side effects from the previous treatment, and a CBC should be obtained before each cycle of chemotherapy. Drug dosages usually must be adjusted for the following conditions: (1) neutropenia, (2) thrombocytopenia, (3) stomatitis, (4) diarrhea, or (5) limited metabolic capacity for the drug. **The advice of an oncologist and precise adherence to a treatment plan are mandatory because of the low therapeutic index of chemotherapeutic agents.**

II. **Route of administration**

A. **Oral drug administration** may be accompanied by nausea and vomiting and may require antiemetic therapy. For some agents, oral absorption is erratic and parenteral administration is preferred.

B. **IV drug administration** should be performed by experienced personnel. Care should be taken to ensure free flow of fluid to the vein, and adequate blood return should be verified before instillation of chemotherapy. Infusions should be through a large-caliber, upper extremity vein. When possible, veins of the antecubital fossa, wrist, dorsum of the hand, and arm ipsilateral to an axillary lymph node dissection should be avoided. In patients with poor peripheral venous access or those who require many doses of chemotherapy, **indwelling venous catheter devices** should be considered (*JAMA* 253:1590, 1985).

C. **Intrathecal chemotherapy** is administered for the treatment of meningeal carcinomatosis or as CNS prophylaxis. Side effects include acute arachnoiditis, subacute motor dysfunction, and progressive neurologic deterioration (leukoencephalopathy). Decreased cognitive function has been found in children. Impaired cognitive function and leukoencephalopathy occur more often when IT chemotherapy is combined with whole-brain radiation. **Methotrexate,** 10–12 mg, is diluted in 5 ml preservative-free nonbacteriostatic isotonic solution. Before administration, 5–10 ml CSF should be allowed to drain; methotrexate is then injected into the spinal canal over 5–10 minutes. To decrease the risk of arachnoiditis, patients should remain in a supine position for 15 minutes after the infusion is completed. To avoid systemic side effects from methotrexate, leucovorin, 5–10 mg PO q6h, should be administered for eight doses beginning 12–24 hours after IT treatment. Slow-release cytarabine, 50 mg, or cytosine arabinoside, 50–100 mg in 5–10 ml diluent, can be administered in a similar manner (*J Clin Oncol* 17:3110, 1999).

D. **Intracavitary instillation** of chemotherapy may be useful in some circumstances. Thiotepa, 30–60 mg, is commonly instilled in the bladder for the treatment of bladder carcinoma. Doxorubicin and cisplatin have been given through an implanted peritoneal catheter for the treatment of peritoneal metastasis.

E. **Intra-arterial chemotherapy** is advocated as a method of achieving high drug concentrations at specific tumor sites. Although it is of theoretical advantage, there are no absolute indications for chemotherapy administered by this route.

III. **Chemotherapeutic agents.** A summary of commonly used chemotherapeutic agents, dosages, and toxicities is given in Table 21-1. Class-specific or unique side effects are described here.

A. **Antimetabolites** exert antitumor activity by acting as pseudosubstrates for essential enzymatic reactions. Their greatest toxicity occurs in tissues that are actively replicating (e.g., GI mucosa, hematopoietic cells).

1. **Ara-C** is an analog of deoxycytidine that is most useful in hematologic neoplasms. In standard doses, myelosuppression and GI toxicity are dose limiting. In high doses, conjunctivitis is common, and prophylaxis with dexamethasone eyedrops, two drops in each eye tid, should be administered. Cerebellar ataxia, pancreatitis, and hepatitis may also develop. If cerebellar dysfunction occurs during treatment, the ara-C must be discontinued.

2. **5-FU** (FU) is a pyrimidine analog that is administered as an injection or as a continuous infusion. When it is administered as a bolus injection,

myelosuppression is dose limiting; with a 4- to 5-day infusion, stomatitis and diarrhea are dose limiting. Cerebellar ataxia has been reported with both schedules and requires discontinuation of the drug. Chest pain ascribed to coronary artery vasospasm may occur with infusions and, if suspected, should be treated with a calcium channel antagonist (e.g., nifedipine) or by discontinuing the chemotherapy (*Cancer* 61:36, 1988). FU can be administered over 6–8 weeks and is limited by the development of a palmar-plantar dermatologic toxicity (the hand-foot syndrome can be palliated with vitamin B_6, 150 mg/day). Leucovorin can be coadministered with FU to potentiate cytotoxicity; diarrhea is dose limiting (*J Clin Oncol* 7:1419, 1989).

3. **Methotrexate** is an inhibitor of dihydrofolate reductase and has numerous toxicities. Mucositis is dose limiting.

   a. **Prolonged reabsorption.** Methotrexate is polyglutamated, and these metabolites accumulate in effusions and may produce substantial toxicity. Patients with effusions that require methotrexate should either have the fluid drained before receiving this drug or have the dosage drastically reduced.

   b. **Interstitial pneumonitis,** unrelated to cumulative dose and associated with a peripheral eosinophilia, may occur. It should be treated with glucocorticoids (e.g., prednisone, 1 mg/kg PO qd or equivalent) and precludes additional use of methotrexate.

   c. **Hepatitis** may occur with long-term oral administration but may also occur after a single high dose.

   d. **High-dose methotrexate** may be associated with crystalline nephropathy and renal failure. Urine alkalinization with sodium bicarbonate should be maintained to minimize this risk. Leucovorin is used to "rescue" normal tissue after high-dose methotrexate. The **leucovorin dose** depends on the amount of methotrexate used, but the usual dosage is 5–25 mg IV or PO q6h for 8–12 doses, or until the serum methotrexate concentration is less than 50 nM.

4. **6-Mercaptopurine** is a purine analog that is partially metabolized by xanthine oxidase. To avoid increased toxicity, patients who take allopurinol should receive 25% of the usual total dose of 6-mercaptopurine. Hepatic cholestasis has been observed.

5. **Fludarabine** is an adenosine monophosphate analog that produces myelosuppression (*J Clin Oncol* 9:175, 1991).

6. **Cladribine (2-chlorodeoxyadenosine)** is a purine substrate analog that is resistant to degradation by adenosine deaminase. Myelosuppression is predictable (*Lancet* 340:952, 1994).

7. **Gemcitabine** is a nucleoside analog that may produce fever, edema, flu-like symptoms, and rash.

B. **Alkylating agents** are useful in a wide variety of malignancies. These drugs cause DNA cross linking and strand breaks. Most alkylating agents are cytotoxic to resting and dividing cells. Patients should be counseled that irreversible sterility may develop after treatment with alkylating agents. Chlorambucil, cyclophosphamide, melphalan, and mechlorethamine have been implicated in the development of acute myeloid leukemia and myelodysplasia 3–10 years after treatment.

   1. **Busulfan** can cause interstitial pneumonitis and gynecomastia, and a reversible syndrome that resembles Addison's disease may develop with long-term daily oral administration.

   2. **Chlorambucil** is a well-tolerated orally administered drug. Myelosuppression is dose limiting and usually readily reversible.

   3. **Cyclophosphamide** may cause hemorrhagic cystitis (see Complications of Treatment, sec. **I.E**). Adequate hydration to maintain urine output should be achieved while administering the drug. Oral cyclophosphamide should be given early in the day to ensure adequate hydration. High-dose

cyclophosphamide is used as a preparative agent before stem cell transplantation; at these doses a hemorrhagic myocarditis may occur.

4. **Dacarbazine** can produce a flu-like syndrome that consists of fever, myalgias, facial flushing, malaise, and marked elevations of hepatic enzymes.

5. **Ifosfamide** is chemically similar to cyclophosphamide, but the incidence of hemorrhagic cystitis is much higher (occurring in 20–30% of treated patients). Administration of 2-mercaptoethanesulfonate (mesna; usually infused with ifosfamide at a dosage of at least 0.6 mg mesna to 1 mg ifosfamide) is recommended to lower the incidence of cystitis (see Complications of Treatment, sec. **I.E**). Ifosfamide can also cause neurologic toxicity, including seizures.

6. **Mechlorethamine (nitrogen mustard)** is a skin irritant; protective gloves and eyewear must be used during drug preparation and administration. Development of a drug rash does not prevent further use of this agent.

7. **Melphalan** is available in oral and injectable forms. An idiosyncratic interstitial pneumonitis may occur, and, although usually reversible, it precludes further use of the drug.

8. **Nitrosoureas [carmustine (BCNU) and lomustine (CCNU)]** are lipid soluble and penetrate the blood-brain barrier. BCNU is usually administered in an ethanol solution, and toxicity from the vehicle, including giddiness, flushing, and phlebitis, may occur. Because delayed myelosuppression occurs 6–8 weeks after treatment and may be cumulative, these agents are commonly given at 8-week intervals.

9. **Thiotepa** can be administered IV with bone marrow rescue. When used intravesically, 60–90 mg is administered in 60–100 ml water and instilled over 2 hours.

C. **Antitumor antibiotics** intercalate adjacent DNA nucleotides, interrupting replication and transcription and causing strand breaks; they are cell cycle nonspecific.

1. **Anthracycline antibiotics** are associated with a cardiomyopathy that consists of **intractable CHF** and dysrhythmias. **With doxorubicin,** this complication is seen in approximately 2% of patients who receive 550 mg/m^2, but the incidence increases dramatically at higher cumulative doses. Concomitant cyclophosphamide or previous chest irradiation may potentiate this toxicity. As the cumulative dose approaches 450–550 mg/m^2, serial radionuclide ventriculography should be performed, and the anthracycline should be discontinued if left ventricular function is compromised. Myocardial damage is related to peak serum concentrations and to cumulative dosage; longer (96-hour) infusions have allowed for higher cumulative dosages. These agents may also produce a radiation recall effect that consists of acute toxicity to previous radiation fields, usually to the heart, GI region, or lungs. The cardioprotectant dexrazoxane has been shown to decrease the incidence and severity of the cardiomyopathy associated with doxorubicin (*Ann Intern Med* 125:47, 1996).

   a. **Daunorubicin** is used in the treatment of acute leukemia. Bone marrow suppression is expected, and the dose-limiting toxicity is usually mucositis. Red urine may be caused by the drug and its metabolites.

   b. **Doxorubicin** toxicity is similar to that of daunorubicin, although this drug has a broader spectrum of activity.

   c. **Mitoxantrone** is structurally similar to doxorubicin and daunorubicin but is associated with less cardiac toxicity. Mucositis and myelosuppression are dose limiting; a bluish discoloration of the urine and sclera may occur.

   d. **Idarubicin** has a more rapid cellular uptake than the other anthracyclines. Toxicity is similar to that of daunorubicin.

   e. **Liposomal doxorubicin** is indicated for Kaposi's sarcoma and has a toxicity profile similar to that of doxorubicin.

2. **Bleomycin** is useful in combination chemotherapy because it is rarely myelosuppressive. **A test dose,** 1–2 mg SC, should be administered before full doses are instituted (especially in patients with lymphoma), because severe allergic reactions with hypotension may occur. Interstitial pneumonitis, which occasionally results in irreversible pulmonary fibrosis, is more common in patients with underlying pulmonary disease or previous lung irradiation or in patients who are receiving a cumulative dose of 200 mg/m^2. Pulmonary symptoms and chest radiographs should be monitored.

3. **Mitomycin-C** is associated with delayed myelosuppression that worsens with repeated use of the drug. Interstitial pneumonitis has been observed. The **hemolytic-uremic syndrome** has been reported, is exacerbated by RBC transfusions, and should be suspected in patients with sudden onset of a microangiopathic hemolytic anemia and renal failure.

4. **2-Deoxycoformycin (Pentostatin)** is isolated from *Streptomyces* and acts as an inhibitor of adenosine deaminase. Myelosuppression is the chief toxicity.

D. **Plant alkaloids** are naturally occurring nitrogenous bases. Most inhibit cell division through inhibition of mitotic spindle formation.

1. **Vincristine** often causes a dose-limiting neuropathy. Paresthesias followed by loss of deep tendon reflexes usually occur. Neuritic pain, jaw pain, diplopia, constipation, abdominal pain, and an adynamic ileus are less likely. Other adverse effects include SIADH and Raynaud's phenomenon.

2. **Vinblastine** is less neurotoxic than vincristine and is usually limited by myelosuppression. In high doses, myalgias, obstipation, and transient hepatitis may occur.

3. **Etoposide (VP-16).** The major dose-limiting toxicity is myelosuppression.

4. **Teniposide (VM-26)** is a semisynthetic derivative of podophyllotoxin. Toxicities include myelosuppression, hypersensitivity reactions, alopecia, and hypotension.

5. **Paclitaxel (Taxol)** has a unique antitubulin mechanism that disrupts microtubule assembly. Because Taxol is dissolved in cremophor, anaphylactoid reactions may occur and are partially related to the rate of infusion. All patients should be premedicated with dexamethasone and H$_1$ and H$_2$ blockers. In addition, myelosuppression, arthralgias, neuropathy, and arrhythmias may occur.

6. **Docetaxel (Taxotere)** can be administered more rapidly than Taxol without anaphylactoid reactions. Dexamethasone, 8 mg bid for 3 days beginning the day before chemotherapy, is administered to prevent third-space fluid collections.

7. **Navelbine** may produce pain in the IV injection site.

E. **Platinum-containing agents** act as intercalators, causing single- and double-strand breaks in DNA.

1. **Cisplatin** produces severe nausea and vomiting; aggressive antiemetic therapy is mandatory (Table 21-2). The patient should be aggressively volume expanded with isotonic saline to prevent renal toxicity. One liter of saline should be administered over 4–6 hours before and after chemotherapy. The dosage of cisplatin should be reduced for patients with renal insufficiency and should be withheld if the serum creatinine is greater than 3 mg/dl. Other toxicities include hypomagnesemia and ototoxicity. Pretreatment with amifostine may reduce the cumulative hematologic, renal, and neurologic toxicities (*J Clin Oncol* 14:2101, 1996).

2. **Carboplatin** is a cisplatin analog with less neurotoxicity, ototoxicity, and nephrotoxicity than cisplatin; myelosuppression is the dose-limiting toxicity.

F. **Other agents**

1. **Hydroxyurea,** an oral agent that inhibits ribonucleotide reductase, is used in the management of the chronic phase of CML and other myelo-

Table 21-2. Recommendations for antiemetic therapy[a]

Phenothiazines[b]

   Prochlorperazine, 5–10 mg PO or IV q4–6h (maximum IU dose, 40 mg/day)

   Prochlorperazine, 25 mg PR q4–6h

   Chlorpromazine, 10 mg PO q4–6h

   Trimethobenzamide, 100 mg PO or IM q4–6h

Serotonin-receptor antagonists

   Granisetron, 10 μg/kg IV or 1 mg PO q12h × 2 doses 15 mins before chemotherapy

   Ondansetron, 8–32 mg IV × 15–30 mins before or 24 mg PO or 8 mg PO tid

   Dolasetron, 1.8 mg/kg IV or 100 mg PO 30 minutes before chemotherapy

Butyrophenone

   Droperidol, 1– 5 mg IV q4–6h

Metoclopramide,[b] 2–3 mg/kg IV before chemotherapy and q2h × 3 doses

Antihistamine

   Diphenhydramine, 50 mg PO or IV q4–6h

Anxiolytic

   Lorazepam, 1–2 mg PO or IV tid–qid

Glucocorticoid

   Dexamethasone, 10–30 mg IV before chemotherapy

[a]See Table 21-1 under the column N&V.
[b]May cause extrapyramidal side effects that can be treated with either diphenhydramine, 25–50 mg PO or IV q4–6h, or benztropine mesylate, 1–2 mg IV or PO q4–6h.

proliferative diseases. The dosage is adjusted according to the peripheral blood neutrophil and platelet count.

2. **L-Asparaginase** hydrolyzes asparagine, depleting cells of an essential substrate in protein synthesis. Allergic or anaphylactic reactions may occur. Other toxicities include hemorrhagic pancreatitis, hepatic failure with depression of clotting factors, and encephalopathy.

3. **Procarbazine** is an oral agent that inhibits DNA, RNA, and protein synthesis. It is a monoamine oxidase inhibitor, and therefore tricyclic antidepressants, sympathomimetic agents, and tyramine-containing foods should be avoided (see Chap. 1). Procarbazine has a disulfiram-like effect, and therefore ethanol should not be ingested while one is taking this medication.

4. **Topotecan** is a topoisomerase I inhibitor for which myelosuppression is dose limiting.

5. **Irinotecan** has a similar mechanism of action to topotecan. It can produce severe diarrhea, which is treated with atropine and loperamide.

G. **Hormonal agents** lack direct cytotoxicity. In general, they have few serious adverse effects. In disseminated disease, eventual resistance to hormonal agents should be anticipated.

1. **Tamoxifen** is a selective ER modulator. It acts as an ER antagonist in some tissues including breast and as an ER agonist on others. The usual dosage is 10 mg PO bid. After 7–14 days of treatment, a **hormone flare** (increasing bone pain, erythema, and hypercalcemia) occurs in approximately 5% of women with ER-positive breast cancer and bone metastases. The symptoms abate over 7–10 days, and 75% of these patients respond to tamoxifen. Palliation of pain, control of hypercalcemia, and continuation of the

drug are recommended. The long-term administration of tamoxifen is not associated with a systemic antiestrogen effect (vaginal atrophy, osteoporosis, or increased risk of heart disease) but is associated with some estrogen effects (endometrial cancer and deep vein thrombosis).

2. **Gonadotropin agonists.** Two LHRH agonists are used in the treatment of metastatic prostate cancer. Leuprolide acetate and goserelin acetate can be given as a monthly SC depot injection, and leuprolide acetate is also available in a daily injection form. The first weeks of treatment may be associated with an initial flare in tumor symptoms, bone pain, fluid retention, hot flashes, sweats, and impotence. Signs of neurologic dysfunction or urinary obstruction should be carefully monitored.

3. **Progestational agents.** Megestrol acetate, 40 mg PO qid, and medroxyprogesterone, 10 mg PO qd, have been used in the treatment of a variety of neoplasms. Principal toxicities include weight gain, fluid retention, hot flashes, and vaginal bleeding with discontinuation of therapy. Both agents have been used in the treatment of cachexia associated with cancer and AIDS (see Complications of Cancer, sec. **II.A.3**).

4. **Antiandrogens.** Flutamide and bicalutamide may produce nausea, vomiting, gynecomastia, and breast tenderness (*Cancer* 71:1083, 1993). In advanced prostate cancer, withdrawal of flutamide results in tumor regression in 25% of patients (*J Clin Oncol* 11:1566, 1993).

H. **Immunotherapy.** Immunotherapeutic agents may be selective or nonspecific.

1. **Selective agents** include monoclonal antibodies, most of which are partially humanized.

   a. **Trastuzumab** (4 mg/kg over 90 minutes week 1 and 2 mg/kg over 30 minutes weekly) should be added to the first-line chemotherapy of patients with metastatic breast cancer whose cancers overexpress her-2 as measured by gene amplification or protein expression. Its use is associated with an improved survival. As a single agent, it has modest activity, and it has a different mechanism of action than chemotherapy (*N Engl J Med* 17:2639, 1999).

   b. **Rituximab,** an unconjugated antibody targeted to CD20, is administered weekly for 1 month as treatment of low-grade non-Hodgkin's lymphomas that are CD20 positive. Toxicities include chills and fevers during administration and rare hypersensitivity reactions (*J Clin Oncol* 16:2825, 1998).

   c. **Campath** is a humanized antibody to CD52 (present on normal B and T cells) and has been used to treat CLL. Because of a high incidence of opportunistic infections, resulting from immunodeficiency, prophylactic antifungals and antivirals are recommended (*Br J Haematol* 93:151, 1996).

2. **Nonspecific immunotherapy**

   a. **Levamisole** is administered with 5-FU as adjuvant therapy in colon cancer (see Approach to the Cancer Patient, sec. **II.B.3**). The dosage of 50 mg PO tid for 3 days every other week is well tolerated and does not appear to add to the toxicity of 5-FU.

   b. **Interferon-alpha** is used for hairy-cell leukemia, CML, and melanoma. Toxicity includes nausea and vomiting, flu-like symptoms, and headaches. Acute toxicity may respond to acetaminophen; with continued administration these symptoms subside.

   c. **Aldesleukin (interleukin-2)** can produce responses in melanoma or renal cell carcinoma. Some of these remissions are durable. At high doses this agent is toxic, producing increased vascular permeability with fluid overload, hypotension, prerenal azotemia, and elevation of liver enzymes.

I. **Chemopreventive agents**

1. **Retinoids** have been used as therapeutic and chemopreventive agents. Isotretinoin (13-cis-retinoic acid), 50–100 mg/m^2 PO qd for 12 months,

Table 21-3. Treatment of extravasation of selected chemotherapeutic agents

Drug	Compress	Antidote
Dacarbazine	Hot	Isotonic thiosulfate IV and SC
Daunorubicin	Cold	DMSO applied topically to vein
Doxorubicin	Cold	DMSO applied topically to vein
Etoposide	Hot	Hyaluronidase (150 units/ml) 1–6 ml SC × 1
Mechlorethamine	—	Isotonic thiosulfate IV and SC
Mitomycin-C	—	Isotonic thiosulfate IV and SC
Vinblastine	Hot	Hyaluronidase (150 units/ml) 1–6 ml SC × 1
Vincristine	Hot	Hyaluronidase (150 units/ml) 1–6 ml SC × 1

DMSO = dimethyl sulfoxide.

has been shown to lower the incidence of second primary tumors in patients who were previously treated for head and neck cancer (*N Engl J Med* 323:795, 1990). Common toxicities include dry skin, cheilitis, hyperlipidemias, and elevation of transaminases (*Cancer* 76:602, 1995).

2. **Tamoxifen,** 20 mg/day administered for 5 years, has been shown to decrease the incidence of breast cancer in women at high risk for the development of breast cancer (*JNCI* 90:1371, 1998).

Complications of Treatment

I. **Chemotherapy** often causes serious or life-threatening toxicity. The most common and predictable toxicities are to rapidly proliferating cells of hematopoietic and mucosal tissue. Because repair of these tissues cannot be accelerated, palliation during the healing process is the primary goal.

A. **Extravasation** of certain chemotherapeutic agents from venous infusion sites may lead to severe local tissue injury. Offending agents are identified as vesicants in Table 21-1. Initial symptoms of pain or erythema may appear within hours or may be delayed for up to 1–2 weeks. When extravasation occurs, the steps described below should be taken.

1. **Stop the chemotherapy infusion.** While the venous catheter is still in place, approximately 5 ml blood should be aspirated to remove any residual drug.

2. **Certain drugs require hot or cold compresses** and may be neutralized by instillation of agents locally through the catheter and subcutaneously into the nearby tissue (Table 21-3).

3. **Observe the area closely** for signs of tissue breakdown; surgical intervention for débridement or skin grafting may be necessary. Because extravasation injuries usually result in severe pain, adequate analgesia should be supplied (*J Clin Oncol* 5:1116, 1987).

B. **Myelosuppression** from most agents reaches its peak 7–14 days after treatment (see Table 21-1).

1. **The risk of infection** increases dramatically with neutropenia (defined as an absolute neutrophil count of less than 500/mm^3) and is directly related to the duration of the neutropenia. In the absence of neutrophils, signs of infection or inflammation may be muted. A febrile neutropenic patient should be presumed to be infected and must be

evaluated and treated promptly. A physical examination must be performed to locate potential sites of infection, with particular attention to indwelling catheter sites, sinuses, and the oral and rectal areas. **Cultures** of blood, urine, stool, sputum, and other foci that are suspected of bacterial infection should be collected, and a chest radiograph should be obtained. **Empiric antimicrobial treatment** should be initiated immediately after cultures are obtained. In the absence of any obvious source, the antimicrobials should provide broad coverage for gram-negative bacilli (including *Pseudomonas aeruginosa*) and gram-positive cocci (including alpha-hemolytic *Streptococcus* species. In choosing a regimen, local susceptibility patterns should also be considered. Empiric therapy may consist of an aminoglycoside and semisynthetic penicillin or a single agent such as cefepime. Vancomycin should not be included in initial empiric regimens unless the patient is clinically unstable or has had a recent oxacillin-resistant *Staphylococcus aureus* infection. Low-risk patients (afebrile after institution of antibiotics, negative cultures, and anticipated to recover from myelosuppression in <1 week) can be discharged on an oral broad-spectrum agent such as a fluoroquinolone or trimethoprim-sulfamethoxazole. **Modification of the antimicrobial regimen** according to the culture data or clinical picture may become necessary. Additional agents to treat *Staphylococcus epidermidis*, *Clostridium difficile*, or anaerobic infections are commonly necessary based on physical examination findings and suspected foci of infection. Persistent fever, in the absence of other data, usually does not warrant an empiric change in the antibacterial therapy. However, empiric antifungal therapy with amphotericin B (starting at 0.5 mg/kg and advanced to 1.0 mg/kg qd) should be added if the fever continues for longer than 72 hours (see Chap. 14). Antimicrobials are continued until the neutrophil count is greater than $500/mm^3$. Neutropenic patients should be maintained in modified reverse isolation. Those who enter the room should wash their hands thoroughly with antiseptic soap or an alcohol-based hand-cleaning solution. Visitors with colds should wear a mask, and those with fevers should not enter. Due to the risk of fungal infection, live plants should not be allowed in the room.

2. **Thrombocytopenia** below $10,000/mm^3$ that is the result of chemotherapy should be treated with platelet transfusions to minimize the risk of spontaneous hemorrhage (see Chap. 19). When prolonged thrombocytopenia is anticipated, histocompatibility testing should be performed before therapy so that HLA-matched single-donor platelets can be provided when alloimmunization makes the patient refractory to random-donor platelets.

3. **RBC transfusions** are indicated for patients who have symptoms of anemia, active bleeding, or a hemoglobin concentration below 7–8 g/dl (see Chap. 19). Because of anecdotal reports of graft-versus-host disease (GVHD) associated with transfusions, radiation of all blood products is generally recommended for immunosuppressed marrow transplant patients.

4. **Growth factors** include many cytokines that may ameliorate the myelosuppression associated with cytotoxic chemotherapy. They act on hematopoietic cells, stimulating proliferation, differentiation, commitment, and some functional activation. Because they can increase myelosuppression, they should not be given within 24 hours of chemotherapy and radiation.

   a. **Granulocyte colony-stimulating factor (G-CSF)**, given at an initial dose of 5 µg/kg SC or IV beginning the day after the last dose of cytotoxic chemotherapy, may reduce the incidence of febrile neutropenic events. Blood counts should be monitored twice a week during therapy. Bone pain is a common toxicity that is usually managed with nonnarcotic analgesics.

      b. Granulocyte-macrophage colony-stimulating factor (GM-CSF), given subcutaneously at a dose of 250 μg/m^2/day beginning the day after the last dose of cytotoxic chemotherapy, shortens the period of neutropenia after stem cell transplant.

      c. Erythropoietin given at a starting dose of 150 units/kg SC three times a week has been shown to improve anemia and decrease transfusion requirements in cancer patients in whom the anemia is predominantly caused by cytotoxic chemotherapy. Hematocrit should be monitored weekly during therapy, and the dose should be adjusted accordingly.

      d. Interleukin-11 was approved to reduce the duration and severity of thrombocytopenia after chemotherapy. However, limited efficacy and significant toxicity (fluid retention and atrial arrhythmias) have limited its use.

C. GI toxicity

    1. Stomatitis is an unpleasant consequence of many chemotherapeutic agents (see Table 21-1) and is commonly the dose-limiting toxicity of methotrexate and FU. With simultaneous administration of radiation therapy, the toxicity is more severe. Healing generally occurs within 7–10 days of the development of symptoms. The severity of stomatitis ranges from mild (oral discomfort) to severe (ulceration, impaired oral intake, and hemorrhage). In mild cases, oral rinses (chlorhexidine, 15–30 ml swish and spit tid, or the combination of equal parts diphenhydramine elixir, saline, and 3% hydrogen peroxide) may provide relief. In severe cases, IV morphine is appropriate. **IV fluids** should be used to supplement oral intake as needed. Aspiration may develop in patients with moderate or severe stomatitis; precautions should include elevation of the head of the bed and availability of a hand-held suction apparatus. In severe or prolonged episodes, superinfection with *Candida* or herpes simplex requires appropriate diagnosis and antimicrobial intervention.

    2. Diarrhea is the result of cytotoxicity to proliferating cells of the intestinal mucosa. In some cases, IV fluids are necessary to avoid intravascular volume depletion. The use of oral opioid agents as antidiarrheals is commonly limited by abdominal cramping. Severe diarrhea associated with 5-FU and leucovorin has been reported to respond to octreotide, 150–500 μg SC tid. Diarrhea secondary to irinotecan is treated with loperamide, 4 mg PO then 2 mg q2h while awake, and 4 mg q4h during the night.

    3. Nausea and vomiting may develop in varying degrees and frequency. Suggestions for antiemetic agent(s) are listed in Table 21-2 according to the severity of nausea and vomiting outlined in Table 21-1.

D. Interstitial pneumonitis may develop as a dose-related, cumulative toxicity or as an idiosyncratic reaction. The implicated agent should be discontinued, and institution of glucocorticoids (e.g., prednisone, 1 mg/kg PO qd or equivalent) may be of some benefit. The long-term outcome is unpredictable.

E. Hemorrhagic cystitis may develop with either cyclophosphamide or ifosfamide and is best anticipated and treated with prophylactic mesna. If it develops, continuous bladder irrigation with isotonic saline should continue until the hematuria resolves.

F. Tumor lysis syndrome occurs in patients with rapidly proliferating neoplasms that are highly sensitive to chemotherapy. Rapid tumor cell death releases intracellular contents and causes hyperkalemia, hyperphosphatemia, and hyperuricemia. Although reported in the treatment of a variety of malignancies, it is usually associated with **high-grade non-Hodgkin's lymphoma** and **acute leukemia.** During induction chemotherapy, prophylactic measures should include allopurinol, 300–600 mg PO qd, and aggressive IV volume expansion (e.g., 3000 ml/m^2/day). The addition of sodium bicarbonate, 50 mEq/1000 ml IV fluid, to alkalinize the urine above pH 7 may prevent uric acid nephropathy and acute renal failure. When hyperphosphatemia accompanies hyperuricemia, urine alkalinization should be avoided because calcium phosphate precipitation may result in renal failure. Despite these preventive measures, hemodialysis may be needed for hyperkalemia, hyperphosphatemia, acute renal failure, or fluid overload.

II. **Radiation therapy** toxicity is related to the location of the therapy, total dose delivered, and rates of delivery. Large dose fractions of radiation are associated with greater toxicity to the normal tissues encompassed in the radiation field.

A. **Acute toxicity** develops within the first 3 months of therapy and is characterized by an inflammatory reaction. Such toxicity may respond to antiinflammatory agents such as glucocorticoids. Local irritations or burns in the treatment field generally resolve with time. Close observation and treatment of any infections and palliation of symptoms such as pain, dysphagia, dysuria, or diarrhea (depending on the site of treatment) are the mainstays of supportive care until healing has occurred.

B. **Subacute toxicities** between 3 and 6 months of therapy and chronic toxicity after 6 months are less amenable to therapy, as fibrosis and scarring are present. Daily amifostine before head and neck radiation therapy decreases the incidence of xerostomia (*J Clin Oncol* 13:490, 1996).

Hematopoietic Stem Cell Transplantation

Hematopoietic stem cell transplantation involves IV infusion of either hematopoietic progenitors collected from the bone marrow by aspiration from the iliac crests in the operating room or peripheral blood stem cells collected by apheresis after treatment of the donor with G-CSF or GM-CSF. Allogeneic stem cells are collected from another person (the donor), whereas autologous stem cells are collected from the patient. For autologous transplant, peripheral blood stem cells have largely replaced bone marrow as the source of progenitors because hematologic recovery is more rapid.

I. **Allogeneic stem cell transplant.** HLA-matched siblings are the most common donors, but matched unrelated donors can be identified for many patients through the National Bone Marrow Donor Registry. Allogeneic transplants are performed to restore normal hematopoiesis or immune function in patients with aplastic anemia, immunodeficiency, or hemoglobinopathies and is also used to treat resistant leukemia and lymphoma. For patients with resistant acute leukemia, allogeneic transplant is generally favored, whereas for those with resistant lymphoma, autologous transplant is usually preferred. The "preparative regimen" is given immediately before transplant and includes chemotherapy with or without total body irradiation. For patients with nonmalignant conditions, the preparative regimen provides immunosuppression, which is needed for engraftment. For patients with resistant malignancy, the preparative regimen is designed to promote engraftment and to kill tumor cells. Unlike autologous transplant, allogeneic transplants may be accompanied by a graft-versus-tumor effect, which appears to be a very important part of curing leukemia or lymphoma (see sec. **III.B**).

II. **Autologous stem cell transplantation.** Eradication of malignancy is entirely the result of the preparative regimen, because no graft-versus-tumor effect can occur. The major advantage of autologous transplant is that GVHD (see sec. **III.B**) does not occur; therefore, the risk of death from transplant-related complications is less than 5%. Most autologous transplants are performed for relapsed lymphoma. In patients with relapsed large-cell lymphoma who achieve at least a partial response to salvage chemotherapy, cure can be achieved in 30–50%. Autologous transplant also prolongs the survival of patients with multiple myeloma and is a viable option for individuals with acute leukemia in first remission who lack a compatible sibling donor.

III. Complications of transplantation may be the result of high-dose therapy, pancytopenia, immunodeficiency, or GVHD.

    A. Infections. After the preparative regimen, 7–10 days of profound pancytopenia (absolute neutrophil count <100, platelets <10,000) develop in all patients. During this time nearly all patients experience fever and require empiric broad-spectrum antibiotics. Patients who are seropositive for herpes simplex virus receive acyclovir prophylaxis until neutrophil recovery. G-CSF or GM-CSF is usually given starting on the day after transplant until neutrophil recovery. Patients who have undergone autologous transplant recover immune function within 3–6 months. However, patients who undergo allogeneic transplant have profound and prolonged impairment of humoral and cell-mediated immunity that persists until GVHD resolves. Therefore, patients who are febrile after allogeneic transplant should be cultured and immediately receive IV broad-spectrum antibiotics even if they are not neutropenic. After allogeneic transplant, patients receive long-term prophylaxis for varicella-zoster virus with acyclovir and for *Pneumocystis* with trimethoprim-sulfamethoxazole. Patients are at risk for reactivation and systemic infection with cytomegalovirus (CMV). One strategy for preventing overt infection is to perform shell vial cultures or polymerase chain reaction assays on blood weekly or biweekly during the period of maximal risk (1–6 months posttransplant). Ganciclovir or foscarnet is given if testing is positive for CMV. Patients who have undergone allogeneic transplant require reimmunization.

    B. GVHD is an immunologic response by the donor to recipient antigens and is the major complication of allogeneic transplantation. GVHD within the first 100 days of transplant (acute GVHD) produces a skin rash, diarrhea, and liver dysfunction. Despite prophylaxis with cyclosporine and methotrexate, significant acute GVHD occurs in 30–50% of transplants from matched sibling donors. Chronic GVHD occurs more than 90–100 days after transplant and resembles an autoimmune disorder, with protean manifestations that include keratoconjunctivitis sicca, lichenoid changes of the buccal mucosa, and sclerodermatous skin changes. Overall, GVHD accounts for most of the 20–30% mortality that accompanies matched sibling transplant, with death usually resulting from infection. After allogeneic transplant, donor T cells can mediate immunologic destruction of residual tumor cells. This "graft-versus-tumor effect" is unique to allogeneic transplant and plays a key role in eradicating residual malignancy.

    C. Veno-occlusive disease occurs in 1–5% of patients, usually within 21 days of treatment. Risk factors include extensive prior therapy and elevated transaminase values before transplant. Manifestations include hyperbilirubinemia, ascites, tender hepatomegaly, and fluid retention.

    D. Pulmonary complications. CMV pneumonia usually occurs within 6 months of transplant in patients who are seropositive or who receive transplants from seropositive donors. CMV pneumonia is uncommon after autologous transplant. Treatment is with ganciclovir or foscarnet. Interstitial pneumonitis may complicate total body radiation or high-dose chemotherapy and is manifested by cough, dyspnea, and interstitial infiltrates that present 1–3 months after transplant. Prior chest radiotherapy is a risk factor; treatment with prednisone usually results in rapid and long-term improvement.

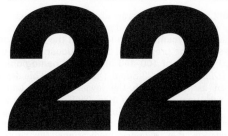

Diabetes Mellitus and Related Disorders

Sam Dagogo-Jack

Diabetes Mellitus

Diabetes mellitus (DM) is a group of metabolic disorders that results in hyperglycemia. These disorders have different etiologies, but their common manifestation, hyperglycemia, is associated with acute and chronic complications regardless of underlying etiology.

I. **Classification of diabetes and related disorders** [*Diabetes Care* 23(Suppl 1):S4, 2000].

    A. **DM** is classified into two broad types and a third, miscellaneous category.

        1. **Type 1 diabetes** accounts for fewer than 10% of all cases of DM, occurs in younger persons, and is caused by severe insulin deficiency that results from an immune-mediated destruction of the pancreatic islet β cells. Exogenous insulin is required to control blood glucose, prevent diabetic ketoacidosis (DKA), and preserve life. A transient period of insulin independence ("honeymoon phase") or reduced insulin requirement may occur early in the course of type 1 DM.

        2. **Type 2 diabetes** accounts for more than 90% of all cases of DM. Usually a disease of adults, type 2 DM is being diagnosed increasingly in younger age groups. Obesity, insulin resistance, and relative insulin deficiency are characteristic findings. Insulin secretion may be sufficient to prevent ketosis under basal conditions, but DKA can develop during severe stress.

        3. **Other specific types** of DM include those that result from genetic defects in insulin secretion or action, exocrine pancreatic disease, pancreatectomy, endocrinopathies (e.g., Cushing's syndrome, acromegaly), drugs, and other syndromes.

    B. **Gestational DM** complicates approximately 4% of all pregnancies and usually resolves after delivery, although affected women remain at an increased risk for development of type 2 DM later in life.

    C. **Impaired glucose tolerance (IGT) and impaired fasting glucose (IFG)** refer to intermediate states between normal glucose tolerance and DM. IFG and IGT appear to be risk factors for type 2 diabetes.

II. **Diagnosis**

    A. **The diagnosis of DM** can be established using any of the following criteria:

        1. **Plasma glucose of 126 mg/dl or greater** after an overnight fast. This should be confirmed with a repeat test.

        2. **Symptoms of diabetes** and a random plasma glucose of **200 mg/dl** or greater.

        3. **Oral glucose tolerance test** that shows a plasma glucose of **200 mg/dl** or greater at 2 hours after a 75-g glucose load.

    B. **IGT** is defined by a 2-hour oral glucose tolerance test plasma glucose greater than 140 mg/dl but less than 200 mg/dl.

    C. **IFG** is defined by a fasting plasma glucose of 110 mg/dl or greater but less than 126 mg/dl. Lifestyle modifications may be appropriate for persons with IGT or IFG, but the rationale for drug therapy has not been established.

III. **Principles of management of DM.** The therapeutic goals are alleviation of symptoms, achievement of metabolic control, and prevention of acute and long-term complications of diabetes. **Glycemic control is set at the same goal for type 1 and type 2 diabetes: average preprandial blood glucose values of 80–120 mg/dl, bedtime blood glucose of 100–140 mg/dl, and hemoglobin A1c (HbA1c) of 7% or lower** [*Diabetes Care* 23(Suppl 1):S4, 2000]. This degree of glycemic control has been associated with the lowest risk for long-term complications in patients with type 1 (*N Engl J Med* 329:978, 1993) as well as type 2 diabetes (*Lancet* 352:837, 1998). An individualized, comprehensive diabetes care plan is necessary to accomplish these goals. The mnemonic **MEDEM** (monitoring, education, diet, exercise, medications) can be used to recall the modalities of diabetes care.

A. **Monitoring** of diabetes control consists of the following.

1. **HbA1c** provides an integrated measure of blood glucose profile over the preceding 2–3 months; it should be obtained approximately every 3 months.

2. **Self-monitoring of blood glucose** is an important tool of diabetes management and is recommended for all patients.

3. **Urine glucose** correlates poorly with blood glucose, is dependent on renal glucose threshold (150–300 mg/dl), and should only be used for monitoring diabetes therapy if self-monitoring of blood glucose is impractical.

4. **Ketonuria** grossly reflects ketonemia. All DM patients should monitor urine ketones using Ketostix or Acetest tablets during febrile illness or persistent hyperglycemia, or if signs of impending DKA (e.g., nausea, vomiting, abdominal pain) develop.

B. **Patient education** is integral to successful management of diabetes. Diabetes education should be reinforced at every opportunity, particularly during hospitalization for diabetes-related complications.

C. **Dietary modification.** A balanced diet that provides adequate nutrition and maintains a healthy weight is desirable. Caloric restriction is recommended for overweight persons. An allowance of 10–20% of total caloric intake as protein and less than 30% as total fat (less than 10% saturated fat) is appropriate. Patients with diabetic nephropathy usually are allowed a protein intake of 0.8 g/kg/day. With deterioration in renal function, further restriction in protein intake (0.6 g/kg) can be considered in selected patients. Carbohydrate allowance should be individualized based on glycemic control, plasma lipids, and weight goals.

D. **Exercise** improves insulin sensitivity, reduces fasting and postprandial blood glucose, and offers numerous metabolic, cardiovascular, and psychological benefits in diabetic patients.

E. **Medications** that are used for treating diabetes include insulin and oral agents (see Type 1 Diabetes and Diabetic Ketoacidosis, and Type 2 Diabetes and Nonketotic Hyperosmolar Syndrome). Patients with type 1 DM require lifelong insulin therapy, whereas type 2 DM patients respond initially to oral antidiabetic agents but may require insulin as the disease progresses. Medications for diabetes are most effective if instituted as part of a comprehensive management approach that includes dietary and exercise counseling.

Diabetes Mellitus in Hospitalized Patients

I. **Indications for hospitalization.** Hospital admission can be considered for stabilization of newly diagnosed diabetes, newly recognized diabetes in pregnancy, and management of complications of diabetes or other acute medical conditions. Inpatient care is particularly appropriate in the following situations:

A. DKA, as indicated by a plasma glucose of 250 mg/dl or greater in association with an arterial pH of less than 7.35 (venous pH <7.30) or serum bicarbonate level of less than 15 mEq/L and ketonuria or ketonemia.

B. Hyperosmolar nonketotic state, usually suggested by marked hyperglycemia (≥400 mg/dl) and elevated serum osmolality (>315 mOsm/kg), often accompanied by impaired mental status.

C. Hypoglycemia (<50 mg/dl), especially if induced by a sulfonylurea drug or resulting in coma, seizures, or altered mentation.

II. Management of diabetes in hospitalized patients (*Diabetes Care* 18:870, 1995). Glycemic control seldom receives priority attention when diabetic patients are hospitalized for reasons other than diabetes, despite evidence linking hyperglycemia to (1) decreased cerebral blood flow, (2) impaired wound healing, (3) infections, and (4) delayed drug clearance (especially narcotic analgesics). Even in previously stable patients, glycemic control tends to deteriorate during hospitalization because of the stress of illness, erratic insulin absorption, effects of medications, and inappropriate dietary practices. Hospital admission, regardless of its indication, is an opportunity to reinforce the elements of diabetes management and optimize glycemic control (see Diabetes Mellitus in Surgical Patients).

A. Patients hospitalized for reasons other than diabetes who are eating normally should continue their usual diabetes treatment, unless specifically contraindicated. The common practice of **sliding scale** administration of regular insulin alone, q6h, based on bedside capillary blood glucose levels, seldom gives satisfactory results; regimens that include intermediate-acting insulin give superior glycemic control (*Arch Intern Med* 157:545, 1997).

    1. Monitoring. Blood glucose should be monitored at least two to four times a day, especially in patients treated with insulin. Extreme values (>300 mg/dl or <60 mg/dl) from bedside capillary blood glucose meters should be confirmed using laboratory measurements. After confirmation, urine ketone reaction should be determined using dipstick (Ketostix) or Acetest tablets if persistent hyperglycemia is observed in febrile or sick patients. HbA1c should be measured if no recent result is available.

    2. Education regarding optimal diabetes care should be reinforced at every opportunity. Many patients admitted for reasons other than diabetes have suboptimal diabetes control (i.e., HbA1c >7%) and will benefit from such reinforcement.

    3. Dietary intervention. A balanced diet should be provided to ensure adequate nutrition. Restriction of total and saturated fat intake, with augmentation of complex carbohydrates and dietary fiber, is appropriate.

    4. Exercise. Physical activity should be encouraged, as appropriate.

    5. Medications for diabetes should be reviewed with regard to potential toxicities. **Metformin** (see Type 2 Diabetes and Nonketotic Hyperosmolar Syndrome, sec. **I.B**) should be withheld 1 day before planned surgical procedures or diagnostic evaluation that involves the use of iodinated radiocontrast dyes. Metformin can be restarted after recovery from surgical procedures, provided that normal renal function is established and oral intake is resumed. Similarly, metformin can be restarted 48 hours after radiocontrast exposure and documentation of normal renal function. Suspension of metformin therapy also is appropriate in the presence of sepsis, CHF, renal dysfunction, or other conditions that predispose to lactic acidosis. **Thiazolidinediones** should not be administered to patients with hepatic dysfunction, as indicated by elevated serum transaminases.

B. Patients hospitalized for reasons other than diabetes who are required to fast should discontinue oral antidiabetic medications. Depending on the circumstances, such patients can be treated with SC or IV insulin, together with IV infusion of 5% dextrose in water (D5W) or dextrose in saline, to maintain plasma glucose at an acceptable range. Blood glucose should be monitored at least four times a day, as well as during episodes of suspected hypoglycemia.

C. **Newly diagnosed type 1 DM** and **newly recognized DM in pregnancy** may be indications for hospitalization, even in the absence of ketoacidosis. Significant hyperglycemia is the rule in patients who meet criteria for admission, and insulin therapy is almost always required. Intensive patient education in self-monitoring, dietary modification, and self-management skills is mandatory.

D. Patients with **newly diagnosed type 2 DM** who meet the criteria for hospitalization often have severe hyperglycemia and may require insulin therapy for initial stabilization, even in the absence of ketoacidosis or hyperosmolar syndrome. The opportunity to teach self-care skills, dietary modification, the role of exercise, and general diabetes principles must not be missed. After achieving glycemic control with exogenous insulin, the response to oral antidiabetic agents can be assessed in-house or as an outpatient. **The initial choice of oral medication** is a matter of clinical judgment (see Type 2 Diabetes and Nonketotic Hyperosmolar Syndrome, sec. **I**).

Type 1 Diabetes and
Diabetic Ketoacidosis

A comprehensive approach, including monitoring, education, dietary and exercise counseling, and insulin therapy, is necessary for successful management of type 1 DM (see Diabetes Mellitus, sec. **III**). The glycemic goals are average preprandial blood glucose values of 80–120 mg/dl, bedtime blood glucose of 100–140 mg/dl, and HbA1c of 7% or lower. A team approach, tailored to the individual patient's needs, that uses the expertise of diabetes educators, dietitians, and other members of the diabetes care team offers the best chances of success.

I. **Treatment of type 1 DM** requires lifelong insulin replacement.

A. **Insulin preparations.** After SC injection, there is individual variability in the duration and peak activity of insulin preparations and day-to-day variability in the same subject (Table 22-1).

1. **Rapid-acting insulins** include regular insulin, semilente, and lispro. Regular insulin can be administered intravenously, intramuscularly, or by the more familiar SC route. Absorption of IM injection is variable and undependable, especially in hypovolemic patients. IV regular insulin is given as a bolus, usually followed by continuous infusion, for the treatment of hyperglycemic crises. An IV bolus of regular insulin exerts maximum effect in 10–30 minutes and is quickly dissipated. SC injection of regular insulin or semilente has an onset of action within 1 hour. **Lispro** is a human regular insulin analog that is absorbed quickly (within 15 minutes) at SC sites, reaches peak plasma levels within 1 hour, and has a shorter duration of action than regular insulin ($\approx$ 3–4 hours).

2. **Intermediate-acting insulins** include NPH (isophane) and lente (zinc). These insulins are released slowly from SC sites and reach peak activity after 6–12 hours, followed by gradual decline.

3. **Long-acting insulins.** Ultralente insulin and protamine zinc insulin are absorbed more slowly than the intermediate-acting preparations. **Glargine** is a bioengineered human insulin analog with an extended duration of activity. Long-acting insulins provide a steady "basal" supply of circulating insulin when administered once or twice a day.

4. **Concentration.** Most insulins now contain 100 units/ml (U-100). A U-500 preparation is available for the rare patient with severe insulin resistance.

5. **Mixed insulin therapy.** Rapid-acting insulins (regular and lispro) can be mixed with intermediate-acting (NPH and lente) or long-acting (ultralente) insulins in the same syringe for convenience. The rapid-

Table 22-1. Approximate kinetics of human insulin preparations after subcutaneous injection

Insulin type	Onset of action (hrs)	Peak effect (hrs)	Duration of activity (hrs)
Rapid acting			
Lispro	0.25–0.50	0.50–1.50	3–5
Regular	0.50–1.00	2–4	6–8
Intermediate acting			
NPH	1–2	6–12	18–24
Lente	1–3	6–12	18–26
Long acting			
Ultralente	4–6	10–16	24–48
PZI	3–8	14–24	24–40
Glargine	4–6	6–24*	>24

PZI = protamine zinc insulin.
*Insulin dosage and individual variability in absorption and clearance rates affect pharmacokinetic data. Human insulins may peak earlier and be dissipated faster than porcine or bovine insulins. Duration of insulin activity is prolonged in renal failure. After a lag time of approximately 5 hrs, glargine has a flat peakless effect over a 24-hr period.

acting insulin should be drawn first, cross contamination should be avoided, and the mixed insulin should be injected immediately. **Protamine zinc insulin should not be mixed with other types of insulin.** Commercial premixed insulin preparations do not allow for dose adjustment of individual components but may be convenient for patients who are unable or unwilling to do the mixing themselves.

6. **SC insulin delivery** is accomplished using disposable syringes with fine hypodermic needles; less widely used devices include insulin pens and pumps. The anterior abdominal wall, thighs, buttocks, and arms are the preferred sites for SC insulin injection. Absorption is fastest from the abdomen, followed by the arm, buttocks, and thigh, probably as a result of differences in blood flow. Injection sites should be rotated within the regions rather than randomly across separate regions, to minimize erratic absorption. Clean techniques should be adopted, and areas of scarring, ulceration, or infection should be avoided. Exercise or massage over the injection site may accelerate insulin absorption.

B. **Initial insulin dosage** for optimal glycemic control is approximately 0.5–1.0 units/kg/day for the average nonobese patient. A conservative total daily dose is given initially; the dose is then adjusted, using blood glucose values.

1. **The conventional insulin regimen** uses a mixture of short- and intermediate-acting (so-called split-mixed) insulins administered before breakfast and before the evening meal. Approximately two-thirds of the total daily dose is injected in the morning and one-third in the evening. Approximately two-thirds of each injection comprises intermediate-acting insulin and one-third is rapid-acting insulin ("rule of thirds"). These proportions should be modified for patients with unusual work schedules or eating patterns. The units of individual insulin components of each injection are then adjusted using data from preprandial and bedtime blood glucose monitoring.

2. **The multiple daily insulin injections regimen** provides approximately 40–50% of the total daily dose of insulin as basal insulin supply, using

one or two injections of long-acting or intermediate-acting insulin. The remainder is given as three doses of rapid-acting insulin divided across the main meals, empirically or in proportion to the carbohydrate content. An allowance of 1.0 unit/10 g carbohydrate consumed is typical.

3. **Continuous SC insulin infusion** is a tool for intensive diabetes control in selected patients. It provides 50% of total daily insulin as basal insulin and the remainder as multiple preprandial boluses of insulin, using a programmable insulin pump. As with the multiple daily insulin injections regimen, the premeal insulin doses are estimated from the carbohydrate content of each meal.

4. **Sliding scale** administration of regular insulin alone to hospitalized patients, based on bedside capillary blood glucose levels, rarely achieves satisfactory glycemic control; regimens that include intermediate-acting insulin give superior results *(Arch Intern Med* 157:545, 1997).

5. **Monitoring.** Blood glucose should be monitored at least four times a day (preprandially and at bedtime) in hospitalized patients with type 1 diabetes. The HbA1c should be obtained if no recent result is available. Urine should be tested for ketones whenever hyperglycemia (>300 mg/dl) persists.

II. **DKA,** a potentially fatal complication, occurs in up to 5% of patients with type 1 diabetes annually; it is seen less frequently in type 2 diabetes. DKA is a manifestation of severe insulin deficiency, often in association with stress and activation of counterregulatory hormones (e.g., catecholamines, glucagon).

A. **Precipitating factors** for DKA include inadvertent or deliberate interruption of insulin therapy, sepsis, trauma, myocardial infarction, and pregnancy. DKA may be the first presentation of type 1, and rarely even type 2, diabetes.

B. **Diagnosis.** A high index of suspicion is warranted, because clinical presentation may be nonspecific.

1. **Clinical features** include nausea, vomiting, and vaguely localized abdominal pain. Prominent GI symptoms may give rise to suspicion for intra-abdominal pathology. Dehydration is invariable, and respiratory distress, shock, and coma can occur.

2. **Laboratory evaluation** shows an increased ion gap metabolic acidosis and positive serum ketones. Plasma glucose usually is elevated, but the degree of hyperglycemia may be moderate ($\approx$ 300 mg/dl or lower) in 10–15% of patients in DKA. Pregnancy and alcohol ingestion are associated with "euglycemic DKA." The urine ketone reaction correlates poorly with ketonemia but is usually positive in DKA. Hyponatremia, hyperkalemia, azotemia, and hyperosmolality are other findings. Serum amylase and transaminases may be elevated, again raising suspicion for intra-abdominal pathology. A focused search for a precipitating infection is always prudent.

C. **Management of DKA** should preferably be conducted in an ICU. For treatment conducted in a non-ICU setting, close monitoring by a physician is mandatory until ketoacidosis resolves and the patient's condition is stabilized. The therapeutic priorities are fluid replacement, adequate insulin administration, and potassium repletion. Administration of bicarbonate, phosphate, magnesium, or other therapies may be advantageous in selected patients but is not a first-line consideration.

1. **IV access and supportive measures** should be instituted without delay.

2. **Fluid** deficits of several liters are common in DKA patients and can be estimated by subtracting the current weight from a recently known dry weight. Hypotension indicates a loss of at least 10% of body fluids.

a. **Initially,** restoration of circulating **volume** using isotonic (0.9%) saline should be accomplished. The first liter should be infused rapidly (if cardiac function is normal) and should be followed by additional fluids at 1 L/hour until the volume deficit is corrected. Hypotonic saline (0.45%) can be used as initial fluid in patients with severe hypernatremia (>155 mEq/L).

    b. The next goal is to replenish total body water deficits; this can be accomplished using a 0.45% saline infusion at 150–500 ml/hour, depending on degree of dehydration and cardiac and renal status.

    c. Maintenance fluid replacement is continued at a tapered rate until the fluid intake/output records indicate an overall positive balance of approximately 6 L. Complete fluid replacement in a typical DKA patient may require 12–24 hours to accomplish.

3. Insulin therapy. Sufficient insulin must be administered to turn off ketogenesis and correct hyperglycemia.

    a. An IV bolus of regular insulin, 10–15 units, can be administered. This should be followed by continuous infusion of regular insulin at an initial rate of 5–10 units/hour (or 0.1 unit/kg/hour). A solution of regular insulin, 100 units in 500 ml 0.9% saline, infused at a rate of 50 ml/hour, delivers 10 units of insulin per hour. It is not necessary to add albumin routinely to the solution to prevent adsorption of insulin to the glass bottle and infusion tubing. Instead, running the initial 50–100 ml of the solution down the sink should saturate adsorption sites in the infusion apparatus and ensure proper delivery of insulin to the patient.

    b. IM injection of regular insulin, 5–10 units q1h, is an alternative to IV infusion, but absorption from this route is unreliable in hypotensive patients.

    c. A decrease in blood glucose of 50–75 mg/dl/hour is an appropriate response; lesser decrements suggest insulin resistance, inadequate volume repletion, or a problem with insulin delivery. If insulin resistance is suspected, the hourly dose of regular insulin should be increased progressively by 50–100% until an appropriate glycemic response is observed.

    d. Excessively rapid correction of hyperglycemia at rates much greater than 100 mg/dl/hour must be avoided to reduce the risk of osmotic encephalopathy.

    e. Maintenance insulin infusion rates of 1–2 units/hour are appropriate when serum bicarbonate rises to 15 mEq/L or higher and the anion gap has closed. Once oral intake resumes, insulin can be administered SC and the parenteral route can be discontinued. It is prudent to give the first SC injection of insulin approximately 30 minutes before stopping the IV route.

4. Dextrose (5%) in saline should be infused once plasma glucose decreases to 250 mg/dl to prevent dangerous hypoglycemia.

5. Potassium deficit should always be assumed or anticipated, regardless of plasma levels on admission. Insulin therapy results in a rapid shift of potassium into the intracellular compartment.

    a. The goal is to maintain plasma potassium in the normal range and thereby prevent potentially fatal cardiac effects of hypokalemia. Potassium status should be documented from the outset; this includes ECG to rule out rare life-threatening hyperkalemia.

    b. Potassium should be added routinely to the IV fluids at a rate of 10–20 mEq/hour except in patients with hyperkalemia (>6.0 mmol/L and/or ECG evidence), renal failure, or oliguria confirmed by bladder catheterization.

    c. Patients who present with hypokalemia should receive higher doses of potassium, 40 mEq/hour or greater, depending on severity.

    d. Potassium chloride is an appropriate initial choice, but this can later be changed to potassium phosphate to reduce chloride load.

6. Monitoring of therapy. Blood glucose should be monitored hourly, serum electrolytes every 1–2 hours, and arterial blood gases as often as necessary. Serum sodium tends to rise as hyperglycemia is corrected; failure to observe this trend suggests that the patient is being overhydrated with free water. Serial serum ketone assays are not necessary, because ketonemia lags behind clinical recovery; closure of the anion gap is a more reliable index of metabolic recovery. Use of a flowchart is an efficient method of tracking clinical data (e.g., weight, fluid balance, mental status) and laboratory results during the management of DKA. Continuous ECG monitoring may be required for proper management of dyskalemia in patients with oliguria or renal failure.

7. **Bicarbonate therapy** is not routinely necessary and may be deleterious if given injudiciously. However, **bicarbonate therapy may be appropriate** and should be considered for DKA patients who develop (1) shock or coma, (2) severe acidosis (pH ≤7.1), (3) severe depletion of buffering reserve (plasma bicarbonate <5 mEq/L), (4) acidosis-induced cardiac or respiratory dysfunction, or (5) severe hyperkalemia. **Sodium bicarbonate, 50–100 mEq in 1 L** of 0.45% saline infused over 30–60 minutes, may be appropriate in these situations. Bicarbonate treatment should be guided by arterial pH measurement and continued until the indications are no longer present. Care should be taken to avoid hypokalemia; an additional dose of potassium, 10 mEq, should be included with each infusion of bicarbonate unless hyperkalemia is present.

8. **Phosphate and magnesium** stores are subnormal in DKA patients, and plasma levels (particularly phosphate) decline further during insulin therapy. The clinical significance of these changes is unclear, and routine replacement of phosphate or magnesium is not necessary. In hypophosphatemic patients with compromised oral intake, the use of potassium phosphate in maintenance IV fluids can be considered (see Chap. 3). Magnesium therapy is indicated in patients with ventricular arrhythmia and can be administered as magnesium sulfate (50%) in doses of 2.5–5.0 ml (10–20 mEq magnesium) IV.

9. **IV antimicrobial therapy** should be started promptly for documented bacterial, fungal, and other treatable infections. Empiric-broad spectrum antibiotics can be started in septic patients, pending results of blood cultures (see Chap. 14).

D. **Complications of DKA** include life-threatening conditions that must be recognized and treated promptly.

1. **Lactic acidosis** may result from prolonged dehydration, shock, infection, and tissue hypoxia in DKA patients. Lactic acidosis should be suspected in patients with refractory metabolic acidosis and persistent anion gap despite optimal therapy for DKA. Adequate volume replacement, control of sepsis, and judicious use of bicarbonate constitute the approach to management.

2. **Arterial thrombosis** manifesting as stroke, myocardial infarction, or an ischemic limb occurs with increased frequency in DKA. However, routine anticoagulation is not indicated in DKA patients except as part of the specific therapy for a thrombotic event.

3. **Cerebral edema,** a dire complication of DKA, is observed more frequently in children than adults. Symptoms of raised intracranial pressure (e.g., headache, altered mental status, papilledema) or sudden deterioration in mental status after initial improvement in a patient with DKA should raise suspicion for cerebral edema. Overhydration with free water and excessively rapid correction of hyperglycemia are known risk factors. A fall in serum sodium or failure to rise during therapy of DKA is a clue to imminent or established overhydration with free water. Neuroimaging with CT can establish the diagnosis. Prompt recognition and treatment with IV mannitol is helpful and may prevent neurologic sequelae in patients who survive cerebral edema.

E. **Prevention of DKA.** Every episode of DKA suggests a breakdown in clinical communication. Diabetes education should therefore be reinforced at every opportunity, with special emphasis on (1) self-management skills during prodromal sick days; (2) the body's need for more, rather than less, insulin during such illnesses; (3) testing of urine for ketones; and (4) procedures for obtaining timely and preventive medical advice.

Type 2 Diabetes and Nonketotic Hyperosmolar Syndrome

The glycemic goals for patients with type 2 DM are average preprandial blood glucose values of 80–120 mg/dl, bedtime blood glucose of 100–140 mg/dl, and HbA1c of 7% or lower [*Diabetes Care* 23(Suppl 1):S32, 2000].

I. **Treatment of type 2 diabetes** requires a comprehensive approach that incorporates lifestyle and pharmacologic interventions (see Diabetes Mellitus, sec. **III**). As in the management of type 1 DM, a treatment plan tailored to the individual patient's needs that uses the expertise of diabetes educators, dietitians, and other members of the diabetes care team offers the best chances of success. The choice of **oral antidiabetic agents** (Table 22-2) for control of hyperglycemia in patients with type 2 diabetes is a matter of clinical judgment. Monotherapy with maximum doses of insulin secretagogues, metformin, or thiazolidinediones yields comparable glucose-lowering effects. Insulin secretagogues such as sulfonylureas and repaglinide exert their glucose-lowering effects within days, but approximately 20% of patients do not respond to these agents ("primary failure"). The maximum effects of metformin or thiazolidinediones may not be observed for several weeks. Because residual pancreatic beta-cell function is required for the glucose-lowering effects of sulfonylureas, repaglinide, metformin, and thiazolidinediones, many patients with advanced type 2 DM do not respond satisfactorily to these agents. Insulin therapy may thus be an early choice for such patients. Moreover, the toxicity profile of some oral agents may preclude their use in patients with pre-existing illnesses.

A. **Insulin secretagogues**

    1. **Sulfonylureas** lower blood glucose by augmenting insulin secretion. Treatment with equivalent doses of different sulfonylurea drugs gives similar results; the mean decrease in fasting blood glucose is approximately 60 mg/dl. Sulfonylureas should be taken 30–60 minutes before food and should never be administered to patients who are observing a voluntary or imposed fast. Therapy should be initiated with the lowest effective dose and increased gradually over several days or weeks to the optimal dose. Hypoglycemia and weight gain are notable adverse effects of sulfonylureas.

    2. **Repaglinide** is a meglitinide analog that augments food-stimulated insulin secretion. It can be used as a single agent or in combination with metformin in patients with type 2 DM. The dose range is 0.5–4.0 mg PO with two to four meals daily. The drug should be taken within 30 minutes before meals and skipped if no meal is planned. Adverse effects include hypoglycemia and weight gain.

    3. **Nateglinide** (*Diabetes Care* 23:202, 2000), a D-phenylalanine derivative chemically distinct from other insulin secretagogues, acts directly on the pancreatic β cells to stimulate early insulin secretion. A dose of 120 mg PO taken 10 minutes before breakfast, lunch, and dinner leads to significant insulin secretion within 15 minutes a return to baseline in 3–4 hours. Nateglinide is effective in controlling postprandial hyperglycemia. The drug is well tolerated and the risk of hypoglycemia appears minimal.

B. **Metformin,** the only biguanide in current clinical use, inhibits hepatic glucose output and stimulates glucose uptake by peripheral tissues. Metformin is taken with food and, beginning with a single 500-mg or 850-mg tablet, the dose is increased slowly every 1–2 weeks until optimal glycemic effect is achieved or the maximum dose (2550 mg/day) is reached. GI symptoms occur

Table 22-2. Characteristics of oral antidiabetic agents

Drug	Daily dosage range	Dose(s) /day	Duration of action (hrs)	Main adverse effects
Sulfonylureas				
First generation				Hypoglycemia, weight gain
Tolbutamide	0.5–2.0 g	2–3	12	
Acetohexamide	0.25–1.5 g	1–2	12–24	
Tolazamide	0.1–0.5 g	1–2	12–24	
Chlorpropamide	1.25–20.0 mg	1	36–72	
Second generation				
Glyburide	5–40 mg	1–2	16–24	
Glipizide	1.8 mg	1–2	12	
Glimepiride		1	24	
Meglitinide	1–16 mg	2–4	1–2	Hypoglycemia, weight gain
Repaglinide				
Biguanide				GI intolerance, lactic acidosis
Metformin	1.0–2.5 g	2–3	6–12	
Alpha-glucosidase inhibitors				GI intolerance
Acarbose	75–300 mg	3	N/A	
Miglitol	75–300 mg	3	N/A	
Thiazolidinediones				Fluid retention, hepatotoxicity
Rosiglitazone	2–8 mg	1–2	12–24	
Pioglitazone	15–45 mg	1	24	

N/A = not applicable because agents do not act systemically.

frequently but are seldom serious. Lactic acidosis, the most serious adverse effect, has an incidence of approximately three cases per 100,000 patient-years and a significant mortality rate. Risk factors for lactic acidosis in patients who are taking metformin include renal dysfunction, hypovolemia, tissue hypoxia, infection, alcoholism, and cardiorespiratory disease. **A serum creatinine level of 1.5 mg/dl in men (1.4 mg/dl in women) or higher is a contraindication to metformin use.** Elderly patients with a glomerular filtration rate of less than 70 ml/minute are not candidates for metformin therapy.

C. **Alpha-glucosidase inhibitors** block carbohydrate digestion and decrease postprandial hyperglycemia when administered with food. Two members of this class, **acarbose** and **miglitol,** exert maximal effects at a dosage of approximately 150 mg/day. Each drug should be initiated at low doses (25 mg PO qd–tid, with food) and increased slowly in weekly steps of 25 mg to minimize GI intolerance. Monotherapy with these agents seldom gives satisfactory results, but their addition to other drugs can improve glycemic control. Dose-related adverse effects are symptoms of carbohydrate malabsorption. Acarbose has been associated with elevation in liver enzymes, and therefore periodic monitoring of transaminases is recommended. Hypoglycemia in patients who are receiving regimens that include alpha-glucosidase inhibitors should be treated with glucose, not sucrose.

D. **Thiazolidinediones** increase tissue sensitivity to insulin. The risk of drug-induced hepatotoxicity with this class mandates close monitoring of liver function, particularly during the initial 12 months of drug exposure. Edema and cytopenia, from increased plasma volume, also occur with these agents. Resumption of ovulation may occur in some premenopausal women with anovulatory cycles after thiazolidinedione therapy. Therefore, contraceptive practice should be reviewed to prevent unintended pregnancy. Two thiazolidinediones are in clinical use.

1. **Rosiglitazone** is used alone as an adjunct to diet and exercise or in combination with metformin or a sulfonylurea. The usual starting dosage is 4 mg PO qd (or 2 mg PO bid) taken with or without food. This can be advanced to 8 mg PO qd (or 4 mg PO bid) after 12 weeks if glycemic response is inadequate. Rosiglitazone should be used with caution in patients with significant heart disease (New York Heart Association class 3 and 4 cardiac status) because of the risk of CHF from fluid retention. Although preapproval clinical trials data suggest a low propensity for hepatotoxicity, regular monitoring of hepatic transaminases is required in patients treated with rosiglitazone.

2. **Pioglitazone** is used as a single agent (as an adjunct to diet and exercise) or in combination with a sulfonylurea, metformin, or insulin. The initial dosage is 15 mg or 30 mg PO qd, taken with or without food; this can be increased after several weeks to 45 mg PO qd for optimal effect. Pioglitazone should be used with caution in patients with significant heart disease (New York Heart Association class 3 and 4 cardiac status) because of the risk of CHF from fluid retention. Although preapproval clinical trials data suggest a low risk for hepatotoxicity, regular monitoring of hepatic transaminases is required during pioglitazone therapy.

E. **Insulin therapy in type 2 DM** is indicated for refractory hyperglycemia, DKA, and nonketotic hyperosmolar crisis during pregnancy and other situations in which oral antidiabetic agents are contraindicated. Effective insulin regimens for patients with type 2 diabetes include multiple daily injections of various proportions of short- and intermediate- or long-acting insulins. Large doses of insulin (>100 units/day) usually are required for optimal glycemic control because of the prevailing insulin resistance. The risk of insulin-induced hypoglycemia is low in this population, but weight gain can be considerable.

F. **Drug combinations.** Concurrent use of two or more medications from different classes often is necessary to achieve optimal glycemic control. Widely used regimens include a sulfonylurea plus metformin, and a thiazolidinedione plus a sulfonylurea or insulin.

II. **Nonketotic hyperosmolar syndrome (NKHS)** results from severe dehydration and hyperglycemia in type 2 DM patients. Ketoacidosis is absent because residual insulin secretion, though inadequate for glycemic control, effectively inhibits lipolysis and ketogenesis. Precipitating factors include stress, infection, stroke, noncompliance with medications, and dietary indiscretion. Impaired glucose excretion is a contributory factor in patients with renal insufficiency or prerenal azotemia.

A. **Diagnosis**

1. **Clinical manifestations.** NKHS often develops in patients who are manifestly ill and obtunded. Clinical evidence of severe dehydration is the rule. Focal neurologic deficits may be found at presentation or may develop during therapy. Therefore, repeated neurologic assessment is recommended.

2. **Laboratory** findings include (1) hyperglycemia, often greater than 600 mg/dl; (2) plasma osmolality of greater than 320 mOsm/L; and (3) absence of ketonemia. Prerenal azotemia and lactic acidosis can develop.

B. Management of NKHS consists of (1) fluid replacement, (2) insulin therapy, and (3) correction of electrolyte deficits. An IV access line should be secured promptly, and supportive measures should be provided. A focused search for precipitating factors (e.g., infection) is appropriate, but such efforts should not delay fluid replacement and insulin therapy.

1. **Fluid replacement** initially should aim to restore intravascular volume and later correct total body water deficit.

   a. **Initial fluid therapy** can be given as isotonic (0.9%) saline. In the absence of cardiac or renal compromise, a rapid infusion rate of 1 L/hour or greater can be used until intravascular volume is restored.

   b. **Free water deficits** can be corrected using infusion of 0.45% saline at a rate guided by serum sodium level and osmolarity, after repletion of intravascular volume (see Chap. 3). Caution should be exercised when replacing fluids in the elderly and in patients with cardiac or renal dysfunction.

   c. **Dextrose (5%)** should be added to the 0.45% saline infusion once plasma glucose decreases to 250–300 mg/dl. If plasma sodium is greater than 150 mmol/L, D5W can be infused instead.

   d. **Maintenance fluids** should be infused at a rate guided by clinical status, especially urine output and evidence of volume repletion or overload. Patients with NKHS may require as much as 10–12 L positive fluid balance over 24–36 hours to restore total deficits.

2. **Insulin therapy** is indicated for all patients with NKHS. In patients with marked hyperglycemia (>600 mg/dl), regular insulin, 5–10 units IV, should be given immediately, followed by continuous infusion. Lower doses of a regular insulin bolus can be used for less severe hyperglycemia. An initial insulin infusion rate of 5–10 units/hour, depending on severity of hyperglycemia, is appropriate. Once plasma glucose decreases to 250–300 mg/dl, insulin infusion can be decreased to 1–2 units/hour. After full rehydration and clinical recovery, insulin can be given SC and patients can thereafter resume their usual diabetes therapy.

3. **Electrolyte management.** Hypokalemia following initiation of IV insulin therapy should be anticipated and corrected. Lactic acidosis requiring bicarbonate therapy may develop as a complication of NKHS or metformin therapy.

4. **Monitoring of therapy.** Use of a flowchart is helpful for tracking clinical data and laboratory results. Initially, blood glucose should be monitored every 30–60 minutes and serum electrolytes every 1–2 hours; frequency of monitoring can be decreased during recovery. Neurologic status must be reassessed frequently; persistent lethargy or altered mentation indicates inadequate therapy. On the other hand, relapse after initial improvement in mental status suggests too-rapid correction of serum osmolarity.

5. **Other considerations.** The clinician should be alert to predisposing factors and possible complications of NKHS.

   a. **Diabetes education** should be reinforced, with emphasis on self-management skills during intercurrent illness.

   b. **IV antimicrobial therapy** should be started promptly for documented bacterial, fungal, and other treatable infections. Empiric broad-spectrum antibiotics can be started in septic patients, pending results of blood cultures.

   c. **Acute renal failure** may result from severe and prolonged hypovolemia. Therefore, evaluation by a nephrologist may be required if oliguria persists despite correction of volume deficit.

   d. **Coagulopathy** that presents either with thrombotic or bleeding episodes requires specialist evaluation and management.

Diabetes Mellitus in
Surgical Patients

Patients with DM undergo surgical procedures at a higher rate than nondiabetic persons (*Arch Intern Med* 159:2405, 1999). Major surgical operations require a period of fasting during which oral antidiabetic medications cannot be used. The stress of surgery itself results in metabolic perturbations that impair glucose regulation, and persistent hyperglycemia is a risk factor for postoperative sepsis. It is therefore important that careful attention be paid to the DM patient who is undergoing a surgical procedure. Elective surgery in patients with uncontrolled DM should preferably be scheduled after acceptable glycemic control has been achieved. If possible, the operation should be scheduled for early morning to minimize prolonged fasting.

 I. **Patients managed with diet alone** may require no special intervention if diabetes is well controlled. Fasting and intraoperative blood glucose should be monitored. If fasting plasma glucose is 200 mg/dl or greater, small doses of SC short-acting insulin (regular or lispro), or IV infusion of insulin and D5W, should be considered, depending on the duration and extent of surgery.

 II. **Patients treated with oral antidiabetic agent.** Sulfonylureas should be discontinued 1 day before surgery; other oral agents should be withheld on the operative day. Blood glucose should be monitored before and after surgery, and during surgery, for extensive procedures. Perioperative hyperglycemia (>200 mg/dl) can be managed with small SC doses of short-acting insulin (regular or lispro). Care must be taken to avoid hypoglycemia. For minor procedures, diabetes medications can be restarted once the patient starts eating. In patients who are exposed to iodinated radiocontrast dyes, metformin therapy is withheld for 48 hours postoperatively and restarted after documentation of normal serum creatinine and absence of contrast-induced nephropathy (see Diabetes Mellitus in Hospitalized Patients, sec. **II.A.5**). For extensive or stressful major procedures, hyperglycemia can be managed using IV insulin infusion (see sec. **IV**).

 III. **Insulin-treated patients can** skip the morning dose of SC insulin on the day of surgery, depending on the nature of the operation. Patients treated with long-acting insulin can be switched to intermediate-acting forms 1–2 days before elective surgery. Close perioperative blood glucose monitoring is crucial to avoid extremes of glycemia.

   A. **Patients undergoing minor surgery** of short duration require no special intervention if fasting plasma glucose is 100–200 mg/dl. Glucose levels should be monitored, q1h, intraoperatively and immediately after surgery. Perioperative hyperglycemia can be managed with small SC doses of short-acting insulin (regular or lispro). The usual insulin treatment can be resumed once oral intake is established.

   B. **Patients undergoing major surgery** should have preoperative measurement of blood glucose, serum electrolytes, and urine ketones. Ideally, metabolic and electrolyte abnormalities (e.g., hyponatremia, dyskalemia, acidosis) should be corrected before surgery. For patients treated with conventional insulin regimens, one-third to one-half of the total daily dose of insulin can be administered SC before surgery, depending on ambient glucose levels. Patients treated with multiple doses of short-acting insulin can have one-third of their usual preprandial dose of insulin, whereas patients who are using the insulin pump can continue their usual basal rate of infusion.

 IV. **IV insulin infusion** is an alternative to SC insulin for the management of diabetes in patients who are undergoing major procedures.

   A. **Initial insulin infusion rate** can be estimated as one-half of the patient's total daily insulin dose expressed as units/hour. Regular insulin, 0.5–1.0 unit/hour, is an appropriate starting dose for most patients with type 1 diabetes; D5W (or D10W), 100 ml/hour, should also be started. An initial infusion rate of 1–2 units/hour can be used in patients treated with oral antidiabetic agents who require perioperative insulin infusion.

B. Maintenance infusion rates for insulin and dextrose are determined using hourly blood glucose measurements; the goal is to maintain intraoperative plasma glucose in the 100- to 200-mg/dl range.

C. Potassium chloride, 10 mEq, is added to each 500 ml dextrose to maintain normokalemia in patients with normal renal function.

D. The duration of insulin and dextrose infusions depends on the clinical status of the patient. The infusions should be continued postoperatively until oral intake is secure, after which the usual diabetes treatment can be resumed. It is prudent to give the first dose of SC insulin 30 minutes before disconnecting the IV route.

Chronic Complications
of Diabetes Mellitus

Prevention of long-term complications is one of the cardinal goals of diabetes management. Appropriate treatment of established complications may delay their progression and improve quality of life.

I. **Microvascular complications** include diabetic retinopathy, nephropathy, and neuropathy. These complications are directly related to hyperglycemia and can be prevented by maintaining scrupulous glycemic control.

A. **Diabetic retinopathy** includes background retinopathy (microaneurysms, retinal infarcts) and proliferative retinopathy.

1. **Background retinopathy** usually is not associated with loss of vision. However, the development of macular edema or proliferative retinopathy (particularly new vessels near the optic disk) requires elective laser photocoagulation therapy to preserve vision. Vitrectomy is indicated for patients with vitreous hemorrhage or retinal detachment.

2. **Annual examination by an ophthalmologist** is recommended from the outset for all type 2 DM patients and beginning at puberty or after 5 years of diagnosis for patients with type 1 DM.

3. **Other ocular abnormalities** associated with diabetes include cataract formation, dyskinetic pupils, glaucoma, optic neuropathy, extraocular muscle paresis, floaters, and fluctuating visual acuity. The latter is related to changes in blood glucose. The presence of floaters may be indicative of preretinal or vitreous hemorrhage; immediate referral for ophthalmologic evaluation is warranted.

B. **Diabetic nephropathy** is preceded by microalbuminuria (30–300 mg albumin/24 hours), a potentially reversible state.

1. **Microalbuminuria precedes overt proteinuria (>300 mg albumin/day) by several years** in type 1 and type 2 diabetes. The mean duration from diagnosis of type 1 diabetes to development of overt proteinuria is 17 years, and the time from the occurrence of proteinuria to end-stage renal failure averages 5 years.

2. **Annual screening for microalbuminuria** should be performed from the outset in type 2 DM patients and beginning at puberty or after 5 years of diagnosis in patients with type 1 DM. Measurement of microalbumin:creatinine ratio (normal, <30 mg albumin/g creatinine) in a random urine sample is acceptable for screening.

3. **Intensive control of diabetes and hypertension** and angiotensin-converting enzyme inhibitors are effective interventions for incipient or established diabetic nephropathy. The angiotensin II–receptor blockers

are being evaluated in clinical trials for a similar purpose. Dietary protein restriction may be beneficial in some patients.

C. Diabetic neuropathy may result in sensory, motor, autonomic, or combined deficits. Sensorimotor diabetic peripheral polyneuropathy is a major risk factor for foot trauma, ulceration, Charcot's arthropathy, and limb amputation. Sensation in the lower extremities should be documented at least annually, using either a light-touch monofilament or a tuning fork.

1. **Painful peripheral neuropathy** responds variably to treatment with tricyclic antidepressants (e.g., amitriptyline, 10–150 mg PO qhs), topical capsaicin (0.075% cream), or anticonvulsants (e.g., carbamazepine, 100–400 mg PO bid). Patients should be warned about adverse effects: sedation and anticholinergic symptoms (tricyclics), burning sensation (capsaicin), and blood dyscrasias (carbamazepine).

2. **Orthostatic hypotension** is a manifestation of autonomic neuropathy, but common etiologies (e.g., dehydration, anemia, medications) should be excluded. Treatment is symptomatic: postural maneuvers, use of compressive garments (e.g., Jobst stockings), and intravascular expansion using sodium chloride, 1–4 g PO qid, and fludrocortisone, 0.1–0.3 mg PO qd. Hypokalemia, supine hypertension, and CHF are some adverse effects of fludrocortisone.

3. **Intractable nausea and vomiting** in diabetes may be due to gastroparesis or enteropathy, both of which are manifestations of impaired GI motility from autonomic neuropathy. **Surveillance for incipient DKA is warranted in insulin-treated patients with nausea and vomiting,** because misguided interruption of insulin therapy is widespread among such patients. Other causes of nausea and vomiting, including intra-abdominal pathologies, should be excluded.

   a. **Management of diabetic gastroenteropathy** can be challenging. Frequent, small meals (6–8/day) of soft consistency that are low in fat and fiber provide relief for some patients. Parenteral nutrition may become necessary in some individuals. Improvement in glycemic control also is beneficial, because hyperglycemia delays gastric emptying.

   b. **Pharmacologic therapy** includes the prokinetic agent metoclopramide, 10–20 mg PO (or as a suppository) before meals and qhs, and erythromycin, 125–500 mg PO qid. Extrapyramidal side effects (tremor and tardive dyskinesia), from the antidopaminergic actions of metoclopramide, may limit therapy.

   c. **Cyclical vomiting** that is unrelated to a GI motility disorder or other clear etiology may also occur in DM patients and appears to respond to amitriptyline, 25–50 mg PO qhs.

4. **Diabetic cystopathy,** or bladder dysfunction, results from impaired autonomic control of detrusor muscle and sphincteric function. Manifestations include urgency, dribbling, incomplete emptying, overflow incontinence, and urinary retention. Recurrent urinary tract infections are common in patients with residual urine. Treatment is unsatisfactory; intermittent self-catheterization may be required to relieve retention.

5. **Diabetic diarrhea** should only be diagnosed after exclusion of other causes of diarrhea. The pathogenesis of diabetic diarrhea is unclear: Impaired parasympathetic control of peristalsis, intestinal stasis, colonic overgrowth, bacterial deconjugation of bile acids, and resultant cathartic effects are some of the mechanisms that have been suggested. Treatment is empiric. Repeated courses of broad-spectrum antibiotics (e.g., azithromycin, tetracycline, cephalosporins) may be beneficial; octreotide, 50–75 µg SC bid, can be effective in patients with intractable diarrhea.

II. Macrovascular complications of DM include coronary artery disease, stroke, and peripheral vascular disease. Risk factors for macrovascular disease include insulin resistance, hyperglycemia, hypertension, hyperlipidemia, cigarette smoking, and obesity. Glycemic control should be optimized; hypertension should be controlled to a target blood pressure of 130/85 mm Hg or lower, and hyperlipidemia should be treated appropriately, with a target low-density lipoprotein cholesterol level of 100 mg/dl or lower. Cigarette smoking should be actively discouraged, and weight loss should be promoted in obese patients. Aspirin, 81–325 mg/day, is of proven benefit in secondary prevention of myocardial infarction or stroke in DM patients.

A. **Coronary artery disease** occurs at a younger age and may have atypical clinical presentations in patients with diabetes. Myocardial infarction carries a worse prognosis, and angioplasty gives less satisfactory results in diabetic patients compared with nondiabetic individuals. **ECG** should be obtained yearly, and there should be a low threshold for ordering periodic stress tests in patients aged 35 years or older.

B. **Management of diabetes after acute myocardial infarction.** Optimization of glycemic control during and after admission for acute myocardial infarction improves survival. Routine IV infusion of regular insulin and glucose to improve glycemic control in the hospital, followed by intensive insulin therapy at home, significantly reduces acute and long-term mortality (*BMJ* 314:1512, 1997).

   1. **Initial insulin infusion** rates of 1–4 units/hour and dextrose infusion of 5 g/hour (100 ml/hour D5W) can be used and adjusted, as necessary, to maintain plasma glucose in the 100- to 150-mg/dl range.

   2. **Potassium chloride,** 10–20 mEq, can be added to each liter of insulin-glucose infusion to prevent hypokalemia in patients with normal renal function.

   3. **Close supervision of therapy** is mandatory, because hypoglycemia triggers release of counterregulatory hormones, some of which (e.g., catecholamines) may be arrhythmogenic.

III. **Miscellaneous complications** such as erectile dysfunction and diabetic foot ulcers have multiple etiologies.

A. **Erectile dysfunction** may result from diabetic neuropathy, vascular insufficiency, adverse drug effects, endocrinopathy, psychological factors, or a combination of these etiologies. Glycemic control should be intensified, and specialist referral should be considered if the problem persists. If endocrinologic evaluation proves negative and other treatable causes have been excluded, a trial of the phosphodiesterase V inhibitor, sildenafil, 50–100 mg PO precoitally, may be appropriate. **Sildenafil should not be used concurrently with nitrates** to prevent severe and potentially fatal hypotensive reactions.

B. **Diabetic foot ulcers** result from chronic neuropathy, vascular insufficiency, and polymicrobial infection. Poorly managed foot ulcers result in limb loss through amputation. Patient education should emphasize prevention: daily foot examination, application of moisturizing lotion, use of proper footwear, and caution with self-pedicure. The exposed feet should be inspected and palpated at every patient encounter; significant findings, such as calluses, hammertoes, other deformities, and soft tissue lesions, should be evaluated by foot care specialists. Patients with active foot ulcers should be treated aggressively; hospitalization for parenteral antibiotic therapy and local wound care often is necessary.

Hypoglycemia

Hypoglycemia is uncommon in the general population but is a significant problem among patients with diabetes. Iatrogenic factors usually account for hypoglycemia in the setting of diabetes, whereas spontaneous hypoglycemia in the nondiabetic populace has multiple etiologies.

I. Iatrogenic hypoglycemia complicates therapy with insulin or sulfonylureas and is a limiting factor to aggressive efforts to achieve optimal glycemic control in patients with DM. Severe hypoglycemia is a frequent problem during intensive insulin therapy in type 1 DM but occurs in only about 2% of patients with type 2 DM who are undergoing intensive therapy. All patients with diabetes should be familiar with the warning symptoms of hypoglycemia and be taught to respond appropriately to such episodes.

   A. Risk factors for iatrogenic hypoglycemia include skipped or insufficient meals, unaccustomed physical exertion, misguided therapy, alcohol ingestion, and drug overdose. Recurrent episodes of hypoglycemia impair recognition of hypoglycemic symptoms, thereby increasing the risk for severe hypoglycemia.

   B. Symptoms of mild hypoglycemia usually are handled competently by an experienced patient, whereas severe hypoglycemia often requires external intervention (e.g., glucagon injection, IV dextrose) or results in altered mentation, seizure, or coma.

   1. Autonomic (or neurogenic) symptoms of hypoglycemia include tremulousness, sweating, palpitations, and hunger. Increased secretion of counterregulatory hormones (e.g., epinephrine) accounts for these symptoms.

   2. Neuroglycopenic symptoms develop as blood glucose decreases further. These symptoms include impaired concentration, irritability, blurred vision, lethargy, and development of seizure or coma. Usually, autonomic warning symptoms occur earlier (and at higher blood glucose levels) than do neuroglycopenic symptoms; this allows corrective measures to be instituted before the occurrence of severe hypoglycemia and disabling neuroglycopenia.

   3. Patients with hypoglycemia unawareness and defective glucose counterregulation have a blunting of autonomic symptoms and counterregulatory hormone secretion during hypoglycemia. Seizures or coma may develop in such patients without the usual warning symptoms of hypoglycemia.

   4. Plasma or capillary blood glucose should be obtained, whenever feasible, to confirm hypoglycemia.

   C. Treatment of hypoglycemia. Isolated episodes of mild hypoglycemia may not require specific intervention. Recurrent episodes require a review of lifestyle factors; adjustments may be indicated in the content, timing, and distribution of meals, as well as medication dosage and timing. Severe hypoglycemia is an indication for supervised treatment, which should be guided by the patient's mental status.

   1. Readily absorbable carbohydrates (e.g., glucose and sugar-containing beverages) can be administered orally to conscious patients for rapid effect. Alternatively, milk, candy bars, fruit, cheese, and crackers may be adequate in some patients with mild hypoglycemia. Hypoglycemia associated with acarbose or miglitol therapy should preferentially be treated with glucose, because these alpha-glucosidase inhibitors block the digestion of disaccharides and complex carbohydrates. Glucose tablets and carbohydrate supplies should be readily available to patients with DM at all times.

   2. IV dextrose is indicated for severe hypoglycemia, in patients with altered consciousness, and during restriction of oral intake. An initial bolus, 20–50 ml 50% dextrose, should be given immediately, followed by infusion of D5W (or D10W) to maintain blood glucose above 100 mg/dl. Aggressive and prolonged IV dextrose infusion, together with close clinical observation, is warranted in sulfonylurea overdose, in the elderly, and in patients with defective counterregulation.

   3. Glucagon, 1 mg IM (or SC), is an effective initial therapy for severe hypoglycemia in patients who are unable to maintain oral intake or in whom an IV access cannot be secured immediately. Vomiting is a frequent side effect, and therefore care should be taken to prevent the risk of aspiration of gastric contents. A glucagon kit should be available to patients with a history of severe hypoglycemia; family members and roommates should be instructed in its proper use.

4. **Education** regarding etiologies of hypoglycemia, preventive measures, and appropriate adjustments to medication, diet, and exercise regimens are essential tasks to be addressed during hospitalization for severe hypoglycemia.

5. **Hypoglycemia unawareness** can develop in patients who are undergoing intensive diabetes therapy. Inability to sense the autonomic warning symptoms of hypoglycemia predisposes to the development of neuroglycopenia, lethargy, stupor, seizures, and coma. These patients should be encouraged to monitor their blood glucose frequently and take timely measures to correct low values (<60 mg/dl). In patients with very tightly controlled diabetes, slight relaxation in glycemic control and scrupulous avoidance of hypoglycemia can restore the lost warning symptoms. Perception of hypoglycemic symptoms can also be attenuated by concurrent therapy with β-adrenergic blockers, but these agents are not contraindicated in diabetic patients who have a genuine need for them.

II. **Spontaneous hypoglycemia,** unrelated to diabetes therapy, is an infrequent problem in general medical practice. Major categories include fasting and postprandial hypoglycemia.

A. **Fasting hypoglycemia** can be caused by inappropriate insulin secretion (e.g., insulinoma), toxic effects of alcohol, severe hepatic or renal insufficiency, hypopituitarism, glucocorticoid deficiency, or surreptitious injection of insulin or ingestion of a sulfonylurea.

1. **Episodic autonomic symptoms** suggestive of hypoglycemia may be present, but, more commonly, neuroglycopenic symptoms predominate.

2. **Recurrent seizures, dementia, and bizarre behavior** may occasion referral for neuropsychiatric evaluation, which may delay timely diagnosis of hypoglycemia.

3. **Definitive diagnosis** of fasting hypoglycemia requires hourly blood glucose monitoring during a supervised fast lasting up to 72 hours and measurement of plasma insulin, C-peptide, and sulfonylurea metabolites if hypoglycemia (<50 mg/dl) is documented.

4. **Patients who develop hypoglycemia** and have measurable plasma insulin and C-peptide levels without sulfonylurea metabolites require further evaluation for an insulinoma.

B. **Postprandial hypoglycemia** often is suspected, but seldom proven, in patients with vague symptoms that occur 1 or more hours after meals.

1. **Alimentary hypoglycemia** is a tenable consideration in a patient with a history of partial gastrectomy or intestinal resection in whom recurrent symptoms develop 1–2 hours after eating. Typically, symptoms are similar to those reported by patients with mild insulin-induced hypoglycemia. The mechanism is thought to be related to too-rapid glucose absorption, resulting in a robust insulin response. Thus, frequent small meals with reduced carbohydrate content may ameliorate symptoms. Theoretically, inhibition of carbohydrate digestion using alpha-glucosidase inhibitors and the resultant limitation of postprandial glucose excursions could also be beneficial.

2. **Functional hypoglycemia.** Symptoms that are possibly suggestive of hypoglycemia, which may or may not be confirmed by plasma glucose measurement, occur in some patients who have not undergone GI surgery. This condition is referred to as "functional hypoglycemia." The symptoms tend to develop 3–5 hours after meals. Current evaluation and management of functional hypoglycemia are imprecise; some patients show evidence of IGT and may respond to dietary therapy.

23

Endocrine Diseases

William E. Clutter

Evaluation of Thyroid Function

The major hormone secreted by the thyroid is **thyroxine (T_4)**, which is converted in many tissues to the more potent **triiodothyronine (T_3)**. Both are bound reversibly to plasma proteins, primarily **thyroxine-binding globulin (TBG)**. Only the unbound (free) fraction enters cells and produces biological effects. T_4 secretion is stimulated by **thyroid-stimulating hormone (TSH)**. In turn, TSH secretion is inhibited by T_4, forming a **negative feedback** loop that keeps free T_4 levels within a narrow normal range. Diagnosis of thyroid disease is based on clinical findings, palpation of the thyroid, and measurement of plasma TSH and thyroid hormones (*Clin Chem* 45:1377, 1999*)*.

I. **Thyroid palpation** determines not only the size and consistency of the thyroid but the presence of nodules, tenderness, or a thrill.

II. **Plasma TSH assay is the initial test of choice in most patients with suspected thyroid disease.** TSH levels are elevated even in mild primary hypothyroidism and are suppressed to less than 0.1 µU/ml even in subclinical hyperthyroidism (i.e., thyroid hormone excess too mild to cause symptoms). Thus, **a normal plasma TSH level excludes hyperthyroidism and primary hypothyroidism.** However, TSH levels usually are within the reference range in secondary hypothyroidism and are not useful for detection of this rare form of hypothyroidism. Because even slight changes in thyroid hormone levels affect TSH secretion, **abnormal TSH levels are not specific for clinically important thyroid disease,** which should usually be confirmed by plasma thyroid hormone measurement.

   A. **Plasma TSH is mildly elevated** (up to 20 µU/ml) in some euthyroid patients with nonthyroidal illnesses and in subclinical hypothyroidism.

   B. **TSH levels may be suppressed to less than 0.1 µU/ml** in nonthyroidal illness, in subclinical hyperthyroidism, in some euthyroid elderly patients, and during treatment with dopamine or high doses of glucocorticoids. Also, TSH levels remain lower than 0.1 µU/ml for some time **after hyperthyroidism is corrected.**

III. **An estimate of plasma free T_4** confirms the diagnosis of clinical hypothyroidism in patients with elevated plasma TSH and confirms the diagnosis and assesses the severity of hyperthyroidism when plasma TSH is less than 0.1 µU/ml. Plasma free T_4 concentrations can be measured by immunoassay or by calculation of the T_4 index (the product of plasma T_4 and T_3 resin uptake). The T_3 resin uptake varies inversely with plasma thyroid hormone–binding capacity. Measurement of total plasma T_4 alone is not adequate, because TBG levels are altered in many circumstances (increased with estrogen therapy, pregnancy, acute or chronic active hepatitis, and familial

Table 23-1. Effects of drugs on thyroid function tests

Effect	Drug
Decreased T$_4$	
True hypothyroidism (TSH elevated)	Iodine (amiodarone, radio-graphic contrast)
	Lithium
Decreased TBG (TSH normal)	Androgens
Inhibition of T$_4$ binding to TBG (TSH normal)	Furosemide (high doses)
	Salicylates
Inhibition of TSH secretion	Glucocorticoids
	Dopamine
Multiple mechanisms (TSH normal)	Phenytoin
Increased T$_4$	
True hyperthyroidism (TSH <0.1 µU/ml)	Iodine (amiodarone, radiographic contrast)
Increased TBG (TSH normal)	Estrogens, tamoxifen
Inhibited T$_4$ to T$_3$ conversion (TSH normal)	Amiodarone
	Propranolol (high doses)
	Oral cholecystographic agents

T$_3$ = triiodothyronine; T$_4$ = thyroxine; TBG = thyroxine-binding globulin; TSH = thyroid-stimulating hormone.

TBG excess; decreased with severe liver disease, malnutrition, nephrotic syndrome, androgen therapy, and familial TBG deficiency).

  IV. **Free T$_4$ measured by equilibrium dialysis** is the most reliable measure of clinical thyroid status, but results seldom are rapidly available. It is needed only in rare cases in which the diagnosis is not clear from measurement of plasma TSH and an estimate of free T$_4$.
  V. **Effect of nonthyroidal illness on thyroid function tests** (*Thyroid* 7:125, 1997). Many illnesses alter thyroid tests without causing true thyroid dysfunction (erythroid sick syndrome). These changes must be recognized to avoid mistaken diagnosis and therapy.
    A. The **low T$_3$ syndrome** occurs in many illnesses, during starvation, and after trauma or surgery. Conversion of T$_4$ to T$_3$ is decreased, and plasma T$_3$ levels are low. Plasma T$_4$ and TSH levels are normal. It may be an adaptive response to illness, and thyroid hormone therapy is not beneficial.
    B. The **low T$_4$ syndrome** occurs in severe illness. It may be due to decreased TBG levels, inhibition of T$_4$ binding to TBG, or suppressed TSH secretion. **TSH levels decrease early in severe illness,** sometimes to less than 0.1 µU/ml. **During recovery they rise, sometimes to levels higher than the normal range** (although rarely higher than 20 µU/ml).
  VI. **The effects of drugs on thyroid function tests vary** (Table 23-1) (*N Engl J Med* 333:1688, 1995). Iodine-containing drugs (amiodarone and radiographic contrast media) may cause hyperthyroidism or hypothyroidism in susceptible patients. Many drugs alter thyroid function tests, especially plasma T$_4$, without causing true thyroid dysfunction. In general, plasma TSH levels are a reliable guide to determining whether true hyperthyroidism or hypothyroidism is present.

Hypothyroidism

I. **Etiology** (*Lancet* 349:413, 1997). **Primary hypothyroidism** (due to disease of the thyroid itself) accounts for more than 90% of cases. **Chronic lymphocytic thyroiditis (Hashimoto's disease)** is the most common cause and may be associated with Addison's disease and other endocrine deficits (*N Engl J Med* 335:99, 1996). Its prevalence is greatest in women and increases with age. **Iatrogenic hypothyroidism** due to thyroidectomy or radioactive iodine (RAI, ^{131}I) therapy also is common. Transient hypothyroidism occurs in postpartum thyroiditis and subacute thyroiditis, usually after a period of hyperthyroidism. Drugs that may cause hypothyroidism include iodine, lithium, interferon-alpha, and interleukin-2. **Secondary hypothyroidism** due to TSH deficiency is uncommon but may occur in any disorder of the pituitary or hypothalamus. However, it rarely occurs without other evidence of pituitary disease.

II. **Clinical findings.** Most symptoms of hypothyroidism are nonspecific and develop gradually. They include cold intolerance, fatigue, somnolence, poor memory, constipation, menorrhagia, myalgias, and hoarseness. Signs include slow tendon-reflex relaxation, bradycardia, facial and periorbital edema, dry skin, and nonpitting edema (myxedema). Mild weight gain may occur, but hypothyroidism does not cause marked obesity. Rare manifestations include hypoventilation, pericardial or pleural effusions, deafness, and carpal tunnel syndrome. Laboratory findings may include hyponatremia and elevated plasma levels of cholesterol, triglycerides, and creatine kinase. The ECG may show low voltage and T-wave abnormalities.

III. **Diagnosis.** Hypothyroidism is readily treatable and should be suspected in any patient with compatible symptoms, especially in the presence of a goiter or a history of RAI therapy or thyroid surgery.

    A. **In suspected primary hypothyroidism, plasma TSH is the best initial diagnostic test.** A normal value excludes primary hypothyroidism, and a markedly elevated value (>20 µU/ml) confirms the diagnosis. If plasma TSH is elevated moderately (<20 µU/ml), plasma free T_4 should be measured. A low free T_4 confirms clinical hypothyroidism. A clearly normal free T_4 with an elevated plasma TSH indicates subclinical hypothyroidism, in which thyroid function is impaired but increased secretion of TSH maintains plasma T_4 levels within the reference range. These patients may have nonspecific symptoms that are compatible with hypothyroidism and a mild increase in serum cholesterol and low-density lipoprotein cholesterol levels (see sec. **IV.D**). They develop clinical hypothyroidism at a rate of 2.5% per year.

    B. **If secondary hypothyroidism is suspected** because of evidence of pituitary disease, plasma free T_4 should be measured. Plasma TSH levels are usually within the reference range in secondary hypothyroidism and cannot be used alone to make this diagnosis. Patients with secondary hypothyroidism should be evaluated for other pituitary hormone deficits and for a mass lesion of the pituitary or hypothalamus (see Anterior Pituitary Gland Dysfunction).

    C. **In severe nonthyroidal illness,** the diagnosis of hypothyroidism may be difficult. Plasma total T_4 and T_4 index often are low. The validity of free T_4 immunoassays in such patients has not been clearly established (*Clin Chem* 42:188, 1996).

        1. **Plasma TSH still is the best initial diagnostic test.** Marked elevation of plasma TSH (>20 µU/ml) establishes the diagnosis of primary hypothyroidism. A normal TSH value is strong evidence that the patient is euthyroid, except when there is evidence of pituitary or hypothalamic disease or in patients treated with dopamine or high doses of glucocorti-

coids. Moderate elevations of plasma TSH (<20 µU/ml) may occur in euthyroid patients with nonthyroidal illness and are not specific for hypothyroidism.

2. **Plasma free T$_4$ by equilibrium dialysis** should be measured in the few cases in which it is unclear whether the patient is hypothyroid based on plasma TSH. Normal free T$_4$ levels exclude hypothyroidism, and patients with low plasma free T$_4$ should be treated for hypothyroidism.

IV. **Therapy. Thyroxine** is the drug of choice (*N Engl J Med* 331:174, 1994). The usual replacement dose is 100–125 µg PO qd, and most patients require doses between 75 and 150 µg qd. In elderly patients, the average replacement dose is somewhat lower. The need for lifelong treatment should be emphasized.

A. **Initiation of therapy.** Young, otherwise healthy adults should be started on 100 µg qd. This regimen gradually corrects hypothyroidism, as several weeks are required to reach steady-state plasma levels of T$_4$. Symptoms begin to improve within a few weeks. In otherwise healthy **elderly patients,** the initial dose should be 50 µg qd. Patients with **cardiac disease** should be started on 25 µg qd and monitored carefully for exacerbation of cardiac symptoms.

B. **Dose adjustment and follow-up**

1. **In primary hypothyroidism, the goal of therapy is to maintain plasma TSH within the normal range.** Plasma TSH should be measured 2–3 months after initiation of therapy. The dose of thyroxine then should be adjusted in 12- to 25-µg increments at intervals of 6–8 weeks until plasma TSH is normal. Thereafter, annual TSH measurement is adequate to monitor therapy and to ensure compliance. Overtreatment, indicated by a subnormal TSH, should be avoided, as it may increase the risk of osteoporosis (*J Clin Endocrinol Metab* 81:4278, 1996) and atrial fibrillation (*Endocrinol Metab Clin North Am* 27:51, 1998).

2. **In secondary hypothyroidism, plasma TSH cannot be used to adjust therapy.** The goal of therapy is to maintain the **plasma free T$_4$** near the middle of the reference range. The dose of thyroxine should be adjusted at 6- to 8-week intervals until this goal is achieved. Thereafter, annual measurement of plasma free T$_4$ is adequate to monitor therapy.

3. **Coronary artery disease** may be exacerbated by treatment of hypothyroidism. The dose of thyroxin should be increased slowly in patients with coronary artery disease, with careful attention to worsening angina, heart failure, or arrhythmias. If cardiac symptoms worsen despite medical therapy, coronary revascularization (which can be done safely in hypothyroid patients) should be considered.

C. **Difficulty in controlling hypothyroidism** is most often due to **poor compliance** with therapy. Observed therapy may be necessary in some cases. Other causes of increasing thyroxine requirement include (1) **malabsorption** due to intestinal disease or **drugs that interfere with thyroxine absorption** (e.g., cholestyramine, sucralfate, aluminum hydroxide, ferrous sulfate); (2) **other drug interactions** that increase thyroxine clearance (e.g., rifampin, carbamazepine, phenytoin) or block conversion of T$_4$ to T$_3$ (amiodarone); (3) **pregnancy,** in which thyroxine requirement increases in the first trimester; and (4) gradual failure of remaining endogenous thyroid function after treatment of hyperthyroidism.

D. **Subclinical hypothyroidism** (see sec. III.A) should be treated with thyroxine if any of the following are present: (1) symptoms compatible with hypothyroidism, (2) a goiter, or (3) hypercholesterolemia that warrants treatment (*Ann Intern Med* 129:141, 1998). Untreated patients should be monitored annually, and thyroxine should be started if symptoms develop or serum TSH increases to more than 20 µU/ml.

E. **Perioperative management.** Although hypothyroidism increases the risk of minor perioperative complications, there is little increase in the risk of serious complications or mortality. Emergency surgery need not be delayed, but treatment of hypothyroidism should be started (see sec. **IV.A**); the initial doses can be given IV. Elective surgery should be postponed until hypothyroidism has been treated for several weeks.

F. Urgent therapy is rarely necessary for hypothyroidism. Most patients with hypothyroidism and concomitant illness can be treated in the usual manner (see secs. **IV.A** and **B**). However, hypothyroidism may impair survival in critical illness by contributing to hypoventilation, hypotension, hypothermia, bradycardia, or hyponatremia. Little evidence supports the contention that severe hypothyroidism alone causes coma or shock; most reports of alleged "myxedema coma" predate recognition that nonthyroidal illness itself lowers thyroid hormone levels.

1. **Hypoventilation** and **hypotension** should be treated intensively, along with any concomitant diseases. **Confirmatory tests should be obtained before thyroid hormone therapy is started** in a severely ill patient, including serum TSH and free T_4 by equilibrium dialysis.

2. **Thyroxine,** 50–100 µg IV, can be given q6–8h for 24 hours, followed by 75–100 µg IV qd until oral intake is possible. Replacement therapy should be continued in the usual manner if the diagnosis of hypothyroidism is confirmed. No clinical trials have determined the optimum method of thyroid hormone replacement, but this method rapidly alleviates thyroxine deficiency while minimizing the risk of exacerbating underlying coronary disease or heart failure. **Such rapid correction is warranted only in extremely ill patients. Vital signs and cardiac rhythm should be monitored carefully** to detect early signs of exacerbation of heart disease.

3. **Hydrocortisone,** 50 mg IV q8h, usually is recommended during rapid replacement of thyroid hormone, because such therapy may precipitate adrenal failure.

Hyperthyroidism

I. Etiology (*Lancet* 349:339, 1997). **Graves' disease** causes most cases of hyperthyroidism, especially in young patients. This autoimmune disorder also may cause **proptosis** (exophthalmos) and **pretibial myxedema**, both of which are not found in other causes of hyperthyroidism. **Toxic multinodular goiter (MNG)** is a common cause of hyperthyroidism in older patients. Other unusual etiologies include **iodine-induced hyperthyroidism** (usually precipitated by drugs such as amiodarone or radiographic contrast media), thyroid adenomas, subacute thyroiditis (painful tender goiter with transient hyperthyroidism), postpartum thyroiditis (nontender goiter with transient hyperthyroidism), and surreptitious ingestion of thyroid hormone. TSH-induced hyperthyroidism is extremely rare.

II. Clinical findings. Symptoms include heat intolerance, weight loss, weakness, palpitations, oligomenorrhea, and anxiety. Signs include brisk tendon reflexes, fine tremor, proximal weakness, stare, and eyelid lag. Cardiac abnormalities may be prominent, including sinus tachycardia, atrial fibrillation, and exacerbation of coronary artery disease or heart failure. In the **elderly,** hyperthyroidism may present with only atrial fibrillation, heart failure, weakness, or weight loss, and a high index of suspicion is needed to make the diagnosis.

III. Diagnosis. Hyperthyroidism should be suspected in any patient with compatible symptoms, as it is a readily treatable disorder that may become highly debilitating.

A. Plasma TSH is the best initial diagnostic test, as a TSH level higher than 0.1 µU/ml excludes clinical hyperthyroidism. If plasma TSH is lower than 0.1 µU/ml, plasma free T_4 should be measured to determine the severity of hyperthyroidism and as a baseline for therapy. If plasma free T_4 is elevated, the diagnosis of clinical hyperthyroidism is established.

Table 23-2. Differential diagnosis of hyperthyroidism

Signs	Diagnosis
Diffuse, nontender goiter	Graves' disease (rarely postpartum silent thyroiditis)
Multiple thyroid nodules	Toxic multinodular goiter
Single thyroid nodule	Thyroid adenoma
Tender painful goiter	Subacute thyroiditis
Normal thyroid gland	Graves' disease (rarely postpartum thyroiditis or factitious hyperthyroidism)

  B. **If plasma TSH is lower than 0.1 μU/ml but free T$_4$ is normal,** the patient may have clinical hyperthyroidism due to **elevation of plasma T$_3$ alone;** therefore, plasma T$_3$ should be measured in this case. Another etiology includes suppression of TSH by **nonthyroidal illness** (see Evaluation of Thyroid Function, sec. **V**). A third-generation TSH assay with a detection limit of 0.01 μU/ml may be helpful in patients with suppressed TSH and nonthyroidal illness. Most patients with clinical hyperthyroidism have plasma TSH levels that are lower than 0.01 μU/ml in such assays, whereas nonthyroidal illness rarely suppresses TSH to this degree. Finally, **subclinical hyperthyroidism** may lower TSH to less than 0.1 μU/ml, and therefore suppression of TSH alone does not confirm that symptoms are due to hyperthyroidism.
  C. **Differential diagnosis** (Table 23-2). The etiology of the hyperthyroidism affects the choice of therapy. Differentiating features include (1) the presence of **proptosis** or **pretibial myxedema,** seen in Graves' disease (although many patients with Graves' disease lack these signs); (2) a **diffuse nontender goiter** on palpation of the thyroid, consistent with Graves' disease; or (3) a history of recent **pregnancy, neck pain,** or **iodine administration,** suggesting causes other than Graves' disease. In rare cases, **24-hour RAI uptake (RAIU)** is needed to distinguish Graves' disease or toxic MNG (in which RAIU is elevated) from postpartum thyroiditis, iodine-induced hyperthyroidism, or factitious hyperthyroidism (in which RAIU is very low). **Thyroid imaging with ultrasound or radionuclide scan is not useful in diagnosing hyperthyroidism.**
 IV. **Therapy** (*Ann Intern Med* 122:281, 1994). Some forms of hyperthyroidism (subacute or postpartum thyroiditis) are transient and require only symptomatic therapy. Three methods (none of which controls hyperthyroidism rapidly) are available for definitive therapy: RAI, thionamides, and subtotal thyroidectomy. **During treatment, patients are followed by clinical evaluation and measurement of plasma T$_4$.** Plasma TSH is useless in assessing the initial response to therapy, as it remains suppressed until after the patient becomes euthyroid. Regardless of the therapy used, all patients with Graves' disease require lifelong follow-up for recurrent hyperthyroidism or development of hypothyroidism.
  A. **Symptomatic therapy. β-Adrenergic antagonists** are used to relieve symptoms of hyperthyroidism, such as palpitations, tremor, and anxiety, until hyperthyroidism is controlled by definitive therapy or until transient forms of hyperthyroidism subside. Atenolol (25–50 mg qd) or propranolol (20–40 mg PO qid) is adjusted to alleviate symptoms and tachycardia. β-Adrenergic antagonist therapy should be reduced gradually, then stopped as hyperthyroidism is controlled. Verapamil at an initial dose of 40–80 mg PO tid can be used to control tachycardia in patients with contraindications to β-adrenergic antagonists.

B. **Choice of definitive therapy**
   1. **In Graves' disease, RAI therapy is the treatment of choice for almost all patients.** It is simple and highly effective and causes no life-threatening complications. However, it **cannot be used in pregnancy. Propylthiouracil (PTU) should be used to treat hyperthyroidism in pregnancy;** however, long-term control of hyperthyroidism is achieved in fewer than half of patients. PTU carries a small risk of life-threatening side effects (see sec. **IV.D.3**). Thyroidectomy should be used only in patients who refuse RAI therapy and who relapse or develop side effects with thionamide therapy.
   2. **Other causes of hyperthyroidism.** Toxic MNG and toxic adenoma should be treated with RAI (except in pregnancy). Transient forms of hyperthyroidism due to thyroiditis should be treated symptomatically with atenolol. Iodine-induced hyperthyroidism is treated with thionamides and atenolol until the patient is euthyroid.

C. **RAI therapy.** A single dose permanently controls hyperthyroidism in 90% of patients, and further doses can be given if necessary. A **pregnancy test** is done immediately before therapy in potentially fertile women. A 24-hour RAIU is usually measured and used to calculate the dose. Thionamides interfere with RAI therapy and should be stopped at least 3 days before treatment. If iodine treatment has been given, it should be stopped at least 2 weeks before RAI therapy. Most patients with Graves' disease are treated with 8–10 mCi, although treatment of toxic MNG requires higher doses.
   1. **Follow-up.** Usually, several months are needed to restore euthyroidism. Patients are evaluated at 4- to 6-week intervals, with assessment of clinical findings and plasma free T_4.
      a. **If thyroid function stabilizes within the normal range,** the interval between follow-up visits is increased gradually to annual intervals.
      b. **If symptomatic hypothyroidism develops,** thyroxine therapy is started (see Hypothyroidism, sec. **IV**). Mild hypothyroidism after RAI therapy may be transient, and asymptomatic patients can be observed for a further 4–6 weeks to determine whether hypothyroidism will resolve spontaneously.
      c. **If symptomatic hyperthyroidism persists** after 6 months, RAI treatment is repeated.
   2. **Side effects. Hypothyroidism** occurs in about 30% of patients within the first year and continues to develop at a rate of approximately 3% per year thereafter. Because of the release of stored hormone, a slight rise in plasma T_4 may occur in the first 2 weeks after therapy. This development is important only in patients with **severe cardiac disease,** which may worsen as a result. Such patients should be treated with thionamides to restore euthyroidism and to deplete stored hormone before treatment with RAI. No convincing evidence has been found that RAI has a clinically important effect on the course of Graves' eye disease. It does not increase the risk of malignancy. No increase in congenital abnormalities has been found in the offspring of women who conceive after RAI therapy, and the radiation exposure to the ovaries is low, comparable to that from common diagnostic radiographs. Concern for potential teratogenic effects should not influence physicians' advice to patients.

D. **Thionamides.** Methimazole and PTU inhibit thyroid hormone synthesis. PTU also inhibits extrathyroidal conversion of T_4 to T_3. Once thyroid hormone stores are depleted (after several weeks to months), T_4 levels decrease. These drugs have no permanent effect on thyroid function. **In the majority of patients with Graves' disease, hyperthyroidism recurs** within 6 months after therapy is stopped. Spontaneous remission of Graves' disease occurs in approximately one-third of patients during thionamide therapy and, in this minority, no other treatment may be needed. Remission is more likely in mild, recent-onset hyperthyroidism.

1. **Initiation of therapy.** Before starting therapy, patients must be warned of side effects and precautions. Usual starting doses are PTU, 100–200 mg PO tid, or methimazole, 10–40 mg PO qd; higher initial doses can be used in severe hyperthyroidism.

2. **Follow-up.** Restoration of euthyroidism takes up to several months. Patients are evaluated at 4-week intervals with assessment of clinical findings and plasma free T_4. If plasma free T_4 levels do not fall after 4–8 weeks, the dose should be increased. Doses as high as PTU, 300 mg PO qid, or methimazole, 60 mg PO qd, may be required. Once the plasma free T_4 level falls to normal, the dose is adjusted to maintain plasma free T_4 within the normal range. No consensus exists on the optimal duration of therapy, but periods of 6 months to 2 years are used most commonly. Regardless of the therapy's duration, patients must be monitored carefully for recurrence of hyperthyroidism after the drug is stopped.

3. **Side effects** are most likely to occur within the first few months of therapy. **Minor side effects** include rash, urticaria, fever, arthralgias, and transient leukopenia. **Agranulocytosis** occurs in 0.3% of patients treated with thionamides. Other life-threatening side effects include hepatitis, vasculitis, and drug-induced lupus erythematosus. These complications usually resolve if the drug is stopped promptly. **Patients must be warned to stop the drug immediately if jaundice or symptoms suggestive of agranulocytosis develop** (e.g., fever, chills, sore throat) and to contact their physician promptly for evaluation. Routine monitoring of the WBC is not useful for detecting agranulocytosis, which develops suddenly.

E. **Subtotal thyroidectomy.** This procedure provides long-term control of hyperthyroidism in most patients.

1. **Surgery** may trigger a perioperative exacerbation of hyperthyroidism, and patients should be prepared for surgery by one of two methods.

   a. **A thionamide** is given until the patient is nearly euthyroid (see sec. IV.D). **Supersaturated potassium iodide (SSKI),** 40–80 mg (1–2 drops) PO bid, is then added 1–2 weeks before surgery. Both drugs are stopped postoperatively.

   b. **Atenolol** (50–100 mg qd) is started 1–2 weeks before surgery. The dose of atenolol is increased, if necessary, to reduce the resting heart rate below 90 beats/minute and is continued for 5–7 days postoperatively.

2. **Follow-up** includes patient evaluation at 4–6 weeks after surgery, with assessment of clinical findings and plasma free T_4 and TSH. If thyroid function is normal, the patient is seen at 3 and 6 months, then annually. If symptomatic hypothyroidism develops, thyroxine therapy is started (see Hypothyroidism, sec. IV). Mild hypothyroidism after subtotal thyroidectomy may be transient, and asymptomatic patients can be observed for a further 4–6 weeks to determine whether hypothyroidism will resolve spontaneously. Hyperthyroidism persists or recurs in 3–7% of patients.

3. **Complications** of thyroidectomy include **hypothyroidism** in 30–50% of patients and **hypoparathyroidism** in 3%. Rare complications include permanent vocal cord paralysis, due to recurrent laryngeal nerve injury, and perioperative death. The complication rate appears to depend on the experience of the surgeon.

F. **Subclinical hyperthyroidism** is present when the plasma TSH is suppressed to less than 0.1 µU/ml but the patient has no symptoms that are definitely caused by hyperthyroidism, and plasma levels of T_4 and T_3 are normal (*Endocrinol Metab Clin North Am* 27:37, 1998). Subclinical hyperthyroidism increases the risk of atrial fibrillation in the elderly and predisposes to osteoporosis in postmenopausal women; it should be treated in these groups of patients (see sec. **IV.C**). Whether other patients should be treated is unclear (*Ann Intern Med* 129:144, 1998).

G. **Urgent therapy** is warranted when hyperthyroidism exacerbates heart failure or coronary artery disease and in rare patients with severe hyperthyroidism complicated by fever and delirium (*Endocrinol Metab Clin North Am* 22:263, 1993). Concomitant diseases should be treated intensively, and confirmatory tests should be obtained before therapy is started, including serum TSH and free T_4. The following treatment regimen is recommended.

1. **PTU,** 300 mg PO q6h, should be started immediately.
2. **Iodide (SSKI,** 1–2 drops PO q12h) should be started approximately 2 hours after the first dose of PTU, to inhibit thyroid hormone secretion rapidly.
3. **Propranolol,** 40 mg PO q6h (or an equivalent dose IV), should be given to patients with **angina or myocardial infarction,** and the dose should be adjusted to prevent tachycardia. Propranolol may benefit some patients with heart failure and marked tachycardia but can further impair left ventricular function. In patients with clinical heart failure, it should be given only during invasive monitoring of left ventricular filling pressure.
4. **Plasma free T_4** is measured every 3–4 days, and the doses of PTU and iodine gradually are decreased when free T_4 approaches the normal range. RAI therapy should be scheduled 2 weeks after iodine is stopped (see sec. **IV.C**).

H. **Hyperthyroidism in pregnancy.** If hyperthyroidism is suspected, plasma TSH should be measured. Plasma TSH declines in early pregnancy, but rarely to less than 0.1 μU/ml. If TSH is less than 0.1 μU/ml, the diagnosis should be confirmed by measurement of plasma free T_4. **RAI is contraindicated in pregnancy,** and therefore patients should be treated with **PTU** (see sec. **IV.D**). The dose should be adjusted to maintain the plasma free T_4 near the upper limit of the normal range. The dose required often decreases in the later stages of pregnancy. Atenolol, 25–50 mg PO qd, can be used to relieve symptoms while awaiting the effects of PTU. The fetus and neonate should be monitored carefully for hyperthyroidism.

Euthyroid Goiter

The diagnosis of euthyroid goiter is based on palpation of the thyroid and on evaluation of thyroid function. If the thyroid is enlarged, the examiner should determine whether the enlargement is diffuse or multinodular or whether a single nodule is present. All three forms of euthyroid goiter are common, especially in women. Imaging studies, such as thyroid scans or ultrasonography, provide no useful information in addition to palpation of the thyroid and should not be performed. Furthermore, 20–50% of people have nonpalpable thyroid nodules that are detectable by ultrasound. These nodules rarely have any clinical importance, but their incidental discovery may lead to unnecessary diagnostic testing and treatment (*Endocrinol Metab Clin North Am* 29:187, 2000).

I. **Diffuse goiter.** Almost all euthyroid diffuse goiters in the United States are due to **chronic lymphocytic thyroiditis** (Hashimoto's thyroiditis) (*N Engl J Med* 335:99, 1996). As Hashimoto's disease may also cause hypothyroidism, plasma TSH should be measured even in patients who are clinically euthyroid. Small diffuse goiters usually are asymptomatic, and therapy seldom is required. Symptomatic diffuse goiters may shrink with suppression of plasma TSH to the lower limit of the normal range by thyroxine therapy. If thyroxine is not given, the patient should be monitored regularly for the development of hypothyroidism.

II. **Multinodual goiter (MNG)** is common in older patients, especially women. Most patients are asymptomatic and require no treatment. In a few patients, hyperthyroidism (toxic MNG) develops (see Hyperthyroidism, sec. **I**). In rare patients, the gland compresses the trachea or esophagus, causing dyspnea or dysphagia, and treatment is required (*N Engl J Med* 338:1438, 1998). Thyroxine treatment has little, if any, effect on the size of MNGs and rarely is indicated. **RAI therapy** reduces gland size and relieves symptoms in most patients. Subtotal thyroidectomy can also be used to relieve compressive symptoms. The risk of malignancy in MNG is low, comparable to the frequency of incidental thyroid carcinoma in clinically normal glands. Evaluation for thyroid carcinoma with needle biopsy is warranted only if one nodule enlarges disproportionately.

III. **Single thyroid nodules** are usually benign, but a small number are thyroid carcinomas (*N Engl J Med* 338:297, 1998). Clinical findings that increase the likelihood of carcinoma include the presence of cervical lymphadenopathy, a history of radiation to the head or neck in childhood, and a family history of medullary thyroid carcinoma or multiple endocrine neoplasia syndromes type 2A or 2B. A hard fixed nodule, recent nodule growth, or hoarseness due to vocal cord paralysis also suggests malignancy. However, most patients with thyroid carcinomas have none of these risk factors, and **nearly all single thyroid nodules should be evaluated with needle aspiration biopsy.** Patients with thyroid carcinoma should be managed in consultation with an endocrinologist. Nodules with benign cytology should be re-evaluated periodically by palpation. Thyroxine therapy has little or no effect on the size of single thyroid nodules and is not indicated (*Ann Intern Med* 128:386, 1998). **Imaging studies cannot distinguish benign from malignant nodules and should not be performed.**

Adrenal Failure

I. **Etiology.** Adrenal failure may be due to disease of the adrenal glands **(primary adrenal failure, Addison's disease),** with deficiency of cortisol and aldosterone and elevated plasma adrenocorticotropic hormone (ACTH), or to ACTH deficiency caused by disorders of the pituitary or hypothalamus **(secondary adrenal failure),** with deficiency of cortisol alone (*N Engl J Med* 335:1206, 1996).

A. **Primary adrenal failure** most often is due to **autoimmune adrenalitis,** which may be associated with other endocrine deficits (e.g., hypothyroidism). Infections of the adrenal gland such as **tuberculosis** and **histoplasmosis** also may cause adrenal failure. **Hemorrhagic adrenal infarction** may occur in the postoperative period, in coagulation disorders and hypercoagulable states, and in sepsis. Adrenal hemorrhage often causes abdominal or flank pain and fever; CT scan of the abdomen reveals high-density bilateral adrenal masses. Adrenoleukodystrophy causes adrenal failure in young males. Adrenal failure may develop in patients with **AIDS,** caused by disseminated cytomegalovirus, mycobacterial or fungal infection, adrenal lymphoma, or treatment with ketoconazole, which inhibits steroid hormone synthesis.

B. **Secondary adrenal failure** is due most often to **glucocorticoid therapy;** ACTH suppression may persist for a year after therapy is stopped. Any disorder of the pituitary or hypothalamus can cause ACTH deficiency, but usually other evidence of these disorders can be seen.

II. **Clinical findings.** Findings in adrenal failure are nonspecific, and, without a high index of suspicion, the diagnosis of this potentially lethal but readily treatable disease is missed easily. Symptoms include **anorexia, nausea, vomiting, weight loss,** weakness, and fatigue. **Orthostatic hypotension** and **hyponatremia** are common. Usually, symptoms are chronic, but **shock** may suddenly develop that is fatal unless treated promptly. Often, this **adrenal crisis** is triggered by illness, injury, or surgery. All these symptoms are due to cortisol deficiency and occur in primary and in secondary adrenal failure. **Hyperpigmentation** (due to marked ACTH excess) and **hyperkalemia and**

volume depletion (due to aldosterone deficiency) occur only in primary adrenal failure.

III. **Diagnosis.** Adrenal failure should be suspected in patients with hypotension, weight loss, hyponatremia, or hyperkalemia.

   A. **The short cosyntropin (Cortrosyn) stimulation test** is used for diagnosis (*Clin Endocrinol* 44:147, 1996). Cosyntropin, 250 µg, is given IV or IM, and **plasma cortisol is measured 30 minutes later.** The normal response is a stimulated plasma cortisol higher than 20 µg/dl. This test detects primary and secondary adrenal failure, except within a few weeks of onset of pituitary dysfunction (e.g., shortly after pituitary surgery; see Anterior Pituitary Gland Dysfunction, sec. **III**).

   B. **The distinction between primary and secondary adrenal failure** usually is clear. Hyperkalemia, hyperpigmentation, or other autoimmune endocrine deficits indicate primary adrenal failure, whereas deficits of other pituitary hormones, symptoms of a pituitary mass (e.g., headache, visual field loss), or known pituitary or hypothalamic disease indicate secondary adrenal failure. If the cause is unclear, the **plasma ACTH** level distinguishes primary adrenal failure (in which it is elevated markedly) from secondary adrenal failure. Most cases of primary adrenal failure are due to autoimmune adrenalitis, but other causes should be considered. Radiographic evidence of adrenal enlargement or calcification indicates that the cause is infection or hemorrhage. Patients with secondary adrenal failure should be tested for other pituitary hormone deficiencies and should be evaluated for a pituitary or hypothalamic tumor (see Anterior Pituitary Gland Dysfunction).

IV. **Therapy for adrenal failure**

   A. **Adrenal crisis** with hypotension must be treated immediately. Patients should be evaluated for an underlying illness that precipitated the crisis.

      1. **If the diagnosis of adrenal failure is known, hydrocortisone, 50 mg IV q8h,** should be given, and **0.9% saline with 5% dextrose** should be infused rapidly until hypotension is corrected (*N Engl J Med* 337:1285, 1997). The dose of hydrocortisone is decreased gradually over several days as symptoms and any precipitating illness resolve, then is changed to oral maintenance therapy. Mineralocorticoid replacement is not needed until the dose of hydrocortisone is less than 100 mg/day.

      2. **If the diagnosis of adrenal failure has not been established,** a single dose of **dexamethasone, 10 mg IV,** should be given, and a rapid infusion of **0.9% saline with 5% dextrose** should be started. A **Cortrosyn stimulation test** should be performed (see sec. **III.A**). Dexamethasone is used because it does not interfere with subsequent measurements of cortisol. After the 30-minute plasma cortisol measurement, hydrocortisone, 50 mg IV q8h, should be given until the test result is known.

   B. **Maintenance therapy** in all patients with adrenal failure necessitates cortisol replacement with prednisone; most patients with primary adrenal failure also require replacement of aldosterone with fludrocortisone.

      1. **Prednisone,** 5 mg PO every morning and 2.5 mg PO every evening, should be started. The dose is adjusted to eliminate symptoms and signs of cortisol deficiency or excess, with most patients requiring between 5 mg PO every morning and 5 mg PO bid. Concomitant therapy with rifampin, phenytoin, or phenobarbital accelerates glucocorticoid metabolism and increases the dose requirement (see Appendix C).

      2. **During illness, injury, or the perioperative period, the dose of prednisone must be increased.** For minor illnesses, the patient should double the dose for 3 days. If the illness resolves, the maintenance dose is resumed. Vomiting requires immediate medical attention, with IV glucocorticoid therapy and IV fluid. Patients can be given a prefilled syringe of dexamethasone, 4 mg, to be self-administered IM for vomiting or severe illness if medical care is not immediately available. **For severe illness or injury,** hydrocortisone, 50 mg IV q8h, should be given,

with the dose tapered as severity of illness wanes (*N Engl J Med* 337:1285, 1997). The same regimen is used in **patients undergoing surgery,** with the first dose of hydrocortisone given preoperatively. Usually, the dose can be reduced to maintenance therapy 3–4 days after uncomplicated surgery.

3. **In primary adrenal failure, fludrocortisone,** 0.1 mg PO qd, should be given, along with liberal salt intake. The dose is adjusted to maintain BP (supine and standing) and serum potassium within the normal range; the usual dosage is 0.05–0.3 mg PO qd.

4. **Patients should be educated** in management of their disease, including adjustment of prednisone dose during illness. They should wear a medical identification tag or bracelet.

Cushing's Syndrome

Cushing's syndrome (the clinical effects of increased glucocorticoid hormone) is most often **iatrogenic,** due to therapy with glucocorticoid drugs. **ACTH-secreting pituitary microadenomas (Cushing's disease)** account for 80% of cases of endogenous Cushing's syndrome. **Adrenal tumors** and **ectopic ACTH secretion** account for the remainder.

I. **Clinical findings** include truncal obesity, rounded face, fat deposits in the supraclavicular fossae and over the posterior neck, hypertension, hirsutism, amenorrhea, and depression. More specific findings include thin skin, easy bruising, reddish striae, proximal muscle weakness, and osteoporosis. Diabetes mellitus develops in some patients. Hyperpigmentation or hypokalemic alkalosis suggests Cushing's syndrome due to ectopic ACTH secretion.

II. **Diagnosis** is based on increased cortisol excretion and lack of normal feedback inhibition of ACTH and cortisol secretion.

A. The **overnight dexamethasone suppression test** (1 mg dexamethasone given PO at 11:00 PM; plasma cortisol measured at 8:00 AM the next day; normal plasma cortisol level <2 µg/dl) or **24-hour urine cortisol** measurement can be done as a screening test. Both tests are very sensitive, and a normal value virtually excludes the diagnosis.

B. **An abnormal screening test** indicates the need to perform a **low-dose dexamethasone suppression test.** Dexamethasone, 0.5 mg PO q6h, is given for 48 hours, and urine cortisol is measured during the last 24 hours. Failure to suppress urine cortisol to less than the normal reference range is diagnostic of Cushing's syndrome. Testing should not be done during severe illness or depression, which may cause false-positive results. Phenytoin therapy also causes false-positive dexamethasone suppression test results by accelerating metabolism of dexamethasone. Random plasma cortisol levels are not useful for diagnosis, because the wide range of normal values overlaps those of Cushing's syndrome. After the diagnosis of Cushing's syndrome is made, tests to determine the cause are best done in consultation with an endocrinologist (*N Engl J Med* 332:791, 1995).

Incidental Adrenal Nodules

Adrenal nodules are a common incidental finding on abdominal imaging studies. Most incidentally discovered nodules are benign adrenocortical tumors that do not secrete excess hormone, but the differential diagnosis includes adrenal adenomas causing Cushing's syndrome or primary hyperaldosteronism, pheochromocytoma, adrenocortical carcinoma, and metastatic cancer.

I. Evaluation. The imaging characteristics of the nodule may suggest a diagnosis but are not specific enough to obviate further evaluation (*Endocrinol Metab Clin North Am* 29:27, 2000).

A. Patients who have potentially resectable cancer elsewhere and in whom an adrenal metastasis must be excluded may require needle biopsy of the nodule. Pheochromocytoma should be excluded with measurement of 24-hour urine catecholamines before biopsy.

B. In patients without known malignancy, the diagnostic issues are whether a syndrome of hormone excess or an adrenocortical carcinoma is present. Patients should be evaluated for symptoms suggestive of pheochromocytoma (episodic headache, palpitations, and sweating) and signs of Cushing's syndrome (see Cushing's Syndrome, sec. I). Plasma potassium and dehydroepiandrosterone sulfate and 24-hour urine catecholamines should be measured, and an overnight dexamethasone suppression test or 24-hour urine cortisol should be performed.

II. Management. Patients with hypertension and hypokalemia should be evaluated for primary hyperaldosteronism in consultation with an endocrinologist. Abnormalities of cortisol secretion should be evaluated further (see Cushing's Syndrome, sec. **II.B**). If clinical or biochemical evidence of a pheochromocytoma is found, the nodule should be resected after appropriate α-adrenergic blockade with phenoxybenzamine. Elevation of plasma dehydroepiandrosterone sulfate or a large nodule suggests adrenocortical carcinoma. A policy of resecting all nodules greater than 4 cm in diameter appropriately treats the great majority of adrenal carcinomas while minimizing the number of benign nodules that are removed unnecessarily (*Endocrinol Metab Clin North Am* 29:159, 2000). Most incidental nodules are less than 4 cm in diameter, do not produce excess hormone, and do not require therapy. At least one repeat imaging procedure 3–6 months later is recommended to ensure that the nodule is not enlarging rapidly (which would suggest an adrenal carcinoma).

Anterior Pituitary
Gland Dysfunction

The anterior pituitary gland secretes prolactin, growth hormone, and four trophic hormones: corticotropin (ACTH), thyrotropin (TSH), and the gonadotropins, luteinizing hormone and follicle-stimulating hormone. Each trophic hormone stimulates a specific target gland. Anterior pituitary function is regulated by hypothalamic hormones that reach the pituitary via portal veins in the pituitary stalk. **The predominant effect of hypothalamic regulation is to stimulate secretion of pituitary hormones, except for prolactin,** which is inhibited by hypothalamic dopamine production. Secretion of trophic hormones is also regulated by **negative feedback** by their target gland hormone, and the normal pituitary response to target hormone deficiency is increased secretion of the appropriate trophic hormone.

I. Anterior pituitary dysfunction can be caused by disorders of either the pituitary or hypothalamus.

A. Pituitary adenomas are the most common pituitary disorder. They are classified by size and function. **Microadenomas** are less than 10 mm in diameter and cause clinical manifestations only if they produce excess hormone. They are too small to produce hypopituitarism or mass effects. **Macroadenomas** are greater than 10 mm in diameter and may produce any combination of pituitary hormone excess, hypopituitarism, and mass effects. **Secretory adenomas** produce prolactin, growth hormone, or ACTH. **Nonsecretory macroadenomas** may cause hypopituitarism or mass effects. **Nonsecretory microadenomas** are common incidental radiographic findings, seen in approximately 10% of the normal population, and do not require therapy (*Endocrinol Metab Clin North Am* 29:205, 2000).

   B. Other pituitary or hypothalamic disorders, such as head trauma, pituitary surgery or radiation, and postpartum pituitary infarction (Sheehan's syndrome) may cause hypopituitarism. Other tumors of the pituitary or hypothalamus (e.g., craniopharyngioma, metastases), inflammatory disorders (e.g., sarcoidosis, histiocytosis X), and infections (e.g., tuberculosis) may cause hypopituitarism or mass effects.

II. Clinical findings. Pituitary and hypothalamic disorders may present in several ways.

   A. In hypopituitarism (deficiency of one or more pituitary hormones), gonadotropin deficiency is most common, causing amenorrhea in women and androgen deficiency in men. Secondary hypothyroidism or adrenal failure rarely occurs alone. Secondary adrenal failure causes deficiency of cortisol but not of aldosterone; hyperkalemia and hyperpigmentation do not occur, although life-threatening adrenal crisis may develop.

   B. Hormone excess most commonly results in **hyperprolactinemia,** which can be due to a secretory adenoma or to nonsecretory lesions that damage the hypothalamus or pituitary stalk. Growth hormone excess **(acromegaly)** and ACTH and cortisol excess **(Cushing's disease)** are caused by secretory adenomas.

   C. Mass effects due to pressure on adjacent structures, such as the optic chiasm, include **headaches** and **loss of visual fields or acuity.** Hyperprolactinemia also may be due to mass effect. **Pituitary apoplexy** is sudden enlargement of a pituitary tumor due to hemorrhagic necrosis.

   D. Asymptomatic pituitary adenomas

   1. If a microadenoma is found on imaging done for another purpose, the patient should be evaluated for clinical evidence of hyperprolactinemia (see sec. **VI**), Cushing's disease (see Cushing's Syndrome), or acromegaly (see sec. **VII**). Plasma prolactin should be measured, and tests for acromegaly and Cushing's syndrome should be performed if symptoms or signs of these disorders are evident. If no pituitary hormone excess exists, therapy is not required. Whether such patients need repeat imaging is not established, but the risk of enlargement is clearly small (*Arch Intern Med* 155:181, 1995).

   2. Incidental discovery of a macroadenoma is unusual. Patients should be evaluated for hormone excess (see sec. **II.D.1**) and hypopituitarism (see sec. **III**). Most tumors should be treated, as they are likely to grow further.

III. Diagnosis of hypopituitarism. Hypopituitarism may be suspected in the presence of clinical signs of target hormone deficiency (e.g., hypothyroidism) or pituitary mass effects.

   A. Laboratory evaluation for hypopituitarism begins with evaluation of **target hormone function,** including **plasma free T_4** and a **Cortrosyn stimulation test** (see Adrenal Failure, sec. **III.A**). If recent onset of secondary adrenal failure is suspected (within a few weeks of evaluation), the patient should be treated empirically with glucocorticoids (see Adrenal Failure, sec. **IV**) and should be tested later. In men, **plasma testosterone** should be measured. The best evaluation of gonadal function in women is the **menstrual history.**

   B. If a target hormone is deficient, its trophic hormone is measured to determine whether target gland dysfunction is secondary to hypopituitarism. An elevated trophic hormone level indicates primary target gland dysfunction. In hypopituitarism, trophic hormone levels are not elevated and usually are not below the reference range. Thus, **pituitary trophic hormone levels can be interpreted only with knowledge of target hormone levels, and measurement of trophic hormone levels alone is useless in the diagnosis of hypopituitarism.** If pituitary disease is obvious, target hormone deficiencies may be assumed to be secondary, and trophic hormones need not be measured.

IV. Anatomic evaluation of the pituitary gland and hypothalamus is done best by MRI. However, hyperprolactinemia and Cushing's disease may be caused by

Table 23-3. Major causes of hyperprolactinemia

Pregnancy and lactation
Prolactin-secreting pituitary adenoma (prolactinoma)
Idiopathic hyperprolactinemia
Drugs
    Dopamine antagonists (phenothiazines, metoclopramide, methyldopa)
    Others (verapamil, cimetidine, some antidepressants)
Interference with synthesis or transport of hypothalamic dopamine
    Hypothalamic lesions
    Pituitary macroadenomas
Primary hypothyroidism
Chronic renal failure

---

microadenomas too small to be seen with current techniques. The prevalence of incidental microadenomas should be kept in mind when interpreting MRIs (see sec. **I.A**). **Visual acuity** and **visual fields** should be tested when imaging suggests compression of the optic chiasm.

V. Treatment of hypopituitarism. Deficient target hormones should be replaced. Secondary adrenal failure should be treated immediately, especially if patients are to undergo surgery (see Adrenal Failure, sec. **IV.B**). Infertility due to gonadotropin deficiency may be correctable, and patients who wish to conceive should be referred to an endocrinologist. Treatment of pituitary macroadenomas generally requires transsphenoidal surgical resection, except for prolactin-secreting tumors (see sec. **VI.C.2**).

VI. Hyperprolactinemia. In women, the most common causes of pathologic hyperprolactinemia are prolactin-secreting pituitary **microadenomas** and **idiopathic hyperprolactinemia** (Table 23-3). **In men,** the most common cause is a prolactin-secreting **macroadenoma.** Hypothalamic or pituitary lesions that cause deficiency of other pituitary hormones often cause hyperprolactinemia.

  A. Clinical findings. In women, hyperprolactinemia causes **amenorrhea** or irregular menses and **infertility.** Only approximately half of these women have **galactorrhea.** Prolonged estrogen deficiency increases the risk of osteoporosis. In men, hyperprolactinemia causes **androgen deficiency** and infertility but not gynecomastia; **mass effects and hypopituitarism** are common.

  B. Diagnosis. Hyperprolactinemia is common in young women, and plasma prolactin should be measured in women with amenorrhea, whether or not galactorrhea is present. Mild elevations should be confirmed by repeat measurements. The history should include medications and symptoms of pituitary mass effects (see sec. **II.C**) or hypothyroidism. Laboratory evaluation should include **plasma TSH** and a **pregnancy test.** Prolactin levels of greater than 200 ng/ml occur only in prolactinomas, and levels between 100 and 200 ng/ml strongly suggest this diagnosis. Levels lower than 100 ng/ml may be due to any cause except prolactin-secreting macroadenoma, and such levels in a patient with a large pituitary mass do not indicate that it is a prolactinoma. Testing for hypopituitarism (see sec. **III**) is needed only in patients with a macroadenoma or hypothalamic lesion. **Pituitary imaging** should be performed in most cases, as nonfunctional pituitary or hypothalamic tumors may present with hyperprolactinemia.

  C. Therapy (*Endocrinol Metab Clin North Am* 28:143, 1999)

    1. Microadenomas and idiopathic hyperprolactinemia. Most patients are treated because of **infertility** or to prevent **estrogen deficiency** and **osteoporosis.** Some women may be observed without therapy by periodic follow-up of prolactin levels and symptoms. In most patients, hyperprolactinemia does not worsen, and prolactin levels sometimes return to normal. Enlargement of microadenomas is rare.

   a. The **dopamine agonists bromocriptine** and **cabergoline** suppress plasma prolactin and restore normal menses and fertility in most women. Initial dosages are bromocriptine, 1.25–2.5 mg PO qhs with a snack, or cabergoline, 0.25 mg twice a week. Plasma prolactin levels are initially obtained at 2- to 4-week intervals, and doses are adjusted until the lowest dose required to maintain prolactin in the normal range is reached. Maximally effective doses are 2.5 mg bromocriptine tid and 1.5 mg cabergoline twice a week. Initially, patients should use barrier contraception, as fertility may be restored quickly. **Side effects** include **nausea** and **orthostatic hypotension,** which can be minimized by increasing the dose gradually, and usually resolve with continued therapy. Side effects are less severe with cabergoline.

   b. **Women who want to become pregnant** should be managed in consultation with an endocrinologist.

   c. **Women who do not want to become pregnant** should be followed with clinical evaluation and plasma prolactin levels every 6–12 months. Every 2 years, plasma prolactin should be measured after bromocriptine has been withdrawn for several weeks, to determine whether the drug is still needed. Follow-up imaging studies are not warranted unless prolactin levels increase substantially.

   d. **Transsphenoidal resection** of prolactin-secreting microadenomas is used only in the rare patients who do not respond to or cannot tolerate bromocriptine. Prolactin levels usually return to normal, but up to one-half of patients experience relapse.

2. **Prolactin-secreting macroadenomas.** Such lesions should be treated with a **dopamine agonist** (see sec. **VI.C.1.a**), which usually suppresses prolactin levels to normal, reduces tumor size, and improves or corrects abnormal visual fields in 90% of cases. If mass effects are present, the dose should be increased to maximally effective levels over a period of several weeks. Visual field tests, if initially abnormal, should be repeated 4–6 weeks after therapy is started. Pituitary imaging should be repeated 3–4 months after initiation of therapy. If tumor shrinkage and correction of visual abnormalities are satisfactory, therapy can be continued indefinitely, with periodic monitoring of plasma prolactin levels. The full effect on tumor size may take more than 6 months. Repeat imaging probably is not warranted unless prolactin levels rise despite therapy.

   a. **Transsphenoidal surgery** is indicated to relieve mass effects and to prevent further tumor growth if the tumor does not shrink or if visual field abnormalities persist during dopamine agonist therapy. However, the likelihood of surgical cure of hyperprolactinemia due to a macroadenoma is low, and most patients require further therapy with a dopamine agonist.

   b. **Women with prolactin-secreting macroadenomas should not become pregnant** unless the tumor has been resected surgically, as the risk of symptomatic enlargement during pregnancy is 15–35%. Barrier contraception is essential during dopamine agonist treatment.

VII. **The acromegaly syndrome** is caused by growth hormone excess in adults and is due to a growth hormone–secreting pituitary adenoma in the vast majority of cases. Clinical findings include thickened skin and enlargement of hands, feet, jaw, and forehead. Arthritis or carpal tunnel syndrome may develop, and the pituitary adenoma may cause headaches and vision loss. Mortality from cardiovascular disease is increased.

   A. **Diagnosis. Plasma somatomedin-C** (insulin-like growth factor I), which mediates most effects of growth hormone, is the best diagnostic test. Marked elevations establish the diagnosis. If somatomedin-C levels are elevated only moderately, the diagnosis can be confirmed by giving 75 mg glucose orally and measuring serum growth hormone q30min for 2 hours. Failure to suppress growth hormone to less than 2 ng/ml confirms the diagnosis of acromegaly. Once the diagnosis is made, the pituitary should be imaged.

B. **Therapy.** The treatment of choice is transsphenoidal resection of the pituitary adenoma. Most patients have macroadenomas, and complete tumor resection with cure of acromegaly often is impossible. If somatomedin-C levels remain elevated after surgery, radiotherapy is used to prevent regrowth of the tumor and to control acromegaly; the full effect of radiotherapy on growth hormone secretion may take up to 10 years. The somatostatin analog octreotide in depot form can be used to suppress growth hormone secretion while the effect of radiation is being awaited. A dose of 10–30 mg IM monthly suppresses somatomedin-C to normal in most patients (*Endocrinol Metab Clin North Am* 28:171, 1999). Side effects include cholelithiasis, diarrhea, and mild abdominal discomfort.

Metabolic Bone Disease

I. **Osteomalacia** is characterized by defective mineralization of osteoid. Bone biopsy reveals increased thickness of osteoid seams and decreased mineralization rate, assessed by tetracycline labeling. **Causes of osteomalacia** include (1) vitamin D deficiency (rare except in the housebound elderly); (2) **malabsorption** of vitamin D and calcium (the most common cause in the United States) due to gastrectomy, or to intestinal, hepatic, or biliary disease; (3) disorders of vitamin D metabolism (e.g., renal disease, vitamin D–dependent rickets); (4) vitamin D resistance; (5) chronic hypophosphatemia; (6) renal tubular acidosis; (7) hypophosphatasia; and (8) therapy with anticonvulsants, fluoride, etidronate, or aluminum compounds.

A. **Clinical manifestations** include diffuse skeletal pain, proximal muscle weakness, waddling gait, and propensity to fractures. Radiographic findings include osteopenia and radiolucent bands perpendicular to bone surfaces (pseudofractures or Looser's zones). Serum alkaline phosphatase is elevated. Serum phosphorus, calcium, or both may be decreased.

B. **Diagnosis.** Osteomalacia should be suspected in a patient with osteopenia, elevated serum alkaline phosphatase, and either hypophosphatemia or hypocalcemia. **Serum 25-hydroxyvitamin D [25(OH)D]** levels may be low, establishing the diagnosis of vitamin D deficiency or malabsorption. Radiography of the chest, pelvis, and hips may reveal characteristic pseudofractures. If neither serum 25(OH)D nor radiography is diagnostic, a bone biopsy may be required for diagnosis.

C. **Treatment**
1. **Dietary vitamin D deficiency** can initially be treated with vitamin D, 50,000 IU PO weekly for several weeks, to replete body stores, followed by long-term therapy with 400–1000 IU/day. Preparations include calcium supplements that contain vitamin D (Os-Cal + D, 125 IU/250- or 500-mg tablet), many multivitamins (400 IU/tablet), and vitamin D drops (200 IU/drop or 8000 IU/ml).
2. **Malabsorption of vitamin D** may require therapy with high doses, ranging from 50,000 IU PO per week to 50,000 IU PO qd. The dose should be adjusted to maintain serum 25(OH)D levels within the normal range. Calcium supplements, 1 g PO qd–tid, may also be required. Serum 25(OH)D, serum calcium, and 24-hour urine calcium should be monitored every 3–6 months to avoid hypercalcemia. Calcifediol [25(OH)D], 20–100 μg PO qd, can also be used. If the underlying disease responds to therapy, the dose of vitamin D must be reduced accordingly.

II. **Paget's disease of bone** (*J Bone Miner Res* 13:1061, 1998) is a focal skeletal disorder characterized by rapid, disorganized bone remodeling. It usually occurs after age 40 and most often affects the pelvis, femur, spine, and skull. Clinical manifestations include bone pain and deformity, degenerative arthritis, pathologic fractures, neurologic deficits due to nerve root or cranial nerve compression (including deafness), and, rarely, high-output heart failure and osteogenic sarcoma. Most patients are asymptomatic, with disease discovered incidentally because of elevated serum alkaline phosphatase or an x-ray taken for other reasons.

A. **Diagnosis.** The radiographic appearance is usually diagnostic, and biopsy is rarely necessary. Serum alkaline phosphatase is elevated, reflecting the activity and extent of disease. Serum and urine calcium are usually normal but may increase with immobilization, as after a fracture.

B. **Management. Bisphosphonates** inhibit excessive bone resorption and are the mainstay of therapy. Newer, more potent bisphosphonates relieve symptoms and restore serum alkaline phosphatase and bone deposition to normal in most patients. Indications for therapy include (1) bone pain due to Paget's disease, (2) nerve compression syndromes, (3) pathologic fracture, (4) elective skeletal surgery, (5) progressive skeletal deformity, (6) immobilization hypercalcemia, (7) hypercalciuria with nephrolithiasis, (8) high-output heart failure, and (9) asymptomatic involvement of weight-bearing bones or the skull. The effectiveness of therapy is monitored by measuring serum alkaline phosphatase. Patients are treated with a course of therapy with **alendronate,** 40 mg/day for 6 months, or **risedronate,** 30 mg/day for 2–3 months. Serum alkaline phosphatase is monitored. If it returns to normal, monitoring is continued. If it remains elevated 3–6 months after the first course of therapy, a second course is given. Therapy can be repeated when serum alkaline phosphatase rises to more than 20% of the upper limit of normal [*J Bone Miner Res* 14(Suppl 2):70, 1999].

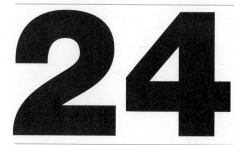

Arthritis and Rheumatologic Diseases

Leslie E. Kahl

Therapeutic Approaches to Rheumatic Disease

The etiology of most rheumatologic disorders is unknown. Therapeutic approaches in rheumatology are, therefore, largely palliative. Such approaches involve either local or systemic administration of analgesic, anti-inflammatory, immunomodulatory, or immunosuppressive drugs. Because the same procedures and medications are used for most of the rheumatologic disorders, they are discussed as a group rather than separately under each disorder.

I. **Joint aspiration and injection**
   A. **Indications.** Joint aspiration should be performed (1) when an effusion is present in a single joint and its etiology is unclear, (2) for symptomatic relief in a patient with a known arthritis diagnosis, and (3) to monitor the response to therapy in patients with infectious arthritis. Analysis of synovial fluid should include a cell count, microscopic examination for crystals, Gram stain, and culture. Intra-articular glucocorticoid therapy can be used to suppress inflammation when only one or a few peripheral joints are inflamed and infection has been excluded. The joint should be aspirated to remove as much fluid as possible before glucocorticoid injection.
   B. **Contraindications. Infection** overlying the site to be injected is an **absolute contraindication;** significant hemostatic defects and bacteremia are relative contraindications to joint aspiration and injection.
   C. **Technique.** The site of aspiration should be cleansed with povidone-iodine solution. Topical ethylchloride spray can be used as a local anesthetic. The site can also be infiltrated with local anesthetic in preparation for the procedure, particularly if there is little or no joint effusion, or if there is notable joint space narrowing.
      1. **Knee** (Fig. 24-1). The leg should be positioned by gently flexing the knee 10–15 degrees. A rolled towel can be placed in the popliteal fossa to support the knee and allow the quadriceps to relax. The joint is then entered either medially or laterally, immediately beneath the undersurface of the patella.
      2. **Ankle** (Fig. 24-2). Aspiration should be performed with the patient supine and the foot perpendicular to the leg. Medial aspiration is performed immediately medial to the extensor hallucis longus tendon, which can be identified by alternately flexing and extending the great toe. A lateral approach can also be used by introducing the needle just distal to the fibula.
      3. **Wrist** (Fig. 24-3). Aspiration is performed on the dorsum of the wrist between the distal radius and carpus with the wrist joint flexed slightly. The point of entry for lateral aspiration is just distal to the end of the radius, between the extensor tendons of the thumb. Medial aspiration can also be performed between the distal ulna and the carpus.

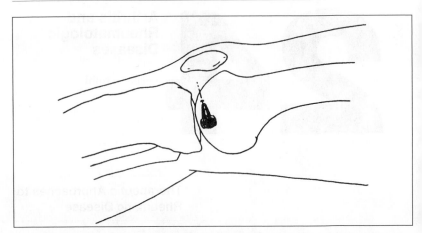

Fig. 24-1. Arthrocentesis of the knee: medial approach. [Reproduced with permission from JR Beary III, CL Christian, NA Johanson (eds), *Manual of Rheumatology and Outpatient Orthopedic Disorders* (2nd ed). Boston: Little, Brown, 1987.]

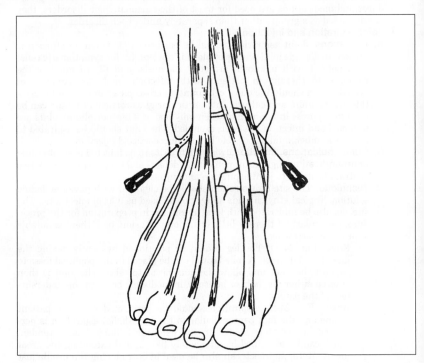

Fig. 24-2. Arthrocentesis of the ankle: medial and lateral approaches. [Reproduced with permission from JR Beary III, CL Christian, NA Johanson (eds), *Manual of Rheumatology and Outpatient Orthopedic Disorders* (2nd ed). Boston: Little, Brown, 1987.]

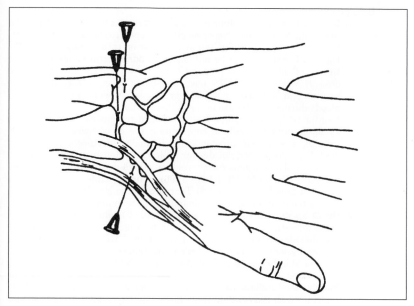

Fig. 24-3. Arthrocentesis of the wrist: medial, dorsal, and lateral approaches. [Reproduced with permission from JR Beary III, CL Christian, NA Johanson (eds), *Manual of Rheumatology and Outpatient Orthopedic Disorders* (2nd ed). Boston: Little, Brown, 1987.]

    4. Joints of the hands and feet. Small joints of the hands and feet are entered similarly by introducing the needle from the dorsal surface immediately beneath the extensor tendon from either the medial or the lateral side. Because these joints yield only very small amounts of fluid, flushing aspirate from the syringe with saline may increase the yield when analysis for crystals is attempted.

  D. Complications. Postinjection synovitis may develop rarely as a result of phagocytosis of glucocorticoid ester crystals. Such reactions usually resolve within 48–72 hours. More persistent symptoms suggest the possibility of iatrogenic infection, which occurs very rarely (in fewer than 0.1% of patients). Localized skin depigmentation and atrophy may result after glucocorticoid injection. Accelerated deterioration of bone and cartilage also may occur when frequent injections are administered over an extended period. Therefore, any single joint should be injected no more frequently than every 3–6 months.

  E. Glucocorticoid preparations. Preparations include methylprednisolone acetate, triamcinolone acetonide, and triamcinolone hexacetonide. The dose used is arbitrary, but the following guidelines based on volume are useful: large joints (knee, ankle, shoulder), 1–2 ml; medium joints (wrists, elbows), 0.5–1.0 ml; small joints of the hands and feet, 0.25–0.5 ml. Lidocaine (or its equivalent), up to 1 ml of a 1% solution, can be mixed in a single syringe with the glucocorticoid to promote immediate relief.

II. Nonsteroidal anti-inflammatory drugs (NSAIDs)

  A. Therapeutic effects. These drugs exert their effects principally by inhibiting the constitutive (COX-1) and inducible (COX-2) isoforms of cyclooxygenase. This inhibition produces a mild to moderate anti-inflammatory and analgesic effect via peripheral and central actions. Individual responses to these agents are variable; if one drug is not effective during a 2- to 3-week trial, another should be tried.

B. Side effects

1. **GI toxicity** manifests clinically as **dyspepsia, nausea, vomiting, or GI bleeding.** Nausea and dyspepsia often respond to the addition of an H_2 blocking agent or proton pump inhibitor or to a change in NSAID. Direct GI irritation can be minimized by administration after food, by the use of enteric-coated preparations, and by use of the lowest effective dose. However, all NSAIDs have a systemic effect on the GI mucosa, resulting in increased permeability to gastric acid. Most serious GI bleeds during NSAID use occur without prior GI symptoms. Risk factors for GI bleed include a history of duodenal-gastric ulceration, age, smoking, ethanol use, and concomitant use of corticosteroids. **Misoprostol,** a synthetic prostaglandin E analog, decreases the risk of NSAID-induced gastric or duodenal ulceration but may cause diarrhea and is an abortifacient. An alternative is high-dose **famotidine,** 40 mg PO bid (*N Engl J Med* 334:1435, 1996), or **omeprazole,** 20 mg qd [*Am J Med* 104(Suppl 3A):67S, 1998]. Diarrhea due to NSAIDs is rare except for the fenamates (e.g., meclofenamic acid, mefenamic acid).

2. **Renal toxicity,** including acute renal failure, nephrotic syndrome, and acute interstitial nephritis, may occur. Risk factors for acute renal failure include pre-existing renal dysfunction, CHF, and cirrhosis with ascites. Periodic monitoring of renal function is recommended, particularly in elderly patients. **Sulindac** is relatively less nephrotoxic than other NSAIDs.

3. **Platelet dysfunction** can be caused by all NSAIDs, and particularly aspirin, which is a covalent inhibitor of cyclooxygenase. NSAIDs should be used cautiously or avoided in patients with a bleeding diathesis or those who are taking warfarin, and should be discontinued 5–7 days before surgical procedures.

4. **Hypersensitivity reactions** are often seen in patients with a history of asthma, nasal polyps, or atopy. NSAIDs may cause a variety of type I hypersensitivity-like reactions, including urticaria, asthma, and anaphylactoid shock, presumably by increasing leukotriene synthesis. Patients with a hypersensitivity reaction to one NSAID should avoid all NSAIDs.

5. **Other side effects.** CNS toxicity (headaches, dizziness, dysphoria, confusion, aseptic meningitis) is uncommon. Tinnitus and deafness can complicate NSAID use, particularly with high-dose salicylates. Blood dyscrasias including aplastic anemia have been observed as isolated case reports with ibuprofen, piroxicam, indomethacin, and phenylbutazone. Dermatologic reactions and elevations in transaminases have been described. Acid-base imbalance is seen with high doses of salicylates. Nonacetylated salicylates have been reported to have less toxicity but also may be less effective.

III. Selective COX-2 inhibitors

A. Therapeutic effects. These agents exhibit selective inhibition of COX-2, thereby inhibiting inflammation while preserving the homeostatic functions of constitutive COX-1–derived prostaglandins. Their anti-inflammatory and analgesic efficacy is similar to that of traditional NSAIDs.

B. Dosage. Two new agents in this class are currently available. **Celecoxib** is indicated for osteoarthritis (OA; 100 or 200 mg qd) and rheumatoid arthritis (RA; 100 or 200 mg bid). **Rofecoxib** is indicated for OA (12.5 or 25 mg qd) and acute pain (50 mg qd for up to 5 days). Both drugs will likely be used for a variety of additional anti-inflammatory conditions.

C. Side effects. GI symptoms and GI ulcerations are reduced with these agents in comparison to NSAIDs (*Med Lett Drugs Ther* 41:11, 1999). **Platelet function** is not impaired, making selective COX-2 inhibitors a good anti-inflammatory option for patients with thrombocytopenia, hemostatic defects, or chronic anticoagulation. In patients who are taking warfarin, however, the international normalized ratio should be monitored after the addition of a

Table 24-1. Corticosteroids and immunomodulatory and immunosuppressive drugs

Generic name	Tablet size (mg)	Starting dose (mg)	Dose interval	Maximum daily or interval dose (mg)
Prednisone	1, 2.5, 5, 10, 20, 50	5–20 (low) 1–2 mg/kg (high)	qd	—
Methylprednisolone (IV)	—	500	bid for 3–5 days	—
Methotrexate	2.5	7.5	Weekly	25
Sulfasalazine	500	500	bid	3000
Hydroxychloroquine	200	200	bid	400
Leflunomide	10, 20	—	20 qd	20[a]
Aurothioglucose (IM)	—	10 (test dose)	Weekly	50
Auranofin (PO)	3	3	bid	9
Penicillamine	125, 250	250	qd	1000
Azathioprine	50 (scored)	1.5 mg/kg	qd	2.5–3.0 mg/kg[b]
Cyclophosphamide	25, 50	1.0–1.5 mg/kg	qd	2.5–3.0 mg/kg[a]
Cyclophosphamide (IV)	—	0.5–1.0 g/m^2	Monthly	—[b,c]
Cyclosporin	25, 50, 100	2–3 mg/kg	qd	5 mg/kg

[a]Treatment is begun with a loading dose of 100 mg/day for 3 days.
[b]Titrate peripheral WBC count to 3500–4500 cells/µl (with neutrophils >1000).
[c]The addition of 2-mercaptoethanesulfonate (mesna) is recommended.

COX-2 inhibitor, as with any medication change. **Fluid retention** has been noted with high-dose rofecoxib therapy, and renal function should be monitored in patients at risk of NSAID-induced acute renal failure (see sec. **II.B.2**).

IV. Glucocorticoids (Table 24-1)

- **A. Therapeutic effects.** Glucocorticoids exert a pluripotent anti-inflammatory effect via the inhibition of inflammatory mediator gene transcription.
- **B. Preparations, dosages, and routes of administration.** The goal of glucocorticoid therapy is to suppress disease activity with the minimum effective dosage. Prednisone (PO) and methylprednisolone (IV) are generally the preferred drugs because of cost and half-life considerations. IM absorption is variable and therefore is not advised. The dose, route, and frequency of administration are determined by the type of disease and the severity of the disease manifestations. The following are relative anti-inflammatory potencies of common glucocorticoid preparations: cortisone, 0.8; hydrocortisone, 1; prednisone, 4; methylprednisolone, 5; dexamethasone, 25.
- **C. Side effects.** Adverse effects are related to dosage and duration of administration and, except for cataracts and osteopenia, can be minimized by alternate-day administration once the disease is controlled (twice the daily dose given every other day).
  - **1. Adrenal suppression.** Glucocorticoids suppress the hypothalamic-pituitary-adrenal axis. Patients who have received more than 10 mg prednisone (or the equivalent) daily for several weeks may have some degree of axis suppression for up to 1 year following cessation of therapy. Adrenal suppression is minimized by dosing in the morning, using

a single daily low dose of a short-acting preparation, such as prednisone, for a short period. In patients receiving chronic glucocorticoid therapy, hypoadrenalism (anorexia, weight loss, lethargy, fever, and postural hypotension) may occur at times of severe stress (e.g., infection, major surgery) and should be treated with stress doses of glucocorticoids (see Chap. 23). Mineralocorticoid activity, however, is preserved. These patients should wear a medical-alert bracelet or carry identification.

2. **Immunosuppression.** Glucocorticoid therapy reduces resistance to infections. Bacterial infections in particular are related to the dosage of glucocorticoids and are a major cause of morbidity and mortality. Thus, minor infections may become systemic, quiescent infections may be activated, and organisms that usually are nonpathogenic may cause disease. Local and systemic signs of infection can be masked partially, although fever associated with infection generally is not suppressed completely by glucocorticoids. When possible, a skin test for tuberculosis should be placed before glucocorticoid therapy is instituted, and, if it is positive, appropriate prophylaxis is indicated (see Chap. 14).

3. **Endocrine abnormalities.** Possible endocrine abnormalities include a **cushingoid habitus** and **hirsutism. Hyperglycemia** may be induced or aggravated by glucocorticoids but usually is not a contraindication to therapy. Insulin therapy may be required, although ketoacidosis is rare. **Fluid and electrolyte abnormalities** include hypokalemia and sodium retention, which may induce or aggravate hypertension.

4. **Musculoskeletal problems. Osteopenia** with vertebral compression fractures is common among patients who are receiving long-term glucocorticoid therapy. Supplemental calcium, 1.0–1.5 g/day PO, should be given along with vitamin D, 800 units, as soon as steroid therapy is begun (*Arthritis Rheum* 39:1791, 1996). Estrogen, bisphosphonates, or calcitonin may be indicated in postmenopausal women or in those at high risk for osteopenia. Determination of baseline bone density is appropriate in these patients. A judicious exercise program may be beneficial in stimulating bone formation. **Steroid myopathy** generally involves the hip and shoulder girdle musculature. Muscles are weak but not tender and, in contrast to inflammatory myositis, serum creatine kinase and aldolase and electromyography are normal. The myopathy should resolve slowly with a reduction in glucocorticoid dosage and an aggressive exercise program. **Ischemic bone necrosis** (aseptic necrosis, avascular necrosis) caused by glucocorticoid use often is multifocal, most commonly affecting the femoral head, humeral head, and tibial plateau. Early changes can be demonstrated by bone scan or MRI. Early surgical intervention with core decompression remains controversial.

5. **Other adverse effects.** Changes in **mental status** ranging from mild nervousness, euphoria, and insomnia to severe depression or psychosis may occur. **Ocular effects** include increased intraocular pressure (sometimes precipitating glaucoma) and the formation of posterior subcapsular cataracts. **Hyperlipidemia, menstrual irregularities,** increased perspiration with **night sweats,** and **pseudotumor cerebri** also may occur.

V. **Immunomodulatory and immunosuppressive drugs.** These agents can be used to treat rheumatologic disorders (see Table 24-1). This group of drugs includes a number of pharmacologically diverse agents that exert anti-inflammatory or immunosuppressive effects. Often, such agents are referred to as disease-modifying antirheumatic drugs (DMARD). These agents are characterized by a delayed onset of action and the potential for serious toxicity. Consequently, they should be prescribed with the guidance of a rheumatologist or other physician who is experienced in their use and given only to well-informed, cooperative patients who are willing to comply with meticulous follow-up.

A. **Methotrexate,** a purine inhibitor and folic acid antagonist, is used to treat synovitis and myositis and may improve the leukopenia of Felty's syndrome.

    1. **Dosage and administration.** Typically, methotrexate is administered as a single PO dose once a week starting with 7.5 mg. Clinical response is usually noted in 4–8 weeks. If no response is attained after 6–8 weeks of therapy, the dosage can be increased by 2.5- to 5.0-mg increments every 2–4 weeks to a maximum of 25 mg/week or until improvement is observed. Dosages above 20 mg/week are generally given by SC injection to promote absorption. Methotrexate in a dose of 7.5–17.5 mg/week is also used in a treatment regimen for RA in combination with sulfasalazine, 500 mg bid, and hydroxychloroquine, 200 mg bid (*N Engl J Med* 16:1287, 1999).

    2. **Contraindications and side effects.** Methotrexate is **teratogenic** and should not be used during pregnancy. It should also be avoided in patients with significant hepatic or renal impairment. Folic acid supplementation at a dosage of 1–2 mg qd may reduce methotrexate toxicity without impeding its efficacy. Concomitant use of trimethoprim-sulfamethoxazole should be avoided.

        a. **Minor side effects** include GI intolerance, stomatitis, rash, headache, and alopecia.

        b. **Bone marrow suppression** may occur, particularly at higher doses. Blood and platelet counts should be obtained before initiation, monthly during the first 3–4 months and every 6–8 weeks thereafter. Macrocytosis may herald serious hematologic toxicity and is an indication for folate supplementation or dose reduction, or both.

        c. **Cirrhosis** may occur rarely with long-term use. Aspartate aminotransferase (AST), alanine aminotransferase, and serum albumin should be measured every 4–8 weeks. Liver biopsy should be performed if the AST is elevated in five of nine determinations or if the serum albumin level falls below the normal range (*Arthritis Rheum* 37:316, 1994). Alcohol consumption increases the risk of methotrexate hepatotoxicity.

        d. **Hypersensitivity pneumonitis** may occur but usually is reversible. Patients with pre-existing pulmonary parenchymal disease may be at increased risk.

        e. **Rheumatoid nodules** may develop or worsen, paradoxically, in some patients on methotrexate.

B. **Sulfasalazine** is useful for treating synovitis in the setting of **RA** and the **seronegative spondyloarthropathies.**

    1. The initial **dosage** is 500 mg PO qd, with increases in 500-mg increments weekly until a total daily dose of 2000–3000 mg (given in evenly divided doses) is reached. Clinical response usually occurs in 6–10 weeks.

    2. **Contraindications and side effects. Sulfasalazine should not be used in patients with glucose 6-phosphate dehydrogenase deficiency or sulfa allergy.** Nausea is the principal adverse effect and can be minimized by the use of the enteric-coated preparation of the drug. Hematologic toxicity including a reduction in any cell line and aplastic anemia rarely occurs. However, periodic monitoring of blood and platelet counts is warranted.

C. **Hydroxychloroquine** is an antimalarial agent that is used to treat dermatitis, alopecia, and synovitis in systemic lupus erythematosus (SLE), and mild synovitis in RA.

    1. **Dosage.** Hydroxychloroquine typically is given at a dose of 200–400 mg PO qd after meals to minimize dyspepsia and nausea.

    2. **Contraindications and side effects. Hydroxychloroquine should not be used in patients with porphyria, glucose 6-phosphate dehydrogenase deficiency, or significant hepatic or renal impairment.** It should be avoided during pregnancy. The most common side effects are allergic

skin eruptions and nausea. Serious ocular toxicity occurs but is rare with currently recommended dosages. Ophthalmologic evaluation should be performed every 6 months.

D. Leflunomide is a pyrimidine inhibitor that has been approved for the treatment of **RA.**

   1. Dosage and administration. Treatment is begun with a loading dose of 100 mg/day for 3 days, followed by maintenance therapy of 20 mg/day. Clinical response is generally seen within 4–8 weeks (*Arthritis Rheum* 38:1595, 1995).

   2. Contraindications and side effects. Leflunomide is **teratogenic** and has a very long half-life. Women who plan to become pregnant must discontinue the drug and complete a course of elimination therapy including cholestyramine, 8 g three times a day for 11 days. Plasma levels should then be verified to be less than 0.02 mg/L on two separate tests at least 14 days apart before pregnancy is considered. Leflunomide is contraindicated in patients with significant hepatic dysfunction or patients who are receiving rifampin. **GI side effects** are the most common. **Diarrhea** occurs in up to 20% of patients. Dosage reduction to 10 mg/day may provide relief while maintaining efficacy. **Elevations in serum transaminase levels** may occur, and transaminase levels should be measured at baseline and then monitored monthly. The dosage should be reduced for confirmed twofold elevations, and greater elevations should be treated with cholestyramine and discontinuation of leflunomide. **Rash** and **alopecia** may occur during therapy.

E. Gold salts are rarely used now and are administered principally for the synovitis of RA but can be used for other arthritides.

   1. Dosage and administration

   a. Parenteral gold salts are administered either as aurothioglucose or gold sodium thiomalate given by deep IM injection. A test dose of 10 mg should be given first and, if it is tolerated, 50 mg should be given weekly thereafter. After a total cumulative dose of 1000 mg, the interval between injections can be increased gradually to every 4–8 weeks.

   b. Oral gold (auranofin) is less effective than parenteral gold but is less toxic. The recommended initial dosage is 3 mg PO bid. If the response is inadequate after 6 months of therapy, an increase to 3 mg tid for 3 more months can be attempted.

   2. Contraindications and side effects. Gold is contraindicated in patients with history of a severe toxic reaction and should be used cautiously, if at all, in patients with **impaired renal or hepatic function.** Adverse reactions can occur at any time during therapy and, with the exception of diarrhea, are much more common with parenteral therapy.

   a. Nitritoid (nitrate-like) reactions (sweating, faintness, flushing, headache) can occur with the initiation of parenteral gold therapy, particularly gold sodium thiomalate.

   b. Dermatitis, typically pruritic, is the most common manifestation of parenteral gold toxicity. Injections should be discontinued but can be restarted carefully at a lower dosage.

   c. Gold nephropathy is manifest by proteinuria and occurs in up to 25% of patients receiving IM gold and 1% of patients receiving PO gold. A urinalysis should be performed before each gold injection and monthly in patients taking oral gold. Gold therapy should be discontinued for patients with proteinuria of greater than 1.5 g/24 hours.

   d. The most serious adverse effects of parenteral gold are cytopenias **(thrombocytopenia, leukopenia, agranulocytosis, and aplastic anemia).** Blood and platelet counts should be performed every 1–2 weeks for the first few months of parenteral therapy and at increasing intervals up to every 6–8 weeks thereafter. **Gold therapy should not be restarted in patients in whom cytopenias develop.**

e. **GI side effects,** including diarrhea, abdominal pain, nausea, and vomiting, are common with auranofin (in up to 50% of patients) and usually require dosage reduction, discontinuation of therapy, or a change to parenteral gold therapy. Stomatitis or enterocolitis can complicate parenteral gold therapy.

F. Penicillamine can be used for RA synovitis. This agent has a toxicity profile similar to that of gold, and concurrent use with gold preparations is not recommended.

1. **Dosage.** Penicillamine is begun at a dosage of 250 mg PO qd for 4–6 weeks and is increased by 125 or 250 mg every 4–8 weeks until clinical improvement occurs or a daily dose of 1000 mg is reached.

2. **Contraindications and side effects**

   a. **Penicillamine is teratogenic** and should not be used during pregnancy. Allergy to penicillin does not predict potential reactions to penicillamine.

   b. **Dermatitis** is the most common side effect of treatment. If rash occurs with fever, rechallenge should be avoided.

   c. **Hematologic toxicity** and proteinuria occur as in gold therapy and require the same close laboratory monitoring.

G. Azathioprine is an antimetabolite used to treat refractory synovitis or myositis. It can also be used as a steroid-sparing agent.

1. **Dosage.** Therapy is initiated at 1.5 mg/kg/day PO, given as a single dose or in two divided doses. The dosage can be increased (8- to 12-week intervals) to a maximum of 2.5–3.0 mg/kg/day as long as the WBC count remains at or above 3500–4500 cells/µl, with more than 1000 neutrophils. The dosage of azathioprine should be reduced by 60–75% if it is given concomitantly with allopurinol, which blocks its metabolic degradation.

2. **Side effects.** Adverse effects of azathioprine include an increased incidence of **infection, nausea,** rare **hepatotoxicity,** and potential long-term **oncogenicity.**

H. Cyclophosphamide, an alkylating agent, is used to treat life-threatening manifestations of SLE and vasculitis.

1. **Dosage and administration.** Cyclophosphamide can be administered either daily (low-dose PO therapy) or intermittently (high-dose IV bolus therapy). The latter route is probably less toxic but also less immunosuppressive. Oral therapy is initiated at a daily morning dose of 1.0–1.5 mg/kg and can be increased to a maximum of 2.5–3.0 mg/kg/day to obtain a WBC count of 3500–4500 cells/µl, with more than 1000 neutrophils. Peripheral WBC counts should be checked 10–14 days after each dosage change and monthly when on a stable dose. IV therapy is initiated at a dose of 0.5–1.0 g/m^2 every 1–3 months. The goal of therapy is to achieve a nadir WBC count of 3500–4500 cells/µl, with more than 1000 neutrophils, 10–14 days after infusion.

2. **Side effects.** Adverse effects include an increased incidence of **infection,** hemorrhagic cystitis, GI toxicity (nausea, vomiting), gonadal suppression and **sterility, alopecia, pulmonary interstitial fibrosis,** and **oncogenicity** (particularly bladder carcinoma). Patients should be encouraged to take the medication in the morning with a lot of fluid, to void frequently, and to void before going to bed to minimize the risk of hemorrhagic cystitis. With IV therapy, sodium 2-mercaptoethane-sulfonate **(mesna)** and large volumes of fluid can be given concomitantly to minimize the risk of hemorrhagic cystitis. Mesna can be given with the cyclophosphamide infusion and repeated 4 and 8 hours later. Each mesna dose should be 20% of the total cyclophosphamide dose. **Antiemetics** may be necessary with high-dose IV therapy.

    I. Cyclosporin is occasionally used to treat refractory **synovitis.** Therapy is initiated at a dose of 2–3 mg/kg/day PO. The dose can be increased as high as 5 mg/kg/day, but **renal toxicity** is usually limiting. The dosage should be reduced if the serum creatinine level increases more than 30% or if hypertension develops. Other toxicities include hirsutism, anemia, liver dysfunction, and oncogenicity.

VI. Tumor necrosis factor (TNF) inhibitors have been approved for treatment of RA.

  A. Etanercept is a fusion protein consisting of the ligand-binding portion of the human TNF receptor linked to the Fc portion of human immunoglobulin G. Etanercept binds to TNF, blocking its interaction with cell surface receptors and, hence, inhibiting the inflammatory and immunoregulatory properties of TNF. The effect on RA synovitis can be dramatic, with responsive patients reporting the onset of symptomatic benefit within 1–2 weeks [*J Rheumatol* 26(S57):7, 1999].

    1. Dosage and administration. Etanercept is indicated for patients with moderately to severely active RA who have had inadequate response to one or more disease-modifying antirheumatic drugs. The drug is given by SC injection at a dosage of 25 mg twice a week. Methotrexate, corticosteroids, NSAIDs, and COX-2 inhibitors can be continued during treatment if needed.

    2. Contraindications and side effects

      a. Serious infections and **sepsis,** including fatalities, have been reported during the use of etanercept. Etanercept is contraindicated in patients with acute or chronic infections, and if serious infection or sepsis occurs, the drug should be stopped. Those with a history of recurrent infections, and those with underlying conditions that may predispose to infection, should be treated with caution and counseled to be vigilant for signs and symptoms of infection. Upper respiratory and sinus infections are most common. Tuberculosis has also been noted. Patients who are undergoing elective surgical procedures can omit the last dose of the drug that is scheduled to be given before surgery, as well as the next dose scheduled to follow the surgery.

      b. Local injection site reactions are common, particularly during the first month of therapy. These reactions are generally self-limited and do not require discontinuation of therapy. Serious systemic allergic reactions are rare.

  B. Infliximab is a chimeric monoclonal antibody that binds specifically to human TNF-α, blocking its proinflammatory and immunomodulatory effects. As with etanercept, the effect on RA synovitis can be profound and very rapid in onset (*Arthritis Rheum* 41:1552, 1998).

    1. Dosage and administration. The indications for infliximab are the same as those for etanercept. Infliximab is given by IV infusion, in conjunction with weekly PO methotrexate to reduce production of antibodies against infliximab. The recommended treatment regimen is methotrexate given at a dose of at least 7.5 mg/week along with infliximab infusions of 3 mg/kg given at initiation, 2 and 6 weeks, and every 8 weeks thereafter.

    2. Contraindications and side effects are the same as for etanercept (see sec. **VI.A.2**). In addition, **systemic hypersensitivity reactions** have occurred, and a **drug-induced lupus-like syndrome** has been reported.

VII. Plasmapheresis. Until concomitant therapy with glucocorticoids or immunosuppressives has taken effect, plasmapheresis has been used on an investigational basis in life-threatening situations to control various rheumatic diseases. It is an impractical long-term therapy, and its short-term use remains controversial. A new approach, pheresis across a column bound with staphylococcal protein A, the **Prosorba** column, has been approved for treatment of RA (*Arthritis Rheum* 42:2153, 1999).

Approach to the Patient
with a Single Painful Joint

The first step for diagnosis for a patient with a single painful joint is to **identify the structure involved.** Pain that arises from periarticular (e.g., tendon, bursa), muscular, and neurologic structures may be perceived as joint pain. If the pain arises in the joint itself and a single joint is involved, the major disorders in the differential diagnosis are **trauma, infection,** and **crystalline arthritis** (*Arthritis Rheum* 39:1, 1996).

I. **Diagnostics studies**
   A. **Radiographs** of the joint may be useful in documenting trauma or pre-existing joint disease. The presence of chondrocalcinosis on x-ray suggests pseudogout but is not diagnostic (see Crystal-Induced Synovitis). Radiographs are usually normal in acute infectious or crystalline arthritis.
   B. **Synovial fluid** should be aspirated in all patients with a monoarticular arthritis who do not have a pre-existing diagnosis that is consistent with the clinical picture. Polyarticular disorders such as RA or lupus (SLE) occasionally present initially as monoarthritis, but when a single joint is inflamed out of proportion to other joints in this setting, infection must be excluded. Synovial fluid cell counts above 5000 nucleated cells/µl suggest an inflammatory etiology. Counts above 50,000 cells/µl may indicate infection, particularly if 75% of cells or more are polymorphonuclear.

II. **Management** is based on the results of radiographs and synovial fluid analysis. Trauma or internal derangement of the joint can be managed by immobilization of the joint and consultation with an orthopedic surgeon. The treatment of infectious arthritis and crystalline disorders is detailed in the following sections.

Infectious Arthritis
and Bursitis

Infectious arthritis is generally categorized into gonococcal and nongonococcal disease. The usual presentation is with fever and an acute monarticular arthritis, although multiple joints may be affected by hematogenous spread of pathogens. **Nongonococcal infectious arthritis** in adults tends to occur in patients with previous joint damage or compromised host defenses. In contrast, **gonococcal arthritis** causes one-half of all septic arthritis in otherwise healthy, sexually active young adults.

I. **General principles of treatment**
   A. **Joint fluid examination,** including Gram stain of a centrifuged pellet, and culture are mandatory to make a diagnosis and to guide management. A joint fluid leukocyte count is useful diagnostically and as a baseline for serial studies to evaluate response to treatment. Cultures of blood and other possible extra-articular sites of infection also should be obtained.
   B. **Hospitalization** is indicated to ensure drug compliance and careful monitoring of the clinical response.
   C. **IV antimicrobials** provide good serum and synovial fluid drug concentrations. Oral or intra-articular antimicrobials are not appropriate as initial therapy.
   D. **Repeated arthrocenteses** should be performed daily or as often as necessary to prevent reaccumulation of fluid. Arthrocentesis is indicated to (1) remove destructive inflammatory mediators, (2) reduce intra-articular pressure and promote antimicrobial penetration into the joint, and (3) monitor response to therapy by documenting sterility of synovial fluid cultures and steadily decreasing leukocyte counts.

E. Surgical drainage or arthroscopic lavage and drainage is indicated for (1) septic hip; (2) joints in which either the anatomy, large amounts of tissue debris, or loculation of pus prevent adequate needle drainage (most commonly the shoulder); (3) septic arthritis with coexistent osteomyelitis; (4) joints that do not respond in 4–6 days to appropriate therapy and repeated arthrocenteses; and (5) prosthetic joint infection.

F. General supportive measures include splinting of the joint, which may help to relieve pain. However, prolonged immobilization can result in joint stiffness. An NSAID or selective COX-2 inhibitor (see Therapeutic Approaches to Rheumatic Disease, sec. II) is often useful to reduce pain and to increase joint mobility but should not be used until response to antimicrobial therapy has been demonstrated by symptomatic and laboratory improvement.

II. Nongonococcal septic arthritis is caused most often by *Staphylococcus aureus* (60%) and *Streptococcus* species. Gram-negative organisms are less common, except with IV drug abuse, neutropenia, concomitant urinary tract infection, and postoperatively. Initial therapy is based on the clinical situation and a carefully performed Gram stain, which reveals the organism in approximately 50% of patients (*N Engl J Med* 330:769, 1994). With a positive Gram stain, antibiotic coverage can be focused accordingly. With a nondiagnostic Gram stain, antibiotics should be chosen to cover *S. aureus* and *Streptococcus* species and *Neisseria gonorrhoeae* in otherwise healthy patients, whereas broad-spectrum antibiotics are appropriate in immunosuppressed patients. IV antimicrobials usually are given for at least 2 weeks, followed by 1–2 weeks of oral antimicrobials, with the course of therapy tailored to the patient's response.

III. Gonococcal arthritis is more common than nongonococcal septic arthritis. The clinical spectrum of disease often includes migratory or additive polyarthralgias, followed by tenosynovitis or arthritis of the wrist, ankle, or knee, and asymptomatic dermatitis on the extremities or trunk. In contrast to nongonococcal septic arthritis, Gram staining of synovial fluid and cultures of blood or synovial fluid often are negative. Bacteriologic assessment of the throat, cervix, urethra, and rectum may aid in establishing the diagnosis. Treatment is begun with an IV antibiotic for the first 1–3 days, generally ceftriaxone, 1 g qd, or ceftizoxime, 1 g q8h. Response to IV antibiotics is usually noted within the first 24–36 hours of treatment. After initial clinical improvement, therapy is continued with an oral antibiotic to complete 7–10 days of treatment. Ciprofloxacin, 500 mg bid, or amoxicillin/clavulanate, 500–850 mg bid, can be used. Treatment of coexisting *Chlamydia* infection should also be considered.

IV. Nonbacterial infectious arthritis is common with many viral infections, especially hepatitis B, rubella, mumps, infectious mononucleosis, parvovirus, enterovirus, and adenovirus. It is generally self-limited, lasting for less than 6 weeks, and responds well to a conservative regimen of rest and NSAIDs. Arthralgias (often severe) or a reactive arthritis can be a manifestation of HIV infection. A variety of fungi and mycobacteria can cause septic arthritis and should be considered in patients with chronic monarticular arthritis.

V. Septic bursitis, usually involving the olecranon or prepatellar bursa, can be differentiated from septic arthritis by localized, fluctuant superficial swelling and by relatively painless joint motion (particularly extension). Most patients have a history of previous trauma to the area or an occupational predisposition (e.g., "housemaid's knee," "writer's elbow"). *S. aureus* is the most common pathogen. Septic bursitis should be treated with aspiration, which can be repeated if fluid reaccumulates. Oral antibiotics and outpatient management are usually appropriate, and surgical drainage is rarely indicated. Preventive measures (e.g., knee pads) should be used in patients with occupational predispositions.

VI. Lyme disease is caused by the tick-borne spirochete *Borrelia burgdorferi*. Typical manifestations begin with an erythematous annular rash (erythema migrans) and flu-like symptoms. Arthralgias, myalgias, meningitis, neuropathy, and cardiac conduction defects may follow in weeks to a few months. Months later, untreated patients may develop an intermittent or chronic arthritis in one or a few joints, characteristically including the knee. The diagnosis is based on the clinical picture, exposure in an endemic area, and serologic studies. Unfortunately, serologic studies often give false-negative or false-positive results (*JAMA* 268:891, 1992), and patients may remain seropositive for years following treatment. Antibiotic therapy is required (see Chap. 14). NSAIDs are a useful adjunct for arthritis. Vaccination should be considered for people living in high-risk areas who have frequent tick exposures.

Crystal-Induced Synovitis

Deposition of microcrystals in joints and periarticular tissues results in **gout, pseudogout,** and **apatite disease.** A definitive diagnosis of gout or pseudogout is made by finding intracellular crystals in joint fluid examined with a compensated polarized light microscope. Urate crystals, which are diagnostic of gout, are needle-shaped and strongly negatively birefringent. Calcium pyrophosphate dihydrate crystals seen in pseudogout are pleomorphic and weakly positively birefringent. Hydroxyapatite complexes, diagnostic of apatite disease, and basic calcium phosphate complexes can be identified only by electron microscopy and mass spectroscopy. In most cases, the arthritides associated with these compounds are suspected clinically but never confirmed.

I. **Primary gouty arthritis** is characterized by hyperuricemia usually due to underexcretion of uric acid, rather than overproduction (90% of cases). Urate crystals may deposit in the joints, SC tissues (tophi), and kidneys. Men are much more commonly affected than are women; most premenopausal women with gout have a family history of the disease. The clinical phases of gout can be divided into (1) asymptomatic hyperuricemia, (2) acute gouty arthritis, and (3) chronic arthritis.

   A. **Asymptomatic hyperuricemia** (uric acid levels >8 mg/dl in men and >7 mg/dl in women) is not routinely treated because of expense, potential drug toxicity, and the low risk for adverse outcome from the hyperuricemia itself.

   B. **Acute gouty arthritis** presents as an excruciating attack of pain, usually in a single joint of the foot or ankle. Occasionally, a polyarticular onset can mimic RA. Attacks can be precipitated by surgery, dehydration, fasting, binge eating, or heavy ingestion of alcohol. Although the acute gouty attack will subside spontaneously over several days, prompt treatment can abort the attack within hours. The serum uric acid level is normal in 30% of patients with acute gout and, if elevated, should not be manipulated until an attack has resolved.

   1. **NSAIDs** are the treatment of choice for acute gout, due to ease of administration and low toxicity. Clinical response may require 12–24 hours, and initial doses should be high, followed by rapid tapering over 2–8 days (see Therapeutic Approaches to Rheumatic Disease, sec. **II**). One approach is to use indomethacin, 50 mg PO q6h for 2 days, followed by 50 mg PO q8h for 3 days, and then 25 mg PO q8h for 2–3 days. The long-acting NSAIDs generally are not recommended for acute gout. Selective COX-2 inhibitors have not been critically evaluated for treatment of gout but should also be effective.

   2. **Glucocorticoids** are useful when NSAIDs are contraindicated. An intra-articular injection of glucocorticoids produces rapid dramatic relief. Alternatively, prednisone, 40–60 mg PO qd, can be given until a response is obtained and then can be tapered rapidly.

   3. **Colchicine** is most effective if given in the first 12–24 hours of an acute attack and usually brings relief in 6–12 hours. In view of the efficacy and tolerability of a short course of NSAID, colchicine is not commonly used to treat gout.

      a. **Oral administration** is often associated with severe GI toxicity. The dosage is 0.5–0.6 mg (1 tablet) q1–2h or 1.0–1.2 mg q2h until symptoms abate, GI toxicity develops, or the maximum dose of 6 mg in a 24-hour period is reached. The dosage should be reduced in elderly patients and in those who have renal or hepatic impairment. No more than 1.2 mg/day should be used after the loading dose.

   b. IV colchicine produces faster relief with fewer GI side effects but can cause severe myelosuppression and is rarely used. The drug is diluted in 10–20 ml normal saline and is given slowly over 3–5 minutes through a freely flowing IV to **avoid extravasation** and tissue necrosis. **Colchicine should not be diluted with or injected into IV tubing that contains 5% dextrose because precipitation will occur.** The initial dose is 2 mg, followed by another 1–2 mg in 6 hours if necessary, to a maximum dose of 4 mg in 24 hours. The dosage should be reduced in the elderly, patients who have been receiving chronic oral colchicine, and those with significant renal or hepatic disease. No further colchicine should be given PO or IV for 7 days.

C. Chronic gouty arthritis. With time, acute gouty attacks occur more frequently, asymptomatic periods are shorter, and chronic joint deformity may appear. Colchicine (0.5–0.6 mg PO qd or bid) can be used prophylactically for acute attacks. Aspirin (uricoretentive), diuretics, large alcohol intake, and foods high in purines (sweetbreads, anchovies, sardines, liver, and kidney) should be avoided. The serum uric acid level should be lowered if arthritic attacks are frequent, renal damage is present, or serum or urine uric acid levels are elevated consistently. **Maintenance colchicine, 0.5–0.6 mg PO bid, should be given a few days before manipulation of the uric acid level to prevent precipitation of an acute attack.** If no attacks occur after the uric acid has been maintained in the normal range for 6–8 weeks, colchicine can be discontinued.

   1. Allopurinol, a xanthine oxidase inhibitor, is effective therapy for hyperuricemia in most patients.

   a. Dosage and administration. The initial dose is usually 300 mg PO qd. Daily doses can be increased by 100 mg every 2–4 weeks to achieve the minimum maintenance dosage that will keep the uric acid level within the normal range. In patients with impaired renal function, the daily dose should be reduced by 50 mg for each 20-ml/minute decrease in the creatinine clearance. For patients with a creatinine clearance below 20 ml/minute, the starting dose is 100 mg every other or every third day. The daily dose should be decreased also in patients with hepatic impairment. The concomitant use of a uricosuric agent may hasten the mobilization of tophi. If an acute attack occurs during treatment with allopurinol, it should be continued at the same dosage while other agents are used to treat the attack.

   b. Side effects. Hypersensitivity reactions from a minor skin rash to a diffuse exfoliative dermatitis associated with fever, eosinophilia, and a combination of renal and hepatic injury occur in up to 5% of patients. Patients who have mild renal insufficiency and are receiving diuretics are at greatest risk. **Severe cases are potentially fatal** and usually require glucocorticoid therapy. Allopurinol may potentiate the effect of oral anticoagulants. Allopurinol blocks metabolism of azathioprine and 6-mercaptopurine, necessitating a 60–75% reduction in dosage of these cytotoxic drugs.

   2. Uricosuric drugs lower serum uric acid levels by blocking renal tubular reabsorption of uric acid. A 24-hour measurement of creatinine clearance and urine uric acid should be obtained before therapy is started. Uricosuric agents are **ineffective with glomerular filtration rates of less than 50 ml/minute.** They are not recommended for patients who already have high levels of urine uric acid (800 mg/24 hours) because of the risk of urate stone formation. This risk can be minimized by maintaining a high fluid intake and by alkalinizing the urine. If these drugs are being used when an acute gouty attack begins, they should be continued while other drugs are used to treat the acute attack.

  a. Probenecid is given at an initial dosage of 500 mg PO qd, which can be raised in 500-mg increments every week until serum uric acid levels normalize or urine uric acid levels exceed 800 mg/24 hours. The maximum dose is 3000 mg/day. Most patients require a total of 1.0–1.5 g/day in two to three divided doses. Salicylates and probenecid are antagonistic and should not be used together. Probenecid decreases renal excretion of penicillin, indomethacin, and sulfonylureas. Side effects are minimal.

  b. Sulfinpyrazone has uricosuric efficacy similar to that of probenecid, but sulfinpyrazone also inhibits platelet function. The initial dosage of 50 mg PO bid can be increased in 100-mg increments weekly until serum uric acid levels normalize, to a maximum dose of 800 mg/day. Most patients require 300–400 mg/day in three to four divided doses.

II. **Secondary gout,** like primary gout, can be caused by either defective renal excretion or overproduction of uric acid. Intrinsic renal disease, diuretic therapy, low-dose aspirin, nicotinic acid, cyclosporine, and ethanol all interfere with renal excretion of uric acid. Starvation, lactic acidosis, dehydration, preeclampsia, and diabetic ketoacidosis also can induce hyperuricemia. Overproduction of uric acid occurs in myeloproliferative and lymphoproliferative disorders, hemolytic anemia, polycythemia, and cyanotic congenital heart disease. Management includes treatment of the underlying disorder and allopurinol therapy.

III. **Pseudogout** results when calcium pyrophosphate dihydrate crystals deposited in bone and cartilage are released into synovial fluid and induce acute inflammation. Risk factors include older age, advanced OA, neuropathic joint, gout, hyperparathyroidism, hemochromatosis, diabetes mellitus, hypothyroidism, and hypomagnesemia. The disease may present as an **acute monoarthritis or oligoarthritis** mimicking gout or as a **chronic polyarthritis** resembling RA or OA. Usually the **knee or wrist** is affected, although any synovial joint can be involved. Dehydration, acute illness, and surgery (especially parathyroidectomy) are common precipitants of an acute attack of pseudogout. As in gout, the therapy of choice for most patients is a brief high-dose course of an NSAID (see sec. **I.B.1**). As with acute gouty arthritis, **oral corticosteroids** can be used (see sec. **I.B.2**), and **colchicine** (PO or IV; see sec. **I.B.3**) also may relieve symptoms promptly, but toxicity limits its use. Maintenance daily PO colchicine may diminish the number of recurrent attacks. Aspiration of the inflammatory joint fluid often results in prompt improvement, and **intra-articular injection of glucocorticoids** may hasten the response. Allopurinol or uricosuric agents have no role in treating pseudogout.

IV. **Apatite disease** may present with periarthritis or tendonitis, particularly in patients with chronic renal failure. An episodic oligoarthritis also may occur, and apatite disease should be suspected when no crystals are present in the synovial fluid. Erosive arthritis may be seen, particularly in the shoulder ("Milwaukee shoulder"). The treatment of apatite disease is similar to that for pseudogout.

Rheumatoid Arthritis

RA is a systemic disease of unknown etiology and characterized by symmetric inflammatory polyarthritis, extra-articular manifestations (rheumatoid nodules, pulmonary fibrosis, serositis, vasculitis), and serum rheumatoid factor in up to 80% of patients. **Felty's syndrome,** the triad of RA, splenomegaly, and granulocytopenia, occurs in a subset of patients who are at risk for recurrent bacterial infections and nonhealing leg ulcers. **Sjögren's syndrome,** characterized by failure of exocrine glands, also occurs in a subset of patients with RA, producing sicca symptoms (dry eyes and mouth), parotid gland enlargement, dental caries, and recurrent tracheobronchitis. The course of RA is variable but tends to be chronic and progressive. Most patients can benefit from an early aggressive treatment program that combines medical, rehabilitative, and surgical services designed with three distinct goals: (1) early suppression of inflammation in the joints and other tissues, (2) maintenance of joint and muscle function and prevention of deformities, and (3) repair of joint damage to relieve pain or improve function. **Patients with RA and a single joint that is inflamed out of proportion to the rest of the joints must be evaluated for coexistent septic arthritis.** This complication occurs with increased frequency in RA and carries a 20–30% mortality.

I. **Medical management** usually is provided in a "stepped" approach (*Arthritis Rheum* 39:713, 1996).

   A. **NSAIDs or selective COX-2 inhibitors** (see Therapeutic Approaches to Rheumatic Disease, secs. **II** and **III**) are used for the initial therapy for RA and as an adjunct to immunomodulatory-immunosuppressive therapy. A longer-acting NSAID may facilitate patient compliance.

   B. **Glucocorticoids** are not curative and probably do not alter the natural history of RA; however, they are among the most potent anti-inflammatory drugs available (see Therapeutic Approaches to Rheumatic Disease, sec. **IV**). Unfortunately, once systemic glucocorticoid therapy has been initiated, few RA patients are able to discontinue it completely.

      1. **Indications** for glucocorticoids include (1) symptomatic relief while waiting for a response to a slow-acting immunosuppressive or immunomodulatory agent, (2) persistent synovitis despite adequate trials of NSAIDs and immunosuppressive or immunomodulatory agents, and (3) severe constitutional symptoms (e.g., fever and weight loss) or extra-articular disease (vasculitis, episcleritis, or pleurisy).

      2. **Oral administration** of 5–20 mg qd usually is sufficient for the treatment of synovitis, whereas severe constitutional symptoms or extra-articular disease may require up to 1 mg/kg PO qd. Although alternate-day glucocorticoid therapy reduces the incidence of undesirable side effects, some patients do not tolerate the increase in symptoms that may occur on the off day. **Intra-articular administration** may provide temporary symptomatic relief when only a few joints are inflamed (see Therapeutic Approaches to Rheumatic Disease, sec. **I**). The beneficial effects of intra-articular steroids may persist for days to months and may delay or negate the need for systemic glucocorticoid therapy.

   C. **Immunomodulatory and immunosuppressive agents** appear to alter the natural history of RA by retarding the progression of bony erosions and cartilage loss. Because RA may lead to substantial long-term disability (and is associated with increased mortality), the current trend is to initiate therapy with such agents early in the course of RA (see Therapeutic Approaches to Rheumatic Disease, sec. **V**). Once a clinical response has been achieved, the chosen drug usually is continued indefinitely at the lowest effective dosage to prevent relapse.

      1. **Indications** for the use of immunomodulatory or immunosuppressive agents include (1) active synovitis that does not respond to conservative management (e.g., NSAIDs); (2) rapidly progressive, erosive arthritis; and (3) dependence on steroids to control synovitis.

      2. **Selection** of an immunomodulatory or immunosuppressive agent is tailored to the character of the patient's disease, taking into account the potential toxicity of these agents (see Therapeutic Approaches to Rheumatic Disease, sec. **V.A.1**, and Table 24-1). **Methotrexate** typically is the initial choice for moderate to severe RA. **Hydroxychloroquine or sulfasalazine** can be used as the initial choice in mild RA. If response to the initial agent is unsatisfactory after an adequate trial (or if limiting toxicity supervenes), an alternate agent, such as **leflunomide, etanercept, infliximab, or azathioprine,** can be used.

3. Combinations of immunomodulatory-immunosuppressive agents can be used if the patient has a partial response to the initial agent. Common combination therapies that are used consist of methotrexate with either hydroxychloroquine, sulfasalazine, or both (see Therapeutic Approaches to Rheumatic Disease, sec. **V.A.1**). For severe RA, methotrexate has been combined with leflunomide, azathioprine, or cyclosporin A (*Arthritis Rheum* 42:1322, 1999; *N Engl J Med* 333:137, 1995; *Arthritis Rheum* 35:849, 1992). Such combinations may lead to synergistic or unexpected toxicities and should be used with appropriate caution.

II. Corrective **surgical procedures,** including synovectomy, total joint replacement, and joint fusion, may be indicated in patients with RA to reduce pain and to improve function. Carpal tunnel syndrome is common, and surgical repair may be curative if local injection therapy is unsuccessful. **Synovectomy** may be helpful if major involvement is limited to one or two joints and if a 6-month trial of medical therapy has failed, but usually it is only of temporary benefit. Prophylactic synovectomy and débridement of the ulnar styloid should be considered for patients with severe wrist disease to prevent rupture of the extensor tendons. Other procedures that may be beneficial include **total joint replacement** of the hip, shoulder, and knee joints and resection of metatarsal heads in patients with bunion deformities and subluxation of the toes. Reconstructive hand surgery may be useful in carefully selected patients. **Surgical fusion of joints** usually results in freedom from pain but also in total loss of motion; this is tolerated well in the wrist and thumb. Cervical spine fusion of C1 and C2 is indicated for significant cervical subluxation (>5 mm) with associated neurologic deficits. RA patients undergoing elective surgical procedures should have a lateral cervical spine radiograph in flexion and extensions performed, to screen for this subluxation.

III. Adjunctive measures

   A. Reactive depression and sleep disorders are often encountered in patients with rheumatic diseases. Judicious use of antidepressants and sedatives may improve the functional status of selected patients.

   B. Rehabilitative therapy should be managed by a team of physicians, physical and occupational therapists, nurses, social workers, and psychologists. This approach may benefit patients with any form of arthritis.

   1. Acute care of inflammatory arthritis such as RA involves joint protection and pain relief. Proper joint positioning and splints are important elements in joint protection. Heat is a useful analgesic.

   2. Subacute disease therapy should include a gradual increase in passive and active joint movement.

   3. Chronic care encompasses instruction in joint protection, work simplification, and performance of activities of daily living. Adaptive equipment, splints, orthotics, and mobility aids may be useful. Specific exercises designed to promote normal joint mechanics and to strengthen affected muscle groups are useful. Overall cardiac conditioning also improves functional status.

   C. Sicca symptoms (dry eyes and mouth) can be treated symptomatically with artificial tears and saliva. Assiduous dental and ophthalmologic care is recommended. Drugs that suppress lacrimal-salivary secretion further should be avoided. Pilocarpine in a dosage of up to 5 mg qid may provide symptomatic relief.

   D. Patient education including pamphlets and support groups are available in many communities through local chapters of the Arthritis Foundation.

Osteoarthritis

OA, or **degenerative joint disease,** is characterized by deterioration of articular cartilage, with subsequent formation of reactive new bone at the articular surface. The disease is more common in the elderly but may occur at any age, especially as a sequel to joint trauma, chronic inflammatory arthritis, or congenital malformation. The joints affected most commonly are the distal and proximal interphalangeal joints of the hands, hips, and knees and the cervical and lumbar spine. OA of the spine may lead to spinal stenosis (neurogenic claudication), with aching or pain in the legs or buttocks on standing or walking.

I. **Medical management.** The objectives of therapy include relief of pain and prevention of disability. **Acetaminophen** in a dosage of up to 1000 mg up to qid is the initial pharmacologic treatment (*Arthritis Rheum* 43:1905, 2000). **Low-dose NSAIDs or selective COX-2 inhibitors** are the next step, followed by full-dose treatment (see Therapeutic Approaches to Rheumatic Disease, secs. **II** and **III**). However, because this patient population is often elderly and may have concomitant renal or cardiopulmonary disease, NSAIDs should be used with caution. GI bleeding secondary to NSAIDs also is increased in the elderly population. **Glucosamine sulfate,** 1500 mg/day, may reduce symptoms as well as the rate of cartilage deterioration. **Intra-articular glucocorticoid injections** often are beneficial but probably should not be given more than every 3–6 months (see Therapeutic Approaches to Rheumatic Disease, sec. **I**). Systemic steroids and narcotic analgesics should be avoided, although the mu-opioid agonist **tramadol** may be useful as an alternative analgesic agent. **Topical capsaicin** may provide symptomatic relief with minimal toxicity.

II. **Adjunctive measures.** Nonpharmacologic approaches may complement drug treatment of arthritis (*Arthritis Rheum* 38:1541, 1995). Brief periods of rest for the involved joint relieve pain. Activities that involve excessive use of the joint should be identified and avoided. Similarly, poor body mechanics can be corrected, and such malalignments as pronated feet may be aided by orthotics. When weight-bearing joints are affected, support in the form of a cane, crutches, or a walker can be helpful, and weight reduction may be advised. Wearing soft-soled shoes is advised. An exercise program to prevent or correct muscle atrophy can also provide pain relief. Consultation with occupational and physical therapists may be helpful. When serious disability results from severe pain or deformity, surgery may be indicated. Total hip or knee replacement usually relieves pain and increases function in selected patients. OA of the spine may cause radicular symptoms from pressure on nerve roots and often produces pain and spasm in paraspinal soft tissues. Physical supports (cervical collar, lumbar corset), local heat, and exercises to strengthen cervical, paravertebral, and abdominal muscles may provide relief in some patients. Laminectomy and spinal fusion should be reserved for severe disease with intractable pain or neurologic complications. Lumbar spinal stenosis may require extensive decompressive laminectomy for relief of symptoms.

Spondyloarthropathies

The **spondyloarthropathies** are an interrelated group of disorders characterized by one or more of the following features: (1) spondylitis, (2) sacroiliitis, (3) inflammation at sites of tendon insertion (enthesopathy), and (4) asymmetric oligoarthritis. Extra-articular features of this group of disorders may include inflammatory eye disease, urethritis, and mucocutaneous lesions. The spondyloarthropathies aggregate in families, where they are associated with human leukocyte antigen HLA-B27.

I. **Ankylosing spondylitis (AS)** clinically presents as inflammation and ossification of the joints and ligaments of the spine and of the sacroiliac joints. Hips and shoulders are the peripheral joints that are most commonly involved. Progressive fusion of the apophyseal joints of the spine occurs in many patients and cannot be predicted or prevented. Physical therapy emphasizing extension exercises and posture is recommended to minimize possible late postural defects and respiratory compromise. Patients should be instructed to sleep supine on a firm bed without a pillow and to practice postural and deep-breathing exercises regularly. Cigarette smoking should be discouraged strongly. **Nonsalicylate NSAIDs,** such as indomethacin, are used to provide symptomatic relief, and **selective COX-2 inhibitors** should also be effective (see Therapeutic Approaches to Rheumatic Disease, secs. **II** and **III**). Methotrexate and sulfasalazine provide benefit in some patients (see Therapeutic Approaches to Rheumatic Disease, sec. **V**, and Table 24-1). Glucocorticoids and immunosuppressive therapy have been used occasionally in patients who do not respond to other agents. Many patients develop osteoporosis in the fused spondylitic spine and are at risk of spinal fracture. Surgical procedures to correct some spine and hip deformities may result in significant rehabilitation in carefully selected patients. Acute anterior uveitis occurs in up to 25% of patients with AS and should be managed by an ophthalmologist. Generally, this problem is self-limited, although glaucoma and blindness are unusual secondary complications.

II. **Arthritis of inflammatory bowel disease** occurs in 10–20% of patients with Crohn's disease or ulcerative colitis and is similar to that of AS. It may also occur in some patients with intestinal bypass and diverticular disease. Clinical features include spondylitis, sacroiliitis, and peripheral arthritis, particularly in the knee and ankle. Although peripheral joint disease may correlate with the activity of the colitis, spinal disease does not. Joint aspiration may be useful to exclude an associated septic arthritis, but antimicrobials are not effective in the management of sterile synovitis associated with colitis. As in AS, **NSAIDs** (other than salicylates) are the treatment of choice, and **selective COX-2 inhibitors** should also be effective. However, GI intolerance of NSAIDs may be increased among this group of patients, and misoprostol may cause unacceptable diarrhea (see Therapeutic Approaches to Rheumatic Disease, sec. **II**). **Sulfasalazine** also may be beneficial for this form of arthritis (see Therapeutic Approaches to Rheumatic Disease, sec. **V**, and Table 24-1). Local **injection of glucocorticoids** and **physical therapy** are useful adjunctive measures.

III. **Reiter's syndrome and reactive arthritis.** Reiter's syndrome is seen predominantly in young men and may occur with increased frequency in patients infected with HIV. *Chlamydia* infection has been implicated in some patients. The clinical syndrome consists of asymmetric oligoarthritis, urethritis, conjunctivitis, and characteristic skin and mucous membrane lesions. The syndrome is usually transient, lasting from 1 to several months, but recurrences associated with varying degrees of disability are common. A reactive arthritis may follow dysentery caused by *Shigella flexneri*, *Salmonella* species, *Yersinia enterocolitica*, or *Clostridium difficile* infections. Articular manifestations are identical to those of Reiter's syndrome; extra-articular manifestations may occur but tend to be mild. Conservative therapy is indicated for control of pain and inflammation in these diseases. Spontaneous remissions are common, making evaluation of therapy difficult. **NSAIDs** (especially indomethacin) are often useful, and **selective COX-2 inhibitors** should also provide relief (see Therapeutic Approaches to Rheumatic Disease, secs. **II** and **III**). **Sulfasalazine** or **methotrexate** may be of benefit in some patients (see Therapeutic Approaches to Rheumatic Disease, sec. **V**, and Table 24-1). In unusually severe cases, **glucocorticoid therapy** may be required to prevent rapid joint destruction (see Therapeutic Approaches to Rheumatic Disease, sec. **IV**, and Table 24-1). **Prolonged antibiotic therapy (such as doxycycline, 100 mg bid) may be beneficial in Reiter's syndrome that is related to *Chlamydia*.** Conjunctivitis usually is transient and benign, but ophthalmologic referral and treatment with topical or systemic glucocorticoids are indicated for **iritis.**

IV. **Psoriatic arthritis.** Seven percent of patients with psoriasis have some form of inflammatory arthritis. Five major patterns of joint disease occur: (1) asymmetric oligoarticular arthritis, (2) distal interphalangeal joint involvement in association with nail disease, (3) symmetric rheumatoid-like polyarthritis, (4) spondylitis and sacroiliitis, and (5) arthritis mutilans. **NSAIDs,** particularly indomethacin, are used to treat the arthritic manifestations of psoriasis, in conjunction with appropriate measures for the skin disease. **Selective COX-2 inhibitors** should also be effective (see Therapeutic Approaches to Rheumatic Disease, secs. **II** and **III**). **Intra-articular glucocorticoids** may be useful in the oligoarticular form of the disease, but injection through a psoriatic plaque should be avoided. Severe skin and joint diseases generally respond well to low-dose **methotrexate** (see Therapeutic Approaches to Rheumatic Disease, sec. **V,** and Table 24-1). **Gold, sulfasalazine, TNF-α blockers,** and **hydroxychloroquine** (see Therapeutic Approaches to Rheumatic Disease, sec. **V,** and Table 24-1) may have disease-modifying effects in polyarthritis, but the latter may worsen the skin rash in some patients. When reconstructive joint surgery is performed, colonization of psoriatic skin with *S. aureus* increases the risk of wound infection.

Systemic Lupus Erythematosus

SLE is a multisystem disease of unknown etiology that primarily affects women of childbearing age. Autoantibodies to nuclear and other autoantigens are the hallmark of disease. The course of this disease is highly variable and unpredictable. Disease manifestations are protean, ranging in severity from fatigue, malaise, weight loss, arthritis or arthralgias, fever, photosensitivity, rashes, and serositis to potentially life-threatening thrombocytopenia, hemolytic anemia, nephritis, cerebritis, vasculitis, pneumonitis, myositis, and myocarditis.

I. **Conservative therapy** is warranted if the patient's manifestations are mild.
   A. **General supportive measures** include adequate sleep and avoidance of fatigue especially, as mild disease exacerbations may subside after a few days of bed rest. For patients with photosensitive rashes, sunscreens with a sun protection factor of 20 or greater, protective clothing, and avoidance of sun exposure are recommended. These patients also should wear a hat and long sleeves. Isolated skin lesions may respond to topical glucocorticoids.
   B. **NSAIDs** usually control SLE-associated arthritis, arthralgias, fever, and serositis but not fatigue, malaise, and major organ system involvement. The response to **selective COX-2 inhibitors** should be similar (see Therapeutic Approaches to Rheumatic Disease, secs. **II** and **III**). Hepatic and renal toxicities of the NSAIDs appear to be increased in SLE. NSAIDs should be avoided in patients with active nephritis.
   C. **Hydroxychloroquine** (see Therapeutic Approaches to Rheumatic Disease, sec. **V.C,** and Table 24-1) may be effective in the treatment of **rash, photosensitivity, arthralgias, arthritis, alopecia, and malaise** associated with SLE and in the treatment of **discoid and subacute cutaneous lupus erythematosus.** Skin lesions may begin to improve within a few days, but joint symptoms may require 6–10 weeks to subside. The drug is not effective for treating fever or renal, CNS, and hematologic problems.
II. **Glucocorticoid therapy** (see Therapeutic Approaches to Rheumatic Disease, sec. **IV,** and Table 24-1)
   A. **Indications** for systemic glucocorticoids include (1) life-threatening manifestations of SLE, such as glomerulonephritis, CNS involvement, thrombocytopenia, and hemolytic anemia, and (2) debilitating manifestations of SLE (fatigue, rash) that are unresponsive to conservative therapy.
   B. **Dosage.** Patients with severe or potentially life-threatening complications of SLE should be treated with prednisone, 1–2 mg/kg PO qd, which often is given initially in divided doses. After disease is controlled, prednisone is consolidated to a single daily dose and then is tapered slowly, the dosage being reduced by no more than 10% every 7–10 days. More rapid reduction may result in relapse. Alternate-day therapy may reduce many of the

adverse effects of long-term glucocorticoid therapy. IV pulse therapy has been used in SLE in such life-threatening situations as rapidly progressive renal failure, active CNS disease, and severe thrombocytopenia. IV infusion of 500 mg methylprednisolone is given over 30 minutes q12h for 3–5 days. Patients who do not show improvement with this regimen probably are unresponsive to steroids, and other therapeutic alternatives must be considered. Oral prednisone is begun after completing pulse therapy as above.

III. **Immunosuppressive therapy** (see Therapeutic Approaches to Rheumatic Disease, sec. **V,** and Table 24-1)

    A. Indications for immunosuppressive therapy in SLE include (1) such life-threatening manifestations of SLE as glomerulonephritis, CNS involvement, thrombocytopenia, and hemolytic anemia, and (2) the inability to reduce corticosteroid dosage or severe corticosteroid side effects.

    B. Choice of an immunosuppressive is individualized to the clinical situation. Often, **cyclophosphamide** is used for life-threatening manifestations of SLE. High-dose IV pulse cyclophosphamide may be less toxic but also less immunosuppressive than is low-dose daily PO cyclophosphamide. **Azathioprine** is used more often as a steroid-sparing agent but may not be as effective as cyclophosphamide in treating nephritis.

IV. **Transplantation and chronic hemodialysis** have been used successfully in SLE patients with renal failure. Clinical and serologic evidence of disease activity often disappears when renal failure ensues. The survival rate in these patients is equivalent to that of patients with other forms of chronic renal disease. Recurrence of nephritis in the allograft rarely occurs.

V. **Pregnancy in SLE.** An increased incidence of second-trimester spontaneous abortion and stillbirth has been reported in some women with antibodies to cardiolipin or the lupus anticoagulant. Neonatal lupus may occur in offspring of SSA/Ro-positive mothers. SLE patients may experience an exacerbation in the activity of their disease in the third trimester or peripartum period. Differentiation between active SLE and preeclampsia often is difficult.

Systemic Sclerosis

Systemic sclerosis (scleroderma) is a systemic illness of unknown cause that is characterized by thickening and hardening of the skin and visceral organs. Most of the manifestations of scleroderma have a vascular basis (Raynaud's phenomenon, telangiectasias, nailfold capillary changes, early edematous skin changes, nephrosclerosis), but frank vasculitis rarely is seen. The label *scleroderma* includes diffuse scleroderma and limited scleroderma (formerly known as the **CREST syndrome: c**alcinosis, **R**aynaud's phenomenon, **e**sophageal dysmotility, **s**clerodactyly, **t**elangiectasias). **Diffuse scleroderma** is characterized by extensive skin disease, the potential for hypertensive "renal crisis," and shortened survival. **Limited scleroderma,** in contrast, may be associated with primary pulmonary hypertension or biliary cirrhosis and has skin thickening that is limited to the face and the distal forearms and hands. Up to 70% of patients with limited scleroderma have anticentromere antibody, which is not seen in patients with diffuse scleroderma. No curative therapy for scleroderma exists; instead, treatment focuses on particular organ involvement in a problem-oriented manner.

I. **Raynaud's phenomenon** is a reversible vasospasm of the digital arteries that can result in ischemia of the digits. Patients must be instructed to avoid exposure of the entire body to cold, protect the hands and feet from cold and trauma, and discontinue cigarette smoking. Most pharmacologic approaches have had limited success. **Calcium channel antagonists** (e.g., nifedipine) are the preferred initial agents, although they may exacerbate gastroesophageal reflux and constipation in these patients. Alternative vasodilators, such as prazosin, occasionally are helpful, but significant side effects, especially orthostatic hypotension, may preclude their use. **Sympathetic ganglion blockade** with a long-acting anesthetic agent may be useful when a patient has progressive digital ulceration that fails to improve with conservative therapy. Surgical digital sympathectomy may also be beneficial.

II. **Skin and periarticular changes.** No therapeutic agent is clearly effective for these cutaneous manifestations, although penicillamine or methotrexate is sometimes used. **Physical therapy** is important to retard and reduce joint contractures.

III. **GI involvement.** Reflux esophagitis generally responds to standard therapy (e.g., **H$_2$-receptor antagonists, proton pump inhibitors,** and **promotility agents;** see Chap. 17). Occasionally, esophageal strictures require mechanical esophageal dilatation. Decreased motility of bowel segments can occur, leading to bacterial overgrowth, malabsorption, and weight loss. Treatment with broad-spectrum antimicrobials in a rotating sequence including **metronidazole** often improves the malabsorption. Metoclopramide may reduce bloating and distension.

IV. **Renal involvement.** The appearance of hypertension and renal insufficiency, often associated with a microangiopathic hemolytic anemia, signals a poor prognosis. Aggressive BP control with **angiotensin-converting enzyme inhibitors** may delay or prevent the onset of uremia, particularly in patients with a serum creatinine of less than 3 mg/dl.

V. **Cardiopulmonary involvement.** Patchy myocardial fibrosis can result in CHF or arrhythmias. Coronary artery vasospasm can cause angina pectoris and may respond to calcium channel antagonists. Pulmonary involvement includes pleurisy with effusion, interstitial fibrosis, pulmonary hypertension, and cor pulmonale. Standard therapies for these conditions are used. Patients with rapidly progressive pulmonary parenchymal disease may benefit from a course of cyclophosphamide.

Necrotizing Vasculitis

Necrotizing vasculitis is characterized by inflammation and necrosis of blood vessels leading to tissue damage. This diagnosis includes a broad spectrum of disorders having various causes and involving vessels of different types, sizes, and locations. The immunopathogenic process often involves immune complexes. Although in most cases the inciting antigen has not been identified, vasculitic syndromes have been associated with chronic hepatitis B and C. Table 24-2 summarizes clinical features and diagnostic and treatment approaches to the most common forms of vasculitis.

I. **Clinical features** are diverse and depend, in part, on the size of the vessel involved. Systemic manifestations including fever and weight loss are also common. The response to therapy and the long-term prognosis of these disorders are highly variable. Vasculitis "mimics" should be considered, including bacterial endocarditis, HIV, atrial myxoma, paraneoplastic syndromes, cholesterol emboli, and cocaine and amphetamine use.

II. **Management** should include consultation with a physician experienced in the treatment of these disorders. Treatment should be tailored to the severity of organ system involvement.

A. **Glucocorticoids** are the usual initial therapy and are beneficial in most vasculitides (see Therapeutic Approaches to Rheumatic Disease, sec. **IV,** and Table 24-1). Although vasculitis limited to the skin may respond to lower doses of corticosteroids, the initial dosage for visceral involvement should be high (prednisone, 1–2 mg/kg/day). If life-threatening manifestations are

Table 24-2. Clinical features and diagnostic and treatment approaches to vasculitis

Vasculitic syndrome	Clinical features	Diagnostic approach	Treatment
Large vessel involvement			
Giant-cell arteritis	Headache Jaw claudication	Temporal artery biopsy	Prednisone, 60–80 mg/day
Takayasu arteritis	Finger ischemia Arm claudication	Aortic arch arteriogram	Prednisone, 60–80 mg/day
Medium vessel involvement			
Polyarteritis nodosa	Skin ulcers Nephritis Mononeuritis multiplex Mesenteric ischemia	Skin biopsy Renal biopsy Sural nerve biopsy Mesenteric angiogram Hepatitis B, C testing	Prednisone, 60–100 mg/day Cyclophosphamide, 1–2 mg/kg/day, can be added
Wegener's granulomatosis	Sinusitis Pulmonary infiltrates Nephritis	c-ANCA Lung biopsy	Prednisone, 60–100 mg/day *and* Cyclophosphamide, 1–2 mg/kg/day
Vasculitis in SLE or RA	Skin ulcers Polyneuropathy	Skin or sural nerve biopsy	Prednisone, 60–80 mg/day Cyclophosphamide, 1–2 mg/kg/day, can be added
Small vessel involvement			
Hypersensitivity vasculitis	Palpable purpura	Skin biopsy	Prednisone, 20–60 mg/day Discontinue inciting drug
Henoch-Schönlein purpura	Palpable purpura Nephritis Mesenteric ischemia	Skin biopsy Renal biopsy	Supportive treatment Prednisone, 20–60 mg/day may be needed

c-ANCA = cytoplasmic antineutrophil cytoplasmic antibodies; RA = rheumatoid arthritis; SLE = systemic lupus erythematosus.

present, a brief course of high-dose pulse therapy with methylprednisolone, 500 mg IV q12h for 3–5 days, should be considered.

- **B. Immunosuppressives,** in particular oral cyclophosphamide, often are used in the initial management of necrotizing vasculitis, especially when major organ system involvement (e.g., lung, kidney, or nerve) is present (see Therapeutic Approaches to Rheumatic Disease, sec. **V,** and Table 24-1).
- **C. Trimethoprim-sulfamethoxazole** can be used in variants of Wegener's granulomatosis limited to the upper airway and may also be useful in preventing relapse (*N Engl J Med* 335:16, 1996).

Polymyalgia Rheumatica
and Temporal Arteritis

Polymyalgia rheumatica (PMR) presents in elderly patients as proximal limb girdle pain, morning stiffness, constitutional symptoms, and an elevated erythrocyte sedimentation rate (ESR). Up to 40% of patients with PMR also have temporal arteritis (TA). TA is a form of vasculitis that presents with headache, scalp tenderness, jaw or tongue claudication, vision disturbances (including blindness), stroke, an elevated ESR, and, in up to 40% of patients, symptoms of PMR.

I. **Management of PMR.** If PMR is present without evidence of TA, **prednisone,** 10–15 mg PO qd, usually produces dramatic clinical improvement within a few days. The ESR should return to normal during initial treatment, but subsequent therapeutic decisions should be based on ESR and clinical status. Glucocorticoid therapy can be tapered gradually to a maintenance dosage of 5–10 mg PO qd but should be continued for at least 1 year to minimize the risk of relapse. NSAIDs may facilitate reduction in prednisone dosage.

II. **Management of TA.** Patients suspected of having TA should be treated promptly with **prednisone,** 1–2 mg/kg/day PO qd, to prevent irreversible blindness. The diagnosis of TA should be confirmed by **temporal artery biopsy,** which will not be altered by 3–5 days of prednisone therapy. High-dose steroid therapy should be continued until symptoms have abated and the ESR has returned to normal. The dosage then should be tapered gradually to 10–20 mg, with close monitoring of the ESR and clinical status, and should be maintained for 1–2 years.

Cryoglobulin Syndromes

Cryoglobulins are serum proteins that reversibly precipitate in the cold. Cryoglobulinemia is traditionally categorized as monoclonal (formerly type 1) or polyclonal (mixed; formerly types 2 and 3). Patients with monoclonal cryoglobulinemia usually have an underlying lymphoproliferative disorder such as myeloma or lymphoma. Symptoms are related to hyperviscosity (blurring of vision, digital ischemia, headache, lethargy) and respond to treatment of the underlying disorder, although plasmapheresis can be used in the acute setting. The majority of patients with mixed cryoglobulinemia have hepatitis C; the remainder of cases are found in association with autoimmune disorders such as SLE or RA, or are idiopathic. Clinical manifestations of mixed cryoglobulinemia are mediated by immune complex deposition (arthralgias, purpura, glomerulonephritis, and neuropathy). **Therapy** for secondary cryoglobulinemic states is directed at the underlying disease. Interferon-alpha treatment of hepatitis C effectively reduces cryoglobulins, although they may recur when treatment is stopped (*J Hepatol* 29:848, 1998). Prednisone or immunosuppressive agents can be used to treat cryoglobulinemia due to SLE or RA but may exacerbate hepatitis C (see Chap. 18).

Polymyositis and
Dermatomyositis

Polymyositis (PM) is an inflammatory myopathy that presents as weakness and, occasionally, tenderness of the proximal musculature. Diagnosis is corroborated by an abnormal electromyogram, elevated muscle enzyme levels (creatine kinase, aldolase, AST), and muscle biopsy. **Dermatomyositis (DM)** is, by definition, PM with a concomitant rash. PM-DM can occur in three forms: (1) alone, (2) in association with any of the other autoimmune diseases, or (3) with a variety of neoplasms. Risk factors for malignancy in the setting of myositis include the presence of DM, cutaneous vasculitis, male sex, and advanced age. Screening for common neoplasms, such as colon, lung, breast, and prostate cancer, should be considered in these patients. When PM-DM occurs without associated disease, it usually responds well to prednisone, 1–2 mg/kg PO qd (see Therapeutic Approaches to Rheumatic Disease, sec. **IV**, and Table 24-1). Systemic complaints, such as fever and malaise, respond to therapy first, followed by muscle enzymes and, finally, muscle strength. Once serum enzyme levels normalize, the prednisone dosage should be reduced slowly to maintenance levels of 10–20 mg PO qd or 20–40 mg PO qod. The appearance of steroid-induced myopathy and hypokalemia may complicate therapeutic assessment. IV infusion of immunoglobulin may hasten improvement of severe dysphagia. PM-DM associated with neoplasia tends to be less responsive to glucocorticoid therapy but may improve after removal of an associated malignant tumor. Patients who do not respond or cannot tolerate the side effects of glucocorticoids may respond to methotrexate or azathioprine (see Therapeutic Approaches to Rheumatic Disease, sec. **V**, and Table 24-1). Physical therapy is essential in the management of myositis. Bed rest with active assisted range of motion is appropriate during very active disease, with more active exercise prescribed to improve strength once inflammation has been controlled.

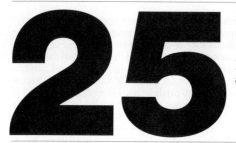

Neurologic Disorders

Kelvin A. Yamada
and Sylvia Awadalla

Alterations in Consciousness

I. **Coma** is a state of complete behavioral unresponsiveness to external stimulation in which the patient lies with the eyes closed. Because some causes of coma may lead to irreversible brain damage, expeditious evaluation and treatment must proceed concurrently. The need for neurosurgical intervention must be determined promptly.

A. **Pathophysiology.** Coma results from diffuse or multifocal dysfunction of **both cerebral hemispheres** or of the **reticular activating system** in the brain stem. Unilateral cerebral lesions (e.g., stroke or tumor) rarely impair consciousness unless they produce sufficient mass effect to compress the opposite hemisphere (midline shift or subfalcine herniation) or the brain stem (transtentorial herniation). Mass lesions in the posterior fossa cause coma by compressing the brain stem. Metabolic disorders impair consciousness by diffuse effects on both cerebral hemispheres. See Table 25-1 for possible etiologies.

B. **Evaluation and management of the comatose patient**

1. The **initial steps** are to control airway and ventilation, administer oxygen, maintain body temperature, and monitor vital signs, including oximetry and continuous ECG.

2. If trauma has or may have occurred, **immobilization of the spine, especially cervical, should be done immediately** with a hard collar until radiographs exclude fracture or instability.

3. An **IV line should be secured,** and adequate circulation should be established. Initial laboratory evaluation should include blood for glucose, electrolytes, BUN, CBC, calcium, ABG, cultures, liver enzymes, ammonia, prothrombin time (PT)/activated partial thromboplastin time (PTT), and blood type and screen. Blood and urine should be sent for toxicologic/drug analysis. A urinalysis should be performed.

4. IV **thiamine** (100 mg), followed by **dextrose,** (50 ml 50% dextrose in water = 25 g dextrose) should be administered.

5. IV **naloxone** (opiate antagonist), 0.01 mg/kg, should be administered if opiate intoxication is suspected (coma, respiratory depression, small reactive pupils). Naloxone may provoke opiate withdrawal syndrome in addicted patients. **Flumazenil** (benzodiazepine antagonist), 0.2 mg IV, may reverse benzodiazepine intoxication, but its duration of action is short. Flumazenil can cause seizures.

6. The **initial assessment** should focus on a **history** of trauma, seizures, medications, alcohol or drug use, and existing medical conditions. The **general physical examination** may reveal a systemic illness associated with coma (e.g., cirrhosis, hemodialysis shunt, rash of meningococcemia) or signs of head trauma (e.g., lacerations, periorbital or mastoid

Table 25-1. Causes of stupor and coma

Diffuse or metabolic

Drugs and toxins

Head trauma

Global cerebral ischemia

CNS infection/inflammation (vasculitis)

Sepsis

Hypoglycemia

Diabetic ketoacidosis

Hypoxemia or hypercapnia

Hyponatremia

Hypernatremia

Hypercalcemia

Liver failure

Renal failure

Thiamine deficiency

Hypertensive encephalopathy

Subclinical seizures/postictal state

Structural lesions, supra- or infratentorial

Hemorrhage/aneurysm

Epidural/subdural hematoma

Tumor

Stroke

Venous occlusion

Abscess

Hydrocephalus

---

ecchymosis, hemotympanum). The **neurologic examination** (see sec. **III**) should localize structural lesions and diagnose brain herniation. Serial examinations should be performed to detect and intervene if clinical deterioration occurs.

7. **Herniation** (see sec. **III.F**) must be recognized and treated immediately. Treatment consists of measures to lower intracranial pressure while surgically treatable etiologies are identified or excluded:

   a. **Hyperventilation** [carbon dioxide tension (PCO_2), 25–30 mm Hg] reduces intracranial pressure by cerebral vasoconstriction, usually within minutes. Reduction of PCO_2 below 25 mm Hg is not recommended because it may reduce cerebral blood flow excessively.

   b. Administration of **mannitol** IV, 1–2 g/kg over 10–20 minutes, osmotically reduces brain free water via the kidneys. The effect peaks at 90 minutes.

   c. **Dexamethasone,** 10 mg IV, followed by 4 mg IV q6h, reduces the edema surrounding a tumor or abscess.

8. As soon as the patient's condition is stable, **a head CT scan** should be obtained to distinguish **operable lesions** (e.g., cerebellar hematoma) from **inoperable lesions** (e.g., pontine hemorrhage). **Coagulopathy** (see Chap. 19) should be corrected if intracranial hemorrhage is diag-

nosed and before surgical treatment or invasive procedures (e.g., lumbar puncture) are performed. Each patient's circumstance should be carefully assessed before therapeutic anticoagulation is reversed.

9. **Lumbar puncture** is indicated whenever CNS infection is considered and when subarachnoid hemorrhage (SAH) is clinically suspected but not confirmed by neuroimaging. **One should not perform lumbar puncture if a mass lesion or midline shift is present on CT scan. In such cases, if CNS infection is suspected, appropriate broad-spectrum antibiotics and acyclovir should be administered without lumbar puncture** (see Chap. 14). If cerebrospinal fluid (CSF) is obtained, it should be sent for cell count, protein, glucose, Gram stain, herpes simplex virus polymerase chain reaction, acid-fast stain, India ink stain, fungal and bacterial cultures, cryptococcal antigen, and bacterial antigens (particularly if antibiotics have been given). If possible, extra CSF should be saved and refrigerated.

10. **Electroencephalogram (EEG) is helpful in the diagnosis of** subclinical electrical seizures (nonconvulsive status epilepticus). Some conditions have characteristic (not necessarily diagnostic) EEG findings, including hepatic encephalopathy, herpes simplex virus encephalitis, and barbiturate or other sedative intoxications.

11. If the initial evaluation yields no diagnosis, a metabolic or toxic etiology is most likely. The patient should be admitted to an ICU with continued supportive care while additional diagnostic studies are pursued.

II. **Acute confusional states (delirium)** result from diffuse or multifocal cerebral dysfunction and are characterized by impaired attention, concentration, and memory; fluctuations of consciousness; disorientation and hallucinations; incoherent speech; and agitation.

A. **Etiologies** include those listed in Table 25-1 and also medication effect or withdrawal, drug intoxication or withdrawal (see sec. **II.C**, and Chap. 1), endocrine disease (i.e., thyroid disorders, diabetes, Cushing's disease), acute intermittent porphyria, confusional migraine, and complex partial seizures. Mild systemic illness commonly produces delirium in an elderly or demented patient, especially in combination with new medications, fever, or sleep deprivation. Structural lesions such as in Table 25-1 can cause acute confusion but must be distinguished from **aphasia** [secondary to transient ischemic attack (TIA), stroke, trauma, seizure, abscess, etc.] and transient global amnesia. Acute psychosis can mimic acute delirium, but confusion and depressed consciousness are usually less prominent.

B. Guidelines for initial **evaluation and management** are similar to those for the comatose patient (see sec. **I.B**).

1. The **history** may suggest one of the above etiologies. One should carefully review medications and available laboratory parameters.

2. The **physical and neurologic examination** may reveal systemic illness (e.g., pneumonia) or neurologic signs (meningismus or paralysis) to narrow the differential diagnosis.

3. **Maintenance of adequate airway, circulation (secure IV access), and oxygenation** is an important initial measure. One should obtain an arterial blood gas and send blood for glucose, electrolytes, BUN, calcium, magnesium, ammonia, thyroid-stimulating hormone, CBC, and cultures. Urine and blood should be sent for drug and toxicologic analysis. Urinalysis and urine porphobilinogens (to screen for porphyria) can be obtained in selected cases.

4. **Head CT scan** quickly identifies intracranial hematoma and may demonstrate other structural lesions such as stroke, SAH, or abscess.

5. **Lumbar puncture** is indicated whenever CNS infection is considered and sometimes to diagnose SAH (see secs. **I.B.8** and **9**).

6. **Additional measures include administration of IV thiamine** (100 mg) **followed by** 50 ml of 50% dextrose. Sedatives should be avoided if possible, but, if necessary, low doses of **lorazepam** (1 mg) or **chlordiazepoxide** (25

mg) can be used. A quiet well-lit room with close observation is necessary. Restraints are sometimes needed for patient safety and should be carefully adjusted and checked periodically to prevent excessive constriction.

C. Alcohol withdrawal typically occurs when illness or hospitalization interrupts alcohol intake and deserves emphasis because severe forms carry significant mortality.

    1. Tremulousness, irritability, anorexia, and nausea characterize **minor alcohol withdrawal.** Symptoms usually appear within a few hours after reduction or cessation of alcohol consumption and resolve within 48 hours. Treatment includes a well-lit room, reassurance, and the presence of family or friends. Thiamine, 100 mg IM, followed by 100 mg PO qd; multivitamins that contain folic acid; and a balanced diet as tolerated should be administered. Chlordiazepoxide (25–100 mg PO q6h) with dosage adjusted until the patient is calm may reduce the incidence of seizures and delirium tremens (*JAMA* 278:144, 1997). Signs of major alcohol withdrawal should be monitored; social circumstances dictate whether this should be done at home or in the hospital.

    2. Alcohol withdrawal seizures, typically one or a few brief generalized convulsions, occur 12–48 hours after cessation of ethanol intake. Antiepileptic drugs are not indicated for typical alcohol withdrawal seizures. Other causes for seizures (see Seizures, sec. **II**) must be excluded. If hypoglycemia is present, thiamine should be administered before glucose.

    3. Severe withdrawal or **delirium tremens** consists of tremulousness, hallucinations, agitation, confusion, disorientation, and autonomic hyperactivity (fever, tachycardia, diaphoresis), typically occurring 72–96 hours after cessation of drinking. Symptoms generally resolve within 3–5 days. Delirium tremens complicates 5–10% of cases of alcohol withdrawal, with mortality up to 15%. Other causes of delirium must be considered in the differential diagnosis (see sec. **II.A**). One should administer supportive management as in sec. **II.C.1.**

        a. Chlordiazepoxide is an effective sedative for delirium tremens, 100 mg IV or PO q2–6h as needed (maximum dose, 500 mg in the first 24 hours). One-half the initial 24-hour dose can be administered over the next 24 hours; the dosage can be reduced by 25–50 mg/day each day thereafter. Longer-lasting benzodiazepines facilitate smoother tapering, but shorter-acting agents (i.e., **lorazepam,** 1–2 mg PO or IV q6–8h as needed) may be desirable in older patients and those with reduced drug clearance. In patients with severe hepatic failure, **oxazepam** (15–30 mg PO, q6–8h as needed), which is excreted by the kidney, can be used instead of chlordiazepoxide.

        b. Maintenance of fluid and electrolyte balance is important. Alcoholic patients are susceptible to hypomagnesemia, hypokalemia, hypoglycemia, and fluid losses, which may be considerable due to fever, diaphoresis, and vomiting.

        c. Other drugs have been used to treat alcohol withdrawal, including clonidine, atenolol, haloperidol, carbamazepine, chlormethiazole, and others. Controlled studies and careful evaluation of the indications for the individual patient must dictate their use for alcohol withdrawal.

III. Neurologic examination of patients with alteration in consciousness

    A. Level of consciousness can be assessed semiquantitatively and followed by all levels of caregivers with the **Glasgow Coma Scale** (Table 25-2). Points are assigned in three categories using the best response and are added together to give scores that range from 3 (unresponsive) to 15 (normal).

    B. Respiratory rate and pattern. Cheyne-Stokes respirations (rhythmic crescendo-decrescendo hyperpnea alternating with periods of apnea) occur in metabolic coma and supratentorial lesions, as well as in chronic pulmonary disease and CHF. **Hyperventilation** is usually a sign of metabolic acidosis, hypoxemia, pneumonia, or other pulmonary disease but may be caused

Table 25-2. Glasgow Coma Scale

Eye opening

Spontaneous	4
To voice	3
To painful stimulation	2
None	1

Best verbal response

Oriented	5
Confused	4
Inappropriate words	3
Unintelligible sounds	2
None	1

Best motor response

Follows commands	6
Localizes pain	5
Withdraws from pain	4
Flexor response	3
Extensor response	2
None	1

by upper brain stem injury. **Apneustic breathing** (long pauses after inspiration), **cluster breathing** (breathing in short bursts), and **ataxic breathing** (irregular breaths without pattern) are signs of brain stem injury and **warn of impending respiratory arrest.**

C. **Pupil size and light reactivity are extremely valuable neurologic signs.**

1. **Anisocoria (asymmetric pupils) in a patient with altered mental status requires diagnosis and treatment, or exclusion, of uncal herniation.** Anisocoria may be physiological or produced by mydriatics (e.g., scopolamine, atropine).

2. **Small but reactive pupils** are seen in narcotic overdose, metabolic encephalopathy, and thalamic or pontine lesions.

3. **Midposition fixed pupils** imply midbrain lesions and occur in transtentorial herniation.

4. **Bilaterally fixed and dilated pupils** are seen with severe anoxic encephalopathy or intoxication with drugs such as scopolamine, atropine, glutethimide, or methyl alcohol.

D. **Eye movements.** The **oculocephalic** (doll's eyes) test is performed (if no cervical injury is present) by quickly turning the head laterally or vertically. In a comatose patient with intact brain stem, the eyes move conjugately opposite the direction of head movement. The **oculovestibular** (cold caloric) test is used if cervical trauma is suspected or if eye movements are absent with the oculocephalic test. To perform the test, the head should be elevated 30 degrees above horizontal and the tympanic membrane visualized to ensure that it is intact and unobstructed. The tympanic membrane should be lavaged with 10–50 ml ice water. In the patient with intact brain stem function, eyes should move conjugately toward the lavaged ear. Vertical gaze can be assessed with simultaneous lavage of both ears.

1. **Absence of all eye movements** indicates a bilateral pontine lesion or drug-induced ophthalmoplegia (e.g., barbiturates, phenytoin, paralytics).

2. **Disconjugate gaze** suggests a brain stem lesion.

3. A **gaze preference** conjugately to one side suggests a unilateral pontine or frontal lobe lesion. An associated hemiparesis and oculocephalic and oculovestibular tests help localize the lesion. In **pontine lesions** gaze preference is **toward** the paretic side, and eyes may move toward but do not cross midline. In **frontal lobe lesions** gaze preference is **away** from the paresis, and eyes move conjugately across midline to both sides.

4. **Loss of vertical gaze** occurs in midbrain lesions, central herniation, and acute hydrocephalus.

E. **Motor responses** help to assess the level of impaired consciousness (see also Table 25-2). **Asymmetric motor responses (spontaneous or stimulus induced) have localizing value.**

F. **Herniation** occurs when mass lesions or edema cause shifts in brain tissue. Prompt diagnosis and treatment are necessary to prevent irreversible brain damage and death (see sec. **I.B.7**).

1. **Nonspecific signs and symptoms of increased intracranial pressure** include headache, nausea, vomiting, hypertension, bradycardia, papilledema, sixth nerve palsy, transient visual obscurations, and alterations in consciousness.

2. **Uncal herniation** is caused by unilateral supratentorial lesions and may progress rapidly. The earliest sign is a dilated pupil ipsilateral to the mass, diminished consciousness, and hemiparesis, first contralateral to the mass and later ipsilateral to the mass (Kernohan's notch syndrome).

3. **Central herniation** is caused by medial or bilateral supratentorial lesions. Signs include progressive alteration of consciousness, Cheyne-Stokes or normal respirations followed later by central hyperventilation, midposition and unreactive pupils, loss of upward gaze, and posturing of the extremities.

4. **Tonsillar herniation** occurs when pressure in the posterior fossa forces the cerebellar tonsils through the foramen magnum, compressing the medulla. Signs include altered level of consciousness and respiratory irregularity or apnea.

Seizures

Generalized convulsive status epilepticus consists of sustained unconsciousness and continuous or intermittent generalized convulsive seizure activity. Convulsive seizure activity lasting 10 minutes continuously, or intermittently without recovery of consciousness, warrants IV anticonvulsant therapy. Diagnostic evaluation and supportive care must proceed concurrently. Important historical information includes pre-existing medical conditions, current medications, drug allergies, and possible precipitating events.

I. **Acute management**

A. Acute management includes placement of a soft plastic oral or nasal airway and administration of maximal supplemental oxygen by mask. Bag-mask ventilation and administration of anticonvulsants are usually preferable to attempting endotracheal intubation in a convulsing patient, which often necessitates neuromuscular blockade, although aggressive measures to control the airway may be required. Vital signs, oximetry, and continuous ECG should be monitored. A large-bore IV line (ideally 2, 1 dextrose free) should be placed. **Thiamine** (100 mg) should be given intravenously **followed by** 50 ml of 50% dextrose. The use of bed padding reduces traumatic injury. **Laboratory analysis** should include glucose, electrolytes, calcium, magnesium, BUN, creatinine, antiepileptic drug levels if indicated, CBC, and urinalysis. Toxicologic analysis of blood and urine is often necessary.

B. **Parenteral anticonvulsants** stop seizures most rapidly but should be reserved for patients with persistent generalized convulsive seizures because of potentially serious adverse effects. If a patient stops convulsing and recovers consciousness, it is safer to administer anticonvulsants orally. The following is one approach to treating persistent convulsive seizures (see also *JAMA* 270:854, 1993; *N Engl J Med* 339:792, 1998).

1. **Lorazepam** (0.1 mg/kg at 2 mg/minute up to 4 mg) or diazepam (0.2 mg/kg at 5 mg/minute up to 10 mg) stops seizures quickly in most patients. The short duration of action of these drugs requires concomitant administration of maintenance anticonvulsants. Respiratory depression may necessitate intubation and assisted ventilation.

2. **Phenytoin** is the preferred maintenance anticonvulsant (combined with benzodiazepines) for convulsive status epilepticus. It can be administered parenterally as phenytoin sodium or **fosphenytoin,** a phosphate ester prodrug of phenytoin. Fosphenytoin is converted in vivo in equimolar concentrations to phenytoin. The loading dose for phenytoin in status epilepticus is 20 mg/kg. The dose of fosphenytoin is expressed as phenytoin equivalents (PE) and should be ordered as such (i.e., **20 mg PE/kg**). The maximum rate of infusion for phosphenytoin is 150 mg PE/minute; the maximum rate of infusion for phenytoin is 50 mg/minute. Fosphenytoin produces less venous irritation and sclerosis than phenytoin. When phenytoin is administered IV, a large-bore IV infusing **dextrose free saline** should be used to prevent precipitation in the line. Alternatively, phenytoin can be mixed with normal saline at the bedside and infused immediately. Although fosphenytoin can be administered IM, this route is less than optimal in an emergent situation because of delayed time to peak concentrations. BP and cardiac rhythm should be monitored continuously for hypotension and heart block, which often resolve when the administration rate is reduced. Phenytoin is contraindicated in heart block.

3. **Phenobarbital** (20 mg/kg at less than 50 mg/minute) should be given if seizures continue after phenytoin loading. Respiratory depression caused by benzodiazepines combined with phenobarbital usually necessitates intubation. When phenobarbital is added to stop recalcitrant seizures, there is no strict dose; it can be administered at 5-mg/kg increments until the seizures are controlled. An IV loading dose of 20 mg/kg generally achieves a serum level of approximately 20 µg/ml within an hour of administration, sufficient to stop most seizures. As with phenytoin, arrhythmias and hypotension may occur during administration, requiring continuous ECG and BP monitoring.

4. **A continuous benzodiazepine infusion** may be preferable over phenytoin and barbiturates in some patients.

5. **Barbiturate coma** or **general anesthesia** with neuromuscular blockade may be required to stop seizures that persist despite the previously mentioned measures. ICU support and appropriate consultations are required at this stage.

II. **A specific etiology** is often associated with status epilepticus, and its treatment may influence successful management of seizures. Structural abnormalities include primary or metastatic CNS tumors, CNS infections (e.g., bacterial meningitis, herpes encephalitis), CNS inflammatory processes (e.g., CNS lupus), cerebral infarction (more commonly embolic), and acute or preexisting brain injury (e.g., trauma, hemorrhage). Nonstructural precipitants include hypoglycemia, electrolyte abnormalities (e.g., hyponatremia, hypocalcemia), uremia, anoxia, drug withdrawal (particularly acute withdrawal of benzodiazepines, barbiturates, antiepileptic drugs), and drug intoxication (e.g., theophylline, cocaine). In epileptic patients subtherapeutic antiepileptic drug levels (noncompliance, drug interaction, etc.) or an acute febrile illness often initiate status epilepticus. Some epileptic patients initially present with status epilepticus. Head CT or MRI and CSF analysis are frequently required to establish a specific diagnosis. EEG is useful to diagnose and treat nonconvulsive status epilepticus (see Alterations in Consciousness), to guide long-term management and support the clinical diagnosis of epilepsy, and sometimes to verify elimination of electrographic seizures after successful initial treatment of convulsive status epilepticus. EEG is not helpful in the acute management of convulsive status epilepticus.

III. **The diagnostic approach** to a patient with **spontaneously terminating seizures** with recovery of consciousness is similar to that described in sec. **II.** Depending on the circumstances, outpatient evaluation may be appropriate. If antiepileptic drugs are indicated, oral loading is typically indicated over IV loading.

IV. **Maintenance therapy.** After status epilepticus has been successfully treated, and causative factors identified and treated, anticonvulsant drugs are usually maintained, except for benzodiazepines (maintenance phenytoin, 4–7 mg/kg/day; phenobarbital, 1–5 mg/kg/day, IV or PO bid), until the patient can capably manage long-term therapy. Conversion to an oral regimen must be individually tailored. Most patients are adequately treated with a single antiepileptic drug, but others may require adjustment of their previous multiple drug regimen.

Cerebrovascular Disease

I. The hallmark of **stroke** is the abrupt onset of symptoms and neurologic deficits that correspond to interruption of vascular supply to a specific brain region. Although stroke is synonymous with **cerebral infarction,** fluctuation of functional deficits after stroke onset and reversible deficits known as **transient ischemic attacks (TIAs)** (deficits resolve within 24 hours) and reversible ischemic neurologic deficits (deficits resolve within a week) suggest that tissue at risk for infarction can be rescued by re-establishing perfusion. **Currently, the most important aspect of stroke management is consideration of stroke as a medical emergency that requires rapid diagnosis and treatment.** Recombinant tissue plasminogen activator **(rt-PA)** is the only proven therapy for acute stroke, but patients must be selected carefully, and administration of rt-PA must commence within 3 hours of stroke onset. Other treatments, including intra-arterial thrombolysis, are available at some centers under research protocols.

A. Important **historical information** includes the onset and progression of symptoms and contributory events (e.g., head trauma or seizure). Prior TIA symptoms (e.g., transient monocular loss of vision, aphasia, dysarthria, paresis, or sensory disturbance) are often associated with atherosclerotic vascular disease, the most common cause for stroke. A history of trauma, even minimal, is important, as extracerebral arterial dissections may cause ischemic strokes. Other medical conditions associated with stroke, such as cardiac arrhythmia or valvular disease, connective tissue disease, and sickle cell anemia, should be identified. Classic migraine can mimic stroke and is a risk factor for stroke. In epileptic patients, ictal paralysis is rare, but postictal paralysis (Todd's paralysis) is common after a focal seizure. The diagnosis may be suggested by stroke risk factors such as hypertension, diabetes, smoking, postpartum state, illicit IV drug use, and medications such as oral contraceptives, and management is influenced by these factors.

B. **Physical examination** should provide clues that indicate specific diagnostic tests and therapy. **Cardiogenic embolism** accounts for about 20% of strokes; physical examination should focus on findings of mitral or aortic stenosis and murmur. Embolic disease affects fundi, conjunctivae, nail beds, fingers, and palms. Urinalysis should be performed to evaluate for hematuria. **Fever** raises concern for infectious etiologies. Meningismus, seizures, or altered mental status suggest **meningitis** or **encephalitis. Septic emboli** from **bacterial endocarditis** can cause meningitis or cerebral or parameningeal abscess. The patient should be examined for evidence of neurocutaneous disease **(neurofibromatosis and tuberous sclerosis)** and vasculitis (e.g., systemic lupus erythematosus).

C. A careful **neurologic examination** reliably establishes the anatomic location of a stroke, which is typically confirmed by neuroimaging. In general, **carotid artery distribution strokes** (anterior circulation) produce combinations of functional deficits (hemiparesis, hemianopsia, cortical sensory loss, often with aphasias or agnosias) contralateral to the affected hemisphere, whereas **vertebral-basilar** strokes (posterior circulation) produce unilateral or bilateral motor/sensory deficits, usually accompanied by cranial nerve and brain stem signs. **Horner's syndrome** (ptosis, miosis, anhidrosis) contralateral to an acute hemiparesis suggests carotid dissection.

II. Initial assessment and management

   A. Vital signs, including oximetry and continuous ECG, should be monitored. Administration of oxygen, placement of IV access, and checking of blood glucose should be done immediately. Laboratory analysis should include CBC with differential and platelet count, PT, activated PTT, and electrolyte panel. ECG (for atrial fibrillation) and a chest radiograph should be obtained.

   B. Immediately after initial assessment and stabilization, a **noncontrast head CT** scan should be performed to identify various hemorrhagic lesions that influence specific management decisions. The CT scan often confirms a suspected ischemic infarct, unless it is very early after onset (hours) or if the stroke is very small (particularly in the brain stem), in which case MRI is more sensitive. A mass lesion may preclude a diagnostic lumbar puncture for meningitis/encephalitis because it may precipitate brain herniation (see Alterations in Consciousness, sec. **III.F**). Appropriate antimicrobial and antiviral drugs should still be administered.

   C. **rt-PA therapy** should be considered when a nonhemorrhagic ischemic infarct has been demonstrated and infectious etiologies are excluded, while one continues to pursue a specific diagnosis. Hemorrhagic transformation of infarcts accompanied by higher mortality was observed with rt-PA; therefore, **strict adherence to the American Academy of Neurology/American Heart Association guidelines is recommended** (*Neurology* 47:835, 1996). **Exclusion criteria include** stroke onset longer than 3 hours; extensive infarction evident on CT scan; recent surgery, head trauma, or GI or urinary hemorrhage; seizure at stroke onset; bleeding disorder or anticoagulation with prolonged PT/PTT; and severe uncontrolled hypertension (systolic >185, diastolic >110 mm Hg). The rt-PA dose is 0.9 mg/kg up to a maximum of 90 mg, with the first 10% (maximum, 9 mg) given IV over 1 minute, then the remaining 90% (maximum, 81 mg) given by infusion pump over 1 hour. Aspirin, heparin, and warfarin are not given during the first 24 hours. Systolic BP should be maintained at less than 185 and diastolic BP at less than 110 mm Hg to reduce the patient's risk for hemorrhagic transformation.

III. Diagnosis and management of specific etiologies

   A. Additional diagnostic tests may be required to establish a specific diagnosis.

      1. MRI scan is more sensitive and accurate than CT in narrowing the differential diagnosis of cerebral lesions, and MR angiography is a useful noninvasive method to evaluate large arteries and veins.

      2. Carotid Doppler studies enable noninvasive estimation of carotid stenosis. Conventional **iodine contrast angiography** may be required to diagnose cerebral aneurysm or isolated CNS angiitis and is usually required when carotid endarterectomy is considered (see sec. **III.B.2**).

      3. Transthoracic two-dimensional echocardiography is helpful to demonstrate intracardiac thrombi, valve vegetations, valvular stenosis or insufficiency, and right-to-left shunting (contrast echocardiogram). In some patients, transesophageal echocardiography is necessary to evaluate the left atrium for thrombi.

4. **CSF analysis** for malignant cells, special cultures, preps (e.g., acid-fast bacilli stain, India ink preparation), or antibody titers (e.g., VDRL) is helpful in the identification of carcinomatous or less common infectious etiologies.
5. **Erythrocyte sedimentation rate, antinuclear antibody, anticardiolipin antibody, hemoglobin electrophoresis, lipid profile,** or other specific tests may be required as indicated to establish a specific diagnosis.

B. **Treatment of atherosclerotic stroke**
1. **Aspirin** reduces the incidence of stroke and vascular mortality. A common aspirin dose is 325 mg/day, but lower and higher doses are effective. The combination of aspirin (25 mg bid) and extended-release dipyridamole (200 mg bid) may be more effective in stroke prevention after TIA or ischemic stroke (*J Neurol Sci* 143:1, 1996). **Clopidogrel** (75 mg qd) and **ticlopidine** (250 mg bid) are alternatives to aspirin for patients who cannot tolerate or have not responded to aspirin therapy (*Chest* 114:683S, 1998).
2. **Carotid endarterectomy** decreases the risk of stroke and death in patients with recent TIAs or nondisabling strokes and ipsilateral high-grade (70–99%) carotid stenosis (*N Engl J Med* 325:445, 1991). Carotid endarterectomy for asymptomatic high-grade carotid stenosis (>60%) reduces the relative risk of stroke provided that the surgical/angiography complication rate is less than 3% (*JAMA* 273:1421, 1995). Stroke risk factor reduction and antiplatelet therapy are important components of postoperative management (*Stroke* 29:554, 1998).
3. **Heparin and warfarin** treatment for atherosclerotic cerebrovascular disease is controversial; use must be individualized, with potential benefits considered with risks for hemorrhagic complications.

C. **Treatment of cardiogenic embolus.** Anticoagulation is indicated to prevent recurrent embolic strokes (see Chap. 19). Anticoagulation with heparin should be initiated. **Warfarin** is used for chronic anticoagulation with a target international normalized ratio of 2–3 for embolic infarcts, the exception being mechanical heart valves, for which an international normalized ratio of between 2.5 and 3.5 is recommended. Systemic hypertension is a relative contraindication to long-term anticoagulation because of increased risk for intracranial hemorrhage.

D. **Modification of risk factors,** including systemic hypertension, diabetes, smoking, illicit IV drug use, and possibly elevated lipids and cholesterol, reduce risk for stroke. Oral contraceptives may need to be discontinued in women with stroke.

IV. **Intracerebral hemorrhage and SAH**
A. **Intracerebral hemorrhage** usually presents with acute onset of focal neurologic deficits that reflect the location and size of the hemorrhage. Headache, vomiting, and altered mental status reflect increased intracranial pressure and often indicate extensive hemorrhage. **Brain herniation and death may occur rapidly.** Head **CT scan** is necessary to differentiate intracerebral hemorrhage from ischemic stroke.
1. **The etiology** is usually chronic systemic hypertension. The locations of hypertensive intracerebral hemorrhage are putamen/thalamus (70%), pons (10%), cerebellum (10%), and cerebral white matter (10%). Less commonly, intracerebral hemorrhage results from trauma, anticoagulant therapy, saccular aneurysm, arteriovenous malformation, tumor, blood dyscrasia, angiopathy, or vasculitis.
2. **Treatment** consists of supportive care and gradual reduction in BP.
   a. **Vascular autoregulation** is unpredictably impaired in patients with chronic hypertension and intracerebral hemorrhage. Higher than normal systemic BP may be required to maintain cerebral perfusion. Therefore, BP is gradually reduced over days, with careful observa-

tion for worsening neurologic deficits, which may reflect cerebral ischemia.

    b. **Surgical consultation** is indicated for **cerebellar** hematomas, because brain stem compression or obstructive hydrocephalus may develop, and immediate hematoma evacuation or ventricular shunting is lifesaving. Evacuation of deep **cerebral** hematomas is rarely beneficial.

B. SAH may present with only **sudden onset of severe headache.** Lethargy or coma, fever, vomiting, seizures and low back pain may also be present. Focal neurologic deficits, nuchal rigidity, and retinal hemorrhages (subhyaloid) suggest SAH. **Complications** of SAH include rebleeding (20% at 2 weeks), vasospasm with ischemic deficits (days 4–14), hydrocephalus, seizures, and hyponatremia.

    1. The most common **etiology of SAH** is a ruptured saccular or "berry" aneurysm, which results from defects in the arterial media and internal elastic lamina of large arteries. Other types of aneurysms include fusiform aneurysms (probably secondary to atherosclerosis) and mycotic aneurysms (from septic embolism). Hypertensive intracerebral hemorrhage, arteriovenous malformation, blood dyscrasia, head trauma, cocaine or amphetamine abuse, and tumor are among the other etiologies.

    2. **Head CT scan is diagnostic** of subarachnoid blood in the sulci and cisternae in 90% of SAH patients in the first 24 hours. In some patients, **lumbar puncture** is necessary to confirm the diagnosis of SAH. Bloody CSF should be centrifuged immediately and examined for xanthochromia (yellow color). **Xanthochromia** results from RBC lysis and takes several hours to develop, indicating SAH rather than traumatic lumbar puncture. Postcontrast head CT or MRI scan may demonstrate vascular abnormalities, but cerebral angiography is often necessary for definitive diagnosis. Angiography is required for presurgical evaluation of saccular aneurysms.

    3. **Treatment** of SAH depends on etiology. Saccular aneurysms are usually treated surgically. The timing of surgery after SAH is controversial and depends on the clinical condition of the patient. Supportive measures while awaiting surgery include bed rest, sedation, analgesia, and laxatives to prevent sudden increases in intracranial pressure or BP. **One should avoid hypotension,** as it may worsen ischemic deficits. Only extreme elevations in BP (diastolic >130 mm Hg) should be treated, and reduction of BP should be gradual, with careful monitoring of BP and the neurologic examination. Nimodipine, a calcium channel blocker, improves outcome in SAH patients and may reduce the incidence of associated cerebral infarction with few side effects. Recommended dosage is 60 mg PO q4h, for 21 days, initiated within 4 days of presentation. Volume expansion, induced hypertension, and balloon dilation can occasionally be used to reverse neurologic deterioration due to vasospasm.

Head Trauma

I. Initial assessment

    A. Adequate airway, oxygenation, ventilation, and circulation should be ensured. The neck should be immobilized in a hard cervical collar to avoid spinal cord injury from manipulating an unstable or fractured cervical spine, and nasal intubation in patients with facial fractures should be avoided. Emergency tracheotomy is sometimes necessary. Hypoventilation and systemic hypotension should also be avoided, as these may reduce cerebral perfusion. One should secure IV access and continuously monitor vital signs, oximetry, and ECG.

B. History should include the temporal course of all symptoms, particularly loss of consciousness, occurrence of a lucid interval (which suggests expanding hematoma), and amnesia (which is related to the severity of the blow).

C. The physical examination should include a careful search for penetrating wounds and other injuries. The neurologic examination should focus on the level of consciousness (see Alterations in Consciousness, sec. **III,** and Table 25-2), focal deficits, and signs of herniation. Serial examinations should be documented to identify neurologic deterioration early.

D. Imaging studies. Head CT is useful in the identification of intracranial hemorrhage; bone window views may be useful in the identification of fractures. Skull and facial radiographs may be necessary to demonstrate some fractures. Cervical radiographs must be performed to exclude fracture or dislocation.

II. Management

A. Awake, alert patients with **concussion** (transient loss of consciousness, confusion, agitation, or amnesia, with normal neurologic examination and radiographic studies) are observed in the hospital for 24 hours with hourly neurologic assessment to detect delayed deterioration. Some patients are observed at home by a reliable adult with instructions for frequent checks and criteria for return. **Neurologic deterioration** after head injury of any severity requires an immediate repeat head CT scan to differentiate between an expanding hematoma that necessitates surgery from diffuse cerebral edema that requires monitoring and reduction of intracranial pressure.

B. Neurosurgical consultation is indicated for patients with contusion, intracranial hematoma, cervical fracture, skull fractures, penetrating injuries, or focal neurologic deficits.

1. **If surgery appears imminent** (severe or multiple injuries, intracranial hematoma), preoperative laboratory analysis should be performed concurrently. In the intubated, comatose patient, modest hyperventilation ($PCO_2 \approx 35$ mm Hg) should be instituted and fluids restricted (avoiding hypotonic fluids). The head should be midline and elevated 30 degrees. Steroids are not indicated. Brain herniation requires immediate countermeasures (see Alterations in Consciousness, sec. **I.B.7**).

2. In **penetrating head trauma,** foreign objects (e.g., knives) should not be moved.

3. Emergency surgical evacuation may be lifesaving in acute **epidural and subdural hematomas.** Epidural hematoma is usually associated with skull fractures across a meningeal artery and may cause precipitous deterioration after a lucid interval. The characteristic noncontrast head CT finding is a lenticular-shaped extra-axial hematoma. Deterioration often follows the classic uncal herniation syndrome (see Alterations in Consciousness, sec. **III.F.2**).

4. **Chronic subdural hematoma** is most common in aged, debilitated, and alcoholic individuals and in anticoagulated patients. Antecedent trauma is often minimal. Symptoms tend to be nonspecific (e.g., headache, confusion, lethargy) and can fluctuate. Surgical intervention is determined by the symptoms and degree of mass effect.

5. **Intracerebral hematomas** may be present initially or develop within a contusion. Surgical intervention versus observation depends on the location and size of the hematoma and the patient's neurologic condition.

6. Skull fractures increase the risk of epidural hemorrhage and meningitis. Clinical diagnosis of **basilar skull fracture** is supported by CSF otorrhea or rhinorrhea, hemotympanum, postauricular hematoma, and periorbital hematoma ("raccoon eyes").

Acute Spinal Cord Dysfunction

The hallmark of spinal cord dysfunction is demonstration of a level below which motor, sensory, and autonomic function is interrupted, due to the spinal cord's segmental functional organization. Rapid diagnosis and treatment may reverse or prevent progression of functional deficits.

I. **Spinal cord compression** typically presents with back pain at the level of compression (some lesions are painless), progressive difficulty in walking, sensory impairment, and urinary retention with overflow incontinence. Rapid deterioration may occur. Etiologies include tumor (primary or metastatic), herniated disk, epidural abscess, hematoma, and vascular malformation. Transverse myelitis or myelopathy presents with symptoms and signs similar to cord compression. **Transverse myelitis** occurs with enteroviruses, herpes zoster, tuberculosis or other granulomatous disease, syphilis, and systemic lupus erythematosus. **Transverse myelopathy** is caused by infarction (cardiogenic, fibrocartilaginous, or gaseous embolus; hypotension; aortic dissection or surgery) and multiple sclerosis.

A. **Examination** helps localize the level of dysfunction, but it should be remembered that lesions may be multiple. **Radicular signs** (lancinating pain, paresthesias, and numbness in the dermatomal distribution of a nerve root, with weakness and decreased tone and reflexes in muscles supplied by the root) imply inflammation or compression of the nerve root. Tenderness to spinal percussion over the lesion may be present. **Myelopathic** signs include a band of dysesthesia at the level of a lesion, with bilateral sensory loss and weakness below the level of the lesion. Tone and reflexes are typically diminished below acute lesions (spinal shock); hypertonia, hyperreflexia, and Babinski's signs are present with slowly progressive lesions. Urinary retention commonly accompanies spinal cord compression. Unilateral cord lesions may result in contralateral pain and temperature loss, with ipsilateral weakness and proprioceptive loss **(Brown-Séquard syndrome)**. **Cauda equina syndrome** from compression of the lower lumbar and sacral roots produces sensory loss in a saddle distribution, flaccid leg weakness, decreased reflexes, and urinary/bowel incontinence.

B. **Imaging studies.** Plain x-rays of the spine may reveal metastatic disease, osteomyelitis, discitis, fractures, or dislocation. MRI scan or myelography with CT scan should be obtained emergently to determine the exact level and extent of the lesion(s). Imaging should include the entire spine. Neurosurgical consultation should be obtained **before** myelography, because occasionally acute postmyelography decompensation occurs with compressive lesions, requiring emergent decompressive laminectomy. For the same reason, **lumbar puncture** for diagnosis of infection, inflammation, or carcinomatous meningitis should follow exclusion of a compressive lesion.

C. **Management**
1. Vital functions should be supported, and preoperative evaluation should be performed.
2. Treatable infections require appropriate antibiotics. Herpes zoster (suggested by a vesicular rash) should be treated with acyclovir.
3. **Dexamethasone,** 10 mg IV followed by 4 mg IV q6h, is given for compressive lesions, and sometimes for transverse myelitis or spinal cord infarction, although benefit has not been proved for all etiologies.
4. **Neurosurgical consultation** should be obtained emergently because many causes for spinal cord compression are surgically treatable.
5. **Emergent radiation therapy** combined with high-dose steroids is usually indicated for cord compression due to malignancy and generally requires a histologic diagnosis.

6. **Anticipatory acute and long-term supportive care** is important for patients with spinal cord dysfunction. Airway security should be confirmed frequently. Pulmonary and urinary infections, skin breakdown at pressure points, joint contractures, and irregular bowel and bladder elimination are common problems. Bladder distention can cause sympathetic overactivity (headache, tachycardia, diaphoresis, hypertension) as a result of autonomic dysreflexia.

II. **Traumatic spinal cord injury** may be obvious from the history or initial examination but must also be excluded in patients who are unconscious, confused, or inebriated when the history regarding trauma is unknown. Penetrating injury, foreign bodies, comminuted fractures, misalignment, and hematoma usually require surgical treatment. **Spinal cord concussion** refers to posttraumatic spinal cord symptoms and signs that resolve rapidly (hours to days).

A. **Immobilization,** especially of the neck, is essential to prevent further injury while the patient's condition is stabilized and radiographic and neurosurgical assessment of the injuries is performed. Vital signs should be continuously monitored, and adequate oxygenation and perfusion should be affirmed. Neurosurgical consultation should be obtained. **Autonomic instability** may lead to fluctuating vital signs and BP. Hypotension may require vasopressors (dopamine or dobutamine). α-Adrenergic agonists increase BP but reduce cardiac output and impair spinal cord perfusion. Fluid resuscitation alone usually results in pulmonary edema.

B. **Respiratory insufficiency** from cervical cord injuries requires immediate airway control and ventilatory assistance, without manipulation of the neck. Bag-mask ventilation, blind nasal intubation, or tracheostomy is typically required.

C. **Examination** may reveal local and radicular pain, local tenderness, weakness in a radicular or myelopathic distribution, sensory loss, absent tone and reflexes, and urinary retention. The presence and extent of injuries should be confirmed with neuroimaging as described previously. One should search for injuries to other systems.

D. **Methylprednisolone,** 30 mg/kg IV bolus, followed by an infusion of 5.4 mg/kg/hour for 24 hours when administered within 3 hours of injury (*N Engl J Med* 322:1405, 1990) and for 48 hours when initiated within 3–8 hours of injury (*JAMA* 277:1597, 1997), may improve neurologic recovery.

Neuromuscular Disease

I. **Guillain-Barré syndrome (GBS, acute idiopathic demyelinating polyneuropathy)**

A. **Presentation** of GBS is typically a rapidly progressive, symmetric ascending paralysis, often following a viral illness (Epstein-Barr virus or cytomegalovirus), gastroenteritis (especially *Campylobacter jejuni*), surgical procedure, or immunization (influenza). Proximal weakness may be pronounced. Cranial nerves, especially the facial nerves, may be involved. Sensory symptoms are usually present and cause discomfort, but objective sensory loss is uncommon. Reflexes are hypoactive or absent. CSF protein is usually elevated, without pleocytosis (lymphocytes may be present but are usually less than $20/\mu l$). Differential diagnosis includes arsenic exposure, acute porphyria, tick paralysis, botulism, and postdiphtheritic paralysis.

B. **Treatment** is supportive. Plasmapheresis and IV immunoglobulin have been shown to be equally effective when carried out early in patients whose conditions are severely compromised or worsening (loss of ambulation, respiratory failure) (*Neurology* 46:100, 1996; *Neurology* 35:1096, 1985). Indications for treatment in mild forms of stable and improving GBS are less clear. Corticosteroids, immunosuppressive drugs, and other agents are not of proven value in GBS.

1. **Respiratory function** must be closely monitored, preferably in an ICU. Respiratory assistance may be necessary.
2. **Autonomic neuropathy** can cause fatal overactivity or underactivity of autonomic functions. No uniform approach to the treatment of autonomic dysfunction is available; only general therapeutic guidelines can be given.
   a. **BP instability.** Paroxysmal hypertension should be managed with short-acting agents that can be titrated against the patient's BP (see Chap. 4). Hypotension is usually caused by decreased venous return and peripheral vasodilatation. Patients on respirators, who already have compromised venous return, are particularly prone to hypotension. Treatment consists of intravascular volume expansion with IV fluids. Occasionally, vasopressors may be required (see Chap. 9).
   b. **Cardiac arrhythmias** have been implicated as a significant cause of mortality in GBS; thus, cardiac monitoring is necessary. Bradyarrhythmias (sinus arrest or complete heart block) as well as tachyarrhythmias are frequent. Hypoxia and electrolyte abnormalities should be excluded as causes of cardiac arrhythmias.

II. **Myasthenia gravis (MG)** is an autoimmune disorder that involves antibody-mediated disruption of neuromuscular junction receptors and is often associated with thymus tumors. Typical symptoms are transient weakness (especially worse after exercise and better after rest), but constant weakness may occur. **Presenting signs** include ptosis, diplopia, dysarthria, dysphagia, extremity weakness, and respiratory difficulty. It is more common in women, and it tends to occur in young women (third decade) and older men (fifth to sixth decade). The clinical course is variable; spontaneous remissions and exacerbations occur. Progressive deterioration is more likely to occur in the first 3 years. The differential diagnosis includes botulism and the Eaton-Lambert syndrome, a neuromuscular defect associated with carcinoma.

A. **The diagnosis** is usually evident from the history and physical examination. Ancillary tests may be useful in confirming the diagnosis.

1. **Edrophonium (Tensilon) test** often produces a marked temporary improvement of strength in myasthenic patients. However, its utility as a diagnostic tool in MG is limited by a high incidence of false positives.
2. **Blood acetylcholine receptor antibody level** remains a highly sensitive and very specific assay and is the diagnostic test of choice.
3. **CT of the thorax** is necessary to exclude thymoma.
4. **Electromyography** may show a decremental response to repetitive nerve stimulation of the myasthenic muscle action potential. In botulism and the Eaton-Lambert syndrome, the response is incremental.

B. **Treatment of MG** follows no specific protocol. The clinician must choose among modalities based on symptoms, lifestyle, and response to treatment. A rapid deterioration in respiratory and swallowing functions necessitates aggressive support, therapy, and correction of precipitating causes (e.g., infection, thyroid dysfunction).

1. **Anticholinesterase drugs** can produce symptomatic improvement in all forms of MG. Pyridostigmine should be started at 30–60 mg PO tid–qid and subsequently titrated to the minimum amount that provides relief of symptoms. Occasional patients require dosing as frequently as q2–3h. Neostigmine methylsulfate as a continuous IV infusion at one–forty-fifth the total daily dose of pyridostigmine over 24 hours can be substituted for patients who are not able to take medications orally.
2. **Thymectomy** is effective treatment for generalized MG and produces complete remission in many patients. However, thymectomy is controversial in children, in adults older than 60 years, and in purely ocular MG. A **thymoma** is an absolute indication for surgery at any age. In general, thymectomy should be performed electively for moderate to

marked generalized MG, early in the course of the disease, and if response to medical treatment is unsatisfactory.

3. **Immunosuppressive drugs** are typically used when additional benefit is needed after cholinesterase inhibitors. High-dose **prednisone** (50 mg qd) is frequently used to achieve rapid improvement, but **hospitalization is advised because initial exacerbation of weakness often occurs.** Initiating therapy at a lower dose (20 mg qd) followed by dose titration may avoid worsening symptoms. The goal is to identify an effective daily dose, maintain stable improvement, and then taper to an alternate-day regimen. Additional dose reductions can be made gradually. Potential risks of steroid treatment need to be weighed against observed clinical benefit on an individual basis. **Azathioprine,** 1–2 mg/kg PO qd, is an alternative drug for patients who do not respond to steroids or cannot take them. Onset of benefit may require months of treatment. **Side effects** include leukopenia, pancytopenia, infection, GI irritation, and abnormal liver function tests. **Cyclosporin A** has been shown to be effective in MG in a double-blind, placebo-controlled clinical trial (*Ann N Y Acad Sci* 681:539, 1993). **Cyclophosphamide** and IV **human immunoglobulin** may be beneficial in selected refractory patients.

4. **Plasmapheresis** is used to treat acute exacerbations, impending crisis, and disabling myasthenia that is refractory to other therapies and is used before surgery when postoperative deterioration is possible (e.g., before thymectomy). Benefits are temporary, and no consensus has been reached about exact indications and protocol. Hypotension and thromboembolism are potential complications.

5. **Precipitating factors** include infection, pregnancy, thyroid dysfunction, and drug reaction. A variety of medications can worsen or even precipitate weakness in myasthenic patients; however, only curariform medications are absolutely contraindicated in MG.

C. **Myasthenic crisis,** the need for assisted ventilation or airway protection, or both, occurs in approximately 10% of patients with MG. Patients with bulbar and respiratory muscle weakness are particularly prone to respiratory failure. Respiratory infection and surgery (e.g., thymectomy) can precipitate crisis. Patients at risk should have pulmonary function monitored closely. Respiratory support follows the guidelines given in Chap. 9. Anticholinesterases should be temporarily withdrawn from patients who are receiving ventilation support; this avoids uncertainties about overdosage ("cholinergic crisis") and avoids cholinergic stimulation of pulmonary secretions. Steroids, IV immunoglobulins, or plasmapheresis may be helpful. Thymectomy is not part of the emergency treatment of MG.

III. **Botulism** is a disorder of the neuromuscular junction caused by ingestion of an exotoxin produced by *Clostridium botulinum*. The exotoxin interferes with release of acetylcholine from presynaptic terminals at the neuromuscular junction. **Symptoms** begin within 12–36 hours of ingestion and include autonomic dysfunction (xerostomia, blurred vision, bowel and bladder dysfunction) followed by cranial nerve palsies and weakness. **Management** includes removing nonabsorbed toxin with cathartics, neutralizing absorbed toxin with equine trivalent antitoxin, one vial IV and one vial IM (after normal intradermal horse serum sensitivity test), and supportive care.

IV. **Rhabdomyolysis** secondary to strenuous exercise or metabolic myopathy or from toxic effects (e.g., alcohol) may produce dramatic and painful muscle weakness. Resultant effects include hyperkalemia, myoglobinuria, and renal failure (see Chap. 12 for management).

V. **Myopathies** (ethanol, steroids, cholesterol-lowering drugs, hypothyroidism) may present with rapidly progressive, proximal muscle weakness. Polymyositis and dermatomyositis should also be considered, particularly if muscle pain is prominent (see Chap. 24).

VI. Neuromuscular disorders with rigidity

   A. Neuroleptic malignant syndrome is associated with drugs such as haloperidol, phenothiazines, lithium, and reserpine. **Typical features** include fever, obtundation, and muscular rigidity, with elevated creatine kinase and myoglobinuria. **Treatment** includes discontinuing precipitating drug(s), cooling, monitoring and supporting vital functions (arrhythmias, shock, hyperkalemia, acidosis, renal failure), and administering dantrolene (2 mg/kg IV; additional doses q5min up to 10 mg/kg total can be given). Oral bromocriptine can be used in mild cases.

   B. High fever, obtundation, and muscular rigidity characterize **malignant hyperthermia syndrome.** Serum creatine kinase is markedly elevated. Renal failure from myoglobinuria and cardiac arrhythmias from electrolyte imbalance can be life threatening. Multiple genetic mutations are associated with malignant hyperthermia syndrome, with a likely common abnormal elevation in intracellular calcium following triggering factors (e.g., halothane anesthesia). Patients with certain muscle disorders (central core disease, Duchenne muscular dystrophy) are particularly at risk. Successful **management** requires prompt recognition of the syndrome, discontinuation of the offending anesthetic agent, aggressive supportive care that focuses on oxygenation/ventilation, circulation, correction of acid-base and electrolyte derangements, and dantrolene sodium, 1–10 mg/kg/day, to reduce muscular rigidity.

   C. Tetanus typically presents with generalized muscle spasm (especially trismus) caused by the exotoxin (tetanospasmin) from *Clostridium tetani.* The organism usually enters the body through wounds; onset typically occurs within 14 days of an injury (range, 2–54 days). Mortality may be as high as 50–60%. **Patients who are unvaccinated or have reduced immunity are at risk, underscoring the importance of prevention by tetanus toxoid boosters following wounds.** Tetanus may occur in drug abusers who inject subcutaneously. **Management** consists of supportive care, particularly airway control (laryngospasm) and treatment of muscle spasms (benzodiazepines, barbiturates, analgesics, and sometimes neuromuscular blockade). Cardiac arrhythmias and fluctuations in BP can occur. The patient should be kept in quiet isolation, sedated but arousable. **Specific measures** include wound débridement; **penicillin G,** 2 million units IV q6h for 10 days (tetracycline, 2 g/day, or erythromycin, 2 g/day, is an alternative in penicillin-allergic patients); and **human tetanus immunoglobulin** (3000–10,000 units) distributed intramuscularly among several sites proximal to the suspected source of exotoxin. **Active immunization is needed after recovery** (see Appendix F, Tables F-1 and F-3).

Headache

Headache may require emergency evaluation when it is debilitating or associated with neurologic deficits.

I. Assessment

   A. Primary headache syndromes include migraines with (classic) or without (common) aura, tension headaches, and cluster headaches. Posttraumatic, exertional, cough- and cold-induced, and fleeting ice pick (stabbing) headaches are also considered within the same category after underlying structural lesions have been excluded. The mechanisms of primary headache syndromes are poorly understood but probably include a disturbance in serotonergic neurotransmission. **Examination** should reveal normal findings during asymptomatic intervals in patients with primary headache syndromes. Persistent neurologic deficits require investigation to rule out an underlying disorder.

   1. Migraines are typically unilateral, pulsating, or throbbing, with nausea, vomiting, and phonophotophobia. Headache severity tends to increase over minutes to hours and lasts 4–72 hours. Protracted episodes constitute intractable migraines or "status migrainosus." The aura of **classic migraine** is a transient visual, motor, sensory, cognitive, or psychic disturbance that usually lasts minutes and precedes or coincides with the headache. **Provocative factors** may be identified and include stress, hunger, fatigue, sleep deprivation or excess, physical exertion, bright light, alcohol, menstruation, pregnancy, oral contraceptives, foods (cheese, chocolate), food additives (monosodium glutamate, nitrites), and nitroglycerin. Most patients who experience migraine are female (18% of females vs. 6% of males) and have their first episode before 30 years of age.

2. **Muscle contraction or tension headache** is often diagnosed when headaches are chronic, bilateral, constricting, nonpulsatile, and associated with neck muscle rigidity. Stress and anxiety are common aggravating factors. Migrainous symptoms frequently overlap and can be difficult to separate from those of tension headache. Tension headaches typically occur daily, begin later in the day, and wax and wane in intensity.

3. **Cluster headaches** are more common in males (6:1 male–female ratio), are excruciatingly painful, are unilateral, are orbital and periorbital or temporal in location, last one-half to 2 hours, and are associated with unilateral autonomic dysfunction (lacrimation, ptosis, miosis, nasal congestion, or conjunctival injection). Alcohol and nitroglycerin are known precipitants of cluster headaches. Most patients who experience cluster headaches assume an upright position to alleviate the discomfort (as opposed to napping in a darkened room with migraines). Periodicity is a hallmark of cluster headache, with pain often recurring daily at about the same hour. "Clusters" last days to weeks and recur at intervals of months to years. In contrast, **chronic cluster headaches** recur at intervals of 4–5 years.

B. **Secondary headache syndromes** can be caused by many disease processes and vary depending on the underlying pathologic cause. For example, SAH causes the abrupt onset of severe pain, whereas cerebral tumors tend to cause a fluctuating, less severe pain of gradual onset, sometimes affected by posture. Age at onset can also be helpful in that the headache of temporal arteritis rarely begins before age 50 years, whereas the onset of migraines is uncommon after age 50 years. Persistent neurologic signs suggest an underlying neurologic disorder. Those signs preceding a headache and resolving before or during the headache suggest classic migraine, rather than a secondary headache syndrome.

1. **Intracranial causes** include subdural hematoma, intracerebral hematoma, SAH, arteriovenous malformation, brain abscess, meningitis, encephalitis, vasculitis, obstructive hydrocephalus, postlumbar puncture, and cerebral ischemia or infarction. Headaches from intracranial disease do not follow any one stereotype.

2. **Extracranial causes** include sinusitis, disorders of the cervical spine, temporomandibular joint syndrome, giant-cell arteritis, glaucoma, optic neuritis, and dental disease.

3. **Systemic causes** include fever, viremia, hypoxia, hypercapnia, systemic hypertension, allergy, anemia, caffeine withdrawal, and vasoactive chemicals, including nitrites and carbon monoxide.

4. **Depression** is a common cause of long-standing, treatment-resistant daily headaches. Specific inquiry should be made about vegetative signs of depression.

II. **Treatment**

A. **Acute treatment** is aimed at aborting headache.

1. **Nonnarcotic analgesics.** Aspirin, acetaminophen, and nonsteroidal anti-inflammatory agents may abort a migraine or tension headache if taken early. Ketorolac tromethamine, 30–60 mg IM; naproxen sodium,

550 mg PO bid or tid; or flurbiprofen, 100 mg PO bid, is effective for migraine and tension headache. Indomethacin, 50 mg PO bid–tid, may be helpful for cluster, cough, and ice pick headache. Drugs with sedative and analgesic properties, such as isometheptene, butalbital with aspirin, or acetaminophen, are primarily helpful in migraine and tension headache.

2. **Prochlorperazine,** 5–10 mg IV, may terminate migraine and helps alleviate nausea. Acute dystonic reactions and hypotension are potential side effects.

3. **Ergotamine** is a vasoconstrictive agent that is effective in aborting migraine headaches, particularly if administered during the prodromal phase. Ergotamine should be taken at symptom onset in the maximum dose tolerated by the patient; nausea often limits the dose. Rectal preparations are better absorbed than oral agents. The initial oral dose is 2–3 mg PO. Additional doses of 1–2 mg can be taken every 30 minutes, up to a total dose of 8–10 mg, but these rarely succeed when an initial dose has failed. Rectal (2 mg) administration should be tried in patients who are unresponsive to oral delivery or when emesis prevents oral administration. Dosages that exceed 16 mg/week should be used cautiously to avoid toxicity, which includes angina pectoris, limb claudication, and ergotamine headache and dependency.

4. **Dihydroergotamine (DHE)** is a potent venoconstrictor with minimal peripheral arterial constriction. Cardiac precautions are indicated in those with a history of angina, peripheral vascular disease, or greater than 60 years of age. A dose of 1–2 mg IM or SC can abort a migraine headache before it reaches peak intensity. If an attack has climaxed, 5–10 mg prochlorperazine can be given IV, followed immediately by 0.2 mg DHE IV given over 3 minutes. If tolerated, another 0.8 mg DHE IV is given. This relieves the primary headache in the majority of cases. For intractable migraines (status migrainosus), DHE can be given q8h with IV metoclopramide (*Neurology* 36:995, 1986; *Neurol Clin* 8:587, 1990). **DHE 45 NS** is administered intranasally, 1 spray in each nostril. It can be repeated in 15 minutes. The maximum recommended dose is 4 sprays/day.

5. **Triptans** are effective abortive medications that are available in multiple formulations and may be effective even in a protracted attack. Sometimes headache recurs within 24 hours after complete resolution. **Triptans should not be used in patients with coronary artery disease, cerebrovascular disease, uncontrolled hypertension, or vertebrobasilar migraine.** Sumatriptan, 6 mg SC, can be repeated in 1 hour (maximum, 2 shots/24 hours), 5 or 20 mg nasal (maximum daily dose, 2 sprays, with minimum interval between doses of 2 hours), or 25–100 mg PO can be repeated in 2 hours (maximum daily dose, 300 mg). Zolmitriptan, 2.5–5.0 mg, can be repeated in 2 hours (maximum dose, 10 mg/24 hours). Naratriptan, 1.0–2.5 mg, can be repeated in 4 hours (maximum dose, 5 mg/24 hours). Rizatriptan, 5–10 mg, can be repeated every 2 hours as needed (maximum dose, 30 mg/24 hours; 50 mg if on a beta-blocker). **Triptans should not be taken within 24 hours of other triptans, isometheptene, or ergot derivatives.**

6. **Opioid** analgesics are sometimes required to abort severe headaches (see Chap. 1). Chronic daily headaches should not be treated with narcotic analgesics to prevent habituation and loss of efficacy.

7. **Caffeine,** in coffee, tea, or a tablet in combination with ergotamine (Cafergot), is a useful adjunct to migraine therapy.

8. **Environment** plays an important role in alleviating headache. A quiet, dark, noise-free environment can speed recovery. Sleep often helps relieve migraines.

B. **Prophylaxis** is used for recurrent headaches, particularly those that are not responsive to acute therapy. **Environmental prophylaxis** includes avoidance of precipitating foods, chemicals, activities, and situations. **Tricyclic antidepressants** are effective in preventing migraine and tension headaches. β-**Adrenergic antagonists** can decrease the frequency of recurrent migraines. **Low-dose ergot preparations** can be used for migraine prophylaxis if **tricyclic antidepressants** and β-**adrenergic antagonists** are ineffective or contraindicated. **Prednisone** is a first-line drug in the treatment of cluster headache. **Methysergide** is effective in the prevention of migraine and cluster headache. Retroperitoneal, pleural, and endocardial fibrosis are severe but reversible complications of chronic methysergide treatment that occur uncommonly (1 in 5000 cases). **Other pharmacotherapy** for refractory migraine includes phenelzine (a monoamine oxidase inhibitor), valproate, and calcium channel antagonists. Indomethacin, verapamil, and valproic acid are useful medications for cluster headache prophylaxis. Lithium and verapamil are used in chronic cluster headache. Relaxation training should be attempted for patients who experience recurrent stress-induced headaches.

26 Medical Emergencies

Daniel Goodenberger

Medical emergencies may not allow time for orderly information gathering and formulation of a narrow differential diagnosis before the initiation of therapy. **The first responsibility** is to provide basic life support (i.e., maintenance of an intact airway, adequate ventilation, and circulation; see Chap. 8).

Acute Upper Airway Obstruction

In the **conscious patient,** manifestations of airway obstruction may include stridor, impaired or absent phonation, sternal or suprasternal retractions, display of the universal choking sign, and respiratory distress. One should look for urticaria, angioedema, fever, or evidence of trauma. The **unconscious patient** may have labored breathing or apnea. One should suspect airway obstruction in a nonbreathing patient who is difficult to ventilate. The **differential diagnosis** includes trauma to the face and neck, foreign body, infection (croup, epiglottitis, Ludwig's angina, retropharyngeal abscess, and diphtheria), tumor, angioedema, laryngospasm, anaphylaxis, retained secretions, or blockage of the upper airway by the tongue (in the unconscious patient). **Therapy** is directed at rapid relief of obstruction to prevent cardiopulmonary arrest and anoxic brain damage.

I. **Partial obstruction in the awake patient with adequate ventilation**
   A. Rapidly take a history, focusing on the causes just listed.
   B. Perform a directed physical examination, looking for airway swelling, trismus, pharyngeal obstruction, respiratory retractions, angioedema, stridor, wheezing, and grossly swollen lymph nodes and masses in the neck.
   C. If the patient is stable, perform indirect laryngoscopy or fiberoptic nasopharyngolaryngoscopy. A careful examination is unlikely to cause acute airway obstruction in an adult.
   D. Soft-tissue radiography of the neck (posteroanterior and lateral views) is less sensitive and specific than is direct examination but may be a valuable adjunct. Such radiography should be performed in the emergency department as a portable study, as the patient should not be left unattended.
   E. Treatment is aimed at the underlying disease process; observe the patient carefully and be prepared to intervene to maintain an airway.

II. **Airway obstruction in the awake patient without ventilation.** The most likely causes are a foreign body (usually food) and angioedema. Other causes include infection or posttraumatic hematoma. History is usually unavailable. One should perform the **Heimlich maneuver** (subdiaphragmatic abdominal thrust) repeatedly until the object is expelled from the airway or the patient becomes unconscious (see Chap. 8).

III. **Airway obstruction in an unconscious patient without intact ventilation.** Such a situation may be due to obstruction by the tongue, or it may be caused by a foreign body, trauma, infection, or angioedema. A history usually is unavailable except from paramedics or relatives. Examination reveals an unresponsive patient with no air movement or paradoxical respiratory efforts.

A. The first maneuver should be a head tilt–chin lift if cervical spine trauma is not suspected. Apply a jaw thrust if cervical spine trauma is suspected.

B. If these maneuvers are effective, place an oral or nasal airway. If they are ineffective, attempt to ventilate the patient with a bag-valve-mask apparatus. If these attempts are also unsuccessful, rapidly examine the oropharynx and hypopharynx. Avoid a blind finger sweep if it is possible to **examine the airway directly** using a laryngoscope and McGill forceps (if necessary) to remove a foreign body.

C. If laryngoscopy cannot be performed immediately and a foreign body is suspected, perform the supine Heimlich maneuver (straddling the supine patient and applying repeated subdiaphragmatic thrusts). Substitute chest thrusts if the patient is very obese or is in late pregnancy.

D. Failure of this maneuver should prompt an attempt at direct laryngoscopy and endotracheal intubation. Establish a surgical airway if the patient cannot be intubated. If a surgeon is not immediately available, perform needle cricothyrotomy using a 12- to 14-gauge over-the-needle catheter with high-flow oxygen (15 L/minute from a 50-psi wall source). Cricothyrotomy (see Chap. 9) is a preferred alternative.

Pneumothorax

Pneumothorax may occur spontaneously or as a result of trauma. Primary spontaneous pneumothorax occurs without obvious underlying lung disease. Secondary spontaneous pneumothorax results from underlying parenchymal lung disease, including chronic obstructive pulmonary disease, interstitial lung disease, necrotizing lung infections, *Pneumocystis carinii* pneumonia, and cystic fibrosis. Traumatic pneumothoraces may occur as a result of penetrating or blunt chest wounds. Iatrogenic pneumothorax occurs after thoracentesis, central line placement, transbronchial biopsy, transthoracic needle biopsy, and barotrauma from mechanical ventilation and resuscitation.

I. The **history** reveals that the patient is complaining of ipsilateral chest or shoulder pain, usually of abrupt onset. Dyspnea is usually present, and the patient sometimes has a cough. Symptoms related to an underlying pulmonary disease process may be seen or a history of recent trauma obtained.

II. Examination of a patient with a small pneumothorax may be normal. With a larger pneumothorax or with underlying lung disease, there is increased dyspnea and tachypnea. The affected hemithorax may be noticeably larger (owing to decreased elastic recoil of the collapsed lung) and relatively immobile during respiration. The patient has decreased breath sounds, decreased vocal fremitus, and a more resonant percussion note. If the pneumothorax is very large, and particularly if it is under tension, the patient may exhibit severe distress, diaphoresis, cyanosis, and hypotension. There may be signs of recent procedures or trauma. In addition, one may see such indications of underlying lung disease as clubbing or fever. If the pneumothorax is the result of penetrating trauma or pneumomediastinum, subcutaneous emphysema may be felt.

III. Diagnosis is confirmed by a chest radiograph, which reveals a separation of the pleural shadow from the chest wall. A small pneumothorax is more easily seen on a film taken during expiration. Air travels to the highest point in a body cavity; thus, a pneumothorax in a supine patient (who often is receiving positive-pressure ventilation) may be detected as an unusually deep costophrenic sulcus and excessive lucency over the upper abdomen caused by the anterior thoracic air. Tension pneumothorax is a clinical diagnosis; radiographic correlates include mediastinal and tracheal shift away from the pneumothorax and depression of the ipsilateral diaphragm. An ECG may reveal diminished anterior QRS amplitude and an anterior axis shift. In extreme cases, tension pneumothorax may cause electromechanical dissociation.

IV. **Treatment** depends on cause, size, and degree of physiologic derangement.

A. **A small, primary, spontaneous pneumothorax** without a continued pleural air leak may resolve spontaneously. Air is resorbed from the pleural space at roughly 1.5% daily, and therefore a small (<15%) pneumothorax is expected to resolve without intervention in approximately 10 days. Confirm that the pneumothorax is stable (repeat the chest radiograph in 6 hours if there is no change in symptoms) and send the patient home if he or she is asymptomatic (apart from mild pleurisy). Obtain follow-up radiographs to confirm resolution of the pneumothorax. Air travel is proscribed during the follow-up period, as a decrease in ambient barometric pressure will result in a larger pneumothorax.

   1. If the pneumothorax is small but the patient is mildly symptomatic or unlikely to cooperate with follow-up, admit the patient and administer high-flow oxygen; the resulting nitrogen gradient will speed resorption.

   2. If the pneumothorax is larger than 15–20% or is more than mildly symptomatic, consider inserting a small pneumothorax tube [No. 8 French (Fr.) over a needle] in the second interspace in the midclavicular line with a one-way valve or, if necessary, connection to suction. If the pneumothorax fails to expand or if there is a continuous large air leak, arrange for insertion of a larger tube with suction (see sec. **IV.B**).

   3. Pleural sclerosis to prevent recurrence is recommended but often is not performed after a first episode. Thoracotomy and resection of apical blebs usually are withheld until the third episode but can be considered after a second episode, given the decreased morbidity of video-assisted thoracoscopic surgery.

B. **Individuals with a secondary spontaneous pneumothorax** usually are symptomatic and require lung re-expansion. Often a bronchopleural fistula persists, and a larger thoracostomy tube and suction are required. If no associated effusion is present, a No. 24–28 Fr. tube is recommended; if fluid is present, choose a larger tube (No. 34–36 Fr.). Attach the thoracostomy tube to a three-bottle suction system or the commercial equivalent and apply 20 cm H_2O suction. Large air leaks may require greater suction. Consult a pulmonologist about pleural sclerosis for persistent air leak and to prevent recurrence. Surgery may be required.

C. **Iatrogenic pneumothorax** generally is caused either by introducing air into the pleural space through the parietal pleura (e.g., thoracentesis, central line placement) or by allowing intrapulmonary air to escape through breach of the visceral pleura (e.g., transbronchial biopsy). Often no further air leak occurs after the initial event.

   1. If the pneumothorax is small and the patient is minimally symptomatic, it can be managed conservatively. If the procedure that caused the pneumothorax required sedation, admit the patient, administer oxygen, and repeat the chest radiograph in 6 hours to ensure the patient's stability. If the patient is completely alert and the chest x-ray shows no change, the patient can be discharged.

   2. If the patient is symptomatic or if the pneumothorax is too large for expectant care, a pneumothorax catheter with a one-way valve usually is adequate and can often be removed the following day.

   3. Iatrogenic pneumothorax due to barotrauma from mechanical ventilation almost always has a persistent air leak and should be managed with a chest tube and suction.

D. **Tension pneumothorax** results from continued accumulation of air in the chest that is sufficient to shift mediastinal structures and impede venous return to the heart, resulting in hypotension, abnormal gas exchange, and, ultimately, cardiovascular collapse. It can occur as a result of barotrauma due to mechanical ventilation, a chest wound that allows ingress but not egress of air, or a rent in the visceral pleura that behaves in the same way ("ball-valve" effect). Suspect tension pneumothorax when a patient experiences hypotension and respiratory distress on mechanical ventilation or after any procedure in which the thorax is pierced by a needle. When the clinical situation and physical examination strongly suggest this diagnosis, decompress the affected hemithorax immediately with a 14-gauge needle attached to a fluid-filled syringe. Release of air with clinical improvement confirms the diagnosis. Seal any chest wound with an occlusive dressing and arrange for placement of a thoracostomy tube as described in sec. **IV.B.**

Heat-Induced Illness

Heat illness is due to exposure to increased ambient temperature under conditions in which the body is unable to maintain appropriate homeostasis. Milder syndromes are exertional; the most severe may occur without exercise.

I. Heat cramps occur in unacclimatized individuals who engage in vigorous exercise in a hot environment; no published evidence has shown unequivocally that they are a result of salt depletion and hypotonic fluid replacement (*Int J Sports Med* 19:S146, 1998). Cramps typically occur in large muscle groups, most often in the legs. On examination, the patient has moist cool skin, a normal body temperature, and minimal distress. **Treatment** includes rest in a cool environment and salt replacement. Administer one-half to 1 teaspoon of salt or a 650-mg sodium chloride tablet in 500 ml water PO or use a commercially available, oral, balanced electrolyte replacement solution. IV therapy rarely is required, but 2 L of normal saline administered over several hours resolves symptoms.

II. Heat exhaustion occurs in unacclimatized individuals who exercise in the heat and is partly a result of loss of both salt and water. The patient complains of headache, nausea, vomiting, dizziness, weakness, irritability, and cramps. On examination, the patient is diaphoretic, demonstrates piloerection, has postural hypotension, and has normal or minimally increased core temperature. **Therapy** consists of rest in a cool environment, acceleration of heat loss by fan evaporation, and fluid repletion with salt-containing solutions. If the patient is not vomiting and has stable BP, an oral, commercial, balanced salt solution is adequate. If the patient is vomiting or hemodynamically unstable, check electrolytes and give 1–2 L 0.9% saline IV. The patient should avoid exercise in a hot environment for 2–3 additional days.

III. Heat syncope affects unacclimatized individuals. Exercise in a hot environment results in peripheral vasodilatation and pooling of blood, with subsequent loss of consciousness. The affected individual regains consciousness promptly when supine, and the body temperature is normal, factors that separate this syndrome from heat stroke. **Treatment** consists of rest in a cool environment, fluid repletion, and a more gradual approach to building exercise endurance.

IV. Heat stroke can occur in the face of high core temperature, which causes direct thermal tissue injury. Secondary effects include acute renal failure from rhabdomyolysis. Even with rapid therapy, mortality may reach 76% for body temperatures of 41.1°C (106°F) or higher.

A. Classic heat stroke occurs after several days of heat exposure. Individuals at risk include those who are chronically ill, dehydrated, elderly, or obese; who have chronic cardiovascular disease; who abuse alcohol; and who use sedatives, hypnotics, β-adrenergic antagonists, diuretics, anticholinergics, or antipsychotics. Abuse of phencyclidine, cocaine, and amphetamines also may contribute. Risk factors include high humidity and lack of air-conditioning. More than 50% may have infection at presentation (*Ann Intern Med* 129:173, 1998). Typically, these patients have core temperatures higher than 40.5°C (105°F) and are comatose and anhidrotic.

B. Exertional heat stroke occurs rapidly in unacclimatized and unfit individuals who exercise in conditions of high ambient temperature and humidity. Those at risk include athletes, soldiers, and laborers, particularly if they lack access to water. Some of the risks associated with classic heat stroke may also be present, and certain congenital diseases that impair sweating may contribute. The core temperature may be lower than 40.5°C; 50% of patients are still sweating at presentation. Individuals with exertional heat stroke are more likely than are those with classic heat stroke to have **disseminated intravascular coagulation (DIC), lactic acidosis, and rhabdomyolysis.**

C. Diagnosis is based on the history of exposure or exercise, a core temperature usually of 40.5°C (105°F) or higher, and changes in mental status ranging from confusion to delirium and coma. Differential diagnosis includes malignant hyperthermia, neuroleptic malignant syndrome, anticholinergic poisoning, severe hyperthyroidism, sepsis, meningitis, cerebral malaria, and Rocky Mountain spotted fever.

D. Therapy

1. Immediate cooling is necessary. The best method of cooling is controversial. No study has directly compared ice water application with tepid spray. However, ice water lowers body temperature twice as quickly and is the procedure chosen when exertional heat stroke is anticipated (long distance races, military training) (*Int J Sports Med* 19:S150, 1998; *Ann Intern Med* 132:678, 2000). Wrap the patient in sheets that are continuously wetted with ice water. If response is insufficiently rapid, submerge the patient in ice water, recognizing that this may interfere with resuscitative efforts. Most emergency facilities that do not care for large numbers of heat illness cases are not equipped for this treatment. In that case, mist the patient continuously with tepid water (20–25°C). Cool the patient with a large electric fan with maximum body surface exposure. Ice packs at points of major heat transfer, such as the groin, axillae, and chest, may further speed cooling. If severely elevated core temperature does not respond to these maneuvers, gastric lavage with ice water may be helpful, although this treatment is controversial (*Crit Care Med* 15:748, 1987). Cold peritoneal lavage is not more effective than evaporative cooling. **Dantrolene sodium does not appear to be effective** (*Crit Care Med* 19:176, 1991). Shivering and vasoconstriction impair cooling and should be prevented by administration of **chlorpromazine,** 10–25 mg IM, or **diazepam,** 5–10 mg IV. Monitor core temperatures continuously by rectal probe. Tympanic membrane thermistor is more likely to be accurate in the emergency facility than in the field. Oral temperatures are unreliable and are frequently incorrectly low. Discontinue cooling measures when the core temperature reaches 39°C (102.2°F), which should ideally be achieved within 30 minutes. A temperature rebound may occur in 3–6 hours and should be retreated.

2. Baseline laboratory studies include CBC; partial thromboplastin time; prothrombin time; fibrin degradation products; electrolytes; BUN; creatinine, glucose, calcium, and creatine kinase levels; liver function tests; arterial blood gases (ABGs); urinalysis; and ECG.

3. For hypotension, administer crystalloids; if refractory, treat with vasopressors and monitor hemodynamics. Avoid pure α-adrenergic agents, as they cause vasoconstriction and impair cooling. Administer crystalloids cautiously to normotensive patients.

4. Treat rhabdomyolysis or urine output of less than 30 ml/hour with adequate volume replacement, mannitol (12.5–25.0 g IV), and bicarbonate (44–100 mEq/L in 0.45% normal saline) to promote osmotic diuresis and urine alkalinization. Despite these measures, **renal failure** may still complicate 5% of cases of classic heat stroke and 25% of cases of exertional heat stroke.

5. Hypoxemia and adult respiratory distress syndrome (ARDS) may occur. Treat as described in Chap. 9.

6. **Other complications** include seizures, which should be treated with diazepam and phenytoin. Provide supportive care for hepatic injury, CHF, and coagulopathy.

Cold-Induced Illness

Exposure to the cold may result in several different forms of injury. An important risk factor is accelerated heat loss, which is promoted by exposure to high wind or by immersion. Extended cold exposure may result from alcohol or drug abuse, injury or immobilization, and mental impairment.

I. **Chilblains** are among the mildest form of cold injury and result from exposure of bare skin to a cold, windy environment (33–60°F). The ears, fingers, and tip of the nose typically are injured, with itchy, painful erythema on rewarming. Treat with rapid rewarming, moisturizing lotions, and analgesics and instruct the patient to avoid re-exposure.

II. **Immersion injury** (trench foot) is caused by prolonged immersion (longer than 10–12 hours at a temperature <50°F). Treat by rewarming followed by dry dressings. Treat secondary infections with antibiotics.

III. **Frostnip** is the mildest form of frostbite and occurs most frequently on the distal extremities, the nose, or the ear. It is marked by tissue blanching and decreased sensitivity. **Rapid rewarming, in a water bath at 104–108°F (40–42°C),** is the treatment of choice for all forms of frostbite. The water temperature should never be hotter than 112°F.

IV. **Superficial frostbite** involves the skin and subcutaneous tissues, which are white, waxy, and anesthetic, have poor capillary refill, and are painful on thawing. The treatment of choice is rapid rewarming. Immerse the affected body part for 15–30 minutes; hexachlorophene or povidone-iodine can be added to the water bath. No deep injury ensues, and healing occurs in 3–4 weeks.

V. **Deep frostbite** involves death of skin, subcutaneous tissue, and muscle (third degree) or deep tendons and bones (fourth degree).
   A. **Diagnosis.** The tissue appears frozen and hard. On rewarming, there is no capillary filling. Healing is very slow, and demarcation of tissue with auto-amputation may occur. Diabetes mellitus, peripheral vascular disease, an outdoor lifestyle, and high altitude are additional risk factors. More than 90% of deep frostbite occurs at temperatures lower than 6.7°C (44°F) with exposures longer than 7–10 hours.
   B. **Treatment.** Treat by rapid rewarming. **Rewarming should not be started until there is no chance of refreezing.** Administer analgesics (IV opioids) as needed. Admit the patient to a surgical service. Elevate the affected extremity, prevent weight bearing, separate the affected digits with cotton wool, prevent tissue maceration by using a blanket cradle, and prohibit smoking. Update tetanus immunization. Intra-arterial vasodilators, heparin, dextran, prostaglandin inhibitors, thrombolytics, and sympathectomy are not routinely justified. Use antibiotics only for documented infection. Amputation is undertaken only after full demarcation has occurred.

VI. **Hypothermia** is defined as a core temperature of less than 35°C (95°F). Classification of severity by temperature is not universal. One scheme defines hypothermia as mild at 34–35°C, moderate at 30–34°C, and severe at less than 30°C. The most common cause of hypothermia in the United States is cold exposure due to alcohol intoxication. Another common cause is cold water immersion. Differential diagnosis and other risk factors include extremes of age, cerebrovascular accident, drug use, diabetic ketoacidosis, uremia, adrenal insufficiency, and myxedema.
   A. **Diagnosis** requires accurate monitoring of core temperature. A standard oral thermometer registers only to a lower limit of 35°C. Monitor the

patient continuously with a rectal probe with a full range of 20–40°C. Equal efficacy of ear thermistor monitoring has not been demonstrated.

B. **Signs and symptoms** vary with the temperature of the patient at presentation. All organ systems can be involved.

1. **CNS effects.** At temperatures below 32°C, mental processes are slowed and the affect is flattened. At less than 32.2°C (90°F), the ability to shiver is lost, and deep tendon reflexes are diminished. At 28°C, coma often supervenes. Below 18°C, the EEG is flat. On rewarming from severe hypothermia, central pontine myelinolysis may develop.

2. **Cardiovascular effects.** After an initial increased release of catecholamines, there is a decrease in cardiac output and heart rate with relatively preserved mean arterial pressure. ECG changes, manifest initially as sinus bradycardia with T-wave inversion and QT interval prolongation, may progress to atrial fibrillation at temperatures of less than 32°C. Osborne waves (J-point elevation) may be visible, particularly in leads II and V6. An increased susceptibility to ventricular arrhythmias occurs at temperatures below 32°C. At temperatures of less than 30°C, the susceptibility to ventricular fibrillation is increased significantly, and unnecessary manipulation or jostling of the patient should be avoided. A decrease in mean arterial pressure may also occur, and, at temperatures of less than 28°C, progressive bradycardia supervenes.

3. **Respiratory complications.** After an initial increase in minute ventilation, respiratory rate and tidal volume decrease progressively with decreasing temperature. **ABGs measured with the machine set at 37°C should serve as the basis for therapy without correction of pH and carbon dioxide tension (PCO$_2$)** (*Ann Emerg Med* 18:72, 1989). Supply supplemental oxygen.

4. **Renal manifestations.** Cold-induced diuresis and tubular concentrating defects may be seen.

C. **Laboratory evaluation** includes CBC; coagulation studies; liver function tests; BUN; electrolytes; creatinine, glucose, creatine kinase, calcium, magnesium, and amylase levels; urinalysis; ABGs; and ECG. Obtain chest, abdominal, and cervical spine radiographs to evaluate all patients with a history of trauma or immersion injury. Electrolyte abnormalities are common. Serum potassium often is increased. Elevated serum amylase may reflect underlying pancreatitis. Hyperglycemia may be noted but should not be treated, as rebound hypoglycemia may occur with rewarming. DIC may also occur.

D. **Therapeutic measures** include maintenance of the airway and oxygen administration. If intubation is required, the most experienced operator should perform it (see Chap. 9, Airway Management and Tracheal Intubation).

1. **CPR.** Conduct CPR in standard fashion. Perform simultaneous vigorous core rewarming; as long as the core temperature is severely decreased, it should not be assumed that the patient cannot be resuscitated. Reliable defibrillation requires a core temperature of 32°C or higher. **Do not begin CPR if an organized ECG rhythm is present,** as inability to detect peripheral pulses may be due to vasoconstriction, and CPR may precipitate ventricular fibrillation. Do not perform Swan-Ganz catheterization, as it may precipitate ventricular fibrillation. If ventricular fibrillation occurs, administer bretylium (5 mg/kg IV) as the agent of choice; lidocaine is an alternative. Avoid procainamide because it may precipitate ventricular fibrillation and increase the temperature that is necessary to defibrillate the patient. Monitor ECG rhythm, urine output, and, possibly, central venous pressure in all patients with an intact circulation.

2. **Rewarming.** The patient should be rewarmed with the goal of increasing the temperature by 0.5 to 2.0°C/hour, although rate of rewarming has not been shown to be related to outcome.

   a. **Passive external rewarming** depends on the patient's ability to shiver and thus generate heat. It is effective only at core temperatures of 32°C or higher. Cover the patient with blankets in a warm environment and monitor.

b. Active external rewarming includes application of heating blankets (40–45°C) or warm bath immersion. This type of therapy has been feared to cause paradoxical core acidosis, hyperkalemia, and decreased core temperature, as cold stagnant blood returns to the central vasculature, although Danish naval research supports arm and leg rewarming as effective and safe (*Aviation Space Environ Med* 70:1081, 1999). Pending further investigation, limit active rewarming to the trunk of a young, previously healthy patient with acute hypothermia and minimal pathophysiologic derangement.

c. Active core rewarming is preferred for treatment of severe hypothermia, although few data are available on outcomes (*Resuscitation* 36:101, 1998).

   (1) Heated oxygen is the initial therapy of choice for the patient whose cardiovascular status is stable. This therapeutic maneuver can be expected to raise core temperatures by 0.5 to 1.2°C/hour (*Ann Emerg Med* 9:456, 1980). Administration through an endotracheal tube results in more rapid rewarming than delivery via face mask. Administer heated oxygen through a cascade humidifier at a temperature of 45°C or lower.

   (2) IV fluids can be heated in a microwave oven or delivered through a blood warmer; give fluids only through peripheral IV lines.

   (3) Heated nasogastric or bladder lavage is of limited efficacy because of low exposed surface area and is reserved for the patient with cardiovascular instability. **Heated peritoneal lavage** with fluid warmed to 40–45°C is more effective than is heated aerosol inhalation, but it should be reserved for patients with cardiovascular instability. Only those who are experienced in its use should perform heated peritoneal lavage, in combination with other modes of rewarming. Closed thoracic lavage with heated fluid by thoracostomy tube has been recommended (*Ann Emerg Med* 19:204, 1990) but is unproved.

   (4) Extracorporeal circulation (cardiac bypass) is used only in hypothermic individuals who are in cardiac arrest; in these cases, it may be dramatically effective. Extracorporeal circulation may raise the temperature as rapidly as 10–12°C/hour but must be performed in an ICU or operating room.

3. Medications. Give thiamine to most patients with cold exposure, as exposure due to alcohol intoxication is common. Administration of antibiotics is a controversial issue; many authorities recommend antibiotic administration for 72 hours, pending cultures. In general, those patients with hypothermia due to exposure and alcohol intoxication are less likely to have a serious underlying infection than are those who are elderly or who have an underlying medical illness.

4. Observation. Admit patients with an underlying disease, physiologic derangement, or core temperature lower than 32°C, preferably to an ICU. Discharge individuals with mild hypothermia (32–35°C) and no predisposing medical conditions or complications when they are normothermic and an adequate home environment can be ensured.

Near-Drowning

Predisposing factors include youth, inability to swim, alcohol and drug use, barotrauma (in scuba diving), head and neck trauma, and loss of consciousness associated with epilepsy, diabetes, syncope, or dysrhythmias. Near-drowning is defined as survival for at least 24 hours after submersion in a liquid medium.

I. **Pathophysiology.** Much has been made of the differences in pathophysiology between fresh- and salt-water drownings. However, the **major insults** (i.e., hypoxemia and tissue hypoxia related to V̇/Q̇ mismatch, acidosis, and hypoxic brain injury with cerebral edema) are common to both. Hypothermia, pneumonia, and, rarely, DIC, acute renal failure, and hemolysis also may occur.

II. **Treatment.** Begin with resuscitation, focusing on airway management and ventilation with 100% oxygen. Establish an IV line with 0.9% saline or lactated Ringer's solution. The Heimlich maneuver is not indicated unless upper airway obstruction is present.

A. **Immobilize the cervical spine,** as trauma may be present.

B. **Treat hypothermia** vigorously (see Cold-Induced Illness).

C. **Manage pulmonary complications.** Administer 100% oxygen initially, titrating thereafter by ABGs. Intubate the patient endotracheally and begin mechanical ventilation with positive end-expiratory pressure (PEEP) if the patient is apneic, is in severe respiratory distress, or has oxygen-resistant hypoxemia. Administer bronchodilators if bronchospasm is present.

D. **Reserve antibiotics for documented infection.** Prophylactic glucocorticoids have no role (*Heart Lung* 16:474, 1987).

E. **Manage metabolic acidosis** with mechanical ventilation, sodium bicarbonate (if the pH is persistently <7.2), and BP support.

F. **Cerebral edema** may occur suddenly within the first 24 hours and is a major cause of death. Treatment of cerebral edema does not appear to increase survival (*Crit Care Med* 14:529, 1986), and intracranial pressure monitoring does not appear to be effective. Nevertheless, if cerebral edema occurs, hyperventilate the patient to a PCO_2 of no less than 25 mm Hg, and administer mannitol (1–2 g/kg q3–4h) or furosemide (1 mg/kg IV q4–6h). Treat seizures aggressively with phenytoin. The routine administration of glucocorticoids is not recommended. Hypothermia or barbiturate "coma" is not indicated. It may be necessary to sedate and paralyze the patient to reduce oxygen consumption and facilitate intracranial pressure management.

III. **Observation.** Admit patients who have survived severe episodes of near-drowning to an ICU. Noncardiogenic pulmonary edema may still develop in those individuals with less severe immersions. Admit any patient with pulmonary signs or symptoms, including cough, bronchospasm, abnormal ABGs or oxygen saturation as measured by pulse oximetry (SpO_2), or abnormal chest radiograph. Observe the asymptomatic patient with a questionable or brief water immersion for 4–6 hours and discharge the patient if the chest radiograph and ABGs are normal (*Ann Emerg Med* 15:1084, 1986). However, if a documented long submersion, unconsciousness, initial cyanosis or apnea, or even a brief requirement for resuscitation has occurred, the patient **must be admitted for at least 24 hours.**

Overdosage

I. **Recognition of poisoning and medication overdose** requires a high index of suspicion and careful clinical evaluation. Up to 50% of all initial poisoning histories may be incorrect. The ingestion of multiple drugs is common. Seek identification of the drug or drugs ingested and their dosages from the patient's family or friends, private physician, pharmacist, and paramedical personnel. Obtain supporting materials (e.g., pill bottles) and clues regarding the timing of ingestion. Recognition of specific toxic syndromes is often helpful in directing initial management (Table 26-1). Vital signs, neurologic status, pupillary reactions, cardiovascular response, abdominal findings, and unusual odors and excreta, as well as evaluation of ABGs, serum electrolytes, and acid-base abnormalities, may suggest a particular toxin. Order baseline screening of liver and kidney function.

Table 26-1. Toxic syndromes and possible causes

Syndrome	Manifestations	Possible causes
Acquired hemo-globinopathies	Dyspnea, cyanosis, confusion or lethargy, headache	Carbon monoxide Methemoglobinemia (nitrites, phenazopyridine) Sulfhemoglobinemia
Anion-gap metabolic acidosis	Variable	Methanol Ethanol Ethylene glycol Paraldehyde Iron Isoniazid Salicylate Vacor Cyanide
Anticholinergic	Dry mouth and skin; blurred vision; mydriasis; tachycardia; generalized sunburn-like rash or flushing of skin; hyperthermia; abdominal distension; urinary urgency or retention; confusion, hallucinations, delusions, excitation, or coma	Atropine and other belladonna alkaloids Antihistamines Tricyclics Phenothiazines Jimson seeds
Cholinergic	Hypersalivation, bronchorrhea, bronchospasm, urination or defecation, neuromuscular failure, lacrimation	Acetylcholine Organophosphate insecticides Bethanechol Methacholine Wild mushrooms
Cyanide	Nausea, vomiting, collapse, coma, bradycardia, no cyanosis, decreased arteriovenous O_2 difference with severe metabolic acidosis	Cyanide Amygdalin
Extrapyramidal	Dysphoria and dysphagia, trismus, oculogyric crisis, rigidity, torticollis, laryngospasm	Prochlorperazine Haloperidol Chlorpromazine and other antipsychotics Other phenothiazines
Narcotic	CNS depression, respiratory depression, miosis, hypotension	Morphine and heroin Codeine Propoxyphene Other synthetic and semisynthetic opiates

Table 26-1. (continued)

Syndrome	Manifestations	Possible causes
Salicylism	Fever, hyperpnea, respiratory alkalosis or mixed acid-base disturbance, hypokalemia, tinnitus	Aspirin Other salicylate products
Sympathomimetic	Excitation, hypertension, cardiac arrhythmias, seizures	Amphetamines Cocaine Caffeine Aminophylline β-Agonists, inhaled or injected

Source: Modified from G Quick, PJ Crocker. Toxic emergency: agent unknown. *Emerg Decisions* 7:44, 1986. Reprinted with permission from Physicians World/Thomson Healthcare, Seacaucus, NJ.

Screening of blood, urine, and gastric aspirate for specific toxic agents is important, but, in most cases, therapy must proceed before such results are available. Abdominal radiography may be useful in detecting retained pills (such as iron). Obtain an ECG and monitor the cardiac rhythm continuously until the ingested agent is identified and thereafter as appropriate. Perform a pregnancy test in women of childbearing years. Although the computerized *Poisindex* (2000) system is helpful, seek additional specific advice from the regional poison control center.

II. Supportive care is crucial.
   A. Maintain a patent airway and adequate ventilation. Intubate the trachea if airway protection is required.
   B. Hypotension usually responds to IV fluids, although vasopressors may be required in refractory cases or in the presence of pulmonary edema. Use dopamine in most situations; choose norepinephrine for overdoses with alpha-antagonists (phenothiazines) and tricyclic antidepressants (due to the proarrhythmic effect of dopamine).
   C. Arrhythmias may be related to cardiac or autonomic effects; treatment depends on the toxin.
   D. CNS depression or coma occurs frequently. When present, administer naloxone (2 mg IV) for possible narcotic overdose, give 50% dextrose in water (50 ml IV) or determine finger-stick glucose immediately, administer thiamine (100 mg IV push) for possible Wernicke-Korsakoff syndrome, and give oxygen for possible carbon monoxide intoxication. Give flumazenil for known or suspected benzodiazepine overdose (see sec. **VII.O.2.b**). However, do not give it for unknown overdoses, as this agent may precipitate seizures in cyclic antidepressant overdose. Also, avoid flumazenil administration in patients who have ingested drugs that are known to cause seizures (cocaine, lithium, theophylline, isoniazid, cyclosporine) or who are known to have a pre-existing seizure disorder (*Clin Ther* 14:292, 1992).

III. Prevention of further drug absorption may be facilitated by gastric emptying (gastric lavage, induced emesis) or by administration of activated charcoal. Gastric emptying procedures, if used, should be initiated within 1 hour of the ingestion. Because most adult overdose patients present several hours after toxic ingestion and because the use of syrup of ipecac may delay subsequent therapy, administration of activated charcoal alone is recommended as the primary GI decontamination procedure for most patients (*Ann Emerg Med* 16:838, 1987). No difference in outcome appears to occur whether gastric emptying plus charcoal or charcoal administration alone is used (*Med J Aust* 163:345, 1995). Theoretical exceptions may include phenothiazine overdose (delayed gastric emptying) and drugs that form gastric concretions. Rapidly absorbed agents such as strychnine and cyanide are unlikely to be affected by charcoal administration.

A. **Activated charcoal** adsorbs most drugs, preventing further absorption from the GI tract. Exceptions include alkalis, arsenic, cyanide, ethanol (EtOH), lithium, ferrous sulfate, carbamate, and mineral acids. Activated charcoal also promotes efflux of selected drugs (theophylline, phenobarbital, and carbamazepine) from the blood into the bowel lumen. Give 50–100 g activated charcoal, diluted in water, as soon as possible after the toxic ingestion; prehospital administration further enhances drug recovery. Do not use it when endoscopy is contemplated. When repeated dosing is used, no more than a single dose of sorbitol or other cathartic should be given. Although multidose charcoal has been shown to increase selected drug elimination significantly, it has not yet been demonstrated in a controlled study to reduce mortality in poisoned patients. It is indicated in ingestions of life-threatening amounts of carbamazepine, phenobarbital, theophylline, dapsone, paraquat, and *Amanita phalloides* (*Clin Toxicol* 37:731, 1999; *BMJ* 319:1414, 1999). It may be of use in overdoses of amitriptyline, dextropropoxyphene, digitoxin, digoxin, disopyramide, nadolol, phenylbutazone, phenytoin, piroxicam, and sotalol. Its use in salicylate overdose is controversial. Give an initial dose of 50–100 g and give 12.5 g/hour until the patient's condition and laboratory parameters improve.

B. **Gastric emptying** can be used in patients who present soon after toxin ingestion and in other situations (see sec. **III**).

1. If the patient is obtunded or has an absent gag reflex, the **airway must be protected;** endotracheal intubation may be necessary.

2. Because there is no evidence to show that administration of **ipecac** improves outcome, and because of its many contraindications, routine use in the emergency center should be abandoned *(Clin Toxicol* 35:699, 1997). **Contraindications** to ipecac use include decreased level of consciousness, absent gag reflex, caustic ingestion, convulsions or exposure to a substance likely to cause convulsions, and medical conditions that make emesis unsafe. Do not give ipecac for ingestion of unknown toxins, as aspiration may occur if coma or seizures develop.

3. **Gastric lavage** should not be used routinely in the management of the poisoned patient. Exceptions include ingestions of a life-threatening amount of toxin when the patient presents within 60 minutes (*Clin Toxicol* 35:711, 1997) or when concretions are believed to be present. Use a large orogastric tube (No. 28–36 Fr.) for these patients. Contraindications include corrosive ingestion. Lavage should not be performed with an unprotected airway if the patient has lost airway protective reflexes or has ingested hydrocarbons with a high aspiration potential. In these cases, lavage should be performed only **after endotracheal intubation.** Lavage with 200-ml boluses of warm saline, repeated until the effluent is clear, and follow this by instillation of activated charcoal. The added efficacy of a **cathartic** is not clear and is not routinely recommended, although the *Poisindex* editorial board continues to recommend a single dose in many overdoses (*Poisindex* 8/2000). If used, give no more than a single dose. Acceptable forms include magnesium citrate, 4 ml/kg (300 ml maximum); sorbitol, 1–2 g/kg (150 g maximum); and magnesium or sodium sulfate, 25–30 g. Do not give magnesium salts to patients with renal failure. Sorbitol premixed with charcoal is available commercially.

4. **Whole-bowel irrigation** with commercially available polyethylene glycol bowel preparation solution should not be used routinely in the management of the poisoned patient (*Clin Toxicol* 35:753, 1997), as there is no conclusive evidence that it improves outcomes. Exceptions can be considered for toxic ingestions of sustained-release drugs such as β-adrenergic

antagonists, calcium channel antagonists, lithium, and theophylline. Evidence is insufficient either to support or exclude its use for iron ingestion with radiographically persistent tablets in the GI tract or body packing with heroin or cocaine. It is contraindicated in the presence of bowel obstruction, ileus, intestinal perforation, and hemodynamic instability and should not be administered to a patient with a compromised unprotected airway. Administer 1–2 L/hour to a total of 10 L; it can be discontinued earlier if the rectal effluent is clear. Obtain an abdominal x-ray to document clearance of iron or drug-containing packets.

IV. **Removal of absorbed drugs** can be achieved by enhancement of renal excretion and extracorporeal methods.

   A. **Use forced diuresis only when specifically indicated** because of the risk of causing acid-base disturbances, electrolyte abnormalities, and cerebral or pulmonary edema. Do not attempt forced diuresis in patients with renal insufficiency, cardiac disease, or existing electrolyte abnormalities. Few data support the efficacy of this procedure in improving survival.

      1. **Forced alkaline diuresis,** achieving a urinary pH of 7.5–9.0, promotes excretion of drugs that are weak acids, such as salicylates, barbital, and phenobarbital. Administer a solution of sodium bicarbonate, 44–100 mEq, added to 1 L of 0.45% saline, at 250–500 ml/hour for the first 1–2 hours. Exercise great care to avoid excessive volume expansion, especially in the elderly. Administer maintenance alkaline solution and diuretics to maintain a urinary output of 2–3 ml/kg/hour.

      2. **Forced acid diuresis** is not recommended for any agent.

   B. **Extracorporeal removal of specific toxins by dialysis or hemoperfusion** is used when (1) clinical deterioration persists despite intensive supportive therapy, (2) blood levels reach potentially lethal concentrations, (3) a risk of lethal delayed effects exists, and (4) renal or hepatic failure impairs clearance of toxin.

V. **Specific antidotes** are available that neutralize or prevent the toxic effect of certain drugs (Table 26-2). For information on the pharmacokinetics of the offending agent and specific treatment guidelines, contact the regional poison control center immediately if the drug that was ingested is known.

VI. **Disposition** must be determined. Observe even those patients with apparently trivial overdoses of potentially toxic agents for at least 4 hours before contemplating their discharge. Do not discharge any patient who has taken an intentional overdose without formal psychiatric consultation and assessment of disposition. Refer individuals who experience inadvertent recreational drug overdose for counseling and, possibly, detoxification. Patients who are considered potentially suicidal require constant one-on-one supervision while on the medical service.

VII. **Specific agents**

   A. **Acetaminophen** is a common ingredient in many analgesic and antipyretic preparations. Hepatic toxicity is due to depletion of hepatic glutathione and subsequent accumulation of a toxic intermediate metabolite, N-acetyl-p-benzoquinonimine. Toxicity usually occurs after acute ingestion of more than 140 mg/kg, or at least 7.5 g. Precise determination of probable toxicity can be obtained by plotting a plasma acetaminophen level (drawn at least 4 hours after ingestion) on a nomogram in relation to the time since ingestion (Fig. 26-1). However, nearly half of hospitalizations for acetaminophen toxicity are due to toxicity from chronic ingestion, which is increased in those with excess alcohol intake (*Acad Emerg Med* 6:1115, 1999). Unfortunately, the nomogram does not provide useful information regarding toxicity of chronic ingestion. It is also of uncertain usefulness in acute overdose of sustained-release products. In this latter situation, the Rocky Mountain Poison Center recommends that a second drug level be obtained 4–8 hours after the first; if either level falls in the toxic range, antidotal therapy is advised (*Poisindex* 8/2000).

      1. **Symptoms** during the first 24 hours include anorexia, vomiting, and diaphoresis. Hepatic enzymes begin to rise 24–36 hours after ingestion and

Table 26-2. Antidotes

Poison or toxic sign	Antidote	Adult dosage
Acetaminophen	N-Acetylcysteine	140 mg/kg PO, followed by 70 mg/kg q4h × 17 doses
Anticholinergics	Physostigmine sulfate	0.5–2.0 mg IV (IM) over 2 mins q30–60min prn
Anticholinesterases	Atropine sulfate	1–5 mg IV (IM, SC) q15min prn to drying of secretions
	Pralidoxime (2-PAM) chloride[a]	1 g IV (PO) over 15–30 mins q8–12h × 3 doses prn
Carbon monoxide	Oxygen	100%, hyperbaric
Cyanide	Amyl nitrite[b] *followed by*	Inhalation pearls for 15–30 secs every min
	Sodium nitrite[b] *followed by*	300 mg (10 ml 3% solution) IV over 3 mins, repeated in half dosage in 2 hrs if persistent or recurrent signs of toxicity
	Sodium thiosulfate	12.5 g (50 ml 25% solution) IV over 10 mins, repeated in half dosage in 2 hrs if persistent or recurrent signs of toxicity
Digoxin	Antidigoxin Fab' fragments	Acute ingestion: Dose (vials) = [ingested digoxin (mg) × 0.8]/0.5
		Chronic ingestion: Dose (vials) = [serum level (ng/ml) × weight (kg)]/100, infused in 0.9% saline over 15–30 mins; repeat if toxicity persists
Ethylene glycol	Ethanol[c]	0.6 g/kg in D5W IV (PO) over 30–45 mins, followed initially by 110 mg/kg/hr to maintain a blood level of 100–150 mg/dl
Extrapyramidal signs	Diphenhydramine hydrochloride	25–50 mg IV (IM, PO) prn
	Benztropine mesylate	1–2 mg IV (IM, PO) prn
Heavy metals (e.g., arsenic, copper, gold, lead, mercury)	Chelators[d]	
	Calcium disodium edetate (EDTA)	1 g IV (IM) over 1 hr q12h
	Dimercaprol (BAL)	2.5–5.0 mg/kg IM q4–6h
	Penicillamine	250–500 mg PO q6h
	2,3-dimercaptosuccinic acid (DMSA, Succimer)	10 mg/kg PO tid × 5 days, then bid × 14 days
Iron	Deferoxamine mesylate	1 g IM (IV at a rate ≤15 mg/kg/hr if hypotension) q8h prn

Table 26-2. (continued)

Poison or toxic sign	Antidote	Adult dosage
Isoniazid (INH)	Pyridoxine	Amount equal to estimated INH ingestion up to 5 g over 30–60 mins; any remainder by IV drip over 1–2 hrs
Methanol	Ethanol[c]	See ethylene glycol
Methemoglobinemia	Methylene blue	1–2 mg/kg (0.1–0.2 ml/kg 1% solution) IV over 5 mins, repeated in 1 hr prn
Opioids	Naloxone hydrochloride	0.4–2.0 mg IV (IM, SC, endotracheally) prn
Warfarin and related drugs	Vitamin K$_1$ (phytonadione)	10 mg IM, SC, or IV[e]
	Fresh frozen plasma	Variable

D5W = 5% dextrose in water.
Note: This table is only a guide. Antidote usage and dosage depend on the specific clinical situation. The regional poison control center should be contacted for specific therapeutic recommendations.
[a]Pralidoxime is indicated in severe organophosphate poisoning with muscle weakness or fasciculations or respiratory depression.
[b]Nitrites may have an antidotal effect in hydrogen sulfide poisoning.
[c]The requisite ethanol dose depends on prior alcohol use, liver function, and dialysis. Consult the regional poison control center for assistance.
[d]The use of a specific chelating agent or combination of agents depends on the heavy metal involved and on the clinical situation.
[e]Caution should be used when giving vitamin K$_1$ IV. It should be given over 20 mins.

peak (aspartate aminotransferase earliest) 72–96 hours after ingestion. Recovery starts after approximately 4 days unless hepatic failure develops.

2. **Treatment** includes supportive measures and GI decontamination. Do not administer ipecac, as its use will delay administration of the specific antidote.

   a. Perform gastric lavage followed by charcoal administration if the patient presents within 1 hour of ingestion. Otherwise, administer activated charcoal (see sec. **II.B.3**). Charcoal appears to provide an additional hepatoprotective effect (*Clin Toxicol* 37:753, 1999).

   b. When the history suggests that a toxic dose has been ingested, do not wait for return of the blood acetaminophen level to administer the first dose of **acetylcysteine (Mucomyst)**, a specific antidote that acts as a glutathione substrate. This antidote is most effective in preventing hepatotoxicity if given within 8 hours of ingestion and is recommended up to 24 hours; it may be helpful when administered up to 36 hours after the event if hepatotoxicity is evident (*Lancet* 335:1572, 1990).

      (1) **The initial dosage** is 140 mg/kg diluted to a 5% solution in a soft drink, juice, or water, given PO or by gastric tube; **it can be given simultaneously with charcoal** without impairment of its efficacy.

      (2) Subsequent administration (70 mg/kg q4h for a total of 17 doses) is directed by the initial plasma acetaminophen level. **If a toxic level is detected, give the full 17 doses;** if not, no further antidote is indicated. If vomiting occurs less than 1 hour after administration of the antidote, repeat the dose.

      (3) If vomiting is repetitive and interferes with acetylcysteine administration, use metoclopramide or droperidol, or administer

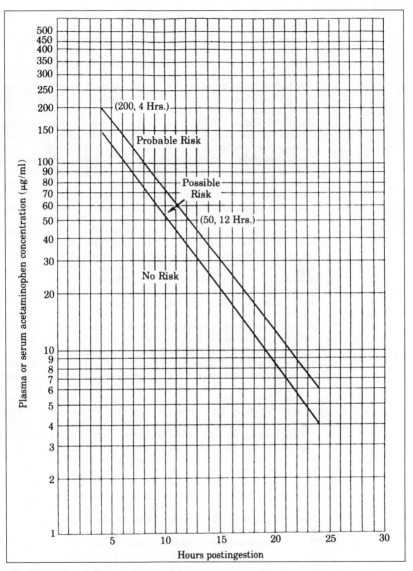

Fig. 26-1. Nomogram for acetaminophen hepatotoxicity. (Adapted from BH Rumack, RC Peterson, GG Koch, IA Amara. Acetaminophen overdose: 662 cases with evaluation of oral acetylcysteine treatment. *Arch Intern Med* 141:380, 1981.)

acetylcysteine via a fluoroscopically placed nasoduodenal tube over a period of 30–60 minutes.

(4) IV acetylcysteine is not Food and Drug Administration (FDA) approved but may be considered for those who cannot or will not take oral acetylcysteine. An IV preparation is not available in the United States but may be prepared from the inhaled formulation. Assistance in preparation and a 48-hour protocol may be obtained by contacting the Rocky Mountain Poison Center, 1-800-525-6115. It appears to be more effective than the oral protocol in preventing hepatotoxicity if begun more than 10 hours after ingestion. The initial dose is 140 mg/kg IV over 1 hour, followed by 70 mg/kg q4h for 48 hours. A 20-hour protocol is equally effective if given less than 10 hours postingestion (National Capitol Poison Center, 202-625-3333). The initial dose is 150 mg/kg IV over 15 minutes in 200 ml 5% dextrose in water (D5W), followed by 50 mg/kg in 500 ml over 4 hours, followed by 100 mg/kg in 500 ml over 16 hours. Side effects include bronchospasm, rash, flushing, and anaphylactoid reaction and are generally dose related. Flushing requires no treatment; treat urticaria with diphenhydramine, and treat angioedema and bronchospasm with diphenhydramine and systemic therapy. Give albuterol and corticosteroids for bronchospasm. Treat angioedema with diphenhydramine, epinephrine, and corticosteroids. Consider administration of IV cimetidine. Administration of acetylcysteine can be safely resumed 1 hour after successful treatment (*Ann Emerg Med* 31:710, 1998).

   c. Obtain baseline aspartate aminotransferase, alanine aminotransferase, bilirubin level, BUN, and prothrombin time, and repeat these readings at least daily for 3 days. Obtain hepatology consultation for consideration of orthotopic liver transplantation if there is biochemical evidence of hepatic failure. Transplantation is considered if the prothrombin time is greater than 100 seconds, there is grade 3–4 coma, or the pH is less than 7.3 after 24 hours.

B. Antidepressants

   1. Cyclic antidepressants. Traditional tricyclic antidepressants include amitriptyline, imipramine, desipramine, nortriptyline, doxepin, and protriptyline. Pharmacologic actions include central and peripheral anticholinergic activity, depression of myocardial contractility, slowing of intraventricular and atrioventricular conduction, and CNS effects that are similar to those of phenothiazines. Next-generation cyclic antidepressants include amoxapine and loxapine (tricyclics with diminished cardiovascular toxicity but increased propensity to severe seizures), maprotiline (a tetracyclic with greater seizure proclivity and cardiovascular toxicity similar to that of older tricyclics), mianserin (a tetracyclic with low propensity for cardiovascular or neurologic toxicity), and trazodone (a noncyclic with minimal cardiovascular and CNS toxicity). Despite the widespread use of the much safer, selective serotonin reuptake inhibitor antidepressants, overdose with cyclic antidepressants is still a leading cause of drug-related death in the United States (*Am J Emerg Med* 17:435, 1999). Overdoses of less than 20 mg/kg cause few fatalities; 35 mg/kg is the approximate median lethal dose, and overdoses in excess of 50 mg/kg are likely to result in death.

   a. Clinical manifestations include evidence of cholinergic blockade (mydriasis, ileus, urinary retention, and hyperpyrexia). **Cardiovascular toxicity** occurs as a result of anticholinergic, catecholamine-related, quinidine-like, and alpha-antagonist effects; these effects result in supraventricular and ventricular arrhythmias, including torsades de pointes, conduction blocks, hypotension, hypoperfusion, and pulmonary edema. **CNS manifestations** range from initial agitation to confusion, stupor, and coma. Seizures may occur, and the resultant metabolic acidosis may worsen cardiac toxicity.

   b. Laboratory evaluation aids in assessing the severity of the condition and in monitoring progress. Plasma levels correlate poorly with severity of symptoms, although blood levels in excess of 1000 ng/ml have a higher risk of cardiac toxicity. ABGs are useful for ensuring adequate gas exchange and for monitoring alkalinization. ECGs showing limb-lead QRS duration of greater than 100 milliseconds are predictive of seizures; duration greater than 160 milliseconds predicts ventricular dysrhythmias; a terminal 40-milliseconds QRS axis that is more rightward than 120 degrees is even more sensitive (*N Engl J Med* 313:474, 1985; *Ann Emerg Med* 18:348, 1989).

  c. **Treatment** includes supportive measures and GI decontamination. Do not administer ipecac syrup, as obtundation may occur rapidly and promote aspiration. Gastric lavage may be performed regardless of the time of presentation, as cyclic antidepressants delay gastric emptying. Repetitive administration of activated charcoal, 50 g PO or per tube q2–4h, is not recommended. Forced diuresis and hemodialysis are not indicated. Resin or charcoal hemoperfusion removes less than 1–3% of body burden, but this reduction may be associated with improvement of life-threatening cardiac or CNS complications.

  (1) **Cardiac toxicity. Continuous cardiac monitoring is mandatory.** Cyclic antidepressants are protein bound in an alkaline environment and are toxic in an acid environment. Cardiac (and CNS) toxicity therefore is enhanced by metabolic or respiratory acidosis. Initiate treatment prophylactically, as toxic complications often are refractory to therapy once they have developed. Induce **alkalinization** with IV sodium bicarbonate, 1–2 mEq/kg, to maintain an arterial pH of 7.45–7.55. Such an alkaline pH is effective in preventing and treating hypotension, arrhythmias (ventricular and supraventricular), and conduction disturbances. If the patient is intubated, hyperventilate to a PCO_2 of no lower than 25 mm Hg and an arterial pH of 7.45–7.55, as this is an effective means of alkalinization and avoids the administration of large amounts of sodium. Do not use physostigmine for arrhythmias. Manage refractory ventricular arrhythmias with lidocaine or phenytoin (see Chap. 7). **Type I antiarrhythmics** (procainamide, quinidine, or disopyramide) **are contraindicated** because of additive toxicity. Treat torsades de pointes with magnesium, isoproterenol, and atrial overdrive pacing (see Chap. 7). Use temporary ventricular pacing for complete heart block. Treat hypotension that is unresponsive to alkalinization with norepinephrine and fluid administration.

  (2) **CNS complications.** Alkalinization does not reverse CNS complications. Physostigmine (2 mg IV over 1 minute) reverses CNS depression rapidly in patients with pure cyclic antidepressant overdose. However, because repeated doses are necessary and physostigmine may cause dysrhythmias and seizures, its use generally is not recommended. Supportive care of coma usually is adequate. Treat seizures with diazepam and phenytoin. Barbiturates are preferred over phenytoin for drug-induced seizures by some but not all authorities. Status epilepticus should be treated aggressively, including the use of high-dose barbiturates, paralysis, and general anesthesia, to prevent permanent neurologic damage. Treat hyperthermia by cooling.

  (3) **Respiratory depression.** Treat this commonly occurring complication with endotracheal intubation and mechanical ventilation. Pulmonary edema and aspiration also are common.

  d. **Disposition.** Patients should be admitted to an ICU if they have a depressed level of consciousness, respiratory depression, hypotension, arrhythmia, conduction blocks (including QRS >100 milliseconds), or seizures. Observe any asymptomatic individual with a normal ECG in the emergency department and perform cardiac monitoring of such a patient for 6 hours. If the patient remains asymptomatic, the ECG remains normal, and bowel sounds are normal, the patient may safely undergo assessment for psychiatric disposition. If any signs or symptoms are present, the patient must be admitted. **Caution is imperative:** Twenty-five percent of fatalities occur in patients who are awake and alert at the time of presentation, and three-fourths of these patients are in normal sinus rhythm. After a patient's admission, criteria for discharge from an ICU include normal mental status, absence of all cyclic antidepressant symptoms, and no ECG abnormalities (including sinus tachycardia) for 24 hours. Significant arrhythmias rarely develop in a patient who meets all these criteria.

2. **Selective serotonin reuptake inhibitors** include fluoxetine, sertraline, paroxetine, fluvoxamine, and citalopram.

   a. **Symptoms.** Symptoms are usually minimal. Patients may become agitated or drowsy or, occasionally, confused. Ataxia, vertigo, tremor, delusions, or hallucinations may occur, as may nausea and emesis. Seizures are rare, occurring most often after fluoxetine or citalopram overdose (*Am J Emerg Med* 10:115, 1992; *Lancet* 347:1602, 1997). Tachycardia is noted frequently; however, ECG changes and significant cardiovascular toxicity are uncommon, although severe citalopram overdose may have QT prolongation. Fatalities are rare [*J Clin Psychiatry* 59(Suppl):42, 1998]. Simultaneous ingestion of these drugs with tricyclic antidepressants may raise plasma levels of the tricyclic. If ingested with other drugs that cause serotonin release, such as clomipramine, monoamine oxidase inhibitors, and L-tryptophan, the serotonin syndrome may result, manifested by restlessness, altered level of consciousness, diaphoresis, hyperthermia, hyperreflexia, nystagmus, and myoclonus, and may result in fatality.

   b. **Treatment. Avoid emesis.** Perform GI lavage if the patient presents less than 1 hour after ingestion, and administer charcoal, particularly if the patient is unconscious. Although cardiovascular and CNS toxicity are rare, obtain an ECG as a baseline. Admit patients who have taken large overdoses to a medical floor, particularly if they are symptomatic or if there is coingestion. Treat seizures with diazepam and phenytoin. If the patient is asymptomatic and medically stable after 6 hours of observation, psychiatric evaluation and disposition assessment can be made safely.

   c. **Serotonin syndrome** occurs most frequently after ingestion of two or more drugs that increase serotonin levels by different mechanisms. Examples include monoamine oxidase inhibitors, L-tryptophan, amphetamines, cocaine, 3,4-methylenedioxymethamphetamine (MDMA), fenfluramine, serotonin reuptake inhibitors, tricyclic antidepressants, sumatriptan, amantadine, levodopa, and bromocriptine. Symptoms include agitation, confusion, hallucinations, myoclonus, diaphoresis, tremor, shivering, diarrhea, and fever. Drowsiness may progress to coma. Seizures may occur. Autonomic effects include tachycardia, hypertension, tachypnea, mydriasis, flushing, salivation, abdominal pain, and diarrhea. **Hyperthermia** is characteristic. Rigidity, trismus, and opisthotonus may be present. Severe complications include DIC, rhabdomyolysis and renal failure, respiratory failure, and ARDS. **Treatment** is supportive with the administration of activated charcoal. Emesis should not be induced. Consider benzodiazepines for agitation and treat hyperthermia with cooling. Diazepam and phenytoin can be given for seizures. Hypertension can be treated with sedation and, if necessary, nitroprusside. If IV saline is unsuccessful for hypotension, administer norepinephrine. Protect the airway and provide ventilatory support for respiratory failure. Consider the administration of cyproheptadine, 4–8 mg q1–4h until improvement occurs or a total of 32 mg is given.

C. Cardiovascular drugs

1. β-Adrenergic antagonists

a. Symptoms. Symptoms of β-adrenergic antagonist overdose usually occur within 2 hours of ingestion. Cardiovascular manifestations include bradycardia, atrioventricular block, hypotension, and depression of cardiac function, which results in CHF. Sotalol may cause QT prolongation and torsades de pointes. Bradycardia occurs early but does not predict more serious cardiac disturbances. Although some β_1-specific agents may have little respiratory effect at the standard dosage in patients with asthma or chronic obstructive pulmonary disease, severe bronchospasm may result from ingestion of any β-adrenergic antagonist, because β_1 selectivity is lost at high doses. CNS manifestations include drowsiness, coma, hypoventilation, and seizures (caused most frequently by propranolol). Nausea and vomiting may occur, and mesenteric ischemia may be severe, particularly with propranolol ingestion, as a result of decreased cardiac output and unopposed alpha-agonist activity. β-adrenergic antagonist overdose may cause hypoglycemia by blockade of counterregulatory mechanisms and may also make more difficult the appreciation of hypoglycemic symptoms. Renal failure may occur as a result of hypotension.

b. Laboratory studies. Measurement of serum drug levels is not useful. Obtain serum glucose and electrolyte levels. Record a baseline ECG and monitor cardiac activity continuously.

c. Therapy

(1) Establish an IV line before any other therapy is undertaken.

(2) Perform gastric lavage if the patient is seen within 1 hour of ingestion and administer activated charcoal. **Do not give syrup of ipecac,** because of the rapidity with which cardiac compromise may occur. Moreover, the increase in vagal tone associated with emesis may promote cardiovascular collapse. If the patient becomes bradycardic or has other manifestations of a vagal reaction, administer up to 2 mg atropine IV. Consider multidose charcoal for sotalol ingestion.

(3) Treat hypotension with IV saline; hemodynamic monitoring may be necessary to gauge optimal fluid resuscitation. **Glucagon** (50–150 µg/kg IV over 1 minute, followed by 1–5 mg/hour in 5% dextrose) increases cardiac contractility and heart rate and is the drug of first choice for β-adrenergic antagonist overdose. Isoproterenol (2–20 mg/minute) may be useful, but high doses (≤200 mg/minute) may be necessary. If the BP does not improve or falls, add norepinephrine. Use epinephrine with caution, particularly with propranolol overdoses, because of the propensity for hypertension and reflex bradycardia. Calcium chloride 10%, 10 ml IV, may also be useful for refractory propranolol overdose. Consider intra-aortic balloon pump for refractory hypotension.

(4) For torsades de pointes associated with sotalol overdose, isoproterenol, magnesium, and overdrive pacing may be useful (see Chap. 7). A pacemaker may be necessary for severe bradycardia or heart block that is unresponsive to medications.

(5) Use β-adrenergic agonists and theophylline for bronchospasm.

(6) Treat seizures with IV benzodiazepine followed by IV phenytoin.

(7) Treat hypoglycemia with IV glucose and, if resistant, IV glucagon.

(8) Severe respiratory depression may require mechanical ventilation.

(9) Dialysis may be useful in removal of nadolol, sotalol, atenolol, and acebutolol but is ineffective for propranolol, metoprolol, and timolol.

d. Disposition. Obtain a baseline ECG and monitor the patient's rhythm for at least 6 hours, even in the absence of symptoms. If any cardiovascular, respiratory, or neurologic symptoms are present, admit the patient to an ICU for therapy and continuous monitoring. If, however, there are no toxic symptoms 6 hours after ingestion, disposition guided by psychiatric consultation can be made safely.

2. Calcium channel antagonists

a. Symptoms. Manifestations of calcium channel antagonist overdose depend on the drug ingested. Hypotension is common, as are nausea and vomiting. Severe bradycardia, atrioventricular block, and asystole are most common after verapamil and diltiazem overdose and less common with the dihydropyridines (e.g., nifedipine, nicardipine, amlodipine), which are more likely to cause reflex tachycardia. Pulmonary edema is most likely to occur after verapamil overdose, as is hypocalcemia. Lethargy, confusion, and coma are common. Seizures are most often due to verapamil, less common with diltiazem, and rare with nifedipine. Hyperglycemia occurs frequently. Cardiovascular manifestations usually are apparent within 1–5 hours postingestion and may persist for more than 24 hours. Sustained-release preparations, particularly verapamil, may cause rhythm disturbances up to 7 days after ingestion.

b. Laboratory studies. These should include serum calcium, magnesium, electrolyte, and glucose levels. Obtain an ECG and monitor the cardiac rhythm.

c. Therapy

(1) Avoid inducing emesis because of the potential for rapid cardiovascular collapse and aspiration. If the patient presents soon after ingestion, consider gastric lavage followed by administration of charcoal. Consider gastroscopy or whole-bowel irrigation with polyethylene glycol solution for removal of retained sustained-release tablets.

(2) Treat hypotension with IV 0.9% saline; if resistant, give IV dopamine. Administer 10% **calcium chloride** (10–20 ml IV) for hypotension, bradycardia, or heart block. Repeat at 10-minute intervals three to four times as necessary. Calcium gluconate (3 g) is preferred when the patient is severely acidotic. **Glucagon** (50–150 µg/kg IV over 1 minute followed by 1–5 mg/hour) may also be useful for heart block and hypotension. If hypotension is resistant to the preceding measures, arrange for placement of an intra-aortic balloon pump.

(3) Atropine (up to 2 mg IV) can also be given for bradycardia or atrioventricular block, although it rarely is successful. Isoproterenol is a less desirable alternative. Place a transvenous pacemaker for medication-resistant heart block.

(4) Treat seizures with an IV benzodiazepine (diazepam or lorazepam; see Chap. 25) and phenytoin. Hemodialysis and hemoperfusion are not useful to accelerate drug removal.

d. Disposition. Admit all patients who have cardiovascular symptoms or seizures or who have ingested a sustained-release preparation to an ICU for continuous cardiovascular monitoring. If the patient has taken a non–sustained-release preparation and is asymptomatic, obtain a baseline ECG and monitor ECG rhythm for at least 8 hours. If, at that point, the patient is completely asymptomatic and has a normal ECG, consider discharge after psychiatric consultation.

3. Digoxin (see Chap. 6 for details; for doses of Fab' fragments, see Table 26-2)

D. Caustic ingestions

1. Alkaline ingestions. These include liquid and crystalline lye, automatic dishwasher detergents, oven cleaners, hair relaxers, Clinitest tablets, and some toilet bowl cleaners. Strong alkali solutions, such as liquid drain cleaner, are the agents most commonly associated with injury.

a. **Symptoms and signs. Deep tissue injury in the aerodigestive tract is common.** Oral burns are common and may cause drooling. A lack of oral burns does not exclude esophageal injury. The overall rate of esophageal injury for alkali ingestions is 30–40%; such injury is suggested by vomiting, drooling, or stridor. Subsequent esophageal stricture may develop. Gastric injury and perforation also may occur and are much more likely with liquid lye ingestions, as the lye passes rapidly into the stomach. Crystalline lye ingestion may lead to severe upper airway injury with stridor and airway obstruction that necessitate rapid intervention. Other symptoms of alkaline ingestion include oral pain, odynophagia, chest pain, abdominal pain, nausea, and vomiting.

b. **Treatment**

   (1) **Immediately rinse the oral cavity** copiously with cold water.

   (2) **Do not induce emesis** because it may increase injury. Charcoal administration, cathartic administration, and gastric lavage are not indicated. Administration of milk obscures anatomic detail for subsequent endoscopy. Diluents are controversial and may induce emesis. *Poisindex* (8/2000) currently recommends administration of diluents (4–8 oz milk or water), although other experts strongly disagree. **Do not attempt to neutralize the alkaline agent with a weak acid,** as this results in an exothermic reaction and increases tissue damage.

   (3) Protect the airway and administer oxygen. Endotracheal intubation or early tracheostomy may be required.

   (4) Establish an IV line and give fluids guided by vital signs.

   (5) Obtain chest and abdominal radiographs for evidence of perforation (pneumomediastinum, pleural effusion, and pneumoperitoneum).

   (6) If the patient exhibits drooling, stridor, or odynophagia, consult a gastroenterologist to arrange for **immediate endoscopy;** otherwise, it can be deferred 12–24 hours. Avoid use of a nasogastric tube.

   (7) Obtain surgical consultation.

   (8) Glucocorticoid treatment of esophageal burns in an attempt to prevent stricture is controversial. Prophylactic antibiotics are not appropriate.

   (9) Obtain a barium swallow after 2–4 weeks to assess for esophageal stricture.

2. **Acids.** Common household acids include most toilet bowl cleaners, drain cleaners, metal cleaners, battery acid, and swimming pool cleaners. Tissue injury is less deep than that produced by alkaline agents. Gastric and esophageal injury, including perforation, are common.

   a. **Symptoms and signs** include oral pain, drooling, odynophagia, and abdominal pain. Occasionally, respiratory distress, DIC, hemolysis, and systemic acidosis occur.

   b. **Therapy**

      (1) The mouth should be washed copiously with cold water. Diluent administration often is recommended but has no demonstrated clinical efficacy.

      (2) Neutralization with a weak base is contraindicated. **Induction of emesis, lavage, or charcoal administration is contraindicated,** and a nasogastric tube should be avoided. Airway involvement is less likely than with alkaline ingestion.

      (3) Establish IV access and administer fluids guided by vital signs.

      (4) Sucralfate (1 g q6h) may decrease symptoms but does not appear to decrease complications or perforation.

      (5) Unsuspected esophageal and gastric burns and duodenal injury are commonly seen with endoscopy, which should be performed within 24 hours. The likelihood of stricture formation (pyloric or esophageal) and perforation depends on the severity of ingestion.

(6) Obtain an upright chest x-ray to detect perforation, and arrange surgical consultation.

(7) The administration of glucocorticoids is controversial, but their use probably is of no added benefit. Prophylactic antibiotics are not recommended.

(8) Obtain an upper GI radiograph after 2–4 weeks.

E. EtOH and other alcohols

1. **EtOH.** The toxicity of EtOH is dose related, but tolerance varies widely, based on prior exposure. Blood levels in excess of 100 mg/dl are associated with ataxia, whereas at 200 mg/dl patients are drowsy and confused. At levels in excess of 400 mg/dl, respiratory depression is common, and death is possible.

   a. **Laboratory studies.** These should include electrolytes, glucose level, serum osmolality, and blood EtOH level. The blood EtOH level may be rapidly estimated by calculating the osmolal gap (measured osmolality minus calculated osmolality) (see Chap. 3). **The blood EtOH level in mg/dl equals 4.6 times the osmolal gap,** in the absence of other low-molecular-weight toxins.

   b. **Treatment.** If the patient's mental status is severely depressed, insert an endotracheal tube before performing gastric lavage if the patient presents less than 1 hour after ingestion. Charcoal is not helpful due to the rapid absorption of EtOH from the stomach. Hemodialysis may be useful for life-threatening overdoses. Administer 100 mg thiamine IV followed by 50 ml 50% dextrose in water IV to any **comatose alcoholic patient.** Admit patients with alcohol intoxication if they have severe underlying illness or significant alcoholic ketoacidosis or if ventilatory support is required. Observe other patients until they are sober (blood alcohol level <100 mg/dl) or can be discharged to the care of a responsible sober adult.

2. **Isopropyl alcohol (IPA).** Most rubbing alcohol is 70% IPA. IPA is more toxic than EtOH at any blood level (50 mg/dl = intoxication, 100–200 mg/dl = stupor and coma). Respiratory depression and hypotension occur at high blood levels. Other symptoms include nausea, vomiting, and abdominal pain.

   a. **Laboratory evaluation.** Workup commonly reveals ketosis without acidosis (IPA is metabolized to acetone). Metabolic acidosis usually is related to associated hypotension. IPA concentration in the blood can be measured directly or can be estimated in the same fashion as for EtOH (see sec. **VII.E.1.a**), substituting a multiplier of 6.0 for 4.6. Absence of an osmolal gap does not exclude IPA ingestion. Measure plasma glucose, as hypoglycemia may occur, particularly in children.

   b. **Therapy.** Do not induce emesis, as mental status may decline rapidly, with subsequent aspiration. Gastric lavage followed by charcoal administration may be useful if performed within 60 minutes of ingestion. For cutaneous exposures, wash the skin and remove contaminated clothes. Maintain an adequate airway and support blood pressure. Hemodialysis is reserved for patients with persistent hypotension despite supportive therapy.

3. **Methanol (MeOH).** MeOH is in gas-line antifreeze, carburetor fluid, duplicator fluid, and windshield washer fluid. Sterno contains EtOH and MeOH, and the EtOH that is present may delay manifestations of MeOH toxicity. The toxicity of MeOH is due to its conversion by alcohol dehydrogenase to formaldehyde and then by acetaldehyde dehydrogenase to formic acid. Initial symptoms may include lethargy and confusion, followed by an apparent hangover. Toxic symptoms, which may be delayed 18–24 hours, include headache, visual symptoms (blurring, diminished acuity, and whiteness in the visual field), nausea, vomiting,

Table 26-3. Fomepizole administration during dialysis

Time from last dose	Dose
	Beginning of dialysis
<6 hrs	None
>6 hrs	Give next scheduled dose
	During dialysis
	Maintenance dose q4h
	At conclusion of dialysis
<1 hr	None
1–3 hrs	One-half of next scheduled dose
>3 hrs	Give next scheduled dose

abdominal pain, tachypnea, and respiratory failure. Coma and convulsions may occur in severe MeOH intoxication.

a. Examination. Typically, examination reveals an uncomfortable patient who may be remarkably tachypneic with decreased visual acuity; optic disk hyperemia may be hard to appreciate. Laboratory studies should include CBC, electrolytes, BUN, creatinine, amylase, urinalysis, EtOH, and MeOH levels, and ABGs, which reveal a severe anion-gap metabolic acidosis. The range of toxic ingestion is 15–400 ml. In general, pH and acid-base status are better predictors of toxicity than is the absolute MeOH level. The MeOH level (in mg/dl) can be estimated in the same way as for EtOH (see sec. **VII.E.a**), substituting a multiplier of 3.2 for 4.6.

b. Treatment. Consider gastric lavage if the patient is seen less than 1 hour after ingestion. Charcoal does not absorb significant amounts of MeOH.

(1) Give **folinic acid** (leucovorin), 1 mg/kg (maximum, 50 mg) IV, followed by folic acid, 1 mg/kg IV q4h for six doses, to increase the metabolism of formate. IV $NaHCO_3$ for severe acidosis may reduce permanent vision damage.

(2) 4-Methylpyrazole (fomepizole; an alcohol dehydrogenase antagonist) (*J Emerg Med* 8:455, 1990) is used routinely in Europe and is available in the United States. It is not FDA approved for the treatment of MeOH toxicity, and no direct comparison with EtOH has been made. Nevertheless, it appears to be effective and is more easily administered than EtOH, although much more expensive. The dosage is 15 mg/kg IV followed by 10 mg/kg IV q12h for four doses. This should be followed by 15 mg/kg IV q12h until the MeOH level is less than 20 mg/dl. During hemodialysis the dosing interval should be changed to q4h (Table 26-3).

(3) EtOH delays metabolism of MeOH to its toxic metabolites by competing for alcohol dehydrogenase. Administer EtOH for the following indications: peak MeOH level in excess of 20 mg/dl, while awaiting levels for an ingestion suspected of being MeOH, or an anion-gap metabolic acidosis after suspicious ingestion. The **loading dose of EtOH** is 7.6–10.0 ml/kg of a 10% solution, given IV, or 0.8–1.0 ml/kg of 95% alcohol, administered PO in orange juice. EtOH (10%) for IV infusion can be prepared by removing 50 ml from a stock 5% EtOH solution and replacing this with 50 ml absolute alcohol, or by removing 100 ml D5W from a 1-L bag and

Table 26-4. Maintenance ethanol dosage regimens for ethylene glycol and methanol intoxication

	10% Ethanol IV (ml/kg/hr)	40% Ethanol PO (ml/kg/hr)	95% Ethanol PO (ml/kg/hr)	Hemodialysis with 10% ethanol IV* (ml/kg/hr)
Moderate drinker	1.4	0.3	0.15	3.3
Chronic drinker	2.0	0.4	0.2	3.9
Nondrinker	0.8	0.2	0.1	2.7

*Dialysate bath concentration of 100 mg/dl preferable.
Source: Modified with permission from E Kuffner, KM Hurlbut. Methanol (management/treatment protocol). In: BH Rumack, DG Spoerke, eds. *Poisindex Information System.* Denver: Micromedex, 2000.

replacing it with 100 ml absolute alcohol. Maintenance dosage varies depending on previous alcohol exposure (Table 26-4). The goal is achievement of a blood alcohol level of 100–150 mg/dl to saturate the available alcohol dehydrogenase and prevent formation of MeOH's toxic metabolites. Check EtOH levels 1 hour after the loading dose and at least two to three times a day during maintenance infusion (some authorities recommend hourly levels). Administer EtOH continuously until the MeOH level is less than 10 mg/dl, the formate level is less than 1.2 mg/dl, there is resolution of acidosis, CNS symptoms abate, and a normal anion gap is restored. If MeOH levels cannot be readily measured, administer EtOH for at least 9 days without dialysis (or 1 day with dialysis) and until clinical findings resolve (*Poisindex* 8/2000).

    (4) Hemodialysis generally is indicated for an MeOH level that exceeds 50 mg/dl, severe and resistant acidosis, renal failure, or visual symptoms.

F. Ethylene glycol (EG) and diethylene glycol are used commonly in antifreeze and windshield deicer. Various metabolites are responsible for toxicity. **Initial symptoms** resemble alcohol intoxication. Vomiting is common. CNS depression, seizures, or coma may occur. CHF and pulmonary edema may occur 12–36 hours after ingestion. Death is most likely in this stage. Oliguric renal failure (from oxalate crystal deposition) may occur 24–72 hours after ingestion. Associated flank pain may be prominent.

    1. Laboratory findings. Obtain electrolyte, BUN, and creatinine levels, serum osmolality, ABGs, urinalysis, and EtOH and EG levels. Findings include a severe metabolic acidosis with an anion gap, an osmolal gap, and oxalate and hippurate crystalluria. Fluorescein often is added to antifreeze, and urine fluorescence detected with a Wood's lamp up to 6 hours after ingestion is diagnostic (*Ann Emerg Med* 19:663, 1990).

    2. Treatment

        a. Neither gastric lavage nor charcoal administration is likely to be effective but should be considered if the patient presents within 1 hour of ingestion, particularly if the ingestion is mixed. Avoid magnesium salt cathartics because of the likelihood of renal failure.

        b. Correct life-threatening acidosis with IV sodium bicarbonate pending dialysis. Administer 1–3 mEq/kg IV and titrate to achieve a normal pH. Monitor the calcium level, as hypocalcemia may result.

        c. Indications for IV EtOH (although not FDA approved and never studied prospectively; see sec. **VII.E.3.b.(3)** and Table 26-4) include an EG level in excess of 20 mg/dl, a suspected EG ingestion (while levels are being awaited), or an anion-gap metabolic acidosis with a history of EG ingestion, regardless of level. It should be continued until the EG level is 0, or less than 20 with no symptoms and a normal pH. An EtOH level of at least 100 mg/dl should be maintained.

  d. Administer pyridoxine (100 mg IV qd) to promote the conversion of glyoxylate to glycine and **thiamine** (100 mg IV qd) to promote the formation of nontoxic alpha-hydroxy-beta-ketoadipic acid.

  e. Dialysis is highly effective in severe cases; EtOH infusion should be continued during dialysis. Indications for dialysis include a glycol level in excess of 50 mg/dl (unless the patient is being given 4-methylpyrazole and the patient is asymptomatic with a normal pH), electrolyte abnormalities that are unresponsive to standard therapy, deteriorating vital signs despite supportive therapy, renal failure, or a pH of less than 7.25–7.30 that is unresponsive to therapy (*Clin Toxicol* 37:537, 1999). Discontinue dialysis when the glycol level is less than 10 mg/dl, the glycolic acid level is undetectable, and the acidosis, clinical status, and anion gap have returned to normal. EG levels can be estimated as for alcohol, using 6.2 as the multiplier of the osmolal gap (see sec. **VII.E.1.a**). When levels cannot be measured easily, continue EtOH administration for at least 3 days without hemodialysis (or for 1 day with hemodialysis) and until clinical findings resolve, whichever is longer (*Poisindex* 8/2000). Measure EtOH levels after the loading dose and two to three times a day during maintenance therapy.

  f. 4-Methylpyrazole (fomepizole) (*N Engl J Med* 340:879, 1998; *N Engl J Med* 340:832, 1998) has been approved by the FDA for use in EG poisoning. It should be strongly considered as an alternative to EtOH therapy when coingestants are causing diminished level of consciousness that might be confounded by EtOH administration, when the ICU facilities or laboratory are inadequate to monitor EtOH therapy, when active hepatic disease is present, or when there are other contraindications to EtOH administration. The dosing is similar to the treatment of MeOH poisoning [see sec. **VII.E.3.b(2)**]. Treatment with 4-methylpyrazole should continue until the EG level is less than 20 mg/dl (*Clin Toxicol* 37:537, 1999).

G. Hydrocarbon ingestions are characterized by GI upset, pulmonary aspiration, and CNS alterations. Morbidity and mortality usually are attributed to pulmonary aspiration. Low viscosity (e.g., kerosene, gasoline, and liquid furniture polish) is associated with greater aspiration potential. Motor oil, transmission oil, mineral oil, baby oil, and suntan oil usually are nontoxic.

  1. Clinical manifestations usually are apparent within the first 6 hours and include vomiting, chest or abdominal pain, cough, dyspnea, low-grade fever, arrhythmias, an altered sensorium, seizures, and radiographic evidence of aspiration pneumonitis or pulmonary edema.

  2. Treatment of nontoxic hydrocarbon ingestion is not required in the absence of symptoms. These agents have high aspiration potential but are associated with little or no GI absorption. Gastric emptying is never necessary. Obtain chest radiographs only if patients have pulmonary symptoms. Such patients can be discharged after 6 hours if they are asymptomatic. Hospitalize patients with an abnormal chest radiograph or ABGs and treat them supportively.

  a. Initiate treatment of toxic hydrocarbon ingestion by removing contaminated clothing and washing the affected skin to prevent dermatitis and percutaneous absorption.

  b. Provide **supplemental oxygen** to patients with significant aspiration injuries.

  c. Gastric emptying, although controversial, is recommended for ingestion of toxic hydrocarbons, particularly halogenated hydrocarbons (trichloroethylene, carbon tetrachloride, methylene chloride) or those that contain toxic additives (e.g., heavy metals, insecticides, nitrobenzene, aniline, or camphor), although some authorities recommend only administration of activated charcoal. Other potentially toxic hydrocarbons (gasoline, benzene, kerosene, lighter fluid, paint thinner, and toluene), except for large suicidal ingestions, do not require gastric emptying. If gastric emptying is performed, this is one of the few potential indications for ipecac, as aspiration appears to be less frequent with the use of ipecac than after gastric lavage. Therefore, in alert patients, induce emesis with ipecac, 30 ml PO. Perform gastric lavage after intubation with a cuffed endotracheal tube in any patient with CNS depression, a depressed gag reflex, or seizures.

  d. Observe the patient for at least 6 hours after gastric decontamination. Hospitalize patients who are lethargic or have pulmonary symptoms or an abnormal pulmonary examination, ABGs, or chest radiograph.

  e. Prophylactic antibiotics or glucocorticoids are not indicated.

H. Lithium is administered as a carbonate or citrate salt for the treatment of psychiatric disease, principally bipolar disorder. Overdose often is suicidal. Excretion is renal. States of dehydration and sodium uptake promote lithium retention and toxicity, as does thiazide diuretic use.

  1. Symptoms are loosely related to blood level in acute overdose. Therapeutic blood levels range between 0.6 and 1.2 mEq/L. At less than 2.5 mEq/L, symptoms are mild and consist of tremor, ataxia, nystagmus, and lethargy. Between 2.5 and 3.5 mEq/L, the patient may be agitated and confused and have fasciculations, nausea, vomiting, and diarrhea. Levels in excess of 3.5 mEq/L are associated with seizures, coma, cardiac arrhythmias, hypotension, noncardiogenic pulmonary edema, nephrogenic diabetes insipidus, and death. Levels associated with severe symptoms may be lower in those with chronic ingestion.

  2. Laboratory studies entail checking electrolytes, creatinine, and lithium level. Obtain an ECG and monitor the patient continuously while he or she is being evaluated and treated. Electrolytes may reveal a low anion gap with elevated bicarbonate, and there may be evidence of diabetes insipidus. Lithium levels should be measured repetitively until at least two sequential levels show continued decline.

  3. Treatment

  a. Consider gastric lavage if the patient presents within 1 hour of ingestion. Charcoal does not bind lithium; sodium polystyrene sulfonate (15 g PO qid or 30–50 g per rectum) can decrease absorption (*Ann Emerg Med* 21:1308, 1992). Sustained-release preparations may form concretions. If levels continue to rise despite treatment, perform whole-bowel irrigation with commercial polyethylene glycol solution, 2 L/hour for 5 hours.

  b. Establish IV access and hydrate with 0.9% saline to achieve euvolemia. Avoid dehydration, as this promotes renal lithium reabsorption. Treat arrhythmias in standard fashion (see Chap. 7).

  c. Criteria for dialysis are inexact. Consult a nephrologist for consideration of hemodialysis (preferably with a bicarbonate rather than acetate bath) for the following indications: blood level that exceeds 3.5–4.0 mEq/L after an acute ingestion, chronic toxicity with a blood level of more than 2.5 mEq/L, worsening mental status, seizures, dysrhythmias, pulmonary edema, and renal failure. The goal is achievement of a sustained level of 1 mEq/L 8 hours after dialysis, which may necessitate prolonged or repeated dialysis.

I. Methemoglobinemia can be caused by nitrites, nitroprusside, nitroglycerin, chlorates, sulfonamides, aniline dyes, nitrobenzene, antimalarials, and phenazopyridine. Methemoglobinemia has also been reported after benzocaine topical anesthesia for endoscopy as well as other topical anesthetics (*Am J Med Sci* 318:415, 1999*)* and after dapsone therapy (*Ann Pharmacother* 32:549, 1998). Symptoms include headache, fatigue, lethargy, dyspnea, tachycardia, and dizziness. The patient may be hypotensive owing to the vasodilating properties of nitrates as well as tissue hypoxia. Seizures may occur.

1. The **diagnosis** is suggested in patients with a normal oxygen tension and generalized cyanosis (suggesting a methemoglobin level of 15%) that does not respond to oxygen. Measured arterial oxygen saturation that is much lower than that calculated for the alveolar oxygen tension also is suspicious for methemoglobinemia. Final confirmation rests with measurement of a methemoglobin level. Blood levels exceeding 50% indicate severe toxicity, often associated with CNS depression, seizures, coma, and arrhythmias; levels higher than 70% are often fatal.

2. **Treatment** includes supplemental oxygen. **Do not give ipecac** because seizures may occur and promote aspiration. Consider gastric lavage (with airway protection) if the patient presents within 1 hour of ingestion or has coma or seizures. Administer activated charcoal. If signs of hypoxia are present or if the methemoglobin level exceeds 30%, administer **methylene blue,** 1–2 mg/kg in a 1% solution IV over 5 minutes. The dose can be repeated in 1 hour if signs of hypoxia persist and q4h thereafter to a maximum dose of 7 mg/kg. Treat seizures with a benzodiazepine and phenytoin. Treat hypotension with IV fluids and, if resistant, with dopamine. Hospitalize the patient in an ICU if he or she is symptomatic or if the methemoglobin level is greater than 20%. Hyperbaric oxygen and exchange transfusion are extreme measures for severely symptomatic patients.

J. **Opioids**

1. **Symptoms** of opioid overdose are respiratory depression, a depressed level of consciousness, and miosis. However, the pupils may be dilated with acidosis or hypoxia or after overdoses with meperidine or diphenoxylate plus atropine. Overdose with alpha-methylfentanyl ("China white") may result in negative toxicology screens. Heroin may be adulterated with scopolamine, cocaine, or caffeine, complicating the clinical picture. Less common complications include hypotension, bradycardia, and pulmonary edema. Be aware of body packers, who smuggle heroin in their intestinal tracts. Deterioration of latex or plastic containers may result in drug release and death (*Am J Forensic Med Pathol* 18:312, 1997).

2. **Treatment** includes airway maintenance, ventilatory and circulatory support, and prevention of further drug absorption. Emesis is contraindicated. Gastric lavage can be considered for oral ingestions that present within 1 hour; administer activated charcoal. Whole-bowel irrigation may be safe and effective for body packers; surgery is not indicated except for obstruction (*Vet Hum Toxicol* 33:353, 1991). **Naloxone hydrochloride** specifically reverses opioid-induced respiratory and CNS depression and hypotension. The initial dose is 2 mg IV; large doses may be required to reverse the effects of propoxyphene, diphenoxylate, buprenorphine, or pentazocine. In the absence of an IV line, naloxone can be administered sublingually (*Ann Emerg Med* 16:572, 1987) or via endotracheal tube. Isolated opioid overdose is unlikely if there is no response to a total of 10 mg naloxone. Repetitive doses may be required (duration of action is 45 minutes), and this should prompt hospitalization despite the patient's return to an alert status. If the patient is alert and asymptomatic for 6 hours after an oral ingestion and a single dose of naloxone, or for 4 hours after treatment for an IV overdose, he or she can be discharged safely. Methadone overdose may require therapy for 24–48 hours, whereas levo-alpha-acetylmethadol may require therapy for 72 hours. A continuous IV drip that provides two-thirds of the initial dose of naloxone hourly, diluted in D5W, may be necessary to maintain an alert state (*Ann Emerg Med* 15:566, 1986). Body packers should be

admitted to an ICU for close monitoring of the respiratory rate and level of consciousness. Ventilatory support should be provided for the patient who is unresponsive to naloxone and for pulmonary edema.

K. Organophosphates are responsible for a number of human poisonings, particularly in developing countries. Parathion and malathion are the most common insecticides involved; they often are contained in hydrocarbon solvent. Suicidal ingestion and agricultural exposure, including dermal absorption, occur.

   1. Diagnosis and routine laboratory measurements. Toxic manifestations are due to inhibition of acetylcholinesterase in the nervous system. **Muscarinic manifestations** include miosis, increased lacrimation, blurred vision, bronchospasm, bronchorrhea, diaphoresis, salivation, bradycardia, hypotension, urinary incontinence, and increased GI motility, manifested by cramps, nausea, vomiting, and diarrhea. Among **the nicotinic manifestations** are fasciculations, muscle weakness, hypotension, cramps, and respiratory paralysis. CNS toxicity is characterized by anxiety, slurred speech, mental status changes (e.g., delirium, coma, and seizures), and respiratory depression. Complications of ingestion include pulmonary edema, aspiration pneumonia, chemical pneumonitis, delayed polyneuropathy, and ARDS. Nonketotic hyperglycemia and glucosuria are common. Hyperamylasemia may reflect pancreatitis. Red cell cholinesterase and plasma pseudocholinesterase levels are decreased; activities of less than 50% of baseline are associated with poor outcome.

   2. Treatment. Apply measures to support ventilation and circulation, decontaminate the skin, and consider gastric lavage if presentation is within 1 hour of ingestion; **induction of emesis is contraindicated.** Administer activated charcoal. Monitor ABGs and ECG; QTc prolongation is associated with a worse prognosis.

     a. Atropine (preservative free) is the drug of choice for organophosphate toxicity. Give an initial dose of 1 mg IV; if the patient experiences no adverse effects, repeat a dose of 2 mg q15min until atropinization (as manifested by drying of secretions, tachycardia, flushing, dry mouth, and dilated pupils) occurs. The average patient requires approximately 40 mg/day, but larger doses (500–1500 mg/day) may be necessary. Intermittent administration may have to be continued for at least 24 hours until the organophosphate is metabolized. Severe cases may require several days or more of therapy, because of slow regeneration of acetylcholinesterase activity. Atropine will not reverse the muscle weakness.

     b. Give **pralidoxime,** 1–2 g IV in 500 ml normal saline over 30 minutes, which reactivates the cholinesterase and counteracts weakness, muscle fasciculations, and respiratory depression. Repeat administration q6–12h to a maximum of 12 g in 24 hours. An alternative is continuous infusion at 500 mg/hour as needed for several days. Unlike organophosphates, carbamate intoxications do not irreversibly inhibit cholinesterase and thus pralidoxime is not usually required and may worsen symptoms.

     c. Treat **seizures** with a benzodiazepine and phenytoin; if severe seizures require muscle relaxants, **do not use succinylcholine,** which may result in prolonged paralysis.

     d. Hemoperfusion should be considered for severe parathion overdoses.

     e. Support respiratory failure with mechanical ventilation.

L. Phencyclidine is a dissociative anesthetic and is available illicitly, mislabeled as LSD, mescaline, psilocybin, and tetrahydrocannabinol.

   1. Symptoms that occur even with small ingestions include agitation, hallucinations, bizarre or violent behavior, hypertension, tachycardia, and horizontal or vertical nystagmus. Patients are relatively impervious to pain and may be catatonic or self-destructive and difficult to subdue. Stupor progressing to coma, hypertension, hyperpyrexia, hypertonicity, and bronchospasm characterizes moderate ingestions. Massive ingestions may lead to hypotension, respiratory failure, rhabdomyolysis, and acute tubular necrosis. Hypoglycemia is common, and death may occur.

2. **Treatment** is primarily supportive. Monitor electrolytes, creatinine, and creatine phosphokinase (CPK). Minimize sensory input and remove potentially injurious objects from the area. Use diazepam to control agitation; give haloperidol if the agitation is severe. Treat dystonic reactions with diphenhydramine. Control adrenergic manifestations (e.g., hypertension) with β-adrenergic blockade if bronchospasm is not present; sodium nitroprusside may be required in severe cases. Ipecac is contraindicated. Gastric lavage may provoke violent behavior and is recommended only in severe poisonings and only after the airway has been protected. In that case, repeated charcoal administration also may interrupt enterogastric and enterohepatic circulations but has not been demonstrated to have an effect on outcome. Acid diuresis no longer is recommended. Avoid restraints, as they may increase rhabdomyolysis. Treat hyperthermia with cooling and hydration. Seizures are uncommon in adults; treat with benzodiazepines and phenytoin. Consider discharging any patient with low-dose intoxication from the emergency department after his or her symptoms resolve and psychiatric consultation has been obtained. Hospitalize patients with more severe intoxication.

M. Neuroleptics

1. Chlorpromazine, thioridazine, prochlorperazine, haloperidol (a butyrophenone), and thiothixene are the most commonly used **phenothiazines.**

   a. **Overdoses** are characterized by agitation or delirium, which may progress rapidly to coma. Pupils may be mydriatic, and deep tendon reflexes are depressed. Seizures and disorders of thermoregulation, particularly hyperthermia, may occur. Frank neuroleptic malignant syndrome may complicate use of these agents. Hypotension (due to strong α-adrenergic antagonism), tachycardia, arrhythmias (including torsades de pointes), and depressed cardiac conduction occur. Measuring blood levels is not helpful. Radiographs may reveal pill concretions present in the stomach despite apparently effective gastric emptying.

   b. **Treatment** includes airway protection, respiratory and hemodynamic support, and administration of activated charcoal. Emesis is contraindicated. Consider gastric lavage, which may be effective hours later owing to delayed gastric emptying caused by the phenothiazines. Monitor the cardiac rhythm and treat ventricular arrhythmias with lidocaine and phenytoin; class Ia agents (e.g., procainamide, quinidine, disopyramide) are contraindicated. Treat hypotension with IV fluid administration and α-adrenergic vasopressors (norepinephrine). Dopamine is an acceptable alternative. Paradoxical vasodilatation may occur in response to epinephrine administration because of unopposed β-adrenergic response in the setting of strong α-adrenergic antagonism. Recurrent torsades de pointes may require magnesium, isoproterenol, or overdrive pacing (see Chap. 7). Treat seizures with diazepam and phenytoin. Treat hyperthermia with cooling. Forced diuresis, hemodialysis, and hemoperfusion are not useful. Admit those patients who have ingested a significant overdose for cardiac monitoring for at least 48 hours.

2. **Clozapine** is an atypical neuroleptic.

   a. **Overdose** is characterized by altered mental status, ranging from somnolence to coma (*Pharm Med* 6:169, 1992). Anticholinergic effects occur, including blurred vision, dry mouth (although hypersalivation may occur in overdose), lethargy, delirium, and constipation. Seizures occur in a minority of overdoses. Coma may occur. Physical manifestations include hypotension, tachycardia, fasciculations, tremor, and myoclonus. Agranulocytosis may result. ECG abnormalities are unusual, but atrioventricular block may occur. Serious dysrhythmias rarely occur.

   b. **Treatment.** Monitor BP and respiratory status, including ABGs if respiratory depression occurs. Obtain an ECG and monitor the cardiac rhythm continuously. Obtain WBC and liver function tests. Induction of emesis is contraindicated. Perform gastric lavage if the patient presents within 1 hour of ingestion. Treat hypotension with crystalloids; if resistant, treat with norepinephrine or dopamine. Treat seizures with benzodiazepines and phenytoin. Provide ventilatory support for respiratory failure. There is no evidence that forced diuresis, hemodialysis, or hemoperfusion is beneficial. Filgrastim can be given for agranulocytosis. Admit and monitor patients with severely symptomatic overdoses for 24 hours or more.

3. **Olanzapine** is an atypical antipsychotic that is similar to clozapine.

   a. **Overdose** is characterized by somnolence, slurred speech, ataxia, vertigo, nausea, and vomiting (*Ann Emerg Med* 34:279, 1999). Anticholinergic effects occur, including blurred vision, dry mouth, and tachycardia. Seizures are uncommon. Coma may occur. Physical manifestations include hypotension, tachycardia, and pinpoint pupils unresponsive to naloxone. Serious dysrhythmias rarely occur.

   b. **Treatment.** Induction of emesis is contraindicated. Consider gastric lavage if presentation is within 1 hour of ingestion. Give activated charcoal. Treat hypotension with fluids and, if ineffective, norepinephrine or dopamine. Give benzodiazepines and phenytoin for seizures. Provide ventilatory support for the unusual manifestation of respiratory failure.

N. **Salicylate** toxicity may result from acute ingestion or chronic intoxication. Toxicity is usually mild after acute ingestions of less than 150 mg/kg, moderate after ingestions of 150–300 mg/kg, and generally severe with overdoses of 300–500 mg/kg. Toxicity from chronic ingestion typically is due to intake of more than 100 mg/kg/day over a period of several days and usually occurs in elderly patients with chronic underlying illness. Diagnosis often is delayed in this group of patients, and mortality is approximately 25%. Significant toxicity owing to chronic ingestion may occur with blood levels lower than those associated with acute ingestions.

   1. **Symptoms.** Nausea, vomiting, tinnitus (implying levels >300 mg/L), hyperpnea, and malaise can occur. Fever suggests a poor prognosis in adults. Severe intoxications are associated with lethargy, convulsions, and coma, which may result from cerebral edema. Noncardiogenic pulmonary edema occurs in up to 30% of adults and is more common with chronic ingestion, cigarette smoking, neurologic symptoms, and older age.

   2. **Laboratory data**

      a. Obtain a CBC, electrolyte, BUN, creatinine, and blood glucose levels and prothrombin and partial thromboplastin times. Prothrombin time prolongation is common.

      b. **ABGs** may reveal an early respiratory alkalosis, followed by metabolic acidosis. Approximately 20% of patients exhibit either respiratory alkalosis or metabolic acidosis alone (*J Crit Illness* 1:77, 1986). Most adults with pure salicylate overdose have a primary metabolic acidosis and a primary respiratory alkalosis. After mixed overdoses, respiratory acidosis may become prominent (*Arch Intern Med* 138:1481, 1978).

      c. **Hypoglycemia,** common in children, is rare in adults.

      d. **Blood levels** must be drawn 6 hours or more after acute ingestion of salicylates to allow prediction of severity of intoxication and patient disposition (Fig. 26-2). Obtaining earlier levels is appropriate in severely intoxicated patients, to guide intervention. Levels in excess of 70 mg/dl at any time represent moderate to severe intoxication;

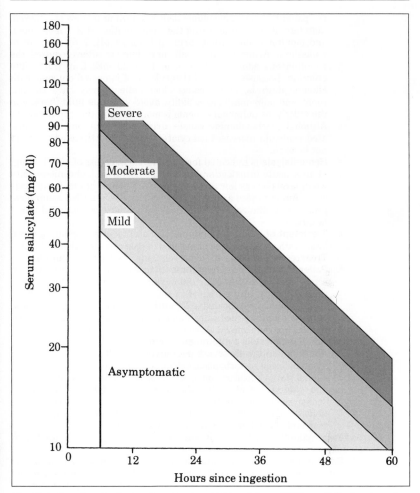

Fig. 26-2. Severity of salicylate intoxication. (Adapted from AK Done. Salicylate intoxication. *Pediatrics* 26:800, 1960.)

levels of more than 100 mg/dl are very serious and often fatal. Blood levels should be repeated daily until they show a decline. This information is useful only for acute overdoses; estimation of severity is invalidated by the use of enteric-coated aspirin or chronic ingestion. Bicarbonate levels and pH are better than salicylate levels as prognostic indicators in chronic intoxication.

3. **Treatment**
   a. Consider **gastric lavage** if presentation is within 1 hour of ingestion. Administer activated charcoal. Multidose charcoal may be useful in severe overdose (*Pediatrics* 85:594, 1990) but is not routinely recommended.
   b. **Alkaline diuresis** is indicated for salicylate blood levels that are higher than 40 mg/dl. Administer 88 or 100 mEq (2 ampules) of sodium bicarbonate in 1000 ml D5W at a rate of 10–15 ml/kg/hour if

the patient is clinically volume depleted until urine flow is achieved. Maintain alkalinization using the same solution at 2–3 ml/kg/hour, and monitor urine output, urine pH (target pH, 7–8), and serum potassium. Achievement of alkaline diuresis often requires the simultaneous administration of at least 20 mEq/L of **potassium chloride.** Because there is little evidence of improved outcome with alkaline diuresis, and because older patients may have cardiac, renal, and pulmonary comorbidity, **avoid vigorous fluid therapy in the elderly,** as pulmonary edema is more likely in this population.

   c. Although acetazolamide causes urine alkalinization, the associated acidemia increases salicylate toxicity, and therefore it must not be used.

   d. **Hemodialysis** is indicated for blood levels in excess of 100–130 mg/dl after acute intoxication but may be useful with chronic toxicity when levels are as low as 40 mg/dl, if other indications for dialysis exist. Among these are refractory acidosis, severe CNS symptoms, progressive clinical deterioration, pulmonary edema, and renal failure.

   e. **Treatment of pulmonary edema** may also require mechanical ventilation with a high fraction of inspired oxygen concentration and PEEP. Treat cerebral edema with hyperventilation and osmotic diuresis.

   f. **Patients with minor symptoms** (nausea, vomiting, tinnitus), an acute ingestion of less than 150 mg/kg, and a first blood level of less than 65 mg/dl can be treated in the emergency department. Blood levels should be repeated q2h until they show a decline. These patients often are medically stable for discharge, and their disposition may be determined based on psychiatric evaluation.

   g. **Admit moderately symptomatic patients** for at least 24 hours.

   h. **Admit patients with severe overdoses to an ICU.** Severe overdoses are manifested by tachypnea, dehydration, pulmonary edema, altered mental status, seizures, coma, or a total dose in excess of 300 mg/kg.

   i. **The elderly are at high risk.** Repeated blood levels that fail to decline should prompt contrast radiography of the stomach; concretions should be subjected to bicarbonate lavage and multidose charcoal, and whole-bowel irrigation should be considered.

O. **Sedative-hypnotics** include a diverse spectrum of frequently abused compounds.

   1. **Barbiturates.** Toxic manifestations of barbiturates vary with the amount of ingestion, type of drug, and length of time since ingestion. Toxicity can occur with lower doses of the short-acting barbiturates (e.g., butabarbital, secobarbital, and pentobarbital) than of the long-acting barbiturates (e.g., phenobarbital, barbital, mephobarbital, and primidone), but fatalities are more common with the latter.

      a. **Clinical manifestations.** Mild intoxication resembles alcohol intoxication. Moderate intoxication is characterized by greater depression of mental status, response only to painful stimuli, decreased deep tendon reflexes, and slow respirations. Severe intoxication causes coma and a loss of all reflexes (except the pupillary light reflex). Plantar reflexes are extensor. Characteristic bullae ("barb burns") may be seen over pressure points and on the dorsum of the fingers (*BMJ* 1:835, 1965). Hypothermia and hypotension may occur. In severe cases, no electrical activity is seen on an EEG.

      b. **Treatment**
         (1) Maintain a patent airway and adequate ventilation.
         (2) Do not induce emesis. Perform **gastric lavage** if presentation occurs within 1 hour of ingestion, and **administer activated charcoal.** Multidose activated charcoal markedly decreases the half-life of phenobarbital.

(3) **Forced alkaline diuresis,** similar to that used for salicylate intoxication, is effective in enhancing phenobarbital excretion, but not that of short-acting barbiturates.

(4) **Hemoperfusion** may be effective for excretion of both phenobarbital and short-acting barbiturates. Reserve charcoal or resin hemoperfusion for stage IV coma with high blood levels and refractory hemodynamic compromise, as it is more effective than hemodialysis.

(5) Treat hypotension with crystalloid administration. If this fails, administer norepinephrine or dopamine.

2. **Benzodiazepines.** These agents depress mental and respiratory function when taken in overdose. Fatalities are rare, but mixed overdoses are common. Flunitrazepam (Rohypnol, "roofies") intoxication has emerged as an increasing problem. Ten times as potent as diazepam, it is mixed with low-quality heroin and used to soften the effects of cocaine. It is also mixed with alcohol as a "date rape" drug. Effects are similar to those of other benzodiazepines. It may cause hallucinations, and mixing with alcohol increases respiratory depression. It often is not detected on standard toxicology screens.

   a. **Symptoms** include drowsiness, dysarthria, ataxia, slurred speech, and confusion.

   b. **Treatment.** Do not induce emesis. Consider gastric lavage if presentation is within 1 hour of ingestion. Administer activated charcoal. Provide general supportive measures for hypotension and bradycardia. Rarely, respiratory depression may require intubation. **Flumazenil,** a benzodiazepine antagonist, reverses toxicity without causing respiratory depression. Administer 0.2 mg (2 ml) IV over 30 seconds, followed by 0.3 mg at 1-minute intervals to a total dose of 3 mg. If no response is observed after such treatment, benzodiazepines are unlikely to be the cause of the patient's sedation. If a partial response has occurred, give additional 0.5-mg increments to a total of 5 mg. Rarely, as much as a 10-mg total dose may be necessary for full reversal. If no IV access is available, the drug can be administered by endotracheal tube. Treat recurrence of sedation or respiratory depression by repeating the preceding regimen or by continuous infusion of 0.1–0.5 mg/hour. **If mixed overdose with cyclic antidepressants is suspected or the patient has a known history of seizure disorder, flumazenil should not be used.** Forced diuresis and hemodialysis are ineffective.

3. **Gamma-hydroxybutyrate.** An endogenous short-chain fatty acid that occurs naturally in the body, this illegal substance is not detected by standard toxicology screens. It has emerged as an important intoxicant. It is often sold to participants at large dance parties ("raves") and has been responsible for mass intoxications (*Prehosp Emerg Care* 3:357, 1999). It has also been used as a "date rape" drug. Synonyms include "liquid Ecstasy," "liquid E," "grievous bodily harm," "Georgia home boy," "soap," "salty water," and "organic Quaaludes."

   a. **Symptoms** include ataxia, nystagmus, somnolence progressing to coma, vomiting, and random clonic movements of the face and extremities. EEG recording supports the belief that these represent myoclonus and not true seizures. Respiratory depression may progress to apnea.

   b. **Treatment.** Absorption is very rapid, and lavage and activated charcoal administration are of little use. Do not induce emesis. The drug is not antagonized by naloxone or flumazenil. Experimental but no clinical evidence has been found for the use of physostigmine, and its use is not recommended. Administer oxygen and protect the airway; monitor oxygenation. Obtain electrolytes and glucose and establish an IV line. Stimulation, including endotracheal intubation, may stimulate violently aggressive behavior. Give atropine for persistent symptomatic bradycardia. Treat hypotension with IV fluids; pressors are rarely necessary. Obtain an ECG and monitor the cardiac rhythm continuously. Intoxication is usually short lived; coma typically lasts for 1–2 hours, and full recovery often occurs within 8 hours. Stable asymptomatic patients can be discharged after 6 hours of observation. Admit any patient who is still clinically intoxicated after 6 hours (*Ann Emerg Med* 31:729, 1998).

P. Stimulants include amphetamines and cocaine.

    1. Amphetamines

        a. Symptoms. Toxicity is manifested by hyperactivity, irritability, delirium, hallucinations, psychosis, mydriasis, hyperpyrexia, flushing, diaphoresis, hypertension, arrhythmias, vomiting, and diarrhea. Less common manifestations include acute renal failure secondary to rhabdomyolysis, seizures, CNS hemorrhage, coma, myocardial infarction, aortic dissection, and circulatory collapse.

        b. Treatment includes early administration of activated charcoal. **Induction of emesis is contraindicated,** as it may induce seizures. Perform gastric lavage only for recent large ingestions. Establish an IV line and monitor electrolytes, renal function, and CPK. Obtain an ECG and monitor the cardiac rhythm. Treat agitation with diazepam; physical restraints may increase the occurrence of rhabdomyolysis. Treat hallucinations and psychosis with haloperidol. Droperidol, 2.5–5.0 mg IV, may be superior to benzodiazepines for sedation (*Eur J Emerg Med* 4:130, 1997). Treat severe hypertension with nitroprusside or a β-adrenergic antagonist; phentolamine can also be considered (see Chap. 4). Diazepam is the initial drug of choice for seizures, followed by phenytoin or phenobarbital. Arrhythmias usually respond to propranolol or lidocaine. Monitor core temperature. Hyperthermia may require cooling blankets, evaporative cooling, or paralysis; if unsuccessful, dantrolene or bromocriptine may be useful. Hemodialysis is not clearly effective. Treat rhabdomyolysis as outlined in Chap. 12. Admit patients with moderate to severe symptoms or with abnormal vital signs.

    2. 3-4 Methylenedioxymethamphetamine ("Ecstasy"). This compound has emerged as a new, very popular drug of abuse associated with "rave" culture. Surveys have shown that nearly 40% of college students have used it at least once. It is often used in association with prolonged vigorous dancing, causing dehydration and contributing to hyperthermia.

        a. Symptoms are due in part to the drug's action as a serotonin releaser. They include hypertension, tachycardia, dilated pupils, diaphoresis, and trismus. Severe intoxications may result in hyperthermia, DIC, muscle rigidity, myoclonus, rhabdomyolysis, acute renal failure, and occasionally the syndrome of inappropriate antidiuretic hormone (SIADH) secretion. Supraventricular and ventricular arrhythmias may occur. Initial confusion and agitation may progress to coma and seizures.

        b. Treatment. Toxicology screens are unreliable. Initiation of therapy is based on presumptive diagnosis according to history and presentation. Therapy at present is based on case reports and reviews (*Pediatrics* 100:705, 1997). Do not induce emesis, as coma and seizures may occur abruptly. Gastric lavage is useful only if initiated within 1 hour of ingestion. Administer activated charcoal. Establish an IV line, and maintain hydration. Treat agitation with benzodiazepines, with preparation to protect the airway and support ventilation. β-Adrenergic antagonists may be useful in treatment of tachycardia and hypertension. Severe hypertension may require nitroprusside. Treat seizures with benzodiazepines followed by phenytoin or phenobarbital. Treat ventricular arrhythmias with lidocaine, phenytoin, or esmolol. Cool the hypothermic patient with evaporative cooling; consider dantrolene administration. Treat rhabdomyolysis supportively (see Chap. 12).

3. Cocaine

a. Symptoms. Cocaine causes short-lived CNS and sympathetic stimulation, hypertension, tachypnea, tachycardia, and mydriasis. Depression of the higher nervous centers ensues rapidly and may result in death. Mortality may also result from drug-induced seizures, subarachnoid hemorrhage, stroke, or direct cardiac effects (e.g., coronary artery spasm, myocardial injury, and precipitation of lethal arrhythmias) (*N Engl J Med* 315:1495, 1986). **Myocardial infarction** may be precipitated in individuals without underlying heart disease. Rhabdomyolysis may occur, precipitating renal failure. **Pulmonary edema** may develop abruptly after an individual smokes the free alkaloid form of cocaine ("free base") or its heated bicarbonate precipitant ("crack"). Pneumomediastinum may occur after smoking crack and may progress to pneumothorax. Other pulmonary complications include alveolar hemorrhage, obliterative bronchiolitis, hypersensitivity pneumonitis, and asthma (*Am J Med* 87:664, 1989). Bowel ischemia and necrosis may occur.

b. Treatment. Maintain a patent airway and support respiration and circulation. Myocardial ischemia and infarction should be managed as outlined in Chap. 5. Avoid β-adrenergic antagonists in patients with myocardial ischemia or infarction, as they allow unopposed α-adrenergic vasospasm (*Ann Intern Med* 112:897, 1990). Labetalol may be preferable, and phentolamine may be useful in selected cases. Nitroglycerin can be used for ischemic pain. Treat ventricular arrhythmias with lidocaine; β-adrenergic antagonists may be useful in those without myocardial ischemia. Use benzodiazepines to decrease the stimulatory effect of cocaine and to treat seizures initially. Follow with phenytoin or phenobarbital for longer-term seizure control. Treat noncoronary manifestations of adrenergic stimulation with labetalol; severe or sustained hypertension may require treatment with nitroprusside. Treat rhabdomyolysis and hypotension supportively. Hyperthermia may require a cooling blanket, evaporative cooling, sedation, or paralysis. Admit patients with marked toxicity to an ICU for observation and cardiac monitoring. **Suspected body packers** should undergo abdominal radiography to rule out cocaine-containing packets in the intestinal tract; noncontrast CT may be more sensitive. If such packets are present, perform gentle catharsis with charcoal and psyllium; mineral oil may dissolve latex packets and precipitate toxicity. Admit such patients to an ICU for monitoring, as rupture may be rapidly fatal. Whole-bowel irrigation and surgery probably are rarely necessary, although they have been recommended; surgery is clearly indicated only for bowel obstruction. With appropriate care, mortality is less than 1% (*Am J Med* 88:325, 1990). The phenomenon of "body stuffing" has been recognized. To avoid arrest, body stuffers may ingest crack cocaine that is unwrapped or wrapped only in a layer of cellophane. Abdominal radiography is almost invariably negative. The course is generally benign, presumably due to poor absorption. Nearly three-fourths of patients remain asymptomatic, and most of the rest have only mild to moderate symptoms, including tachycardia and hypertension. Only 4% have severe toxicity, including seizures, dysrhythmias, and death (*Ann Emerg Med* 29:596, 1999; *J Emerg Med* 18:221, 2000). Close observation is nevertheless warranted.

Q. Theophylline

1. Symptoms. Nausea and vomiting are the most common symptoms of theophylline toxicity and are associated with serum levels exceeding 20 mg/ml. Moderate toxicity is largely due to relative epinephrine excess, and includes tachycardia, arrhythmias, tremors, and agitation. Severe toxicity results in hallucinations, seizures (which may be refractory to standard therapy), dysrhythmias (including sinus tachycardia, atrial fibrillation, supraventricular tachycardia, and ventricular tachycardia and fibrillation), and hypotension. Rhabdomyolysis occurs occasionally (*Intensive Care Med* 18:129, 1992). Severity of intoxication is modified by chronicity, age of the patient, and the presence of comorbid diseases. Severe toxicity is most common at serum levels in excess of 90 mg/ml in the acutely intoxicated, usually younger individual. Seizures and cardiac toxicity are likely at serum levels of more than 60 mg/ml in the chronically intoxicated and might occur at even lower levels.

2. **Laboratory studies.** Obtain theophylline levels q2h until a plateau is reached. The peak level may be delayed significantly after the ingestion of sustained-release theophylline preparations, with toxic levels persisting 50–60 hours after ingestion. Check potassium, electrolyte, glucose, calcium, and magnesium levels; BUN; and ABGs. Obtain a baseline ECG and maintain continuous cardiac monitoring. Acid-base abnormalities include respiratory alkalosis and metabolic acidosis. Hypokalemia, hyperglycemia, hypercalcemia, and hypophosphatemia may be present.

3. **Therapy**

   a. Establish an IV line and perform gastric lavage if the patient has taken a potentially life-threatening acute ingestion. Consider lavage also after a large ingestion of a sustained-release preparation, as a bezoar may form. Avoid the use of ipecac because of the potential for seizures and aspiration. Administer activated charcoal. **Multidose charcoal** decreases the half-life of theophylline by 50%, although it has not been clearly shown to improve outcome. Consider whole-bowel irrigation with polyethylene glycol solution for overdoses with sustained-release preparations and blood levels that continue to rise despite therapy.

   b. Treat severe nausea with metoclopramide, 10–60 mg IV, or ondansetron, 0.15 mg/kg IV (8–10 mg in the average individual) (*Ann Pharmacother* 27:584, 1993). **Do not use phenothiazines because of their propensity to lower the seizure threshold.**

   c. Treat hypotension with **IV crystalloids** and, if resistant, with dopamine.

   d. Phenobarbital is preferred to phenytoin for **seizure prophylaxis** in the severely poisoned patient. The treatment of choice for seizures is a benzodiazepine followed by phenobarbital (10 mg/kg loading dose at 50 mg/minute, followed by up to a total of 30 mg/kg at a rate of 50 mg/minute, followed by 1–5 mg/kg/day to maintain therapeutic plasma levels). Because of the cardiovascular and respiratory depressant activities of barbiturates, careful management of the airway and cardiovascular status is mandatory. For those patients refractory to phenobarbital therapy, obtain anesthesiology consultation for administration of pentobarbital; muscle paralysis and general anesthesia can be considered.

   e. Arrhythmias should be treated as they would be in nonintoxicated patients. β-Adrenergic antagonists may be particularly useful but may precipitate bronchospasm in asthmatics. Because of its short half-life, IV esmolol usually is safer.

   f. **Hemoperfusion** (charcoal or resin) is preferable to hemodialysis because of faster drug removal and is indicated for (1) intractable seizures or life-threatening cardiovascular complications, regardless of drug level; (2) a theophylline level that approaches or exceeds 100 mg/ml after an acute overdose; (3) a theophylline level of more than 60 mg/ml in acute intoxication, with increasing symptoms, and a patient who is intolerant of oral charcoal administration; (4) a theophylline level in excess of 60 mg/ml in chronic intoxication without life-threatening symptoms; and (5) a theophylline level of more than 40 mg/ml in a patient with chronic intoxication and CHF, respiratory insufficiency, hepatic failure (*J Emerg Med* 11:415, 1993), or age older than 60 years.

g. **Disposition.** Admit patients who have chronic intoxication, acute ingestion of sustained-release formulations, or acute ingestions with levels that fail to fall or are rising despite therapy, or who have worsening symptoms. Those with levels that are falling to less than 20 mg/ml and whose symptoms are resolving can be discharged.

Toxic Inhalants

Toxic inhalants comprise a variety of noxious gases and particulate matter capable of producing local irritation, asphyxiation, and systemic toxicity. In the management of exposure victims, identification of the offending agent is critical, and the regional poison control center must be contacted for specific therapeutic guidelines.

I. **Irritant gases** produce cutaneous burns, mucosal irritation, laryngotracheitis, bronchitis, pneumonitis, bronchospasm, and pulmonary edema (which may be delayed up to 24 hours after exposure). The more water-soluble gases (e.g., chlorine, ammonia, formaldehyde, sulfur dioxide, ozone) primarily produce inflammation of the eyes, throat, and upper respiratory tract, whereas the less soluble gases (e.g., phosgene, nitrogen dioxide) tend to cause more damage to the terminal airways and alveoli. Household exposure may result from inadvertent mixture of bleach (sodium hypochlorite) with toilet bowl cleaner (sulfuric acid), which produces chlorine gas, or of bleach with ammonia, which produces chloramine gas.

A. **Treatment.** Maintain a patent airway and adequate oxygenation. Treat bronchospasm with bronchodilators. Treat noncardiogenic pulmonary edema with oxygen, mechanical ventilation, and PEEP as needed (see Chap. 9). Treat skin burns by copious irrigation, removal of contaminated clothing, and tetanus prophylaxis (see Appendix F), if needed. Irrigate the eyes immediately and copiously with water or saline if the patient has had chemical contact. Obtain ophthalmologic consultation for caustic eye burns.

B. **Disposition.** Because the development of pulmonary edema may be delayed, observe asymptomatic patients with normal ABGs and chest radiographs for at least 6 hours. Hospitalize patients with symptoms or signs of upper airway edema or pulmonary involvement.

II. **Simple asphyxiants** (e.g., acetylene, argon, ethane, helium, hydrogen, nitrogen, methane, neon, butane, carbon dioxide, natural gas, and propane) cause hypoxia by displacing oxygen from the inspired air. Morbidity and mortality are related to the extent and duration of the hypoxia. **Treatment** consists of supplemental oxygen and supportive care for symptomatic patients.

III. **Systemic toxic inhalants** are those gases that are capable of producing prominent systemic toxicity, including hydrogen sulfide, methyl bromide, organophosphates (see Overdosage, sec. **VII.K**), carbon monoxide, and hydrogen cyanide. Treatment consists of supportive care and specific therapy directed toward the offending agent.

A. **Carbon monoxide** displaces oxygen from hemoglobin, shifts the oxyhemoglobin dissociation curve to the left, and depresses cellular respiration by inhibiting the cytochrome oxidase system. Direct binding to cardiac myoglobin depresses cardiac function. Toxic manifestations are a consequence of tissue hypoxia. Poisoning usually occurs in poorly ventilated areas in which carbon monoxide is released by fires, combustion engines, or faulty stoves or heating systems. Intoxication is seasonal, with more cases occurring in winter. **Arterial oxygen tension usually is normal; thus, the diagnosis of car-**

bon monoxide poisoning requires a high level of suspicion and direct measurement of arterial oxygen saturation or carbon monoxide (carboxyhemoglobin) levels. Standard pulse oximetry is not reliable.

1. **Symptoms** correlate imperfectly with the carboxyhemoglobin level. Levels of 20–40% are associated with dizziness, headache, weakness, disturbed judgment, nausea and vomiting, and diminished visual acuity. These symptoms and seasonality frequently lead to a misdiagnosis of influenza. Examination may reveal retinal hemorrhages. Levels of 40–60% are associated with tachypnea, tachycardia, ataxia, syncope, and seizures. The ECG may reveal ST segment changes, conduction blocks, and atrial or ventricular arrhythmias. Levels in excess of 60% are associated with coma and death. Cherry-red coloration of the lips or skin is a relatively rare, late manifestation. Late complications include basal ganglia infarction and parkinsonism. Less severe, delayed neuropsychiatric symptoms also may occur.

2. **Treatment** begins with administration of **100% oxygen** by tight-fitting mask or endotracheal tube. The latter ensures tissue oxygen delivery and decreases the half-life of carboxyhemoglobin from 4–5 hours to 90 minutes. Measure carboxyhemoglobin levels q2–4h, and continue oxygen administration until blood levels are less than 10%. Obtain electrolytes, CPK, ABGs, and an ECG, and monitor the cardiac rhythm continuously. **Hyperbaric oxygen** (3 atm) has been strongly recommended for patients who have been unconscious at any time and present with neurologic signs or symptoms, ECG changes consistent with ischemia, severe metabolic acidosis, rhabdomyolysis, pulmonary edema, or shock. Hyperbaric treatment of patients who have minor or no symptoms but who have carboxyhemoglobin levels of greater than 25–30% is controversial, as is treatment in pregnancy. A randomized controlled trial showed no benefit for hyperbaric oxygen therapy as compared to administration of 100% oxygen (*Med J Aust* 170:203, 1999). Consult with an expert in the field when indications are unclear. In no case should patients be transferred to a hyperbaric oxygen facility until their condition is stabilized. Treat seizures with diazepam and phenytoin (see Chap. 25). Arrhythmias and rhabdomyolysis are treated as described elsewhere.

B. **Hydrogen cyanide** may be present in industrial fumigants, insecticides, and products of combustion of synthetics and plastics. It may be generated as a by-product of phencyclidine manufacture. The gas has a characteristic bitter almond odor. Toxic amounts are absorbed rapidly through the bronchial mucosa and alveoli, and symptoms usually appear seconds after inhalation. Concentrations of 0.2–0.3 mg/L of air are almost immediately fatal. Oral exposures to **potassium cyanide** may be due to rodenticides, insecticides, silver polish, artificial fingernail remover (acetonitrile), film developer, laboratory reagents, and amygdalin.

1. **Toxic manifestations** include headache, palpitations, dyspnea, and mental status depression, which may progress quickly to coma, seizures, and death. ECG changes include atrial fibrillation, ventricular ectopy, and abnormal ventricular repolarization. Severe lactic acidosis is present, and venous oxygen content is higher than normal and may approach arterial oxygen content. Do not delay initiation of therapy for measurement of whole-blood cyanide levels.

2. **Therapy** focuses on conversion of hemoglobin to methemoglobin, which binds to the cyanide ion, sparing vital oxidative enzymes.

   a. **Amyl nitrite** (1 broken pearl held under the nostril for 15–30 seconds/minute, repeated every minute, with a new pearl q3min) produces a methemoglobin level of approximately 5%. This should be followed as rapidly as possible with 10 ml of 3% **sodium nitrite** IV

(0.3 g over 3–5 minutes). If the response is inadequate, one-half of the dose of sodium nitrite should be repeated in 30 minutes. The goal is a measured methemoglobin level of 30%.

b. Give **sodium thiosulfate** (50 ml of a 25% solution IV) immediately after the sodium nitrite, as it converts the cyanide into thiocyanate, which is excreted in the urine. Repeat one-half the dose in 30 minutes if the response is inadequate.

c. **Administer 100% oxygen** at all times during treatment to ensure adequate tissue oxygen delivery despite methemoglobinemia. Do not give methylene blue for methemoglobin levels less than 70%, as cyanide may be released. In the event of life-threatening methemoglobinemia, consider exchange transfusion. Monitor the cardiac rhythm continuously.

d. For severe persistent acidosis (pH <7.2), **administer sodium bicarbonate**, 1 mEq/kg, after the preceding measures have been undertaken.

e. In the event of oral ingestion, empty the stomach by gastric lavage after the preceding measures have been undertaken. Do not induce emesis. Rapid absorption makes administration of activated charcoal of dubious utility.

f. The efficacy of hyperbaric oxygen is controversial but can be considered for those who respond poorly to conventional therapy.

g. In Europe, hydroxocobalamin, 4 g IV (10 ml of a 40% solution administered over 20 minutes), is an effective alternative to the above regimen (*Occup Med* 48:427, 1998). The only preparation available in the United States is a 1% solution, and the requirement for infusion of 4 L makes this impractical. Dicobalt ethylenediamine-tetra-acetic acid and dimethylaminophenol are antidotes that are not available in the United States.

C. **Hydrogen sulfide** is a colorless gas with a characteristic rotten-egg odor. It is found in mines and sewers as well as petrochemical, agricultural (liquid manure processing), and tanning industries.

1. **Symptoms.** Exposure to low concentrations of hydrogen sulfide causes mucous membrane and eye irritation and vision changes. Higher concentrations cause cyanosis, confusion, pulmonary edema, coma, and convulsions. Rapid death occurs in approximately 6% of cases.

2. **Treatment.** Therapy is similar to that used for hydrogen cyanide. Oxygen 100% and nitrites are used, but thiosulfate is not. The efficacy of nitrites is controversial (*Vet Hum Toxicol* 39:152, 1997). Flush the mucous membranes with saline or water. Consider hyperbaric oxygenation for severe intoxication.

IV. **Smoke inhalation** is the cause of death in more than 50% of fire-related fatalities. Thermal injury usually is confined to the upper airway because of the rapid cooling of inhaled gases that occurs proximal to the larynx. Toxic gases released by fire include carbon dioxide, carbon monoxide, hydrogen chloride, phosgene, chlorine, benzene, isocyanate, hydrogen cyanide, aldehydes, oxides of sulfur and nitrogen, ammonia, and numerous organic acids. Carbon monoxide accounts for 80% of mortality in the first 12 hours. The other toxins produce epithelial injury that results in airway edema, increased capillary permeability, and mechanical obstruction from desquamated tissue and secretions. Patients who have lost consciousness, have been exposed to a large quantity of smoke in a closed space, have suffered prolonged inhalation or steam exposure, were involved in an explosion, were with other persons who died or were severely injured, or have sustained facial burns or singed nasal vibrissae are at risk for development of respiratory complications, which may be delayed in onset for up to 3 days. High-risk patients should undergo upper airway endoscopy to rule out any life-threatening airway injury immediately; bronchoscopy rarely provides additional therapeutically useful information. A positive xenon scan predicts increased mortality but is rarely justified. Carboxyhemoglobin levels that exceed 15% are indicative of severe exposure.

A. Clinical manifestations. Asphyxiation, expectoration of carbonaceous sputum, hoarseness, dyspnea from upper airway edema, stridor, bronchospasm, and noncardiogenic pulmonary edema are characteristic features of smoke inhalation. Upper airway burns may also be noted. Neurologic manifestations include stupor and coma. Late complications include bacterial pneumonia and pulmonary embolism.

B. Treatment. Scrupulous airway care is essential, with frequent suctioning as needed. Endotracheal intubation is required in patients who display evidence of significant upper airway edema or respiratory insufficiency. Bronchoscopy may be necessary to remove endotracheal debris. Administer **humidified oxygen** to all patients. Give bronchodilators for bronchospasm. Treat ARDS with mechanical ventilation and PEEP. High-frequency flow interruption ventilation has been reported to be effective (*Curr Opin Pulm Med* 3:221, 1997) but is not widely available and requires additional confirmation. Prophylactic antibiotics and glucocorticoids are not indicated. Treat specific intoxications (e.g., cyanide and carbon monoxide poisoning) appropriately. Suspect cyanide intoxication if coma and significant lactic acidosis are present.

C. Disposition. Patients who have experienced minor smoke inhalation, who are asymptomatic at 4–6 hours, and who exhibit none of the risk factors just listed can be safely discharged home. Admit asymptomatic patients who have any risk factors for potential respiratory complications for a minimum of 24 hours. Admit patients who have symptoms, significant laboratory abnormalities, or an abnormal alveolar-arterial oxygen gradient to an ICU.

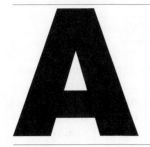

Barnes-Jewish Hospital Laboratory Reference Values

Tom Daly

Reference values for the more commonly used laboratory tests are listed in the following table. These values are given in the units currently used at Barnes-Jewish Hospital and in Systeme International (SI) units, which are used in many areas of the world. Individual reference values can be population and method dependent.

Test	Current units	Factor[a]	SI units
Common serum chemistries			
Albumin	3.6–5.0 g/dl	10	36–50 g/L
Ammonia (plasma)	9–33 µmol/L	1	9–33 µmol/L
Bilirubin			
Total[b]	0.3–1.1 mg/dl	17.1	5.13–18.80 µmol/L
Direct	0–0.3 mg/dl	17.1	0–5.1 µmol/L
Blood gases (arterial)			
pH	7.35–7.45	1	7.35–7.45
PO_2	80–105 mm Hg	0.133	10.6–14.0 kPa
PCO_2	35–45 mm Hg	0.133	4.7–6.0 kPa
Calcium			
Total	8.6–10.3 mg/dl	0.25	2.15–2.58 mmol/L
Ionized	4.5–5.1 mg/dl	0.25	1.13–1.28 mmol/L
CO_2 content (plasma)	22–32 mmol/L	1	22–32 mmol/L
Ceruloplasmin	24–46 mg/dl	0.063	1.5–2.9 µmol/L
Chloride	97–110 mmol/L	1	97–110 mmol/L
Cholesterol[c]			
Desirable	<200 mg/dl	0.0259	<5.18 mmol/L
Borderline high	200–239 mg/dl	0.0259	5.18–6.19 mmol/L
High	≥240 mg/dl	0.0259	≥6.22 mmol/L
HDL cholesterol[b]	>35 mg/dl	0.0259	>0.91 mmol/L
Copper (total)	75–145 mg/dl	0.157	11.8–22.8 mmol/L
Creatinine[b]	0.5–1.7 mg/dl	88.4	44–150 µmol/L
Ferritin			
Male adult	20–323 ng/ml	2.25	45–727 pmol/L
Female adult	10–283 ng/ml	2.25	23–637 pmol/L

Test	Current units	Factor[a]	SI units
Folate			
Plasma	3.1–12.4 ng/ml	2.27	7.0–28.1 nmol/L
Red cell	186–645 ng/ml	2.27	422–1464 nmol/L
Glucose, fasting (plasma)	65–109 mg/dl	0.055	3.58–6.00 mmol/L
Haptoglobin	30–220 mg/dl	0.01	0.3–2.2 g/L
Hemoglobin a1c (estimated)	4.0–6.0%	0.01	0.04–0.06
Iron (total)			
Male	45–160 μg/dl	—	8.1–31.3 μmol/L
Female	30–160 μg/dl	0.179	5.4–31.3 μmol/L
Iron-binding capacity	220–420 μg/dl	0.179	39.4–75.2 μmol/L
Transferrin saturation	20–50%	0.01	0.2–0.5
Lactate (plasma)	0.7–2.1 mmol/L	1	0.7–2.1 mmol/L
Magnesium	1.3–2.2 mEq/L	0.5	0.65–1.10 mmol/L
Osmolality	275–300 mOsm/kg	1	275–300 mmol/kg
Phosphate	2.5–4.5 mg/dl	0.323	0.81–1.45 mmol/L
Potassium (plasma)	3.3–4.9 mmol/L	1	3.3–4.9 mmol/L
Protein, total (plasma)	6.5–8.5 g/dl	10	65–85 g/L
Sodium	135–145 mmol/L	1	135–145 mmol/L
Triglycerides, fasting[c]	<250 mg/dl	0.0113	<2.8 mmol/L
Troponin I			
Normal	≤0.6 ng/ml	100	≤60 ng/L
Indeterminant	0.7–1.4 ng/ml	100	70–140 ng/L
Abnormal	≥1.5 ng/ml	100	≥150 ng/L
Urea nitrogen	8–25 mg/dl	0.357	2.9–8.9 mmol/L
Uric acid[b]	3–8 mg/dl	59.5	179–476 μmol/L
Vitamin B_{12}	187–1057 pg/ml	0.738	138–780 pmol/L
Common serum enzymatic activities			
Aminotransferases			
Alanine (ALT, SGPT)	7–53 IU/L	0.01667	0.12–0.88 μkat/L
Aspartate (AST, SGOT)	11–47 IU/L	0.01667	0.18–0.78 μkat/L
Amylase	25–115 IU/L	0.01667	0.42–1.92 μkat/L
Creatine kinase			
Male	30–200 IU/L	0.01667	0.50–3.33 μkat/L
Female	20–170 IU/L	0.01667	0.33–2.83 μkat/L
MB fraction	0–7 IU/L	0.01667	0–0.12 μkat/L
Gamma-glutamyl transpeptidase (GGT)			
Male	11–50 IU/L	0.01667	0.18–0.83 μkat/L
Female	7–32 IU/L	0.01667	0.12–0.53 μkat/L
Lactate dehydrogenase[b]	100–250 IU/L	0.01667	1.67–4.17 μkat/L
Lipase	<100 IU/dl	0.1667	<1.67 μkat/L

Test	Current units	Factor[a]	SI units
5'-Nucleotidase	2–16 IU/L	0.01667	0.03–0.27 μkat/L
Phosphatase, acid	0–0.7 IU/L	16.67	0–11.6 nkat/L
Phosphatase, alkaline[d]	38–126 IU/L	0.01667	0.63–2.10 μkat/L
Common serum hormone values[e]			
ACTH, fasting (8 AM, supine)	<60 pg/ml	0.22	<13.2 pmol/L
Aldosterone[f]	10–160 ng/L	2.77	28–443 mmol/L
Cortisol (plasma, morning)	6–30 mg/dl	0.027	0.16–0.81 μmol/L
FSH			
Male	1–8 IU/L	1	1–8 IU/L
Female			
Follicular	4–13 IU/L	1	4–13 IU/L
Luteal	2–13 IU/L	1	2–13 IU/L
Midcycle	5–22 IU/L	1	5–22 IU/L
Postmenopausal	20–138 IU/L	1	20–138 IU/L
Gastrin, fasting	0–130 pg/ml	1	0–130 ng/L
Growth hormone, fasting			
Male	<5 ng/ml	1	<5 μg/L
Female	<10 ng/ml	1	<10 μg/L
17-Hydroxyprogesterone			
Male adult	<200 ng/dl	0.03	<6.6 nmol/L
Female			
Follicular	<80 ng/dl	0.03	<2.4 nmol/L
Luteal	<235 ng/dl	0.03	<8.6 nmol/L
Postmenopausal	<51 ng/dl	0.03	<1.5 nmol/L
Insulin, fasting	3–15 mU/L	7.18	≤144 pmol/L
LH			
Male	2–12 IU/L	1	2–12 IU/L
Female			
Follicular	1–18 IU/L	1	1–18 IU/L
Luteal	≤20 IU/L	1	≤20 IU/L
Midcycle	24–105 IU/L	1	24–105 IU/L
Postmenopausal	15–62 IU/L	1	15–62 IU/L
Parathyroid hormone	12–72 pg/ml	—	—
Progesterone			
Male	<0.5 ng/ml	3.18	<1.6 nmol/L
Female			
Follicular	0.1–1.5 ng/ml	3.18	0.32–4.80 nmol/L
Luteal	2.5–28.0 ng/ml	3.18	8–89 nmol/L
First trimester	9–47 ng/ml	3.18	29–149 nmol/L
Third trimester	55–255 ng/ml	3.18	175–811 nmol/L
Postmenopausal	<0.5 ng/ml	3.18	<1.6 nmol/L

Test	Current units	Factor[a]	SI units
Prolactin			
Male	1.6–18.8 ng/ml	1	1.6–18.8 µg/L
Female	1.4–24.2 ng/ml	1	1.4–24.2 µg/L
Renin activity (plasma)[g]	0.9–3.3 ng/ml/hr	0.278	0.25–0.91 ng/(L × secs)
Testosterone, total			
Male	270–1070 ng/dl	0.0346	9.3–37.0 nmol/L
Female	6–86 ng/dl	0.0346	0.21–3.00 nmol/L
Testosterone, free			
Male	9–30 ng/dl	0.0346	0.31–1.00 pmol/L
Female	0.3–1.9 ng/dl	0.0346	0.0013–0.26 pmol/L
Thyroxine, total (T_4)	4.5–12.0 µg/dl	12.9	58–155 nmol/L
Thyroxine, free	0.7–1.8 ng/dl	12.9	10.3–34.8 pmol/L
T uptake[h]	30–46%	0.01	0.3–0.46
Triiodothyronine (T_3)	45–132 ng/dl	0.0154	0.91–2.70 nmol/L
T_4 index[i]	1.5–4.5	1	1.5–4.5
TSH	0.35–6.20 µU/ml	1	0.35–6.20 mU/L
Vitamin D, 1,25-dihydroxy	15–60 pg/ml	2.4	36–144 pmol/L
Vitamin D, 25-hydroxy	10–55 ng/ml	2.49	25–137 nmol/L
Common urinary chemistries			
Delta-aminolevulinic acid	1.5–7.5 mg/day	7.6	11.4–53.2 µmol/day
Amylase	0.04–0.30 IU/min	16.67	0.67–5.00 nkat/min
	60–450 U/24 hrs	—	—
Calcium	50–250 mg/day	0.250	1.25–6.25 mmol/day
Catecholamines	<540 µg/day	—	—
Dopamine	65–400 µg/day	—	—
Epinephrine	<20 µg/day	5.5	<110 nmol/day
Norepinephrine	15–80 µg/day	5.9	88.5–472.0 nmol/day
Copper	15–60 µg/day	0.0157	0.24–0.95 µmol/day
Cortisol, free	9–53 µg/day	2.76	25–146 nmol/day
Creatinine			
Male	0.8–1.8 g/day	8.84	7.1–15.9 mmol/day
Female	0.6–1.5 g/day	8.84	5.3–13.3 mmol/day
5-Hydroxyindoleacetic acid	<6 mg/day	5.23	<47 µmol/day
Metanephrine	<1.3 mg/day	5.46	<7.1 µmol/day
Oxalate			
Male	7–44 mg/day	11.4	80–502 µmol/day
Female	4–31 mg/day	11.4	46–353 µmol/day
Porphyrins			
Coproporphyrin			
Male	≤96 µg/day	1.53	0–110 nmol/day
Female	≤60 µg/day	1.54	0–92 nmol/day

Test	Current units	Factor[a]	SI units
Uroporphyrin			
Male	≤46 µg/day	1.2	0–32 nmol/day
Female	≤22 µg/day	1.2	0–26 nmol/day
Protein	0–150 mg/day	0.001	0–0.150 g/day
Vanillylmandelic acid (VMA)	<8 mg/day	5.05	<40 µmol/day
Common hematologic values			
Coagulation			
Bleeding time[j]	2.5–9.5 mins	60	150–570 secs
Fibrin degradation products	<8 µg/ml	—	—
Fibrinogen[k]	150–360 mg/dl	0.01	1.5–3.6 g/L
Partial thromboplastin time (activated)	21–32 secs	1	21–32 secs
Prothrombin time	8.2–10.3[l] secs	1	8.2–10.3 secs[l]
INR	0.9–1.13	—	—
Thrombin time	11.3–18.5 secs	1	11.3–18.5 secs
CBC			
Hematocrit			
Male	40.7–50.3%	0.01	0.407–0.503
Female	36.1–44.3%	0.01	0.361–0.443
Hemoglobin			
Male	13.8–17.2 g/dl	0.620[m]	8.56–10.70 mmol/L
Female	12.1–15.1 g/dl	0.620	7.50–9.36 mmol/L
Erythrocyte count			
Male	$4.5–5.7 \times 10^6/\mu l$	1	$4.5–5.7 \times 10^{12}/L$
Female	$3.9–5.0 \times 10^6/\mu l$	1	$3.9–5.0 \times 10^{12}/L$
Mean corpuscular hemoglobin	26.7–33.7 pg/cell	0.062	1.66–2.09 fmol/cell
Mean corpuscular hemoglobin concentration	32.7–35.5 g/dl	0.620	20.3–22.0 mmol/L
Mean corpuscular volume	$80.0–97.6 \mu m^3$	1	80.0–97.6 fl
Red cell distribution width	11.8–14.6%	0.01	0.118–0.146
Leukocyte profile			
Total	$3.8–9.8 \times 10^3/\mu l$	1	$3.8–9.8 \times 10^9/L$
Lymphocytes	$1.2–3.3 \times 10^3/\mu l$	1	$1.2–3.3 \times 10^9/L$
Mononuclear cells	$0.2–0.7 \times 10^3/\mu l$	1	$0.2–0.7 \times 10^9/L$
Granulocytes	$1.8–6.6 \times 10^3/\mu l$	1	$1.8–6.6 \times 10^9/L$
Platelet count	$140–440 \times 10^3/\mu l$	1	$140–440 \times 10^9/L$
Erythrocyte sedimentation rate			
Male	<50 y.o.	0–15	—
	>50 y.o.	0–20	—
Female	<50 y.o.	0–20	—
	>50 y.o.	0–30	—

Test	Current units	Factor[a]	SI units
Reticulocyte count			
Adults	0.5–1.5%	0.01	0.005–0.015
Children	2.5–6.5%	—	—
Immunology testing			
Complement (total hemolytic)[n]	118–226 U/ml	—	—
C3	75–165 mg/dl	0.01	0.85–1.85 g/L
C4	12–42 mg/dl	0.01	0.12–0.54 g/L
Immunoglobulin			
IgA	70–370 mg/dl	0.01	0.70–3.70 g/L
IgM	30–210 mg/dl	0.01	0.30–2.10 g/L
IgG	700–1450 mg/dl	0.01	7.00–14.50 g/L
Therapeutic agents			
Amitriptyline (+ nortrip-tyline)	150–250 μg/L	—	—
Carbamazepine	4–12 mg/L	4.23	17–51 μmol/L
Clonazepam	10–50 μg/ml	3.17	32–159 nmol/L
Cyclosporine (whole blood)	183–335 ng/ml		Exact range depends on the type of trans-plant
Digoxin	0.8–2.0 μg/L	1.28	1.0–2.6 nmol/L
Disopyramide	2–5 mg/L	2.95	6–15 μmol/L
Ethosuximide	40–75 mg/L	7.08	283–531 μmol/L
Imipramine			
Imipramine	150–300 μg/L	3.57	536–1071 nmol/L
Desipramine	100–300 μg/L	3.75	375–1125 nmol/L
Lithium	0.6–1.3 mmol/L	1	0.6–1.3 mmol/L
Nortriptyline	50–150 μg/L	3.8	190–665 nmol/L
Phenobarbital	10–40 mg/L	4.3	43–172 μmol/L
Phenytoin (diphenylhydantoin)	10–20 mg/L	3.96	40–79 μmol/L
Primidone			
Primidone	5–15 mg/L	4.58	23–69 μmol/L
Phenobarbital	10–40 mg/L	4.3	45–172 μmol/L
Procainamide			
Procainamide	4–10 mg/L	4.23	17–42 μmol/L
Procainamide + N-acetylprocainamide	6–20 mg/L	—	—
Quinidine	2–5 mg/L	3.08	6.2–15.4 μmol/L
Salicylate[o]	20–290 mg/L	0.0072	0.14–2.10 mmol/L
Theophylline	10–20 mg/L	5.5	55–110 μmol/L
Valproic acid	50–100 mg/L	6.93	346–693 μmol/L

Test	Current units	Factor[a]	SI units
Antimicrobials			
Amikacin			
Trough	1–8 mg/L	1.71	1.7–13.7 μmol/L
Peak	20–30 mg/L	1.71	34–51 μmol/L
5-Fluorocytosine			
Trough	20–60 mg/L	—	—
Peak	50–100 mg/L	—	—
Gentamicin			
Trough	0.5–2.0 mg/L	2.09	1.0–4.2 μmol/L
Peak	6–10 mg/L	2.09	12.5–20.9 μmol/L
Ketoconazole			
Trough	≤1 mg/L	—	—
Peak	1–4 mg/L	—	—
Sulfamethoxazole			
Trough	75–120 mg/L	—	—
Peak	100–150 mg/L	—	—
Tobramycin			
Trough	0.5–2.0 mg/L	2.14	1.1–4.3 μmol/L
Peak	6–10 mg/L	2.14	12.8–21.4 μmol/L
Trimethoprim			
Trough	2–8 mg/L	—	—
Peak	5–15 mg/L	—	—
Vancomycin			
Trough	5–15 mg/L	—	—
Peak	20–40 mg/L	—	—

ACTH = adrenocorticotropic hormone; ALT = alanine aminotransferase; AST = aspartate aminotransferase; CBC = complete blood cell count; fl = femtoliter; fmol = femtomole; FSH = follicle-stimulating hormone; HDL = high-density lipoprotein; INR = international normalized ratio; katal = mole/sec; kPa = kilopascal; LH = luteinizing hormone; μkat = microkatal; nkat = nanokatal; pmol = picomole; TSH = thyroid-stimulating hormone.

[a]A more complete list of multiplication factors for converting conventional units to SI units can be found in *Ann Intern Med* 106:114, 1967, and in *The SI for the Health Professions*. Geneva: World Health Organization, 1977.

[b]Variation occurs with age and gender. This range includes both genders and persons older than 5 yrs.

[c]National Institutes of Health Congress Development Panel on Triglycerides, HDL, and Coronary Artery Diseases (*JAMA* 269:505, 1993).

[d]Higher values (up to 350 μU/ml) can be normal in persons younger than 20 yrs.

[e]Because most hormones are measured by immunologic techniques and because hormones may vary in molecular weight (e.g., gastrin), most are expressed as mass/L. The reference ranges are method dependent.

[f]Supine, normal unit diet; in the upright position, the reference range is 40–310 ng/L.

[g]High-sodium diet, supplemented with sodium, 3 g/day.

[h]Replaces T_3 resin uptake.

[i]$T_4 \times$ (T uptake).

[j]Template modified after Ivy.

[k]Determined by the Clauss method.

[l]Normal ranges for prothrombin times vary according to the reagent used. Therefore, we report an INR with all prothrombin times ordered.

[m]This factor assumes a unit molecular weight of 16,000; assuming a unit molecular weight of 64,500, the multiplication factor is 0.156.

[n]CH_{50} = reciprocal of dilution of sera required to lyse 50% of sheep erythrocytes.

[o]Therapeutic range for treatment of rheumatoid arthritis (see Chap. 24).

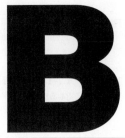

B

Pregnancy and Medical Therapeutics

Lesley Ann Watson

Class of medication	Relatively safe to use in pregnancy	Limited data or fetal risk appear minimal	Evidence of fetal risk[a]	Significant fetal risk; avoid in pregnancy
Analgesics	Acetaminophen	Celecoxib[b] Diclofenac[b] Fentanyl[c] Hydrocodone[c] Hydromorphone[c] Ibuprofen[b] Ketoprofen[b] Meperidine[c] Morphine[c] Naproxen[b] Oxycodone[c] Piroxicam[b] Rofecoxib[b] Sulindac[b]	Aspirin[b] Codeine[c] Etodolac[b] Indomethacin[b] Ketorolac[b] Nabumetone[b] Oxaprozin[b] Propoxyphene[c] Tramadol	
Anticonvulsants[d]	Magnesium sulfate[e]		Carbamazepine Clonazepam Ethosuximide Gabapentin Lamotrigine Tiagabine Topiramate	Fosphenytoin Phenobarbital Phenytoin Primidone Valproic acid
Antidepressants/ antipsychotics		Bupropion Citalopram Fluoxetine Paroxetine Sertraline	Amitriptyline Desipramine Doxepin Haloperidol Imipramine Mirtazapine Nefazodone Nortriptyline Olanzapine Quetiapine	Lithium Monoamine oxidase inhibitors

Class of medication	Relatively safe to use in pregnancy	Limited data or fetal risk appear minimal	Evidence of fetal risk[a]	Significant fetal risk; avoid in pregnancy
			Risperidone	
			Thioridazine	
			Trazodone	
			Venlafaxine	
Antidiabetic agents	Insulin	Acarbose	Glimepiride[f]	
		Metformin	Glipizide[f]	
		Miglitol	Glyburide[f]	
			Pioglitazone	
			Repaglinide[f]	
			Rosiglitazone	
			Troglitazone	
Antiemetics	Doxylamine[f]	Chlorpromazine[g]		
	Meclizine[f]	Dimenhydrinate[f]		
	Metoclopra-mide	Dolasetron		
	Pyridoxine	Granisetron		
		Ondansetron		
		Prochlorpera-zine[g]		
		Promethazine[g]		
		Scopolamine		
		Trimethobenza-mide		
Antihista-mines[f]	Chlorphen-iramine	Astemizole		
	Triprolidine	Bromphen-iramine		
		Cetirizine		
		Clemastine		
		Diphenhy-dramine		
		Fexofenadine		
		Hydroxyzine		
		Loratadine		
Antilipemics		Cholestyramine[h]	Fenofibrate	HMG-CoA reductase inhibitors
		Colestipol[h]	Gemfibrozil	
Antimicro-bials	Amoxicillin	Acyclovir	Amikacin	Fluoroquinolones
	Amoxicillin/ clavulanic acid	Azithromycin	Ethambutol[l]	Streptomycin[l]
		Aztreonam	Fluconazole	Tetracyclines
	Amphoteri-cin B	Chlorampheni-col[f]	Gentamicin	
	Ampicillin	Clarithromycin	Isoniazid[l]	
	Ampicillin/ sulbactam	Clindamycin	Itraconazole	
		Famciclovir	Ketoconazole	
			Miconazole (systemic)	

Class of medication	Relatively safe to use in pregnancy	Limited data or fetal risk appear minimal	Evidence of fetal risk[a]	Significant fetal risk; avoid in pregnancy
	Cephalosporins Clotrimazole (topical)[i] Erythromycin[j] Mezlocillin Miconazole (topical)[i] Nitrofurantoin Nystatin Oxacillin Penicillin Piperacillin/tazobactam Ticarcillin/clavulanic acid	Imipenem/cilastatin Metronidazole[k] Valacyclovir Vancomycin	Pentamidine Pyrazinamide[l] Rifampin[l] Tobramycin Trimethoprim-sulamethoxazole[f]	
Antithrombotics		Clopidogrel Dalteparin[m] Danaparoid[m] Dipyridamole Enoxaparin[m] Heparin[m] Lepirudin[m] Ticlopidine	Aspirin[b]	Warfarin
Cardiovascular drugs		Atenolol[n] Clonidine Digoxin Doxazosin Hydralazine Labetalol[n] Lidocaine Methyldopa Metoprolol[n] Prazosin Procainamide Propranolol[n] Quinidine Terazosin Timolol[n]	Amlodipine Diltiazem Felodipine Nicardipine Nifedipine Nitrates Verapamil	Angiotensin-converting enzyme inhibitors Angiotensin II–receptor antagonists
Cough and cold agents		Dextromethorphan	Guaifenesin Phenylpropanolamine Pseudoephedrine	

Class of medication	Relatively safe to use in pregnancy	Limited data or fetal risk appear minimal	Evidence of fetal risk[a]	Significant fetal risk; avoid in pregnancy
Diuretics[o]		Amiloride Bumetanide Chlorthalidone Chlorthiazide Ethacrynic acid Furosemide Hydrochlorothiazide Indapamide Metolazone Spironolactone Torsemide Triamterene		
Gastrointestinal agents	Antacids[p] Attapulgite Kaolin-pectin Loperamide Metoclopramide Psyllium	Bismuth subsalicylate Casanthranol Cisapride Dicyclomine Docusate H_2-receptor antagonists Lansoprazole Omeprazole Phenolphthalein Senna Simethicone Sucralfate		Misoprostol
Hormonal agents			Glucocorticoids[q] (systemic) Progestins[r]	Estrogens Oral contraceptives
Respiratory agents		Albuterol[s] Beclomethasone (inhalation) Cromolyn Flunisolide (inhalation) Ipratropium Metaproterenol[s] Montelukast Nedocromil Pirbuterol[s] Salmeterol[s] Theophylline Triamcinolone (inhalation) Zafirlukast	Zileuton	

Class of medication	Relatively safe to use in pregnancy	Limited data or fetal risk appear minimal	Evidence of fetal risk[a]	Significant fetal risk; avoid in pregnancy
Sedatives		Buspirone Propofol Zolpidem	Benzodiazepines[c]	Pentobarbital Phenobarbital
Thyroid preparations	Levothyroxine Thyroid		Methimazole Potassium iodide Propylthiouracil[t]	
Miscellaneous	Ferrous sulfate Potassium chloride	Allopurinol Carisoprodol Chlorzoxazone Cyclobenzaprine Etanercept Flavoxate Oxybutynin	Azathioprine Cilostazol Cyclosporine Modafinil Naratriptan Pentoxifylline Sumatriptan Rizatriptan Zolmitriptan	Isotretinoin Leflunomide Quinine Tamoxifen

HMG-CoA = 3-hydroxy-3-methylglutaryl coenzyme A.

[a]These medications have some associated risk when used during pregnancy. The potential benefit should be carefully weighed against possible adverse effects.

[b]Use during the third trimester may cause constriction of the ductus arteriosus, which may result in persistent pulmonary hypertension in the newborn. These agents may also inhibit labor and prolong the length of pregnancy.

[c]Regular use during pregnancy may cause physical dependence in the neonate. Avoid use for prolonged periods or in high doses at term.

[d]The risk to the mother may be greater if anticonvulsant therapy is withheld and seizure control is lost. Epilepsy should be treated with the fewest drugs in the lowest doses that are sufficient to prevent convulsions, and pregnant women should be counseled regarding increased risk of malformations.

[e]Drug of choice for convulsions associated with toxemia of pregnancy.

[f]Avoid during the last few weeks of pregnancy.

[g]Generally recognized as safe for mother and fetus if used occasionally in low doses.

[h]These agents are almost totally unabsorbed, but potential adverse effects on the fetus may occur because of impaired maternal absorption of fat-soluble vitamins.

[i]For self-medication, these drugs should not be used in pregnant women unless otherwise instructed by a physician.

[j]Erythromycin estolate has been associated with an increased risk of reversible subclinical hepatotoxicity in approximately 10% of pregnant women; problems with other erythromycins have not been documented.

[k]Avoid use during the first trimester.

[l]Pregnant women with tuberculosis should be managed in concert with an expert in the management of tuberculosis. Untreated tuberculosis represents a far greater hazard to a pregnant woman and her fetus than does treatment of the disease.

[m]Use in the last trimester may increase the risk of maternal bleeding. Maternal osteopenia may be a complication of long-term therapy.

[n]Fetal and neonatal bradycardia, hypotension, hypoglycemia, and respiratory depression have been reported. Whenever possible, avoid therapy during the first trimester and discontinue therapy 2–3 days before delivery.

[o]Routine use of diuretics in pregnancy is not recommended, except for patients with cardiovascular disorders, as these agents do not prevent or alter the course of toxemia and may decrease placental perfusion.

[p]Antacids are generally considered safe as long as chronic high doses are avoided.

[q]Physiologic replacement doses of glucocorticoids administered for treatment of maternal adrenal insufficiency are unlikely to affect the fetus or neonate adversely. Infants born to mothers who received substantial doses of glucocorticoids during pregnancy should be observed carefully for signs of hypoadrenalism.

[r]Progestational agents have been used to prevent habitual or threatened abortion within the first few months of pregnancy and to treat corpus luteum deficiency in early pregnancy.

[s]β-Adrenergic agonists may cause maternal and, to a lesser extent, fetal tachycardia. Maternal hypotension, hyperglycemia, and neonatal hypoglycemia should be expected.

ᵗConsidered the drug of choice for the medical treatment of hyperthyroidism during pregnancy.
Source: Drugs in Pregnancy, 2nd ed. New York: Chapman & Hall, 1997; *Drugs in Pregnancy and Lactation,* 5th ed. Baltimore: Williams & Wilkins, 1998; *Drug Therapy in Obstetrics and Gynecology,* 3rd ed. St. Louis: Mosby–Year Book, 1992; *Handbook of Medicine of the Fetus and Mother.* Philadelphia: Lippincott, 1995; and *Drug Information for the Health Care Professional* (USP DI, vol I). Rockville, MD: United States Pharmacopeial Convention, 1999.

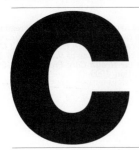

Drug Interactions

S. Troy McMullin

Common drug interactions are summarized in Table C. Because new information on drug interactions is continually emerging, it is impossible to include all current drug interactions in a reference text. Information regarding the metabolic pathway of selected medications is included to assist in the prediction of likely drug interactions with new medications. For example, if a new medication inhibits the 3A4 pathway, it would be anticipated to increase the serum concentration of alprazolam, carbamazepine, cisapride, cyclosporine, and other 3A4 substrates. A key to the abbreviations can be found on page 607.

Table C. Common drug interactions

Medication	Interacting drug	Effect
Adenosine	Carbamazepine	Increased adenosine toxicity
	Dipyridamole	Increased adenosine toxicity
	Theophylline	Decreased adenosine effectiveness
Alendronate	Antacids	Decreased alendronate absorption
	Calcium	Decreased alendronate absorption
	Ferrous sulfate	Decreased alendronate absorption
	Sucralfate	Decreased alendronate absorption
Allopurinol	6-Mercaptopurine	Increased 6-mercaptopurine concentrations
	Azathioprine	Increased azathioprine concentrations
	Cyclophosphamide	Increased cyclophosphamide concentrations
Alprazolam (3A4 substrate)	Clarithromycin	Increased alprazolam/T concentrations
	Diltiazem	Increased alprazolam/T concentrations
	Erythromycin	Increased alprazolam/T concentrations
	Fluconazole	Increased alprazolam/T concentrations
	Fluoxetine	Increased alprazolam/T concentrations
	Fluvoxamine	Increased alprazolam/T concentrations
	Grapefruit juice	Increased alprazolam/T concentrations
	Itraconazole	Increased alprazolam/T concentrations
	Ketoconazole	Increased alprazolam/T concentrations
	Nefazodone	Increased alprazolam/T concentrations
	Quinupristin/dalfopristin	Increased alprazolam/T concentrations
	Verapamil	Increased alprazolam/T concentrations

Medication	Interacting drug	Effect
Amiodarone (2C9 inhibitor)	Barbiturates	Decreased amiodarone concentrations
	Carbamazepine	Decreased amiodarone concentrations
	Cisapride	Increased risk for arrhythmias
	Cyclosporine	Increased cyclosporine concentrations
	Digoxin	Increased digoxin concentrations
	Phenytoin	Increased phenytoin concentrations or decreased amiodarone concentrations
	Rifampin	Decreased amiodarone concentrations
	Warfarin	Increased warfarin concentrations
Amprenavir (3A4 inhibitor)	Atorvastatin	Increased atorvastatin concentrations
	Barbiturates	Decreased amprenavir/I/L/N/R/S concentrations
	Carbamazepine	Decreased amprenavir/I/L/N/R/S concentrations or increased carbamazepine concentrations
	Cerivastatin	Increased cerivastatin concentrations
	Cilostazol	Increased cilostazol concentrations
	Cisapride	Increased cisapride concentrations
	Cyclosporine	Increased cyclosporine concentrations
	Desipramine	Increased desipramine concentrations
	Flecainide	Increased flecainide concentrations
	Lovastatin	Increased lovastatin concentrations
	Phenytoin	Decreased amprenavir/I/L/N/R/S concentrations
	Pimozide	Increased pimozide concentrations
	Propafenone	Increased propafenone concentrations
	Rifampin	Decreased amprenavir/I/L/N/R/S concentrations
	Simvastatin	Increased simvastatin concentrations
	Triazolam	Increased triazolam concentrations
Antacids	Alendronate	Decreased alendronate absorption
	Isoniazid	Decreased isoniazid absorption
	Itraconazole	Decreased itraconazole absorption
	Ketoconazole	Decreased ketoconazole absorption
	Quinolone antibiotics	Decreased quinolone absorption
	Tetracyclines	Decreased tetracycline absorption
Atorvastatin (3A4 substrate)	Clarithromycin	Increased atorvastatin/C/L/S concentrations
	Diltiazem	Increased atorvastatin/C/L/S concentrations
	Erythromycin	Increased atorvastatin/C/L/S concentrations
	Fenofibrate	Increased risk of myopathy or rhabdomyolysis
	Fluconazole	Increased atorvastatin/C/L/S concentrations
	Fluvoxamine	Increased atorvastatin/C/L/S concentrations

Medication	Interacting drug	Effect
	Gemfibrozil	Increased risk of myopathy or rhabdomyolysis
	Grapefruit juice	Increased atorvastatin/C/L/S concentrations
	Itraconazole	Increased atorvastatin/C/L/S concentrations
	Ketoconazole	Increased atorvastatin/C/L/S concentrations
	Nefazodone	Increased atorvastatin/C/L/S concentrations
	Niacin	Increased risk of myopathy or rhabdomyolysis
	Protease inhibitors	Increased atorvastatin/C/L/S concentrations
	Quinupristin/dalfopristin	Increased atorvastatin/C/L/S concentrations
	Verapamil	Increased atorvastatin/C/L/S concentrations
Barbiturates (enzyme inducer)	Antiarrhythmics	Decreased antiarrhythmic concentrations
	Azole antifungals	Decreased antifungal concentrations
	Beta-blockers	Decreased beta-blocker concentrations
	Chloramphenicol	Decreased chloramphenicol concentrations
	Corticosteroids	Decreased corticosteroid concentrations
	Cyclosporine	Decreased cyclosporine concentrations
	Oral contraceptives	Decreased contraceptive concentrations
	Protease inhibitors	Decreased protease inhibitor concentrations
	Theophylline	Decreased theophylline concentrations
	Warfarin	Decreased warfarin concentrations
Calcium salts	Alendronate	Decreased alendronate absorption
	Quinolone antibiotics	Decreased quinolone absorption
	Tetracyclines	Decreased tetracycline absorption
Carbamazepine (enzyme inducer, 3A4 substrate)	Adenosine	Increased adenosine toxicity
	Antiarrhythmics	Decreased antiarrhythmic concentrations
	Azole antifungals	Decreased antifungal concentrations
	Beta-blockers	Decreased beta-blocker concentrations
	Chloramphenicol	Decreased chloramphenicol concentrations
	Clarithromycin	Increased carbamazepine concentrations
	Corticosteroids	Decreased corticosteroid concentrations
	Cyclosporine	Decreased cyclosporine concentrations
	Diltiazem	Increased carbamazepine concentrations
	Erythromycin	Increased carbamazepine concentrations
	Fluconazole	Increased carbamazepine concentrations or decreased antifungal concentrations
	Fluvoxamine	Increased carbamazepine concentrations
	Grapefruit juice	Increased carbamazepine concentrations
	Isoniazid	Increased carbamazepine concentrations
	Itraconazole	Increased carbamazepine concentrations or decreased antifungal concentrations

Medication	Interacting drug	Effect
	Ketoconazole	Increased carbamazepine concentrations or decreased antifungal concentrations
	Nefazodone	Increased carbamazepine concentrations
	Oral contraceptives	Decreased contraceptive concentrations
	Protease inhibitors	Decreased protease inhibitor concentrations
	Quinidine	Decreased quinidine concentrations
	Quinupristin/dalfopristin	Increased carbamazepine concentrations
	Theophylline	Decreased theophylline concentrations
	Verapamil	Increased carbamazepine concentrations
	Warfarin	Decreased warfarin concentrations
Carvedilol (2D6 substrate)	β-Agonists	Decreased β-agonist effectiveness
	Barbiturates	Decreased carvedilol/L/M/P concentrations
	Carbamazepine	Decreased carvedilol/L/M/P concentrations
	Cimetidine	Increased carvedilol/L/M/P concentrations
	Fluoxetine	Increased carvedilol/L/M/P concentrations
	Paroxetine	Increased carvedilol/L/M/P concentrations
	Phenytoin	Decreased carvedilol/L/M/P concentrations
	Quinidine	Increased carvedilol/L/M/P concentrations
	Rifampin	Decreased carvedilol/L/M/P concentrations
	Ritonavir	Increased carvedilol/L/M/P concentrations
Cerivastatin (3A4 substrate)	See atorvastatin	
Chloramphenicol (2C9 inhibitor)	Barbiturates	Decreased chloramphenicol concentrations
	Carbamazepine	Decreased chloramphenicol concentrations
	Phenytoin	Decreased chloramphenicol concentrations
	Rifampin	Decreased chloramphenicol concentrations
	Warfarin	Increased warfarin concentrations
Cilostazol (3A4 substrate)	Clarithromycin	Increased cilostazol concentrations
	Diltiazem	Increased cilostazol concentrations
	Erythromycin	Increased cilostazol concentrations
	Fluconazole	Increased cilostazol concentrations
	Fluvoxamine	Increased cilostazol concentrations
	Grapefruit juice	Increased cilostazol concentrations
	Itraconazole	Increased cilostazol concentrations
	Ketoconazole	Increased cilostazol concentrations
	Nefazodone	Increased cilostazol concentrations
	Omeprazole	Increased cilostazol concentrations
	Protease inhibitors	Increased cilostazol concentrations
	Quinupristin/dalfopristin	Increased cilostazol concentrations
	Verapamil	Increased cilostazol concentrations

Medication	Interacting drug	Effect
Cimetidine (1A2, 2C9, 2D6 inhibitor)	Beta-blockers	Increased beta-blocker concentrations
	Metformin	Increased metformin concentrations
	Phenytoin	Increased phenytoin concentrations
	Procainamide	Increased procainamide concentrations
	Tacrine	Increased tacrine concentrations
	Theophylline	Increased theophylline concentrations
	Tricyclic antidepressants	Increased antidepressant concentrations
	Warfarin	Increased warfarin concentrations
Ciprofloxacin (1A2 inhibitor)	Antacids	Decreased ciprofloxacin absorption
	Calcium	Decreased ciprofloxacin absorption
	Didanosine	Decreased ciprofloxacin absorption
	Ferrous sulfate	Decreased ciprofloxacin absorption
	Sucralfate	Decreased ciprofloxacin absorption
	Theophylline	Increased theophylline concentrations
	Warfarin	Increased warfarin concentrations
Cisapride (3A4 substrate)	Amiodarone	Increased risk for arrhythmias
	Antiarrhythmics	Increased risk for arrhythmias
	Antidepressants	Increased risk for arrhythmias
	Antipsychotics	Increased risk for arrhythmias
	Bepridil	Increased risk for arrhythmias
	Clarithromycin	Increased cisapride concentrations
	Erythromycin	Increased cisapride concentrations
	Fluconazole	Increased cisapride concentrations
	Fluvoxamine	Increased cisapride concentrations
	Grapefruit juice	Increased cisapride concentrations
	Haloperidol	Increased risk for arrhythmias
	Ibutilide	Increased risk of arrhythmias
	Itraconazole	Increased cisapride concentrations
	Ketoconazole	Increased cisapride concentrations
	Nefazodone	Increased cisapride concentrations
	Pimozide	Increased risk for arrhythmias
	Procainamide	Increased risk for arrhythmias
	Protease inhibitors	Increased cisapride concentrations
	Quinidine	Increased risk for arrhythmias
	Quinupristin/dalfopristin	Increased cisapride concentrations
	Sotalol	Increased risk for arrhythmias
	Sparfloxacin	Increased risk for arrhythmias
	Terodiline	Increased risk for arrhythmias
	Zileuton	Increased cisapride concentrations

Medication	Interacting drug	Effect
Citalopram	MAO inhibitors	Serotonin syndrome
	Rizatriptan	Increased risk for serotonin syndrome
	Sumatriptan	Increased risk for serotonin syndrome
Clarithromycin (3A4 inhibitor)	Alprazolam	Increased alprazolam concentrations
	Atorvastatin	Increased atorvastatin concentrations
	Carbamazepine	Increased carbamazepine concentrations
	Cerivastatin	Increased cerivastatin concentrations
	Cilostazol	Increased cilostazol concentrations
	Cisapride	Increased cisapride concentrations
	Cyclosporine	Increased cyclosporine concentrations
	Digoxin	Increased digoxin concentrations
	Disopyramide	Increased disopyramide concentrations
	Lovastatin	Increased lovastatin concentrations
	Pimozide	Increased pimozide concentrations
	Simvastatin	Increased simvastatin concentrations
	Theophylline	Increased theophylline concentrations
	Triazolam	Increased triazolam concentrations
Codeine (2D6 substrate)	Fluoxetine	Decreased codeine effectiveness
	Paroxetine	Decreased codeine effectiveness
	Quinidine	Decreased codeine effectiveness
	Ritonavir	Decreased codeine effectiveness
Corticosteroids	Barbiturates	Decreased corticosteroid concentrations
	Carbamazepine	Decreased corticosteroid concentrations
	Phenytoin	Decreased corticosteroid concentrations
	Rifampin	Decreased corticosteroid concentrations
Cyclosporine (3A4 substrate)	Amiodarone	Increased cyclosporine concentrations
	Barbiturates	Decreased cyclosporine concentrations
	Carbamazepine	Decreased cyclosporine concentrations
	Clarithromycin	Increased cyclosporine concentrations
	Diltiazem	Increased cyclosporine concentrations
	Erythromycin	Increased cyclosporine concentrations
	Fluconazole	Increased cyclosporine concentrations
	Fluoxetine	Increased cyclosporine concentrations
	Fluvoxamine	Increased cyclosporine concentrations
	Grapefruit juice	Increased cyclosporine concentrations
	Itraconazole	Increased cyclosporine concentrations
	Ketoconazole	Increased cyclosporine concentrations
	Nefazodone	Increased cyclosporine concentrations
	Phenytoin	Decreased cyclosporine concentrations
	Protease inhibitors	Increased cyclosporine concentrations
	Quinupristin/dal-fopristin	Increased cyclosporine concentrations

Medication	Interacting drug	Effect
	Rifampin	Decreased cyclosporine concentrations
	Sirolimus	Increased sirolimus concentrations
Dapsone	Didanosine	Decreased dapsone absorption
	H$_2$ antagonists	Decreased dapsone absorption
	Lansoprazole	Decreased dapsone absorption
	Omeprazole	Decreased dapsone absorption
Delavirdine	Alprazolam	Increased alprazolam concentrations
	Cisapride	Increased cisapride concentrations
	Ergot derivatives	Increased ergotamine concentrations
	Rifampin	Decreased delavirdine/efavirenz/nevirapine concentrations
	Triazolam	Increased triazolam concentrations
Dextromethorphan (2D6 substrate)	Fluoxetine	Increased risk of serotonin syndrome
	Paroxetine	Increased risk of serotonin syndrome
Didanosine	Dapsone	Decreased dapsone absorption
	Indinavir	Decreased indinavir absorption
	Itraconazole	Decreased itraconazole absorption
	Ketoconazole	Decreased ketoconazole absorption
	Quinolone antibiotics	Decreased quinolone absorption
Digoxin	Amiodarone	Increased digoxin concentrations
	Clarithromycin	Increased digoxin concentrations
	Erythromycin	Increased digoxin concentrations
	Quinidine	Increased digoxin concentrations
	Verapamil	Increased digoxin concentrations
Diltiazem (3A4 inhibitor)	Alprazolam	Increased alprazolam concentrations
	Atorvastatin	Increased atorvastatin concentrations
	Carbamazepine	Increased carbamazepine concentrations
	Cerivastatin	Increased cerivastatin concentrations
	Cilostazol	Increased cilostazol concentrations
	Cyclosporine	Increased cyclosporine concentrations
	Lovastatin	Increased lovastatin concentrations
	Simvastatin	Increased simvastatin concentrations
	Sirolimus	Increased sirolimus concentrations
	Triazolam	Increased triazolam concentrations
Disopyramide (3A4 substrate)	Antipsychotics	Increased risk for arrhythmias
	Barbiturates	Decreased disopyramide concentrations
	Bepridil	Increased risk for arrhythmias
	Carbamazepine	Decreased disopyramide concentrations
	Clarithromycin	Increased disopyramide concentrations
	Erythromycin	Increased disopyramide concentrations
	Fluconazole	Increased disopyramide concentrations

Medication	Interacting drug	Effect
	Fluvoxamine	Increased disopyramide concentrations
	Grapefruit juice	Increased disopyramide concentrations
	Itraconazole	Increased disopyramide concentrations
	Ketoconazole	Increased disopyramide concentrations
	Phenytoin	Decreased disopyramide concentrations
	Quinupristin/dal-fopristin	Increased disopyramide concentrations
	Rifampin	Decreased disopyramide concentrations
	Sparfloxacin	Increased risk for arrhythmias
	Tricyclic antide-pressants	Increased risk for arrhythmias
Efavirenz	See delavirdine	
Erythromycin (3A4 inhibitor)	Alprazolam	Increased alprazolam concentrations
	Atorvastatin	Increased atorvastatin concentrations
	Carbamazepine	Increased carbamazepine concentrations
	Cerivastatin	Increased cerivastatin concentrations
	Cilostazol	Increased cilostazol concentrations
	Cisapride	Increased cisapride concentrations
	Cyclosporine	Increased cyclosporine concentrations
	Digoxin	Increased digoxin concentrations
	Disopyramide	Increased disopyramide concentrations
	Lovastatin	Increased lovastatin concentrations
	Pimozide	Increased pimozide concentrations
	Simvastatin	Increased simvastatin concentrations
	Theophylline	Increased theophylline concentrations
	Triazolam	Increased triazolam concentrations
Fenofibrate	HMG CoA reduc-tase inhibitors	Increased risk of myopathy or rhabdomyolysis
Ferrous sulfate	Alendronate	Decreased alendronate absorption
	Quinolone antibi-otics	Decreased quinolone absorption
	Tetracyclines	Decreased tetracycline absorption
Flecainide (2D6 substrate)	Fluoxetine	Increased flecainide concentrations
	Paroxetine	Increased flecainide concentrations
	Protease inhibitors	Increased flecainide concentrations
Fluconazole (2C9, 3A4 inhibitor)	Alprazolam	Increased alprazolam concentrations
	Atorvastatin	Increased atorvastatin concentrations
	Carbamazepine	Increased carbamazepine concentrations or decreased fluconazole concentrations
	Cerivastatin	Increased cerivastatin concentrations
	Cilostazol	Increased cilostazol concentrations
	Cisapride	Increased cisapride concentrations
	Cyclosporine	Increased cyclosporine concentrations

Medication	Interacting drug	Effect
	Disopyramide	Increased disopyramide concentrations
	Lovastatin	Increased lovastatin concentrations
	Phenytoin	Increased phenytoin concentrations or decreased fluconazole concentrations
	Simvastatin	Increased simvastatin concentrations
	Triazolam	Increased triazolam concentrations
	Warfarin	Increased warfarin concentrations
Fluoxetine (2D6, 3A4 inhibitor)	Alprazolam	Increased alprazolam concentrations
	Amitriptyline	Increased amitriptyline concentrations
	Benztropine	Increased benztropine concentrations
	Carvedilol	Increased carvedilol concentrations
	Clomipramine	Increased clomipramine concentrations
	Codeine	Decreased codeine effectiveness
	Cyclosporine	Increased cyclosporine concentrations
	Desipramine	Increased desipramine concentrations
	Dextromethorphan	Increased risk for serotonin syndrome
	Diazepam	Increased diazepam concentrations
	Flecainide	Increased flecainide concentrations
	Imipramine	Increased imipramine concentrations
	Labetalol	Increased labetalol concentrations
	MAO inhibitors	Serotonin syndrome
	Metoprolol	Increased metoprolol concentrations
	Nortriptyline	Increased nortriptyline concentrations
	Phenytoin	Increased phenytoin concentrations
	Propafenone	Increased propafenone concentrations
	Propranolol	Increased propranolol concentrations
	Rizatriptan	Increased risk for serotonin syndrome
	Sumatriptan	Increased risk for serotonin syndrome
	Tramadol	Decreased tramadol effectiveness
	Triazolam	Increased triazolam concentrations
Fluvastatin	Fenofibrate	Increased risk of myopathy or rhabdomyolysis
	Gemfibrozil	Increased risk of myopathy or rhabdomyolysis
	Niacin	Increased risk of myopathy or rhabdomyolysis
Fluvoxamine (1A2, 2C9, 3A4 inhibitor)	Alprazolam	Increased alprazolam concentrations
	Amitriptyline	Increased amitriptyline concentrations
	Atorvastatin	Increased atorvastatin concentrations
	Carbamazepine	Increased carbamazepine concentrations
	Cerivastatin	Increased cerivastatin concentrations
	Cilostazol	Increased cilostazol concentrations
	Cisapride	Increased cisapride concentrations
	Clomipramine	Increased clomipramine concentrations
	Clozapine	Increased clozapine concentrations

Medication	Interacting drug	Effect
	Cyclosporine	Increased cyclosporine concentrations
	Diazepam	Increased diazepam concentrations
	Disopyramide	Increased disopyramide concentrations
	Imipramine	Increased imipramine concentrations
	Lovastatin	Increased lovastatin concentrations
	MAO inhibitors	Serotonin syndrome
	Phenytoin	Increased phenytoin concentrations
	Pimozide	Increased pimozide concentrations
	Simvastatin	Increased simvastatin concentrations
	Theophylline	Increased theophylline concentrations
	Triazolam	Increased triazolam concentrations
	Warfarin	Increased warfarin concentrations
Gemfibrozil	HMG CoA reductase inhibitors	Increased risk of myopathy or rhabdomyolysis
Grapefruit juice (3A4 inhibitor)	Alprazolam	Increased alprazolam concentrations
	Atorvastatin	Increased atorvastatin concentrations
	Carbamazepine	Increased carbamazepine concentrations
	Cerivastatin	Increased cerivastatin concentrations
	Cilostazol	Increased cilostazol concentrations
	Cisapride	Increased cisapride concentrations
	Cyclosporine	Increased cyclosporine concentrations
	Disopyramide	Increased disopyramide concentrations
	Lovastatin	Increased lovastatin concentrations
	Pimozide	Increased pimozide concentrations
	Simvastatin	Increased simvastatin concentrations
	Theophylline	Increased theophylline concentrations
	Triazolam	Increased triazolam concentrations
Ibutilide	Antiarrhythmics	Increased risk of arrhythmias
	Bepridil	Increased risk of arrhythmias
	Cisapride	Increased risk of arrhythmias
	Phenothiazines	Increased risk of arrhythmias
	Sparfloxacin	Increased risk of arrhythmias
	Tricyclic antidepressants	Increased risk of arrhythmias
Indinavir	See amprenavir	
Isoniazid	Carbamazepine	Increased carbamazepine concentrations
	Diazepam	Increased diazepam concentrations
	Phenytoin	Increased phenytoin concentrations
Itraconazole (3A4 inhibitor)	Alprazolam	Increased alprazolam concentrations
	Antacids	Decreased itraconazole/K absorption
	Atorvastatin	Increased atorvastatin concentrations

Medication	Interacting drug	Effect
	Carbamazepine	Increased carbamazepine concentrations or decreased itraconazole/K concentrations
	Cerivastatin	Increased cerivastatin concentrations
	Cilostazol	Increased cilostazol concentrations
	Cisapride	Increased cisapride concentrations
	Cyclosporine	Increased cyclosporine concentrations
	Didanosine	Decreased itraconazole/K absorption
	Disopyramide	Increased disopyramide concentrations
	H_2 antagonists	Decreased itraconazole/K absorption
	Lansoprazole	Decreased itraconazole/K absorption
	Lovastatin	Increased lovastatin concentrations
	Omeprazole	Decreased itraconazole/K absorption
	Phenytoin	Increased phenytoin concentrations or decreased itraconazole/K concentrations
	Simvastatin	Increased simvastatin concentrations
	Triazolam	Increased triazolam concentrations
	Warfarin	Increased warfarin concentrations
Ketoconazole (3A4 inhibitor)	See itraconazole	
Labetalol (2D6 substrate)	See carvedilol	
Lansoprazole	Dapsone	Decreased dapsone absorption
	Itraconazole	Decreased itraconazole absorption
	Ketoconazole	Decreased ketoconazole absorption
Linezolid	See MAO inhibitors	
Lopinavir	See amprenavir	
Lovastatin (3A4 substrate)	See atorvastatin	
MAO inhibitors	Amphetamines	Hypertensive crisis
	Meperidine	Hyperpyrexia, agitation, and seizures
	Nefazodone	Serotonin syndrome
	Rizatriptan	Increased rizatriptan concentrations
	SSRIs	Serotonin syndrome
	Sumatriptan	Increased sumatriptan concentrations
	Sympathomimetics	Hypertensive crisis
	Tramadol	Increased toxicity from MAOI/linezolid
	Tricyclic antidepressants	Increased toxicity from MAOI/linezolid
	Venlafaxine	Serotonin syndrome
	Zolmitriptan	Increased zolmitriptan concentrations
Metformin	Cimetidine	Increased metformin concentrations
Metoprolol (2D6 substrate)	See carvedilol	

Medication	Interacting drug	Effect
Metronidazole (2C9 inhibitor)	Disulfiram	Increased disulfiram toxicity
	Warfarin	Increased warfarin concentrations
Nefazodone (3A4 inhibitor)	Alprazolam	Increased alprazolam concentrations
	Atorvastatin	Increased atorvastatin concentrations
	Carbamazepine	Increased carbamazepine concentrations
	Cerivastatin	Increased cerivastatin concentrations
	Cilostazol	Increased cilostazol concentrations
	Cisapride	Increased cisapride concentrations
	Cyclosporine	Increased cyclosporine concentrations
	Lovastatin	Increased lovastatin concentrations
	MAO inhibitors	Increased toxicity from MAOI
	Simvastatin	Increased simvastatin concentrations
	Triazolam	Increased triazolam concentrations
Nelfinavir	See amprenavir	
Nevirapine	See delavirdine	
Niacin	HMG CoA reductase inhibitors	Increased risk of myopathy or rhabdomyolysis
NSAIDs	ACE inhibitors	Increased risk of nephrotoxicity or blunted antihypertensive effects
	Diuretics	Increased risk of nephrotoxicity or blunted antihypertensive effects
	Lithium	Increased lithium concentrations
	Methotrexate	Increased methotrexate concentrations
	Warfarin	Increased risk of bleeding
Omeprazole (1A2 inducer, 2C19 inhibitor)	Dapsone	Decreased dapsone absorption
	Diazepam	Increased diazepam concentrations
	Itraconazole	Decreased itraconazole absorption
	Ketoconazole	Decreased ketoconazole absorption
	Phenytoin	Increased phenytoin concentrations
	Theophylline	Decreased theophylline concentrations
Oral contraceptives	Antibiotics	Decreased contraceptive effectiveness
	Barbiturates	Decreased contraceptive effectiveness
	Carbamazepine	Decreased contraceptive effectiveness
	Phenytoin	Decreased contraceptive effectiveness
	Rifampin	Decreased contraceptive effectiveness
Paroxetine (2D6 inhibitor)	Benztropine	Increased benztropine concentrations
	Carvedilol	Increased carvedilol concentrations
	Codeine	Decreased codeine effectiveness
	Desipramine	Increased desipramine concentrations
	Dextromethorphan	Increased risk for serotonin syndrome
	Flecainide	Increased flecainide concentrations
	Labetalol	Increased labetalol concentrations

Medication	Interacting drug	Effect
	MAO inhibitors	Serotonin syndrome
	Metoprolol	Increased metoprolol concentrations
	Nortriptyline	Increased nortriptyline concentrations
	Propafenone	Increased propafenone concentrations
	Propranolol	Increased propranolol concentrations
	Rizatriptan	Increased risk for serotonin syndrome
	Sumatriptan	Increased risk for serotonin syndrome
	Tramadol	Decreased tramadol effectiveness
Phenytoin (enzyme inducer, 2C9 substrate)	Amiodarone	Decreased amiodarone concentrations or increased phenytoin concentrations
	Antiarrhythmics	Decreased antiarrhythmic concentrations
	Azole antifungals	Decreased antifungal concentrations
	Beta-blockers	Decreased beta-blocker concentrations
	Chloramphenicol	Decreased chloramphenicol concentrations or increased phenytoin concentrations
	Cimetidine	Increased phenytoin concentrations
	Corticosteroids	Decreased corticosteroid concentrations
	Cyclosporine	Decreased cyclosporine concentrations
	Fluconazole	Decreased fluconazole concentrations or increased phenytoin concentrations
	Fluoxetine	Increased phenytoin concentrations
	Isoniazid	Increased phenytoin concentrations
	Itraconazole	Decreased itraconazole concentrations or increased phenytoin concentrations
	Ketoconazole	Decreased ketoconazole concentrations
	Omeprazole	Increased phenytoin concentrations
	Oral contraceptives	Decreased contraceptive effectiveness
	Protease inhibitors	Decreased protease inhibitor concentrations
	Quinidine	Decreased quinidine concentrations
	Theophylline	Decreased theophylline concentrations
	Ticlopidine	Increased phenytoin concentrations
	Warfarin	Decreased warfarin concentrations
Pimozide (3A4 substrate)	Amiodarone	Increased risk for arrhythmias
	Antiarrhythmics	Increased risk for arrhythmias
	Antidepressants	Increased risk for arrhythmias
	Antipsychotics	Increased risk for arrhythmias
	Bepridil	Increased risk for arrhythmias
	Cisapride	Increased risk for arrhythmias
	Clarithromycin	Increased pimozide concentrations
	Erythromycin	Increased pimozide concentrations
	Fluconazole	Increased pimozide concentrations
	Fluvoxamine	Increased pimozide concentrations

Medication	Interacting drug	Effect
	Grapefruit juice	Increased pimozide concentrations
	Haloperidol	Increased risk for arrhythmias
	Ibutilide	Increased risk for arrhythmias
	Itraconazole	Increased pimozide concentrations
	Ketoconazole	Increased pimozide concentrations
	Nefazodone	Increased pimozide concentrations
	Procainamide	Increased risk for arrhythmias
	Protease inhibitors	Increased pimozide concentrations
	Quinidine	Increased risk for arrhythmias
	Quinupristin/dalfopristin	Increased pimozide concentrations
	Sotalol	Increased risk for arrhythmias
	Sparfloxacin	Increased risk for arrhythmias
	Terodiline	Increased risk for arrhythmias
	Zileuton	Increased pimozide concentrations
Pravastatin	Fenofibrate	Increased risk of myopathy or rhabdomyolysis
	Gemfibrozil	Increased risk of myopathy or rhabdomyolysis
	Niacin	Increased risk of myopathy or rhabdomyolysis
Procainamide	Antipsychotics	Increased risk for arrhythmias
	Bepridil	Increased risk for arrhythmias
	Cimetidine	Increased procainamide concentrations
	Cisapride	Increased risk for arrhythmias
	Sparfloxacin	Increased risk for arrhythmias
	Tricyclic antidepressants	Increased risk for arrhythmias
Propafenone (2D6 substrate)	Antipsychotics	Increased risk for arrhythmias
	Bepridil	Increased risk for arrhythmias
	Cisapride	Increased risk for arrhythmias
	Fluoxetine	Increased propafenone concentrations
	Paroxetine	Increased propafenone concentrations
	Protease inhibitors	Increased propafenone concentrations
	Sparfloxacin	Increased risk for arrhythmias
	Tricyclic antidepressants	Increased risk for arrhythmias
Propranolol (2D6 substrate)	See carvedilol	
Quinidine (2D6 inhibitor)	Antipsychotics	Increased risk for arrhythmias
	Barbiturates	Decreased quinidine concentrations
	Bepridil	Increased risk for arrhythmias
	Carbamazepine	Decreased quinidine concentrations
	Cisapride	Increased risk for arrhythmias
	Codeine	Decreased codeine effectiveness

Medication	Interacting drug	Effect
	Desipramine	Increased desipramine concentrations
	Digoxin	Increased digoxin concentrations
	Nortriptyline	Increased nortriptyline concentrations
	Phenytoin	Decreased quinidine concentrations
	Rifampin	Decreased quinidine concentrations
	Sparfloxacin	Increased risk for arrhythmias
	Tramadol	Decreased tramadol effectiveness
	Tricyclic antidepressants	Increased risk for arrhythmias
Quinupristin/dalfopristin (3A4 inhibitor)	Alprazolam	Increased alprazolam concentrations
	Atorvastatin	Increased atorvastatin concentrations
	Carbamazepine	Increased carbamazepine concentrations
	Cerivastatin	Increased cerivastatin concentrations
	Cilostazol	Increased cilostazol concentrations
	Cisapride	Increased cisapride concentrations
	Cyclosporine	Increased cyclosporine concentrations
	Disopyramide	Increased disopyramide concentrations
	Lovastatin	Increased lovastatin concentrations
	Pimozide	Increased pimozide concentrations
	Simvastatin	Increased simvastatin concentrations
	Triazolam	Increased triazolam concentrations
Rifampin (enzyme inducer)	Antiarrhythmics	Decreased antiarrhythmic concentrations
	Azole antifungals	Decreased antifungal concentrations
	Beta-blockers	Decreased beta-blocker concentrations
	Chloramphenicol	Decreased chloramphenicol concentrations
	Corticosteroids	Decreased corticosteroid concentrations
	Cyclosporine	Decreased cyclosporine concentrations
	Oral contraceptives	Decreased contraceptive effectiveness
	Protease inhibitors	Decreased protease inhibitor concentrations
	Theophylline	Decreased theophylline concentrations
	Warfarin	Decreased warfarin concentrations
Ritonavir	See amprenavir	
Rizatriptan	Ergot derivatives	Increased risk of rizatriptan/sumatriptan toxicity
	MAO inhibitors	Increased risk of MAOI toxicity
	SSRIs	Increased risk of serotonin syndrome
Saquinavir	See amprenavir	
Sertraline	MAO inhibitors	Increased toxicity from MAOI
	Rizatriptan	Increased risk for serotonin syndrome
	Sumatriptan	Increased risk for serotonin syndrome
Sildenafil	Nitrates	Increased toxicity from sildenafil

Medication	Interacting drug	Effect
Simvastatin (3A4 substrate)	See atorvastatin	
Sirolimus	Cyclosporine	Increased sirolimus concentrations
	Diltiazem	Increased sirolimus concentrations
Sotalol	Bepridil	Increased risk for arrhythmias
	Cisapride	Increased risk for arrhythmias
	Sparfloxacin	Increased risk for arrhythmias
Sparfloxacin	Antacids	Decreased sparfloxacin absorption
	Antiarrhythmics	Increased risk for arrhythmias
	Bepridil	Increased risk for arrhythmias
	Calcium	Decreased sparfloxacin absorption
	Cisapride	Increased risk for arrhythmias
	Didanosine	Decreased sparfloxacin absorption
	Ferrous sulfate	Decreased sparfloxacin absorption
	Flecainide	Increased risk for arrhythmias
	Procainamide	Increased risk for arrhythmias
	Quinidine	Increased risk for arrhythmias
	Sotalol	Increased risk for arrhythmias
	Sucralfate	Decreased sparfloxacin absorption
Sucralfate	Alendronate	Decreased alendronate absorption
	Quinolone antibiotics	Decreased quinolone absorption
	Tetracyclines	Decreased tetracycline absorption
Sulfamethoxazole	Warfarin	Increased warfarin concentrations
Sumatriptan	See rizatriptan	
Tetracyclines	Antacids	Decreased tetracycline absorption
	Calcium	Decreased tetracycline absorption
	Ferrous sulfate	Decreased tetracycline absorption
	Sucralfate	Decreased tetracycline absorption
Theophylline (1A2 substrate)	Adenosine	Decreased adenosine effectiveness
	Barbiturates	Decreased theophylline concentrations
	Carbamazepine	Decreased theophylline concentrations
	Cimetidine	Increased theophylline concentrations
	Ciprofloxacin	Increased theophylline concentrations
	Clarithromycin	Increased theophylline concentrations
	Erythromycin	Increased theophylline concentrations
	Fluvoxamine	Increased theophylline concentrations
	Grapefruit juice	Increased theophylline concentrations
	Omeprazole	Decreased theophylline concentrations
	Phenytoin	Decreased theophylline concentrations
	Rifampin	Decreased theophylline concentrations
	Tacrine	Increased theophylline concentrations

Medication	Interacting drug	Effect
	Ticlopidine	Increased theophylline concentrations
	Zileuton	Increased theophylline concentrations
Ticlopidine	Phenytoin	Increased phenytoin concentrations
	Theophylline	Increased theophylline concentrations
	Warfarin	Increased warfarin concentrations
Tramadol (2D6 substrate)	Cyclobenzaprine	Increased risk for seizures
	Fluoxetine	Decreased tramadol effectiveness; increased risk for seizures
	Meperidine	Increased risk for seizures
	Paroxetine	Decreased tramadol effectiveness; increased risk for seizures
	Quinidine	Decreased tramadol effectiveness
	SSRIs	Increased risk for seizures
	Tricyclic antidepressants	Increased risk for seizures
Triazolam (3A4 substrate)	See alprazolam	
Verapamil (3A4 inhibitor)	Atorvastatin	Increased atorvastatin concentrations
	Carbamazepine	Increased carbamazepine concentrations
	Cerivastatin	Increased cerivastatin concentrations
	Cilostazol	Increased cilostazol concentrations
	Cyclosporine	Increased cyclosporine concentrations
	Digoxin	Increased digoxin concentrations
	Lovastatin	Increased lovastatin concentrations
	Simvastatin	Increased simvastatin concentrations
	Triazolam	Increased triazolam concentrations
Warfarin (1A2, 2C9 substrate)	Amiodarone	Increased warfarin concentrations
	Aspirin	Increased risk of bleeding
	Barbiturates	Decreased warfarin concentrations
	Carbamazepine	Decreased warfarin concentrations
	Cefamandole	Increased risk of bleeding
	Cefmetazole	Increased risk of bleeding
	Cefoperazone	Increased risk of bleeding
	Cefotetan	Increased risk of bleeding
	Chloramphenicol	Increased warfarin concentrations
	Cimetidine	Increased warfarin concentrations
	Fluconazole	Increased warfarin concentrations
	Fluvoxamine	Increased warfarin concentrations
	Itraconazole	Increased warfarin concentrations
	Ketoconazole	Increased warfarin concentrations
	Metronidazole	Increased warfarin concentrations
	NSAIDs	Increased risk of bleeding

Medication	Interacting drug	Effect
	Phenytoin	Transient increased warfarin effect acutely; decreased warfarin concentrations chronically
	Rifampin	Decreased warfarin concentrations
	Salicylates	Increased risk of bleeding
	Sulfamethoxazole	Increased warfarin concentrations
	Ticlopidine	Increased warfarin concentrations
	Zafirlukast	Increased warfarin concentrations
Zafirlukast	Warfarin	Increased warfarin concentrations
Zileuton (1A2, 3A4 inhibitor)	Cisapride	Increased cisapride concentrations
	Theophylline	Increased theophylline concentrations

ACE = angiotensin-converting enzyme; C/L/S = cerivastatin/lovastatin/simvastatin; HMG-CoA = 3-hydroxy-3-methylglutaryl coenzyme A; I/L/N/R/S = indinavir/lopinavir/nelfinavir/ritonavir/saquinavir; K = ketaconazole; L/M/P = labetalol/metoprolol/propanol; MAO = monoamine oxidase; MAOI = MAO inhibitor; NSAIDs = nonsteroidal anti-inflammatory drugs; SSRIs = selective serotonin reuptake inhibitors; T = triazolam.

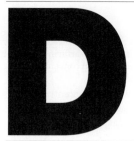

Intravenous Admixture Preparation and Administration Guide[a]

Robyn A. Schaiff

Aminophylline (see Theophylline)

Amiodarone (Cordarone)

Diluent: D5W only (glass or polyolefin containers for maintenance infusion)

Loading dosage: 150 mg over 10 mins (can repeat), then 1 mg/min for 6 hrs

Maintenance concentration: 450 mg/250 ml = 1.8 mg/ml

Infusion rate: 0.5 mg/min (0.5 mg/min = 17 ml/hr)

Amrinone [see Inamrinone (Inocor)]

Diltiazem (Cardizem)

Diluent: NS, D5W

Concentration: 125 mg/125 ml = 1 mg/ml

Initial dosage: 0.25 mg/kg (20 mg) bolus followed by 0.35 mg/kg (25 mg) bolus if necessary

Infusion rate: 5–15 mg/hr; titrate to effect

Dobutamine (Dobutrex)

Diluent: NS, D5W

Concentration: 250 mg/250 ml = 1000 µg/ml

Infusion rate: Usually start at 3 µg/kg/min; titrate up to 20 µg/kg/min

(Example: For a 70-kg patient to receive 3 µg/kg/min, the drip rate should be 13 ml/hr)

Dopamine (Intropin)

Diluent: NS, D5W

Concentration: 800 mg/500 ml = 1600 µg/ml

Infusion rate: Usually start at 3 µg/kg/min; titrate to effect

(Example: For a 70-kg patient to receive 3 µg/kg/min, the drip rate should be 8 ml/hr)

Epinephrine

Diluent: NS or D5W

Concentration: 5 mg/500 ml = 10 µg/ml

Infusion rate: 1–4 µg/min initially; titrate to effect (1 µg/min = 6 ml/hr)

Esmolol (Brevibloc)

Diluent: NS, D5W

Concentration: 2.5 g/250 ml = 10 mg/ml

Initial dosage: Loading dosage 500 µg/kg over 1 min

Infusion rate: Usually start at 50 µg/kg/min (21 ml/hr for a 70-kg patient)

Heparin

Diluent: NS, D5W, $^1\!/_2$ NS

Concentration: 25,000 units/250 ml = 100 units/ml

Initial dose: 60–80 units/kg

Infusion rate: Usually start at 14–18 units/kg/hr

Ibutilide (Corvert)

Diluent: NS or D5W or undiluted

Dosage: 1 mg (if weight <60 kg: 0.01 mg/kg) over 10 mins; can repeat 10 mins after initial infusion

Concentration: Undiluted, 1 mg/10 ml; diluted, 1 mg/50 ml (0.02 mg/ml)

Inamrinone (Inocor)

Diluent: NS only (protect from light)

Concentration: 200 mg/100 ml = 2 mg/ml

Initial dosage: Loading dosage 0.75 mg/kg over 2 mins

Infusion rate: Usually start at 5 µg/kg/min; titrate up to 15 µg/kg/min[b]

Isoproterenol (Isuprel)

Diluent: NS, D5W

Concentration: 2 mg/500 ml = 4 µg/ml

Infusion rate: Initially 2 µg/min; titrate up to 10 µg/min

Lepirudin (Refludan)

Diluent: NS or D5W

Concentration: 100 mg/250 ml

Loading dose: 0.4 mg/kg (0.2 mg/kg if Cl_{Cr} <60 ml/min)

Maintenance dose: 0.15 mg/kg/hr (decrease dose in renal dysfunction, titrate to prothrombin time 2.0–2.5 × normal)[b]

Lidocaine

Diluent: NS, D5W

Concentration: 2 g/500 ml = 4 mg/ml

Infusion rate: 1–4 mg/min (1 mg/min = 15 ml/hr)

Milrinone (Primacor)

Diluent: NS or D5W

Loading dosage: 50 µg/kg diluted over 10 mins

Concentration: 40 mg/200 ml = 0.2 mg/ml

Infusion rate: 0.375–0.750 µg/kg/min (2 mg/hr = 10 ml/hr)[b]

Nicardipine (Cardene)

Diluent: NS, D5W

Concentration: 25 mg/250 ml = 0.1 mg/ml

Infusion rate: 2–15 mg/hr

Nitroglycerin

Diluent: NS, D5W (glass or polyolefin containers only)

Concentration: 50 mg/250 ml = 200 µg/ml

Infusion rate: Initially 10 µg/min; titrate to effect (10 µg/min = 3 ml/hr)

Nitroprusside (Nipride)

Diluent: **D5W only** (protect from light)

Concentration: 50 mg/250 ml = 200 µg/ml

Infusion rate: Initially 0.25 µg/kg/min; titrate to effect (10 µg/min = 3 ml/hr)

Norepinephrine (Levophed)

    Diluent: **D5W only**

    Concentration: 8 mg/500 ml = 16 µg/ml

    Infusion rate: Initially 2 µg/min; titrate to effect (2 µg/min = 8 ml/hr)

Phenylephrine (Neo-Synephrine)

    Diluent: NS, D5W

    Concentration: 10 mg/250 ml = 40 µg/ml

    Infusion rate: Initially 10 µg/min; titrate to effect (10 µg/min = 15 ml/hr)

Procainamide (Pronestyl)

    Diluent: NS, D5W

    Concentration: 2 g/500 ml = 4 mg/ml

    Loading dose: 17 mg/kg

    Infusion rate: 1–4 mg/min (1 mg/min = 15 ml/hr)[b]

Theophylline

    Diluent: D5W, NS

    Concentration: 800 mg/500 ml =1.6 mg/ml

    Initial dosage: Loading dose 5 mg/kg over 20 mins

    Infusion rate: 0.2–0.6 mg/kg/hr (see Table 10-3)

Cl_{Cr} = creatinine clearance; D5W = 5% dextrose in water; NS = normal saline.
[a]To determine infusion rate:

$$\text{Infusion rate (ml/min)} = \frac{\text{Desired concentration infused (µg/kg/min)} \times \text{weight (kg)}}{\text{Concentration of solution (µg/ml)}}$$

[b]Dependent on renal function.

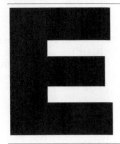

E

Dosage Adjustments of Drugs in Renal Failure

Way Y. Huey
and Daniel W. Coyne

| Medication | Route | Adjusted dosing interval (hrs) or % dose | | | Supplement dose after specific dialysis |
		>50 GFR (ml/min)	10–50 GFR (ml/min)	<10 GFR (ml/min)	
Analgesics—nonnarcotic					
Acetaminophen	H	4	6	8	HD
Aspirin	H, R	4	4–6	A	HD
Celecoxib	H	N	N	N	N
Diclofenac	H	N	N	N	N
Ibuprofen	H	N	N	N	N
Indomethacin	H, R	N	N	N	N
Ketoprofen	H	N	N	N	N
Ketorolac (IM)	H, R	N	N	50%	N
Nabumetone	H	N	N	N	N
Naproxen	H	N	N	N	N
Oxaprozin	H	N	N	N	N
Piroxicam	H	N	N	N	N
Rofecoxib	H	N	N	N	N
Sulindac	H, R	N	N	50%	N
Tramadol	H, R	N	12	12	N
Analgesics—opioid					
Codeine	H	N	75%	50%	N
Meperidine	H	N	75%	50%	N
Morphine	H	N	75%	50%	N
Antiarrhythmics					
Amiodarone	H	N	N	N	N
Bretylium	R, H	N	25–50%	A	?
Digoxin*	R	24	36	48	N
Disopyramide*	R, H	75%	15–50%	10–25%	HD
Flecainide*	R, H	N	50%	50%	N
Lidocaine*	H, R	N	N	N	N
Mexiletine	H, R	N	N	50–75%	HD
Moricizine	H	N	N	50–75%	N

| Medication | Route | Adjusted dosing interval (hrs) or % dose | | | Supplement dose after specific dialysis |
		>50 GFR (ml/min)	10–50 GFR (ml/min)	<10 GFR (ml/min)	
Procainamide*	R, H	4	6–12	12–24	HD
Propafenone	H	N	N	50–75%	N
Quinidine*	H, R	N	N	N	HD, PD
Sotalol	R	N	30%	15%	N
Tocainide*	R, H	N	N	50%	HD
Antibiotic drugs					
Aminoglycosides					
Amikacin*	R	8–12	12	>24	HD, PD
Gentamicin*	R	8–12	12	>24	HD, PD
Tobramycin*	R	8–12	12	>24	HD, PD
Antimycobacterial drugs					
Clofazimine	H	N	N	N	N
Cycloserine	R	12	12–24	24	N
Ethambutol	R	24	24–36	48	HD, PD
Ethionamide	H	N	N	50%	N
Isoniazid	H, R	N	N	N	HD, PD
Pyrazinamide	H, R	N	N	50%	HD, PD
Rifabutin	H	N	N	N	N
Rifampin	H	N	N	N	?
Cephalosporins					
Cefadroxil	R	12	12–24	24–48	HD
Cefazolin	R	8	12	24–48	HD
Cefdinir	R	12	24	48	HD
Cefepime	R	12	16–24	24–48	HD
Cefixime	R	12–24	75%	50%	N
Cefonicid	R	N	50%	25%	N
Cefoperazone	H	N	N	N	N
Cefotaxime	R, H	6–8	8–12	24	HD
Cefotetan	R	12	24	24	HD, PD
Cefoxitin	R	8	8–12	24–48	HD
Cefpodoxime	R	12	16	24–48	HD
Cefprozil	R	12	16	24	HD
Ceftazidime	R	8–12	24–48	48	HD
Ceftibuten	R	24	50%	25%	HD
Ceftizoxime	R	8–12	12–24	24	HD
Ceftriaxone	R, H	N	N	24	N
Cefuroxime	R	8	8–12	24	HD
Cephalexin	R	8	12	12	HD, PD
Cephalothin	R	6	6–8	12	HD, PD

| Medication | Route | Adjusted dosing interval (hrs) or % dose | | | Supplement dose after specific dialysis |
		>50 GFR (ml/min)	10–50 GFR (ml/min)	<10 GFR (ml/min)	
Cephradine	R	6	50% q6h	25% q6h	HD, PD
Loracarbef	R	12	50%	3–5 days	HD
Penicillins					
Amoxicillin/ clavulanate	R, H	8	8–12	12–24	HD
Ampicillin	R, H	6	6–12	12–24	HD
Ampicillin/ sulbactam	R, H	6–8	12	24	HD
Carbenicillin	R, H	8–12	12–24	24–48	HD, PD
Dicloxacillin	R, H	N	N	N	N
Mezlocillin	R, H	4–6	6–8	8–12	HD
Oxacillin	R, H	N	N	N	N
Penicillin G	R, H	N	75%	25–50%	HD
Piperacillin	R	4–6	6–8	12	HD
Piperacillin/ tazobactam	R, H	6	8	12	HD
Ticarcillin	R	8	8–12	24	HD
Ticarcillin/ clavulanate	R, H	3.1 g q4–6h	2g q6–8h	2g q12h	HD
Quinolones					
Ciprofloxacin	R	N	12–24	24	N
Enoxacin	R	N	50%	50% q24h	N
Gatifloxacin	R	N	50%	50%	HD, PD
Levofloxacin	R	8–12	24	48	N
Lomefloxacin	R	N	75%	50%	N
Moxifloxacin	H	N	N	N	N
Norfloxacin	R	N	12–24	A	N
Ofloxacin	R	N	12–24	24	N
Other antibacterial drugs					
Azithromycin	H	N	N	N	N
Aztreonam	R	N	50–75%	25%	HD, PD
Chloramphenicol	R, H	N	N	N	N
Clarithromycin	R, H	N	75%	50%	N
Clindamycin	H	N	N	N	N
Dirithromycin	H	N	N	N	N
Doxycycline	R, H	12	12–18	18–24	N
Erythromycin	H	N	N	N	N
Imipenem	R	N	50%	25%	HD
Meropenem	R	N	50% q12h	50% q24h	HD
Metronidazole	R, H	N	N	50%	HD

Medication	Route	Adjusted dosing interval (hrs) or % dose			Supplement dose after specific dialysis
		>50 GFR (ml/min)	10–50 GFR (ml/min)	<10 GFR (ml/min)	
Pentamidine	?	N	N	24–48	N
Quinupristin/ dalfopristin	H	N	N	N	N
Sulfamethoxazole	R, H	12	18	24	HD
Tetracycline	R, H	12	12–18	18–24	N
Trimethoprim	R, H	12	18	24	HD
Vancomycin* (IV)	R	6–12	24–48	48–96	N
Antifungal drugs					
Amphotericin B	N	24	24	24–36	N
Fluconazole	R, H	N	50%	25%	HD
Flucytosine	R	6	24	24–48	HD, PD
Itraconazole	H, R	N	N	50%	N
Ketoconazole	H	N	N	N	N
Miconazole	H	N	N	N	N
Terbinafine	R, H	N	?	?	?
Antiviral drugs					
Abacavir	H	N	N	N	?
Acyclovir (IV)	R	6	24	48	HD
Acyclovir (PO)	R	N	12–24	24	HD
Amantadine	R	12–24	24–72	72–168	N
Amprenavir	H	N	N	N	?
Cidofovir	R	N	A	A	?
Delavirdine	H	N	?	?	?
Didanosine	R	12	24	48	N
Efavirenz	H	N	N	N	?
Famciclovir	R	8	12–24	48	HD
Foscarnet	R	25 mg/kg q8h	15 mg/kg q8h	6 mg/kg q8h	HD
Ganciclovir	R	12	24	24	HD
Indinavir	H, R	8	?	?	?
Lamivudine	R	12	24	33% q24h	?
Nelfinavir	H	N	N	N	?
Nevirapine	H	N	?	?	?
Rimantadine	H	N	N	50%	?
Ritonavir	H	N	N	N	?
Saquinavir	H	N	N	N	?
Stavudine	H, R	N	50% q12–24h	?	?
Valacyclovir	R	8	12–24	50% q24h	HD
Zalcitabine	R	8	12	24	?
Zidovudine	H	N	N	N	HD

| Medication | Route | Adjusted dosing interval (hrs) or % dose | | | Supplement dose after specific dialysis |
		>50 GFR (ml/min)	10–50 GFR (ml/min)	<10 GFR (ml/min)	
Anticoagulants					
Antithrombin agents					
Argatroban	H	N	N	N	?
Dalteparin	R	N	?	?	N
Enoxaparin	R	N	?	?	N
Heparin	H	N	N	N	N
Lepirudin	R	N	15–50%	A	?
Warfarin	H	N	N	N	N
Platelet glycoprotein IIb/IIIa–receptor antagonists					
Abciximab	—	N	N	N	N
Eptifibatide	R	N	50%	A	A
Tirofiban	R	N	50% if Cl_{Cr} <30	50%	N
Cardiovascular agents					
Angiotensin-converting enzyme inhibitors					
Benazepril	H, R	N	75%	50%	N
Captopril	R, H	N	N	50%	HD
Enalapril	R	N	75%	50%	HD
Fosinopril	H	N	N	N	N
Lisinopril	R	N	50%	25%	HD
Moexipril	R, H	N	50%	50%	?
Quinapril	H, R	N	75%	50%	N
Ramipril	R, H	N	50%	50%	HD
Trandolapril	R, H	N	25–50%	A	N
Angiotensin II–receptor antagonists					
Candesartan	GI	M	50%	50%	N
Irbesartan	H	N	N	N	N
Losartan	H	N	N	N	N
Telmisartan	H	N	N	?	N
Valsartan	R	H	N	N	?
β-Adrenergic antagonists					
Acebutolol	R, H	N	50%	25%	N
Atenolol	R	N	50%	25%	HD
Betaxolol	H, R	N	N	50%	N
Bisoprolol	H, R	N	50%	25%	N
Carteolol	R	24	48	72	?
Carvedilol	H	N	N	N	N
Labetalol	H	N	N	N	N
Metoprolol	H	N	N	N	HD
Nadolol	R	N	50%	25%	HD

| Medication | Route | Adjusted dosing interval (hrs) or % dose | | | Supplement dose after specific dialysis |
		>50 GFR (ml/min)	10–50 GFR (ml/min)	<10 GFR (ml/min)	
Penbutolol	H	N	N	N	N
Pindolol	H, R	N	N	N	?
Propranolol	H	N	N	N	N
Sotalol	R	N	24–48	?	?
Timolol	H	N	N	N	N
Calcium channel antagonists					
Amlodipine	H	N	N	N	N
Diltiazem	H	N	N	N	N
Felodipine	H	N	N	N	N
Isradipine	H	N	N	N	N
Nicardipine	H	N	N	N	N
Nifedipine	H	N	N	N	N
Verapamil	H	N	N	50–75%	N
Diuretics					
Acetazolamide	R	6	12	A	—
Bumetanide	R, H	N	N	N	—
Furosemide	R	N	N	N	—
Indapamide	H	N	N	N	—
Metolazone	R	N	N	N	—
Spironolactone	R	6–12	12–24	A	—
Thiazide	R	N	N	A	—
Torsemide	H, R	N	N	N	—
Other antihypertensives					
Clonidine	R	N	N	N	N
Doxazosin	H	N	N	N	N
Hydralazine (PO)	H	8	8	8–16	N
Methyldopa	R, H	8	8–12	12–24	HD, PD
Minoxidil	H	N	N	N	HD
Nitroprusside	N	N	N	N	N
Prazosin	H, R	N	N	N	N
Terazosin	R	N	N	N	N
CNS agents					
Antidepressants					
Amitriptyline	H	N	N	N	N
Doxepin	H	N	N	N	N
Fluoxetine	H	N	N	N	N
Imipramine	H	N	N	N	N
Nortriptyline	H	N	N	N	N
Paroxetine	H	N	N	N	N
Sertraline	H	N	N	N	N

Medication	Route	Adjusted dosing interval (hrs) or % dose			Supplement dose after specific dialysis
		>50 GFR (ml/min)	10–50 GFR (ml/min)	<10 GFR (ml/min)	
Trazodone	H	N	N	N	N
Venlafaxine	H	N	75%	50%	N
Anticonvulsants					
Carbamazepine*	H, R	N	N	75%	N
Ethosuximide*	H, R	N	N	75%	HD
Phenobarbital*	H, R	N	N	12–16	HD, PD
Phenytoin*	H	N	N	N	N
Primidone*	H, R	8	8–12	12–24	HD
Valproic acid*	H	N	N	75%	N
Sedatives					
Alprazolam	H	N	N	N	N
Chlordiazepoxide	H	N	N	50%	N
Diazepam	H	N	N	N	N
Flurazepam	H	N	N	N	N
Lorazepam	H	N	N	N	N
Midazolam	H	N	N	50%	N
Temazepam	H	N	N	N	N
Zolpidem	H	N	?	?	N
Other psychoactive drugs					
Buspirone	H, R	N	N	25–50%	HD
Chlorpromazine	H	N	N	N	N
Haloperidol	H	N	N	N	N
Lithium*	R	N	50–75%	25–50%	HD, PD
Others					
Antidiabetic drugs					
Acarbose	GI	N	A	A	N
Acetohexamide	H	12–24	A	A	N
Chlorpropamide	?	24–36	A	A	N
Glimepiride	H, R	N	N	N	N
Glipizide	H, R	N	N	N	N
Glyburide	H, R	N	A	A	N
Metformin	R	A	A	A	N
Pioglitazone	H	N	N	N	N
Repaglinide	H	N	N	?	?
Rosiglitazone	H	N	N	N	N
Tolazamide	H	N	N	N	N
Tolbutamide	H	N	N	N	N
Antihistamines					
Azatadine	H	N	N	N	N

Medication	Route	Adjusted dosing interval (hrs) or % dose			Supplement dose after specific dialysis
		>50 GFR (ml/min)	10–50 GFR (ml/min)	<10 GFR (ml/min)	
Cetirizine	H, R	N	50%	50%	?
Fexofenadine	H, R	N	24	24	?
Loratadine	H	N	48	48	N
Antilipemic drugs					
Cholestyramine	N	N	N	N	N
Clofibrate	H	6–12	12–24	24–48	N
Fluvastatin	H	N	N	?	N
Gemfibrozil	R, H	N	50%	25%	N
Lovastatin	H	N	N	N	N
Pravastatin	R, H	N	N	50%	N
Simvastatin	H	N	N	50%	N
Gastrointestinal drugs					
Cimetidine	R	6	8	12	N
Famotidine	R, H	N	N	50%	?
Mesalamine	H	N	N	?	N
Metoclopramide	R, H	N	75%	50%	N
Misoprostol	R	N	N	N	N
Nizatidine	H	N	24	48	N
Omeprazole	H	N	N	N	?
Ranitidine	R	N	18–24	24	HD
Other drugs					
Alendronate	R	N	A	A	?
Allopurinol	R	N	50%	10–25%	?
Colchicine (PO)	R, H	N	N	50%	N
Dipyridamole	H	N	N	N	?
Etidronate	R	N	A	A	?
Finasteride	H, R	N	N	N	N
Glucocorticoids	H	N	N	N	N
Nitrates	H	N	N	N	N
Pentoxifylline	H	N	N	N	N
Risedronate	R	N	A	A	?
Terbutaline	H, R	N	50%	A	?
Theophylline	H	N	N	N	HD, PD
Ticlopidine	H	N	N	N	?
Tiludronate	R	N	A	A	?

A = avoid use; Cl_{Cr} = creatinine clearance; GFR = glomerular filtration rate; H = hepatic; HD = hemodialysis; N = none; PD = peritoneal dialysis; R = renal; % = percentage of normal dose; ? = no data.
*Serum levels should be used to determine exact dosing.
Source: G Aronoff, W Bennett, J Berns, et al. *Drug Prescribing in Renal Failure: Dosing Guidelines for Adults* (4th ed). Philadelphia: American College of Physicians, 1999; CR Gelman, BH Rumack, AJ Hess (eds), *Drugdex System.* Englewood, CO: Micromedex, Inc, 1999; and GK McEvoy (ed), *American Hospital Formulary Service Drug Information.* Bethesda, MD: American Society of Health-System Pharmacists, 2000.

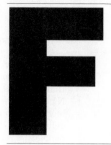

Immunizations and Postexposure Therapies

Alexis M. Elward
and Victoria J. Fraser

Table F-1. Routine adult immunizations

Vaccine	Persons for whom indicated	Dose	Contraindications
Lyme disease	Consider for persons who reside, work, or recreate in areas of high or moderate risk[b] aged 15–70 yrs who engage in activities that result in frequent or prolonged exposure to tick-infested habitats	0.5 ml IM × 3, second dose 1 mo after first, third dose 1 yr after first[c]	Treatment-resistant Lyme arthritis[d]
Hepatitis A[a]	Travelers to endemic areas, homosexual men, military personnel	0.5 ml IM (repeated in 6–18 mos for extended immunity)	
Hepatitis B[a]	Everyone	1 ml IM (in the deltoid) at 0, 1, and 6 mos (higher dose for immunocompromised and dialysis patients)	
Influenza	Everyone ≥50 yrs, high-risk patients, and health care workers (consider offering to everyone)	0.5 ml IM every fall	Anaphylactic hypersensitivity to eggs
Pneumococcus	Everyone ≥65 yrs and high-risk patients	0.5 ml IM once (repeated after 6 yrs for highest-risk patients)	
Tetanus/ diphtheria booster (adult Td)	Everyone	0.5 ml q10yr (or a single booster at age 50 yrs)	Neurologic or hypersensitivity reaction to previous dose

Vaccine	Persons for whom indicated	Dose	Contraindications
Varicella	Children entering child care facilities and elementary schools, all susceptible (1) health care workers, (2) persons who live/work in environments where VZV transmission likely,[e] (3) adolescents and adults living with children, (4) nonpregnant women of childbearing age, (5) international travelers; consider for asymptomatic or mildly symptomatic HIV-infected children in CDC class N1 or A1 with age-specific T lymphocyte ≥25%[f]	0.5 ml SC	Pregnancy, HIV-infected other than CDC class N1 or A1, primary immunodeficiency, neoplasms affecting bone marrow or lymphatic system[g]
Measles	Persons entering college, U.S. travelers to foreign countries, health care workers	0.5 ml SC	Pregnancy, history of sensitivity to eggs or neomycin, severe immunosuppression

CDC = Centers for Disease Control and Prevention; VZV = varicella-zoster virus.

[a]A combined hepatitis A and B vaccine is currently available outside the United States and may have a role in improving administration and compliance of these vaccines to populations in whom both vaccines are indicated.

[b]Ninety percent of cases in 140 counties along Northeastern and Mid-Atlantic seaboard.

[c]Booster may be required for immunity longer than 1 yr after 12-mo dose.

[d]Safety and efficacy unknown in persons with immunodeficiency, musculoskeletal disease, pregnancy, age <15 yrs or >70 yrs, chronic joint or neurologic illness related to Lyme disease, and second- and third-degree atrioventricular block.

[e]Teachers of young children, day care employees, residents/staff in institutional settings, college students, correctional institution inmates/staff members, military personnel.

[f]HIV-infected children in CDC class N1 or A1 should receive 2 doses of varicella vaccine with a 3-mo interval between doses.

[g]Research protocol available through vaccine manufacturer for use in patients with acute lymphocytic leukemia who meet eligibility criteria.

Table F-2. Passive immunization

Disease	Indications and dosage
Diphtheria	Suspected respiratory tract diphtheria: diphtheria antitoxin (DAT-equine source), 20,000–100,000 units IM (IV for serious illness) after cultures taken (given in addition to antibiotics)
Hepatitis A	**Postexposure:** Within 14 days of known exposure of high-risk persons (family and sex partners of infected individual, coworkers of infected food handlers, all staff and children at day care centers where ≥2 cases have occurred, and family members of diapered children who attend such a day care center): immune globulin (IG), 0.02 ml IM. IG not indicated for casual contacts (e.g., office coworkers).
	Pre-exposure: Vaccine prophylaxis preferred (see Table F-1)
Hepatitis B	See Table F-5
Measles	For nonimmune contacts within 6 days of exposure: IG, 0.25 ml/kg (maximum, 15 ml) for normal host; 0.5 ml/kg (maximum, 15 ml) for immunocompromised patients
Rabies	See Table F-4
Tetanus	See Table F-3
Varicella	Vaccine, 0.5 ml SC, within 3 days of exposure (possibly effective up to 5 days postexposure) and varicella-zoster IG (VZIG), 1 vial (125 units) IM for each 10 kg body weight (minimum, 125 units; maximum, 625 units) within 96 hrs of exposure (optimal if given within 48 hrs)

Table F-3. Tetanus prophylaxis

History of tetanus immunization (doses)	Clean, minor wounds		Other wounds	
	Give Td	Give TIG	Give Td	Give TIG
Unknown or <3 doses	Yes	No	Yes	Yes
≥3 doses	No if last dose within 10 yrs; otherwise yes	No	Yes, unless last dose within 5 yrs	No

Td = adult tetanus-diphtheria booster; TIG = tetanus immune globulin, 250 units IM, given concurrently with Td at a separate site.

Management of Rabies

I. **Pre-exposure vaccination** is indicated for persons in high-risk groups, including laboratory workers, veterinarians, animal handlers, international travelers.*
   A. **Dose.** Three 1.0-ml injections of human diploid cell vaccine (HDCV)[†], rabies vaccine adsorbed (RVA), or purified chick embryo cell vaccine (PCEC) IM (deltoid) on days 0, 7, and 21 or 28.
   B. **Contraindications.** Intradermal HDCV should not be given to travelers who are taking antimalarial prophylactics (IM should be used instead).

*If contact with potentially rabid animals and limited access to medical care are likely.
[†]HDCV can also be given intradermally (ID); ID dose is 0.1 ml on days 0, 7, and 21 or 28.

C. **Research laboratory and vaccine production workers** should have serum rabies antibody testing every 6 mos; spelunkers, veterinarians and staff and animal control and wildlife officers in areas where rabies is enzootic, and laboratory workers who perform rabies diagnostic testing should have serum rabies antibody testing every 2 yrs. Pre-exposure booster vaccination should be given to people in the above groups to maintain serum titer corresponding to complete neutralization at a 1:5 serum dilution by rapid fluorescent focus inhibition test.

II. **Postexposure rabies therapy.** See Table F-4. For bats and wild animals, capturing and sacrificing the animal and performing immunofluorescence on brain tissue provide definitive determination of the animal's rabies status. If diagnostic testing on animal brain tissue is negative, no postexposure therapy is necessary. Except in cases of bites/scratches on the head and neck (when postexposure therapy should be instituted immediately because of proximity to the CNS and potentially shorter incubation period) it is reasonable to wait for diagnostic testing on the animal before instituting postexposure therapy.

Table F-4. Postexposure rabies therapy

Species	Condition of animal at time of attack	Treatment of exposed[a] persons
Domestic cat, dog, ferret	Healthy and available for 10 days of observation	None unless animal develops rabies
	Rabid or suspected rabid	RIG and vaccine[b]
	Unknown	Contact public health department
Bat[a]	Any	RIG and vaccine
Wild skunk, fox, coyote, raccoon, or other carnivore	Unknown; to be regarded as rabid unless proved negative by laboratory testing	RIG and vaccine
Wild or domestic rodents (squirrels, rats, mice) and lagomorphs (rabbits, hares)	Unknown: rarely infected with rabies	Contact local health department

RIG = rabies immune globulin.

[a]Exposure: bites or scratches, or animal saliva contaminating abrasions, open wounds, or mucous membranes, except for bats. **Any bat exposure warrants therapy. Potential bat exposures also warrant therapy if there is any possibility of an unobserved bite/scratch (i.e., person sleeping in room, unattended child, demented or obtunded adult).**

[b]RIG: Administer 20 IU/kg once to previously unvaccinated persons; best if done immediately (can be given through seventh day after first dose of vaccine given). The full dose should be infiltrated around wound(s) if anatomically feasible; inject any remaining RIG intramuscularly at site distant from vaccine administration. **Do not** administer RIG in same syringe or at same anatomic site as vaccine. Previously vaccinated persons (those who received one of the recommended regimens of human diploid cell vaccine, rabies vaccine adsorbed, or purified chick embryo cell and had a documented rabies antibody titer) should not receive RIG. They should receive 2 IM 1.0-ml doses of vaccine, days 0 (immediately) and 3.

Vaccine: Five 1-ml doses on days 0, 3, 7, 14, and 28 IM in deltoid (anterolateral aspect of thigh acceptable for children). Gluteal area should **not** be used, as this results in lower neutralizing antibody titers.

Table F-5. Blood-borne pathogen postexposure guidelines[a]

Pathogen	Treatment
HIV[b]	For percutaneous injury (e.g., bloody needle-stick) or prolonged excessive exposure of mucous membrane or nonintact skin to blood, blood-contaminated fluids, or potentially infectious material (e.g., cerebrospinal fluid, amniotic fluid): zidovudine, 200 mg PO tid (or 300 mg PO bid), plus lamivudine (3TC), 150 mg PO bid for 4 wks. For highest-risk exposure (e.g., large blood volumes, high HIV viral load, hollow-bore needle) indinavir, 800 mg PO tid, or nelfinavir, 750 mg PO tid, can be added. Consult with experts in occupational health or infectious diseases[c]; occupational health follow-up is essential [*MMWR Morb Mortal Wkly Rep* 47(RR-7):1–28, 1998].
	For exposures to other material (e.g. urine), therapy not recommended.
Hepatitis B	For percutaneous injury with blood or blood-contaminated fluids:
	1. Health care worker not vaccinated: Administer hepatitis B immune globulin (HBIG), 0.06 ml/kg IM within 96 hrs of exposure; start hepatitis B vaccine series
	2. Health care worker vaccinated: Check hepatitis B surface antibody titer. If ≥10 IU/ml, no therapy. If <10 IU/ml, give HBIG, 0.06 ml/kg, and booster dose of vaccine.
Hepatitis C	Immune globulin not effective. Ensure occupational health follow-up for baseline and subsequent testing.

[a]All blood and body fluid exposures should be reported to occupational health department. Source patients should be tested for HIV (with consent), hepatitis B surface antigen (HbsAg), and hepatitis C antibody (anti-HCV).
[b]For exposure to patients with known HIV or at high risk for HIV. Postexposure prophylaxis should be started as soon as possible (preferably within 1–2 hrs) because less evidence exists for efficacy in preventing transmission after 24–36 hrs.
[c]Other antiretrovirals may be indicated if there is a high likelihood that the source patient has drug resistance to components of the standard regimen. If therapy is started for a patient with suspected HIV, it can be stopped if the patient's HIV antibody test is negative, unless a high suspicion of acute HIV illness exists.

HIV postexposure prophylaxis resources

National Clinicians Postexposure Hotline	Telephone: (888) 448–4911
	(888) 737–4448
	(888) PEP–4HIV
Centers for Disease Control and Prevention (for reporting HIV seroconversions in health care workers who received postexposure prophylaxis)	Telephone: (404) 639–6425
Antiretroviral Pregnancy Registry	Telephone: (800) 258–4263
U.S. Food and Drug Administration (for reporting unusual or severe toxicity to antiretroviral agents)	Telephone: (800) 322–1088

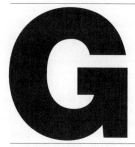

Infection Control and Isolation Recommendations

Victoria J. Fraser
and Alexis M. Elward

I. Standard precautions should be practiced on all patients at all times to minimize the risk of nosocomial infection (previously called body substance isolation or universal precautions).

A. Wash hands between caring for different patients and after removing gloves.

B. Wear gloves when direct contact with moist body substances (e.g., blood, sputum, urine, pus, stool) is anticipated.

C. Wear a gown when clothing is likely to be soiled by a body fluid.

D. Wear a mask and goggles or glasses when splashes of a body fluid are anticipated (e.g., during most invasive procedures).

II. Specific isolation categories. In addition to precautions that should be followed for all patients, certain diseases, depending on their mode of spread, require additional isolation precautions. Categories and indications for their use may vary slightly among different hospitals. An infection control specialist should be contacted if there is any uncertainty about what type of isolation a patient might need. The following categories are those suggested by the Centers for Disease Control and Prevention.

A. Airborne precautions

1. Use a negative-pressure room.
2. **Keep doors closed.**
3. Wear a respirator, grade N95 or better, that is certified by the National Institute for Occupational Safety and Health (not a surgical mask) if entering the room of a patient who is suspected of having tuberculosis.
4. For patients with measles or varicella (e.g., chickenpox) infections, immune persons may enter the room without a mask. Nonimmune persons ideally should not enter the room of such patients but, if it is absolutely necessary that they enter, should wear a mask.
5. If patient transport is absolutely necessary, the patient should wear a surgical mask.
6. Instruct the patient to cover his or her mouth when coughing or sneezing, even if alone.

B. Droplet precautions

1. Keep doors closed.
2. Wear a surgical mask if entering the room.
3. Discard mask after leaving the room.
4. If patient transport is absolutely necessary, the patient should wear a surgical mask.

C. Contact precautions

1. Wear a gown and gloves to enter the room.
2. Use a dedicated stethoscope and thermometer.
3. Remove gown and gloves before leaving the room.
4. Wash hands with antimicrobial soap before leaving the room.

III. Isolation for specific infections and duration of isolation (see Table G-1)

Table G-1. Isolation for specific infections and duration of isolation

Isolation type and diseases	Duration of isolation
Airborne	
Tuberculosis (TB)	Until TB ruled out with three negative acid-fast bacilli smears on consecutive days (If patient has documented or strongly suspected TB, isolation for hospitalized patients should continue for at least 2 wks of therapy with a good clinical response; however, patients can be discharged during this time if proper follow-up has been arranged with the local health department.)
Measles[a]	4 days after start of rash or for duration of illness if patient is immunocompromised
Chickenpox[a]/disseminated zoster[a]	Until all lesions crusted (Note: Nonimmune persons are potentially contagious on days 8–21 after exposure to varicella-zoster virus.)
Droplet	
Adenovirus (pneumonia)	Duration of illness
Diphtheria (pharyngeal)	Until cultures are negative (at least 24 hrs after stopping antibiotics)
Influenza	Duration of illness
Meningitis	24 hrs after start of therapy (for known or suspected *Neisseria meningitidis* or *Haemophilus influenzae*). This is prudent for all meningitis initially.
Mumps[a]	9 days after onset of swelling
Mycoplasma	Duration of illness
Parvovirus B19[b]	7 days for aplastic crisis (or for duration of illness if patient is immunosuppressed)
Pertussis	5 days after start of therapy
Plague (pneumonic)	72 hrs after start of therapy
Rubella[b]	7 days after onset of rash; for congenital rubella place infant on contact precautions during any admission until 1 yr of age unless nasopharyngeal and urine cultures negative after age 3 mos
Streptococcal pharyngitis, pneumonia or scarlet fever in infants and young children	24 hrs after start of therapy
Contact	
Acute infectious diarrhea	Duration of illness
Abscess/draining wound	Duration of illness
Enterovirus	Duration of illness
Herpes simplex (neonatal, primary, or disseminated mucocutaneous, severe)	Duration of illness
Hepatitis A	Until 1 wk after onset of symptoms (for children <age 3 yrs, duration of hospitalization; for children ages 3–14 yrs, 2 wks after onset of symptoms)

Isolation type and diseases	Duration of isolation
Parainfluenza	Duration of illness
Respiratory syncytial virus (infants, young children, and immunocompromised adults)	Duration of illness
Scabies	24 hrs after start of therapy
Viral conjunctivitis ("pink eye")	Duration of illness
Viral hemorrhagic fevers (Ebola, Marburg, Lassa)	Duration of illness
Oxacillin-resistant *Staphylococcus aureus*	Duration of hospitalization and future hospitalizations[c]
Vancomycin-resistant or intermediate-sensitive *S. aureus*	Duration of hospitalization and future hospitalizations[c]
Vancomycin-resistant enterococci	Duration of hospitalization and future hospitalizations[c]
Multidrug-resistant gram-negative bacteria	Duration of hospitalization and future hospitalizations[c]
Clostridium difficile	Duration of hospitalization and future hospitalizations[c]

[a]Nonimmune persons stay out of room if possible.
[b]Nonimmune pregnant women are not to enter room (Barnes-Jewish Hospital policy, not a Centers for Disease Control and Prevention recommendation).
[c]Unless criteria for discontinuing isolation have been met; consult hospital infection control specialists for specifics. See Table G-2 for current Barnes-Jewish Hospital policy.

Table G-2. Criteria for discontinuing contact isolation

Organism	Criteria
Oxacillin-resistant *Staphylococcus aureus*	• Two to three consecutive negative cultures from original infected or colonized site, plus
	• Two to three consecutive negative nasal cultures
	• All cultures to be obtained on separate days at least 24 hrs after last dose of vancomycin
Vancomycin-resistant enterococci (VRE)	• Three consecutive negative stool or perirectal cultures
	• Cultures to be obtained 1 wk apart; first culture at least 24 hrs after last dose of VRE therapy (if any)
Multidrug-resistant gram-negative bacteria	• Two to three consecutive negative cultures from original site
	• Cultures to be obtained on separate days at least 24 hrs after last dose of antibiotics
Clostridium difficile	• One negative toxin assay obtained at least 24 hrs after end of therapy (7 days of therapy minimum)

Source: Barnes-Jewish Hospital, St. Louis, MO.

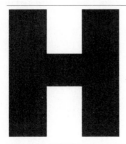

Critical Care Parameters and Formulas

Marin H. Kollef

Hemodynamic parameters

Systemic arterial pressure (SAP)	100–140/60–90 mm Hg
Pulse pressure (PP) = systolic SAP – diastolic SAP	30–50 mm Hg
Mean SAP (MAP) = [systolic SAP + (2 × diastolic SAP)]/3	70–100 mm Hg
Right arterial pressure (RAP)	0–6 mm Hg
Mean RAP	3 mm Hg
Right ventricular pressure (RVP)	17–30/0–6 mm Hg
Pulmonary artery pressure (PAP)	15–30/5–13 mm Hg
Mean PAP	10–18 mm Hg
Mean pulmonary artery occlusive pressure (PAoP) [i.e., pulmonary capillary wedge pressure (PCWP)]	2–12 mm Hg
Heart rate (HR)	60–100 beats/min
Body surface area (BSA; in m^2) = [height (cm)]$^{0.718}$ × [weight (kg)]$^{0.427}$ × 0.007449	
Stroke volume (SV)	60–120 ml/contraction
SV index = SV/BSA	40–50 ml/contraction/m^2
Cardiac output (CO) = SV × HR	3–7 L/min
Cardiac index = CO/BSA	2.5–4.5 L/min/m^2
Systemic vascular resistance (SVR) = (MAP – mean RAP) × 80/CO	800–1200 dynes/sec/cm^{-5}
Pulmonary vascular resistance (PVR) = (mean PAP – PAoP) × 80/CO	120–250 dynes/sec/cm^{-5}

Blood gas values

pH	7.35–7.45
Arterial oxygen tension (PaO_2)	75–100 mm Hg
Arterial carbon dioxide tension ($PaCO_2$)	35–45 mm Hg
Mixed venous oxygen tension ($P\bar{v}O_2$)	38–42 mm Hg
Arterial oxygen saturation (SaO_2)	95–100%
Mixed venous oxygen saturation ($S\bar{v}O_2$)	70–75%

Mixed acid-base equations

Henderson-Hasselbalch equation: $pH = 6.1 + \log([HCO_3^-]/0.03\ PaCO_2)$

Henderson equation for concentration of H+: $[H^+]$ (nM/L) = $24 \times (PaCO_2/[HCO_3^-])$

Metabolic acidosis

Bicarbonate deficit (mEq/L) = $[0.5 \times$ body weight (kg)$] \times (24 - [HCO_3^-])$

Expected $PaCO_2 = 1.5 \times [HCO_3^-] + 8 \pm 2$

Metabolic alkalosis

Bicarbonate excess = $[0.4 \times$ body weight (kg)$] \times ([HCO_3^-] - 24)$

Expected: $PaCO_2 = 0.7 \times [HCO_3^-] + 21 \pm 1.5$ (when $HCO_3^- \leq 40$ mEq/L)

$PaCO_2 = 0.75 \times [HCO_3^-] + 19 \pm 7.5$ (when $[HCO_3^-] > 40$ mEq/L)

Respiratory acidosis

Acute $\Delta pH/\Delta PaCO_2 = 0.008$

Chronic $\Delta pH/\Delta PaCO_2 = 0.003$

Respiratory alkalosis

Acute $\Delta pH/\Delta PaCO_2 = 0.008$

Chronic $\Delta pH/\Delta PaCO_2 = 0.002$

Oxygen transport

Arterial oxygen content $(CaO_2) = (1.39 \times SaO_2 \times Hb) + (0.0031\ PaO_2)$	18–21 ml O_2/dl
Mixed venous oxygen content $(C\bar{v}O_2) = (1.39 \times S\bar{v}O_2 \times Hb) + (0.0031 \times P\bar{v}O_2)$	14.5–15.5 ml O_2/dl
Capillary oxygen content $(C_{cap}O_2) = (1.39 \times S_{cap}O_2 \times Hb) \times (0.0031 \times PaO_2)$ ($S_{cap}O_2$ is assumed to be 1.00)	21 ml O_2/dl
Arterial–mixed venous oxygen content difference $(C_{a-\bar{v}}O_2)$	3.5–5.5 ml O_2/dl
Oxygen consumption $(\dot{V}O_2) = CO \times (C_{a-\bar{v}}O_2)$	200–250 ml/min
Oxygen delivery $(\dot{D}O_2) = CO \times CaO_2$	1000 ml/min
Oxygen extraction ratio = $\dot{V}O_2/\dot{D}O_2$	22–32%
Fick equation: $CO = 10\ \dot{V}O_2/[Hb \times 1.39\ (SaO_2 - S_{\bar{v}}O_2)]$	3–7 L/min

Respiratory parameters

Respiratory quotient (RQ) = $\dot{V}CO_2/\dot{V}O_2$	0.7–1.0
Alveolar oxygen tension $(PAO_2) = FIO_2\ (P_{atm} - P_{H_2O}) - PaCO_2/RQ$ (alveolar air equation)	
Alveolar-arteriolar oxygen gradient $[P(A–a)O_2]$	
For $FIO_2 = 21\%$	5–25 mm Hg
For $FIO_2 = 100\%$	<150 mm Hg
Physiologic shunt (QS/QT) = $(C_{cap}O_2)/(C_{cap}O_2 - C\bar{v}O_2)$, where $S_{cap}O_2$ is assumed to be 1.0	<5%
Minute ventilation $(\dot{V}E) = k\dot{V}CO_2/PaCO_2 = (0.863 \times \dot{V}CO_2)/[PaCO_2\ (1 - \dot{V}D/\dot{V}T)]$	4–6 L/min

Bohr equation of dead space (VD/VT) = ($PaCO_2$ – P expiratory CO_2)/$PaCO_2$ 0.2–0.3

Physiologic dead space (VD/VT) = ($PaCO_2$ – P expiratory CO_2)/$PaCO_2$ 0.2–0.3

Respiratory system compliance (Cstatic, rs) during mechanical ventilation

   Static Crs (Cstatic, rs) = VT/($P_{plateau}$ – PEEP)   70–100 ml/cm H_2O*

   Dynamic Crs (Cdynamic, rs) = VT/(P_{peak} – PEEP)   60–100 ml/cm H_2O

Hb = hemoglobin; PEEP = positive end-expiratory pressure.
*$P_{plateau}$ is obtained by inserting a 0.3-sec pause at end inspiration to give a plateau-pressure value.

Index

Abacavir
  dose adjustment in renal failure, 614
  in HIV infection and AIDS, 330
Abciximab
  dose adjustment in renal failure, 615
  in unstable angina, 104, 105
Abdominal infections, 307–308
Abrasion
  corneal and conjunctival, 21–22
  pleural, in pleural effusion therapy, 221
Abscess
  intra-abdominal, 307, 308
    glomerulonephritis in, 265
  isolation procedures in, 625
  of liver, 388
  of lung, 233–234
  perirectal, 371
Absorption of drugs in overdose and poisoning, 546–548
Acarbose
  in diabetes mellitus, 464
  dose adjustment in renal failure, 617
Acebutolol
  dose adjustment in renal failure, 615
  in hypertension, 80
Acetaminophen
  adverse effects of, 4, 548–552
    antidote in, 549, 550–552
    liver disorders in, 385, 389, 548–552
  in amphotericin B therapy, 292
  dose adjustment in renal failure, 611
  in fever, 3
  in headache, 533, 534
  in osteoarthritis, 508
  in pain relief, 4, 6
  in transfusion therapy, 426, 427
Acetazolamide
  dose adjustment in renal failure, 616
  in glaucoma, 22
  in uric acid nephropathy, 260
Acetohexamide in diabetes mellitus, 464
  dose adjustment in renal failure, 617
Acetylcholine receptor antibody in myasthenia gravis, 530
Acetylcysteine
  in acetaminophen overdose, 549, 550–552
  in radiocontrast nephropathy, 260
Achalasia, 358
Acid-base disorders, 69–75
  compensatory responses in, 70
  equations on, 627–628

in ventilatory support, 206–207
Acid ingestion, 557–558
Acid phosphatase serum levels, 579
Acid secretion, gastric, in peptic ulcer disease, 359, 360
Acidemia, 70, 73–74
  in transfusion therapy, 428
Acidosis
  metabolic, 70, 71–74
    equations on, 628
    hyperkalemia in, 57, 58, 59, 73
    ketoacidosis. See Ketoacidosis
    lactic acid. See Lactic acidosis
    in near-drowning, 544
    in renal failure, 58, 72–73, 262, 268
    in ventilatory support, 206
  in overdose and poisoning, 72, 545
    from antidepressants, 553
    from cyanide, 574, 575
    from ethylene glycol, 560, 561
    from methanol, 559
    from salicylates, 566
  respiratory, 70, 75
    in chronic obstructive pulmonary disease, 222
    equations on, 628
    in respiratory failure, 197
Acromegaly in pituitary adenoma, 486, 488–489
ACTH. See Adrenocorticotropic hormone
Acyclovir, 290
  dose adjustment in renal failure, 614
  in herpes simplex virus infections, 290
    esophageal, 357–358
    genital, 313
    in HIV infection and AIDS, 337
  in varicella-zoster virus infections, 290
    in HIV infection and AIDS, 337
Addison's disease, 482
  hyperkalemia in, 57
  hyponatremia in, 46
Adefovir dipivoxil in hepatitis B, 383
Adenoma of pituitary, 484, 485–486, 487–489
Adenosine
  in arrhythmias, 166, 179–180, 193
  interaction with other drugs, 193, 590
Adenovirus infections, isolation procedures in, 625
Admission orders, 1
Adrenal disorders, 482–485
  cortical hyperfunction, 484